MEDICAL COMPLICATIONS IN PREGNANCY

PRACTICAL PATHWAYS IN OBSTETRICS AND GYNECOLOGY

Sabrina D. Craigo, MD

Chief, Division of Maternal-Fetal Medicine
Department of Obstetrics and Gynecology
Tufts-New England Medical Center
Boston, Massachusetts

Emily R. Baker, MD

Associate Professor of Obstetrics
and Gynecology and of Radiation
Division Director of Maternal-Fetal Medicine
Dartmouth Medical School
Dartmouth-Hitchcock Medical Center
Lebanon, New Hampshire

McGRAW-HILL
Medical Publishing Division

New York   Chicago   San Francisco   Lisbon   London   Madrid   Mexico City   Milan
New Delhi   San Juan   Seoul   Singapore   Sydney   Toronto

Medical Complications in Pregnancy

Copyright © 2005 by The McGraw-Hill Companies, Inc. All rights reserved. Printed in the United States of America. Except as permitted under the United States Copyright Act of 1976, no part of this publication may be reproduced or distributed in any form or by any means, or stored in a data base or retrieval system, without the prior written permission of the publisher.

1 2 3 4 5 6 7 8 9 0   DOC/DOC   0 9 8 7 6 5

ISBN 0-07-141715-X

This book was set in Melior by International Typesetting and Composition.
The editors were Andrea Seils, Daniel Pepper, Nicky Fernando, and Penny Linskey.
The production supervisor was Catherine H. Saggese.
The cover designer was Mary McKeon.
The indexer was Betty Hallinger.
RR Donnelley was printer and binder.

This book is printed on acid-free paper.

Cataloging-in-Publication data for this title is on file with the Library of Congress.

Dedication

We would like to thank all of our teachers of medicine and obstetrics at Tufts-New England Medical Center, West Virginia University, Charleston Area Medical Center, Stanford University, University of Washington, and the University of Chicago.

We would like to dedicate this book to our children Aleksandar Bošković, Paul Beach, and Matthew Beach.

Contents

Contents   vii

SECTION 10 OTHER PREGNANCY COMPLICATIONS

Contributors

Jennifer T. Ahn, MD *(Chapter 4)*
Instructor, Obstetrics and Gynecology
University of Chicago Hospitals
Chicago, Illinois

Emily R. Baker, MD *(Chapter 41)*
Associate Professor of Obstetrics and
  Gynecology and of Radiology
Division Director of Maternal-Fetal
  Medicine
Dartmouth Medical School
Dartmouth-Hitchcock Medical Center
Lebanon, New Hampshire

Dorothy Beazley, DO *(Chapter 16)*
Assistant Professor of Obstetric and
  Gynecology
Division of Maternal-Fetal Medicine
Tufts-New England Medical Center
Boston, Massachusetts

Kim A. Boggess, MD *(Chapter 23)*
Assistant Professor of Obstetrics and
  Gynecology
University of North Carolina School
  of Medicine
Chapel Hill, North Carolina

Jeanine A. Carlson, MD *(Chapter 11)*
Associate Clinical Professor of Medicine
  and Nephrology
Tufts-New England Medical Center
Boston, Massachusetts

Lionel Carmant MD, FRCPC (C)
(Chapter 37)
Associate Professor of Pediatrics
University of Montreal
Hospital Ste-Justine
Division of Neurology
Montreal, Quebec, Canada

Charles Cassidy, MD *(Chapter 32)*
Assistant Professor of Orthopedics
Chief, Hand and Upper Extremity Services
Tufts-New England Medical Center
Boston, Massachusetts

Curtis L. Cetrulo, MD *(Chapter 33)*
Professor, Department of Obstetrics and
  Gynecology
Division of Maternal-Fetal Medicine
Tufts-New England Medical Center
Boston, Massachusetts

Johnny Chang, BS *(Chapter 32)*
Tufts University School of Medicine
Boston, Massachusetts

Jeff B. Chapa, MD *(Chapter 9)*
Assistant Professor, Department of
  Reproductive Biology
Section of Maternal-Fetal Medicine
University MacDonald Women's Hospital
Case School of Medicine
University Hospitals of Cleveland
Obstetrics and Gynecology
Chicago, Illinois

David Chelmow, MD *(Chapter 24)*
Professor of Obstetrics and Gynecology
Department of Obstetrics and Gynecology
Tufts-New England Medical Center
Boston, Massachusetts

Hui Min Cheong, MD *(Chapter 25)*
Obstetrics and Gynecology
Roanoke Carilion Community Hospital
Roanoke, Virginia

Garfield A. Clunie, MD *(Chapter 12)*
Assistant Professor of Obstetrics and
   Gynecology and Women's Health
Division of Maternal-Fetal Medicine
Albert Einstein College of Medicine
Montefiore Medical Center
Bronx, New York

Sabrina D. Craigo, MD *(Chapter 34)*
Associate Professor of Obstetrics and
   Gynecology
Chief, Division of Maternal-Fetal Medicine
Department of Obstetrics and Gynecology
Tufts-New England Medical Center
Boston, Massachusetts

Karen M. Davidson, MD *(Chapter 17)*
Instructor in Obstetrics and Gynecology
   at Harvard Medical School
Division of Maternal-Fetal Medicine
Brigham and Women's Hospital
Boston, Massachusetts

Patricia C. Devine, MD *(Chapter 5)*
Assistant Clinical Professor of Obstetrics
   and Gynecology
Division of Maternal-Fetal Medicine
Columbia University Medical Center
New York, New York

Lisa Dunn-Albanese, MD *(Chapter 8)*
Instructor of Obstetrics, Gynecology, and
   Reproductive Biology
Harvard Medical School
Division of Maternal-Fetal Medicine
Brigham and Women's Hospital
Boston, Massachusetts

Sara H. Garmel, MD *(Chapter 10)*
Co-Director, Maternal-Fetal Medicine
Oakwood Hospital
Dearborn, Michigan

Barbara Rackow Gerling, MD
(Chapter 28)
Associate Professor of Cardiology
Dartmouth-Hitchcock Medical Center
Lebanon, New Hampshire

Laura Goetzl, MD *(Chapter 14)*
Assistant Professor
Medical University of South Carolina
Division of Maternal-Fetal Medicine
Department of Obstetrics and Gynecology
Charleston, South Carolina

Nicholas Guerina, MD
(Chapter 21)
Assistant Professor in Pediatrics
Tufts-New England Medical Center
Boston, Massachusetts

Judith U. Hibbard, MD
(Chapters 4 and 9)
Professor of Obstetrics and Gynecology
Division of Maternal-Fetal Medicine
Department of Obstetrics and Gynecology
University of Illinois at Chicago
Chicago, Illinois

Michael House, MD *(Chapter 1)*
Assistant Professor of Obstetrics and
  Gynecology
Division of Maternal-Fetal Medicine
Tufts-New England Medical Center
Boston, Massachusetts

Gary E. Kaufman, MD *(Chapter 40)*
Assistant Professor of Obstetrics and
  Gynecology
Dartmouth-Hitchcock Medical Center
Lebanon, New Hampshire

Kristine M. King, MD *(Chapter 33)*
Obstetrics and Gynecology
Tufts-New England Medical Center
Boston, Massachusetts

Sahar A. Kinney, MD *(Chapter 18)*
Obstetrics and Gynecology
Cedar-Sinai Medical Center
Los Angeles, California

Michele R. Lauria, MD *(Chapter 27)*
Associate Professor of Obstetrics and
  Gynecology
Dartmouth-Hitchcock Medical Center
Lebanon, New Hampshire

Elizabeth G. Livingston, MD
(Chapter 20)
Associate Professor of Obstetrics and
  Gynecology
Duke University Medical Center
Durham, North Carolina

Jeffery C. Livingston, MD *(Chapter 25)*
Assistant Professor of Obstetrics and
  Gynecology
University of Cincinnati
Cincinnati, Ohio

Teresa Marino, MD *(Chapter 38)*
Assistant Professor of Obstetrics and
  Gynecology
Division of Maternal-Fetal Medicine
Department of Obstetrics and Gynecology
Tufts-New England Medical Center
Boston, Massachusetts

Marjorie C. Meyer, MD *(Chapters 2 and 3)*
Associate Professor of Obstetrics and
  Gynecology
University of Vermont College of Medicine
Burlington, Vermont

Lucie Morin, MD, FRCS (C)
(Chapter 37)
Associate Professor
Department of Obstetrics and Gynecology
McGill University
Montreal, Quebec, Canada

Barbara M. O'Brien, MD *(Chapter 13)*
Clinical Instructor
Division of Maternal-Fetal Medicine
Department of Obstetrics and Gynecology
Tufts-New England Medical Center
Boston, Massachusetts

Karen O'Brien, MD *(Chapter 35)*
Assistant Professor of Obstetrics and
  Gynecology
Division of Maternal-Fetal Medicine
Department of Obstetrics and Gynecology
Tufts-New England Medical Center
Boston, Massachusetts

Kelly Pagidas, MD *(Chapter 6)*
Assistant Professor of Obstetrics and
  Gynecology
Women and Infants Division of Reproductive
  Medicine and Infertility Department of
  Women and Infants Hospital
Providence, Rhode Island

Annette Perez-Delboy, MD
(Chapter 29)
Assistant Professor of Obstetrics and
    Gynecology
Department of Obstetrics and Gynecology
Columbia Presbyterian Medical Center
Columbia University College of Physicians
    and Surgeons
New York, New York

Erika Peterson, MD *(Chapter 31)*
Clinical Instructor, Obstetrics and
    Gynecology
Division of Maternal-Fetal Medicine
Tufts-New England Medical Center
Boston, Massachusetts

Peter G. Pryde, MD *(Chapter 22)*
Department of Anesthesiology
University of Wisconsin
Madison, Wisconsin

Steven J. Ralston, MD *(Chapter 19)*
Assistant Professor of Obstetrics and
    Gynecology
Division of Maternal-Fetal Medicine
Tufts-New England Medical Center
Boston, Massachusetts

Michelle Russell, MD *(Chapters 7 and 8)*
Division of Maternal Fetal-Medicine
Women and Infants Hospital
Providence, Rhode Island

Steven Schwaitzberg, MD, FACS
(Chapter 18)
Associate Professor of Surgery
Department of Surgery
Director of Surgical Research
Tufts-New England Medical Center
Boston, Massachusetts

Kathryn Schwarzenberger, MD
(Chapter 39)
Associate Professor of Medicine
Section of Dermatology
Dartmouth-Hitchcock Medical Center
Lebanon, New Hampshire

Lynn L. Simpson, MD *(Chapter 29)*
Associate Professor of Obstetrics and
    Gynecology
Division of Maternal-Fetal Medicine
Department of Obstetrics and Gynecology
Columbia University Medical Center
College of Physicians and Surgeons
New York, New York

Tanya K. Sorsensen, MD
(Chapter 26)
Associated Clinical Professor
Department of Obstetrics and Gynecology
University of Washington
Division of Perinatal Medicine
Obstetrix Medical Group
Swedish Medical Center
Seattle, Washington

John L. Stanley, MD *(Chapter 36)*
Harbor Medical Associates
Pembroke, Massachusetts

Theresa L. Stewart, MD *(Chapter 30)*
Assistant Professor of Obstetrics and
    Gynecology
Uniformed Services University of Health
    Sciences
Lackland Air Force Base, Texas

Stanley J. Stys, MD *(Chapter 15)*
Professor of Obstetrics and Gynecology
Dartmouth-Hitchcock Medical Center
Lebanon, New Hampshire

Preface

As obstetricians we continue to be surprised at the discomfort physicians have when managing common medical conditions in the pregnant patient. Our goal was to make a clinically useful textbook with chapters which contain current, concise, and practical information. Given the breadth of clinical problems addressed by this textbook, our contributors include clinicians from a variety of disciplines including maternal-fetal medicine, obstetrics, surgery, neonatology, internal medicine, and family medicine. We hope this book to be a resource for the busy obstetrical care provider to use on a day to day basis.

MEDICAL COMPLICATIONS
IN PREGNANCY

Hyperprolactinemia in Pregnancy

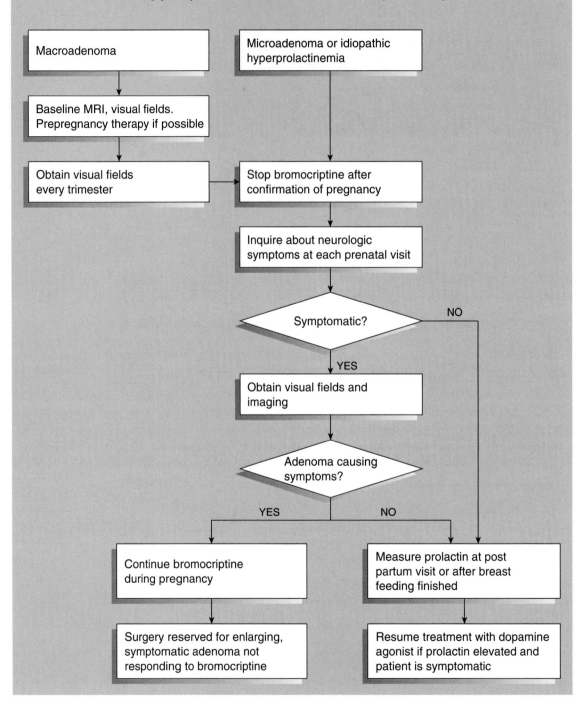

1 Hyperprolactinemia

Michael House

Introduction

Hyperprolactinemia is a common cause of oligomenorrhea and infertility. With treatment, many patients can become pregnant. Several etiologies can cause hyperprolactinemia, but the most common is an adenoma in the anterior pituitary gland. Pregnancy complications are associated with the size of the adenoma. Microadenomas (<10 mm) are rarely linked to problems in pregnancy, whereas macroadenomas (>10 mm) are associated with a significant risk (23%) of symptomatic enlargement. Vigilance for signs and symptoms of an enlarging adenoma is the key to antepartum care for a pregnant patient with hyperprolactinemia. Bromocriptine is the first-line therapy for a symptomatic adenoma. More than 20 years of clinical experience has accumulated with bromocriptine and it is considered safe. In the postpartum period, patients can be counseled that there is no contraindication to breast feeding.

Physiology

Prolactin exists in monomeric and polymeric forms. The biologically active form is a monomer that contains 198 amino acids and has a molecular weight of 22 kDa. Approximately 90% of prolactin circulates as a monomer ("little" prolactin). Other structural variants are "big" prolactin (45–50 kDa) and "big-big" prolactin (>100 kDa). Prolactin heterogeneity is caused by complex structural modifications to little prolactin, including glycosylation and dimerization. Big prolactin and big-big prolactin have less biologic potency compared with little prolactin. However, serum immunoreactivity may remain intact, which can cause clinical confusion in pregnancy.[1,2]

3

The synthesis of prolactin occurs primarily in the lactotroph cells of the anterior pituitary gland. During pregnancy, a second source of prolactin is the maternal decidua, which is thought to be the source of prolactin in the amniotic fluid. Neuroendocrine regulation of prolactin secretion in the pituitary is under control of prolactin inhibiting factors (PIFs) and prolactin releasing factors (PRFs) originating in the hypothalamus.

- Prolactin inhibiting factors: Dopamine is the important PIF and dopamine agonists comprise the primary medical therapy for hyperprolactinemia (see Treatment). Dopamine is released in the hypothalamus and travels to the anterior pituitary through the portal circulation, where it binds to D_2 class dopamine receptors on the lactotroph cell membrane.
- Prolactin releasing factors: Hormones that have been studied as PRFs include thyrotropin releasing hormone and vasoactive intestinal peptide, although their precise physiologic role is unclear.
- Hypothalamus: The hypothalamus receives afferent input from different sources that mediate the balance of PIF and PRF acting on the lactotroph cells. For example, breast feeding activates spinal afferents that travel to the hypothalamus to increase prolactin production by increasing PRFs or decreasing PIFs. Also, psychological stress acts to increase prolactin at the hypothalamic level.
- Anterior pituitary: Estrogen stimulates growth of the lactotroph cells, which increases circulating prolactin.

It is known that the anterior pituitary is under tonic inhibitory control because separation of the pituitary from the hypothalamus increases prolactin levels.[3]

In the nonpregnant state, hyperprolactinemia is defined as greater than 20–25 ng/mL in most clinical laboratories. Pregnancy causes a sustained increase in prolactin levels due to a stimulatory effect of estrogen on the anterior pituitary. Prolactin levels increase throughout gestation, reaching a peak of 200 ng/mL at term. The pituitary also undergoes physiologic enlargement during pregnancy. At term, the volume of the pituitary is at least twice as large as in the nonpregnant state.[4] The increase in prolactin during pregnancy does not cause milk production because estrogen and progesterone inhibit the activity of prolactin in the breast. After delivery, levels of steroid hormones decrease rapidly. Prolactin levels decrease more

KEY POINT

Obtaining prolactin levels is not useful in patients with hyperprolactinemia during pregnancy.

slowly and lactation is initiated because the inhibitory effects of estrogen and progesterone are removed.

Differential Diagnosis

Usually the cause of hyperprolactinemia is known before pregnancy. A high level of prolactin is associated with oligomenorrhea, amenorrhea, and infertility and patients require treatment to achieve pregnancy. The causes of hyperprolactinemia can be divided into five broad categories (Table 1-1).

Table 1-1. CAUSES OF HYPERPROLACTINEMIA

I. **Physiologic**
   A. Pregnancy
   B. Lactation
   C. Chest wall stimulation
   D. Sleep
   E. Stress
II. **Hypothalamic-pituitary stalk damage**
   A. Tumors
       a. Craniopharyngioma
       b. Suprasellar pituitary mass extension
       c. Meningioma
       d. Dysgerminoma
       e. Metastases
   B. Empty sella
   C. Lymphocytic hypophysitis
   D. Adenoma with stalk compression
   E. Granulomas
   F. Rathke's cyst
   G. Irradiation
   H. Trauma
       a. Pituitary stalk section
       b. Suprasellar surgery
III. **Pituitary hypersecretion**
   A. Prolactinoma
   B. Acromegaly
IV. **Systemic disorders**
   A. Chronic renal failure
   B. Hypothyroidism
   C. Cirrhosis
   D. Pseudocyesis
   E. Epileptic seizures

(Continued)

Table 1-1. **CAUSES OF HYPERPROLACTINEMIA (*CONTINUED*)**

V. Drug-induced hypersecretion
- A. Dopamine receptor blocker
  - a. Phenothiazines
  - b. Butyrophenones
  - c. Thioxanthenes
  - d. Metoclopramide
- B. Dopamine synthesis inhibitors
  - a. α-Methyldopa
- C. Catecholamine depletors
  - a. Reserpine
- D. Opiates
- E. H_2 antagonists
  - a. Cimetidine, ranitidine
- F. Imipramines
  - a. Amitriptyline, amoxapine
- G. Serotonin reuptake inhibitors
  - a. Fluoxetine
- H. Calcium channel blockers
  - a. Verapamil
- I. Hormones
  - a. Estrogen
  - b. Antiandrogens

Source: Adapted from Melmed S. Disorders of the anterior pituitary and hypothalamus. In: Braunwald E, Fauci AS, Kasper DL, et al, eds. *Harrison's Principles of Internal Medicine*, 15th ed. New York: McGraw-Hill, 2001; p. 2039. Reproduced with permission of The McGraw-Hill Companies.

- Physiologic hypersecretion: A mildly increased prolactin level (<70 ng/mL) should prompt a repeat test under controlled conditions. Physiologic factors that have been associated with fluctuations of prolactin include psychological stress, chest wall stimulation, and sleep. In many instances, the prolactin will normalize if it is obtained as a fasting specimen under relaxed conditions.[5]
- Drug-induced hypersecretion: Many medications are associated with hyperprolactinemia, usually mediated by an interaction with the dopamine receptor. Estrogen stimulates the growth of lactotroph cells, an effect seen most dramatically in pregnancy.
- Systemic disorders: Hypothyroidism has been associated with hyperprolactinemia, probably because of increased thyrotropin releasing hormone. End-stage renal disease can

decrease prolactin clearance and cause mild increases. Cirrhosis has also been associated with hyperprolactinemia, although the mechanism is unclear.

- Hypothalamic or pituitary disorder: If a healthy nonpregnant woman has no drug history and is not hypothyroid, the etiology of hyperprolactinemia is usually in the hypothalamus or pituitary gland. Marked increases in prolactin are usually caused by a prolactinoma, a functional adenoma of the lactotroph cells (see Prolactinoma). Mechanical compression of a tumor on the hypothalamus or pituitary stalk can interrupt tonic prolactin inhibition and lead to hyperprolactinemia. Lymphocytic hypophysitis is a rare autoimmune, inflammatory disorder that may present with features similar to a pituitary adenoma. Prolactin may be increased or other pituitary hormones may be affected. Most cases occur in association with pregnancy for reasons that are unclear.[6]

- Prolactinoma: Hyperprolactinemia is associated with a prolactin secreting adenoma in almost half of all cases. A markedly high level of prolactin (>100 ng/mL) confers a greater risk of having a prolactinoma. Prolactinomas are classified by size: a microadenoma is defined as a tumor diameter smaller than 1 cm, and a macroadenoma is larger than 1 cm. Most prolactinomas are microadenomas (95%).

If a thorough search for the cause of hyperprolactinemia is unrevealing, the diagnosis of idiopathic (also known as "functional") hyperprolactinemia is made. In many cases, a functioning adenoma is present but too small to be visualized. With time, idiopathic hyperprolactinemia can manifest as a microadenoma. Further, prolactin heterogeneity can confuse the clinical picture. *Macrohyperprolactinemia* refers to hyperprolactinemia caused by high levels of big-big prolactin. Big-big prolactin typically retains its immunoreactivity but not its biologic potency, resulting in a very high serum prolactin out of proportion to the clinical symptoms.[1]

Symptoms of Hyperprolactinemia

It is rare for a case of hyperprolactinemia to present during a spontaneous pregnancy. Rather, hyperprolactinemia is associated with oligomenorrhea, amenorrhea, and infertility. Other symptoms attributable to hypogonadism include vaginal dryness, dyspareunia, and decreased libido. Galactorrhea occurs in one-third of cases of increased prolactin. Longstanding hyperprolactinemia is associated with significant hypoestrogenemia that leads to subsequent loss of bone mineral density.[7]

Just as high levels of circulating estrogen stimulate growth in the anterior pituitary during pregnancy,[4] estrogen directly stimulates a prolactinoma. Symptoms result from a mass effect on adjoining structures. Suprasellar extension can compress the optic chiasm, causing visual field defects.[8] Headache is a common symptom in pregnancy. Local mass effects in the pituitary may also cause hypopituitarism. Although uncommon, inferior or lateral invasion can cause neurologic dysfunction, seizures, or cerebrospinal fluid rhinorrhea.

Workup of Hyperprolactinemia

The workup for suspected hyperprolactinemia begins with confirmation that the prolactin level is truly high. A mildly high level of prolactin may revert to normal if it drawn as a fasting specimen during a calm state. A medical history will point to secondary causes of hyperprolactinemia. A drug history is essential because numerous medications have been linked to hyperprolactinemia (see Table 1-1). When a drug etiology is suspected, a 1-month trial period off the medicine can be attempted with subsequent remeasurement of serum prolactin. Diagnostic challenges can occur in cases when it would be imprudent to stop a medication (i.e., a neuroleptic) and the prolactin level is mildly high.

The laboratory workup of hyperprolactinemia consists of a pregnancy test, thyroid function tests, and serum chemistry. Radiologic imaging is indicated in the setting of unexplained hyperprolactinemia that does not normalize with conservative measures. Prolactinomas are usually associated with markedly increased prolactin (>100 ng/mL), but nonfunctioning adenomas and other tumors are sometimes seen with mildly increased prolactin. Macrohyperprolactinemia should be considered when the prolactin is very high, clinical symptoms are mild, and there is no evidence of a prolactinoma.

Natural History of Prolactinomas in Pregnancy: What's the Evidence?

Data on the natural history of prolactinomas during pregnancy come from reviews of case series from individual institutions. In an early review, Gemzell and Wang[9] reported complications that occurred infrequently in 91 pregnancies with a preexisting microadenoma. Headache was seen in three pregnancies, visual disturbances were seen in one, and diabetes insipidus was seen in one, for an overall complication rate of 5.5%. In contrast, among 56 pregnancies with a preexisting macroadenoma, the complication rate was 35.7% and five patients required surgery during pregnancy.

Molitch[10] combined data from the four most recent case series[8,11–13] and reported on 376 women with microadenoma, 86 patients with an untreated macroadenoma, and 71 patients with a previously treated macroadenoma. Microadenomas were associated with a small risk of significant symptoms from enlargement, which occurred in only 6 of 376 women (1.3%). In contrast, the risk of symptomatic enlargement in the 86 women with an untreated macroadenoma was significantly higher, which occurred in 20 women (23.2%). Treatment of a macroadenoma before conception decreased the risk of symptomatic enlargement during pregnancy because only 2 of 71 patients (2.8%) developed symptoms during pregnancy.

Treatment of Hyperprolactinemia in Pregnancy

Patients with hyperprolactinemia often come to the attention of the obstetrician after a spontaneous pregnancy or after previous treatment for hyperprolactinemia associated infertility. Pregnancy represents a temporary, physiologic hyperprolactinemic state. Whereas clinical symptoms (galactorrhea, anovulation, or hypogonadism) guide therapy decisions outside of pregnancy, these symptoms are not relevant during pregnancy. Moreover, idiopathic hyperprolactinemia and microadenomas rarely cause significant adverse effects. Hence, an enlarging macroadenoma is the most common indication for treatment during pregnancy. The options for treatment during pregnancy include bromocriptine and transsphenoidal surgery.

Bromocriptine (Parlodel) is an ergot derivative with potent dopamine agonist activity. In patients who undergo bromocriptine therapy for hyperprolactinemic anovulation, menses are normalized in 80–90%[14] of cases and many will achieve pregnancy. Side effects can be significant, with nausea and orthostatic hypotension being the most common. Side effects occur most frequently after initiation of therapy. Therapy is begun at a low dose (1.25 mg) at bedtime with a snack. The dose is typically increased to 2.5 mg twice a day over the course of several weeks and the clinical effect is checked over several months. When side effects are not tolerated, vaginal bromocriptine can be tried.[15]

In addition to ameliorating the clinical symptoms of hyperprolactinemia (amenorrhea, galactorrhea, or hypogonadism), bromocriptine shrinks prolactinomas. After summarizing 21 case series that included 248 nonpregnant patients, Molitch[3] reported that 76% of cases had some degree of tumor shrinkage. When the size of the effect was quantified, 40% of cases showed greater than 50% tumor shrinkage in tumor volume.

Safety of Dopamine Agonists in Pregnancy: What's the Evidence?

KEY POINT

First-trimester exposure of the fetus to bromocriptine is safe.

Because many patients with hyperprolactinemic anovulation require treatment to become pregnant, there is a large body of evidence on the fetal effect of first-trimester exposure to bromocriptine. Turkalj[16] reported on the results of a surveillance project conducted by the manufacturer of bromocriptine. Information was gathered on 1410 pregnancies in 1335 women. Bromocriptine was stopped when the pregnancy was recognized, which typically occurred before 8 weeks of gestation. The incidence rates of spontaneous abortions (11.1%), ectopic pregnancies (0.9%), minor malformations (2.5%), and major malformations (1.0%) were low and not different from the expected complication rate in an unselected population. Cabergoline is a more recent dopamine agonist that has a better side effect profile with a clinical efficacy similar to that of bromocriptine.[17] Cabergoline is less commonly used in women being treated for hyperprolactinemic infertility, although small case series do not suggest adverse pregnancy outcome.[18]

A challenging clinical situation arises when a macroadenoma undergoes symptomatic enlargement during pregnancy. The rationale for using bromocriptine during pregnancy for a symptomatic macroadenoma is that (1) bromocriptine shrinks macroadenomas in nonpregnant patients and (2) the fetal and maternal risks of bromocriptine are probably less than the risks of transsphenoidal surgery. The evidence to support the use of bromocriptine for a symptomatic macroadenoma is limited to case reports. The manufacturer of bromocriptine collected a series of case reports[19] in which bromocriptine was reinstituted after a macroadenoma became symptomatic or used continuously throughout pregnancy. Bromocriptine was effective at controlling symptoms and preventing the need for surgery in 44 of 46 patients in whom it was restarted for increasing symptoms attributable to a macroadenoma.

Transsphenoidal surgery in pregnancy is indicated in select circumstances. In nonpregnant patients, dopamine agonists are favored over surgery for the treatment of symptomatic adenomas.[20] When the adenoma does not respond to medical therapy or the patient does not tolerate the side effects, attention is turned to transsphenoidal debulking. In pregnancy, surgery is reserved for cases involving an enlarging macroadenoma that is not responsive to restarting bromocriptine or increasing the dose. These cases are complex and should involve a multidisciplinary team approach involving the obstetrician, endocrinologist, and neurosurgeon. Factors to consider include the gestational age of the pregnancy and the acuity of the patient's symptoms.

A pregnant patient with a microadenoma or idiopathic hyperprolactinemia can be counseled that the risk of an adverse pregnancy outcome is low. If bromocriptine is used to achieve pregnancy, it is stopped when pregnancy is confirmed. With this protocol, the risk of fetal malformation is no higher than the background risk. Patients using bromocriptine for infertility should undergo frequent evaluation for pregnancy to minimize fetal exposure to bromocriptine. Patients with a microadenoma can be counseled that the risk of symptomatic enlargement is close to 1%. At each prenatal visit, the patient is evaluated for the onset of headaches, visual disturbances, or other symptoms attributable to enlarging adenoma. Suspicious symptoms should prompt an imaging study and formal visual field testing. If an enlarging adenoma is found, bromocriptine should be reinstituted.

Patients with macroadenomas are followed more closely because of the relatively high risk of symptomatic enlargement (23%). Baseline magnetic resonance imaging (MRI) and visual field testing should be performed. If the macroadenoma is confined to the sella, it typically follows a course similar to that of a microadenoma. Complications usually occur in patients with a suprasellar macroadenoma. At each visit, the patient is evaluated for symptoms that could be caused by an enlarging macroadenoma. In addition, formal visual field testing is performed every trimester. If symptoms occur or if visual field testing indicates a deficit, imaging is performed and bromocriptine is reinstituted. If bromocriptine has no effect, the dose can be increased. If the patient's symptoms are significant and medical therapy is not working, transsphenoidal debulking surgery is indicated.

Three clinical conditions deserve special mention.

- Pituitary apoplexy: Hemorrhage or necrosis of a pituitary adenoma is an endocrine emergency. The classic, acute syndrome presents over 1–2 days and is characterized by headache, meningeal signs, visual disturbances, and neurologic dysfunction. Recent improvements in MRI technology have revealed a subclinical form of pituitary apoplexy in which a small pituitary hemorrhage causes few symptoms. *Sheehan's syndrome* refers to a postpartum event, although a spontaneous hemorrhage into a prolactinoma can occur during pregnancy.[21] Patients with pituitary apoplexy require intensive support and treatment for hypopituitarism. Worsening visual disturbances or signs of pituitary compression are indications for transsphenoidal decompression.
- Lymphocytic hypophysitis is a rare, autoimmune, inflammatory disorder that is most often associated with pregnancy and can present in a fashion similar to that of a pituitary adenoma. The etiology of lymphocytic hypophysitis is unknown but is associated with other autoimmune disorders.[6] Histologic features include lymphocytic infiltration of the anterior pituitary with associated destruction and fibrosis of the gland. Radiographic features are nonspecific and the appearance mimics that of a pituitary adenoma. The clinical symptoms are attributable to a mass effect on adjoining structures: headache, visual disturbances, or pituitary dysfunction. There is no unique endocrinologic profile associated with lymphocytic hypophysitis. It can present with hyperprolactinemia, diabetes insipidus, or hypopituitarism. The diagnosis is made by transsphenoidal biopsy and steroids are the first-line therapy.[22]
- Macrohyperprolactinemia: When the serum level of prolactin is very high and out of proportion to the clinical symptoms, macrohyperprolactinemia should be considered. Big-big prolactin retains its immunoreactivity but with less biologic potency compared with monomeric prolactin.

Macrohyperprolactinemia is not associated with adverse outcome in pregnancy.[1]

Guiding Questions in Approaching the Patient

- Does the patient have a macroadenoma?
- During the course of the pregnancy, does the patient have any symptoms that can be attributed to an enlarging macroadenoma?

Hyperprolactinemia and Lactation

Lactation has not been reported to cause symptomatic growth of a macroadenoma. Hence, there is no contraindication to breast feeding in these patients. Current recommendations are to measure the serum prolactin at the 6-week postpartum visit or after breast feeding is finished. A dopamine agonist can be resumed if the prolactin is high and the patient is symptomatic. Bromocriptine is no longer used to suppress breast engorgement in women who do not want to lactate.

Conclusion

The key question in the antepartum care of the pregnant patient with a microadenoma or macroadenoma is whether symptomatic enlargement is occurring. The probability of symptomatic enlargement is low with a microadenoma (1%), but the risk is higher with a macroadenoma (23%). If possible, prepregnancy treatment of a macroadenoma is desirable because it decreases the risk of enlargement during pregnancy. The patient with a macroadenoma should be followed with formal visual field testing at each trimester. There should be no hesitation in obtaining an imaging study if the patient has symptoms attributable to an enlarging adenoma. Bromocriptine is the first-line therapy for a symptomatic adenoma. Surgical therapy is reserved for those patients in whom bromocriptine is ineffective.

Discussion of Cases

CASE 1: NULIGRAVIDA WITH OLIGOMENORRHEA DESIRING PREGNANCY

A 30-year-old gravida 0 who desired pregnancy presented with oligomenorrhea and infertility. Laboratory evaluation was normal except for a serum prolactin concentration of 75 ng/mL. Hyperprolactinemia was confirmed with a subsequent fasting specimen. MRI showed a 6-mm microadenoma.

What is the next step?

The patient was counseled to begin bromocriptine therapy. She was told that bromocriptine normalizes menses in 80–90% of patients, with subsequent return to fertility. She was counseled that (1) first-trimester exposure to bromocriptine is not associated with fetal malformations and (2) the risk of symptomatic expansion of a microadenoma in pregnancy is small, about 1–2%. A barrier method of contraception was recommended until menses became regular so that pregnancy could be recognized at the earliest opportunity.

Menses were normalized and the patient became pregnant.

How should she be followed? Should breast feeding be allowed?

Bromocriptine was stopped at 5 weeks of pregnancy. At each prenatal visit, the patient was asked about headaches and visual changes, but she remained asymptomatic. An uneventful term delivery occurred. The patient was counseled that breast feeding is safe in the setting of hyperprolactinemia.

CASE 2: DESIRED PREGNANCY DESPITE HYPERPROLACTINEMIA AND MACROADENOMA

A 28-year-old gravida 0 with hyperprolactinemia, infertility and a known suprasellar macroadenoma desires pregnancy.

How should she be counseled?

Patients with a macroadenoma who want to become pregnant should be counseled about the risk of symptomatic enlargement during pregnancy. Small macroadenomas (confined to the sella) typically behave like a microadenoma and the risk of growth is small. Suprasellar macroadenomas have a 23% chance of symptomatic growth during pregnancy. The risk of growth decreases markedly (from 23% to 3%) if the macroadenoma is treated before pregnancy. Whether transsphenoidal surgery or bromocriptine is used as the first-line therapy is controversial, and treatment decisions should be individualized.

The patient elected to have transsphenoidal surgery. Her prolactin normalized, regular menses began, and she became pregnant.

How should she be followed?

Although the risk of adenoma growth is decreased with surgery, it is still significant. Baseline MRI and visual fields were obtained in the first trimester. At each prenatal visit, the patient was asked about symptoms attributable to a growing macroadenoma. Formal visual field testing was obtained each trimester. The patient remained asymptomatic until 31 weeks, when she presented with significant headaches and new-onset visual field deficits. MRI detected an enlarging macroadenoma. Bromocriptine was started at 5 mg and increased to 7.5 mg with normalization of vision. Delivery occurred at 36 weeks after documenting lung maturity.

REFERENCES

1 Heaney AP, Laing I, Walton L, et al. Misleading hyperprolactinemia in pregnancy. *Lancet* 1999;353:720.

2 Hattori N. The frequency of macroprolactinemia in pregnant women and the heterogeneity of its etiologies. *J Clin Endocrinol Metab* 1996; 81:586–590.

3 Molitch ME. Disorders of prolactin secretion. *Endocrinol Metab Clin* 2001;30:585–610.

4 Gonzalez JG, Elizondo G, Saldivar D, et al. Pituitary gland growth during normal pregnancy: an *in vivo* study using magnetic resonance imaging. *Am J Med* 1988;85:217–220.

5 Muneyyirci-Delale O, Goldstein D, Reyes FI, et al. Diagnosis of stress-related hyperprolactinemia: evaluation of the hyperprolactinemia rest test. *NY State Med J* 1989;89:205.

6 Feigenbaum S, Martin M, Wilson CB, et al. Lymphocytic adenohypophysitis: a pituitary mass lesion occurring in pregnancy. *Am J Obstet Gynecol* 1991;164:1549–1555.

7 Biller BMK, Baum HB, Rosenthal DI, et al. Progressive trabecular osteopenia in women with hyperprolactinemic amenorrhea. *J Clin Endocrinol Metab* 1992;75:692–697.

8 Kupersmith MJ, Rosenberg C, Kleinberg D. Visual loss in pregnant women with pituitary adenomas. *Ann Intern Med* 1994;121:473–477.

9 Gemzell C, Wang CF. Outcome of pregnancy in women with pituitary adenoma. *Fertil Steril* 1979;31:363–372.

10 Molitch M. Management of prolactinomas during pregnancy. *J Reprod Med* 1999;44:1121–1126.

11 Molitch M. Pregnancy and the hyperprolactinemic woman. *N Engl J Med* 1985;312:1365–1370.

12 Rossi A, Vilska S, Heinonen PK. Outcome of pregnancies in women with treated or untreated hyperprolactinemia. *Eur J Obstet Gynecol Reprod Biol* 1995;63:143–146.

13 Musolino N, Bronstein M. Prolactinomas and pregnancy: use of dopamine agonists: bromocriptine and cabergoline. Proceedings of the 6th International Pituitary Congress; Long Beach, California; 1999.

14 Vance ML, Evans WS, Thorner MO. Bromocriptine. *Ann Intern Med* 1984;100:78–91.

15 Ricci G, Giolo E, Nucera G. Pregnancy in hyperprolactinemic infertile women treated with vaginal bromocriptine: report of two cases and review of the literature. *Gynecol Obstet Invest* 2001;51:266–270.

16 Turkalj I, Braun P, Krupp P. Surveillance of bromocriptine in pregnancy. *JAMA* 1982;247:1589–1591.

17 Webster J, Piscitelli G, Polli A, et al. A comparison of cabergoline and bromocriptine in the treatment of hyperprolactinemic amenorrhea. *N Engl J Med* 1994;331:904–909.

18 Robert E, Musatti L, Piscitelli G, et al. Pregnancy outcome after treatment with the ergot derivative, cabergoline. *Reprod Toxicol* 1996;10:333–337.

19 Weil C. The safety of bromocriptine in hyperprolactinemic female infertility: a literature review. *Curr Med Res Opin* 1986;10:172–195.

20 Schlechte JA. Prolactinoma. *N Engl J Med* 2003;349:2035–2041.

21 Freeman R, Wezenter B, Silverstein M. Pregnancy-associated subacute hemorrhage into a prolactinoma resulting in diabetes insipidus. *Fertil Steril* 1992;58:427–429.

22 Kerrison JB, Lee AG. Acute loss of vision during pregnancy due to a suprasellar mass. *Surv Ophthalmol* 1997;41:402–408.

Evaluation for Suspected Hypothyroidism

Suspect iodide dietary deficiency? → Pathway 2 → Follow-up 6 weeks post partum

- History of thyroid disease?
- History of autoimmune disease?
- Abnormal history and physical examination?
- Type I DM?

YES → TSH, fT4

NO → No increased risk

TSH, fT4 branches

- Low TSH
- Normal (nl) fT4

→ Physiologic suppression in 1st trimester; repeat 8 weeks

- nl TSH
- nl fT4

→ Goiter?

YES → Repeat TSH, fT4 8 weeks

NO → Euthyroid; nl f/u

- High TSH
- nl fT4

→ Subclinical hypothyroidism

- High TSH
- Low fT4

→ Overt hypothyroidism

→ Start replacement; check every 4–6 weeks and increase dose until euthyroid

Pathway 1

2 Hypothyroidism

Marjorie C. Meyer

Introduction

KEY POINT

Pregnancy is a thyroid "stress test"; women who are euthyroid before pregnancy may not be able to meet the demands of early pregnancy.

Pregnancy stresses the capacity of the thyroid gland to produce adequate amounts of thyroid hormones. Just as pregnancy can uncover latent insulin resistance and hypertension, it can tip the marginally compensated patient from having euthyroidism to having subclinical or even overt hypothyroidism. Approximately 2.5% of pregnant women have hypothyroidism.[1] Although the association of severe maternal hypothyroidism with neonatal cretinism (severe mental retardation and gait and motor function impairment) is well established,[2] recent evidence suggests that subclinical hypothyroidism may be associated with subtle neurodevelopmental abnormalities.[3] Thus, identification of the pregnant woman with thyroid abnormalities is an essential part of pregnancy care.

Pregnancy-Induced Changes in Thyroid Function

Thyroid disease is difficult to diagnose in early pregnancy because of the influence of pregnancy-related hormones on thyroid function tests. Understanding the physiology of the thyroid gland in pregnancy clarifies the interpretation of these tests (Pathway 1). The thyroid gland is under the control of the hypothalamic-pituitary axis, which regulates the production of the two major thyroid hormones, thyroxine (T_4) and triiodothyronine (T_3). Thyrotropin releasing hormone induces the secretion of thyrotropin (thyroid stimulating hormone, TSH). TSH in turn binds to its receptors on the thyroid gland, the target endocrine organ, to induce the production of T_4 and T_3 (see Pathway 1). An essential micronutrient for this production is iodine, which is stored in the thyroid gland. Once produced and secreted

19

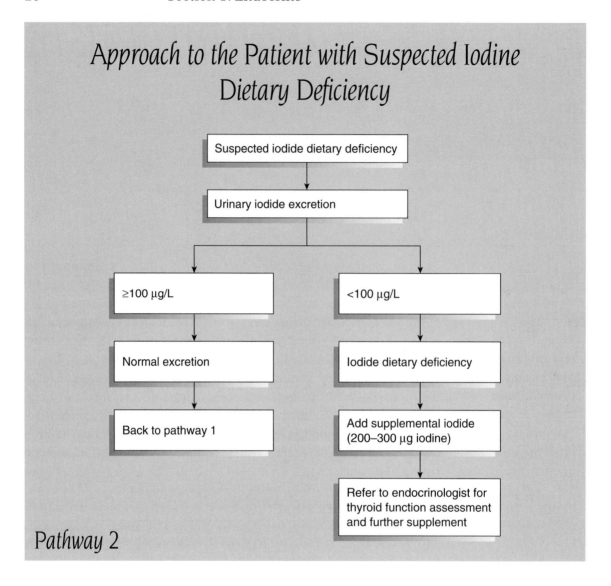

Approach to the Patient with Suspected Iodine Dietary Deficiency

Suspected iodide dietary deficiency

↓

Urinary iodide excretion

≥100 µg/L → Normal excretion → Back to pathway 1

<100 µg/L → Iodide dietary deficiency → Add supplemental iodide (200–300 µg iodine) → Refer to endocrinologist for thyroid function assessment and further supplement

Pathway 2

by the thyroid, T_4 and T_3 are extensively bound to protein primarily by thyroid binding globulin (TBG), with only 0.04% of total T_4 and 0.5% of T_3 available unbound in the serum. The free hormone, primarily T_4, feeds back to the pituitary in a negative loop to down-regulate TSH production.[4]

The stress of pregnancy on thyroid function begins early in gestation, at 6–12 weeks, in the setting of high levels of estrogen and human chorionic gonadotropin (hCG; see Pathway 1). Estrogen increases the

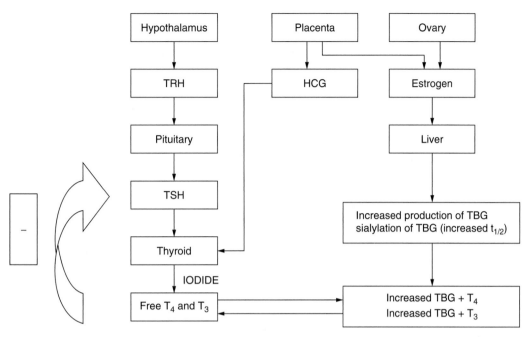

Figure 2-1: Effect of pregnancy on thyroid physiology.

production of TBG by the liver and extends the half-life of TBG, resulting in an increase in TBG by 2.5-fold early in gestation. This increase in such a high affinity binding protein would decrease the availability of free T_4 and increase TSH were it not for the direct stimulation of T_4 production by the thyroid by hCG.[4] There is significant homology between the β-subunits of TSH and hCG, allowing for "spillover," i.e., hCG can bind to the same domain of the TSH receptor used by TSH, thus directly stimulating production of thyroid hormone. Early pregnancy is therefore characterized by the paradox of decreasing TSH in the face of increased production of T_4 and T_3. The net effect of these changes is an increased total pool of thyroid hormone bound to TBG, stable free hormone that is unchanged, and suppressed TSH. By the midtrimester, hCG decreases, and TSH increases back to baseline levels. Hypothyroidism can be difficult to diagnose in early pregnancy because of the hCG-induced maintenance of T_4 production and TSH suppression. Evaluation in the midtrimester will provide a more accurate picture of the hypothalamic-pituitary axis regulation of thyroid hormone production.

Effect of Hypothyroidism on Pregnancy Outcome

Hypothyroidism due to iodine dietary deficiency is the leading cause of preventable mental retardation worldwide. The repletion of iodine on a population basis has had a remarkable effect in preventing this tragic outcome.[2] The success of this program has sparked investigation into the role hypothyroidism may play in other countries that have iodine deficiency. Although there are reports of increased miscarriages and low-birth-weight infants associated with maternal hypothyroidism, the data are inconsistent, with no clear association emerging.[5] Haddow et al.[3] reported on the neurodevelopmental outcome of children born to women with high levels of TSH in mid-gestation. They reported a modest decrease in intelligence quotient scores (4 points) associated with undiagnosed hypothyroidism during pregnancy. The results of this study resulted in calls for universal screening of all pregnant women for subclinical hypothyroidism. Unfortunately, in this study there was a difference in outcome only between women with untreated hypothyroidism and control subjects; there was no difference between those women with untreated hypothyroidism and those with treated hypothyroidism. Because of the interest in this topic and the possible implications of screening and treatment, trials will likely be available soon to answer this important question. Until that time, routine screening is not recommended, but treatment of subclinical disease during pregnancy is prudent,[6] as discussed below.

KEY POINT

Universal screening of all pregnant women for hypothyroidism is not currently recommended because no trials have demonstrated the benefit of this approach.

Congenital hypothyroidism on the basis of maternally derived thyroid blocking antibodies (blocking TSH receptor antibodies or TSH binding inhibitory immunoglobulin) is uncommon, at only 1% of all cases of congenital hypothyroidism (incidence 1 in 4000). The effect on the neonate is transient and, although evaluation of neonatal thyroid function should be performed, thyroxine replacement in the neonate is usually unnecessary.[7]

Iodine Deficiency Disorders

Although uncommon in the United States, iodine deficiency is a major cause of hypothyroidism worldwide. In the United States, iodine intake has been reported to decrease to a point at which examination for iodine excretion for adequacy can be considered.[8] Over the past decade, there has been a focus to eliminate dietary iodine deficiency led by the International Council for the Control of Iodine Deficiency Disorders, which was established in 1986. Unfortunately, 36 countries remain without an iodization program. Because of nutritional trends in the United States and the rapid influx of immigrants into many communities, the prudent clinician should assess each patient's history for potential compromised iodine stores during pregnancy. One-fourth teaspoon of iodized table salt provides iodine 95 µg. A 6-oz portion of ocean fish provides iodine 650 µg. Most people are able to meet their iodine requirements by eating seafood, seaweed, iodized salt, and plants grown in iodine-rich soil. In the evaluation of thyroid function tests, a high level of T_3 in the face of normal levels of TSH and T_4 is characteristic for iodine deficiency in the general population, but pregnancy-specific data are not available. Nonetheless, urinary iodine excretion is the best test for adequacy of iodine intake for all individuals because it is more sensitive and specific than thyroid function tests alone for the diagnosis of iodine dietary deficiency. Urinary iodine excretion less than 100 µg/L suggests a need for repletion (according to criteria of the World Health Organization).[8]

KEY POINT

Iodine deficiency is the leading cause of treatable mental retardation worldwide. Daily recommended iodine intakes are 175 µg during pregnancy and 200 µg during lactation.

Treatment of Hypothyroidism During Pregnancy

All women should be carefully evaluated for the potential for hypothyroidism early in gestation by history and physical examination. The American College of Obstetrics and Gynecology[9] recommends screening for all "high-risk" women, i.e., those with a strong family history of thyroid disease or autoimmune disease. Although testing is not required for mild thyroid enlargement associated with pregnancy, any marked enlargement should be evaluated according to recommendations by the American College of Obstetrics and Gynecology. Iodine intake should be assessed by history, with urinary iodine excretion measured for those at risk for iodine deficiency. Although it is reasonable to recommend the use of iodized salt for these women, further iodine supplementation should be performed with the aid of an endocrinologist. Care must be taken to avoid over supplementation because this can result in hyperthyroidism and attendant complications (see Chap. 3, Hyperthyroidism).

In the United States, most women will have hypothyroidism on the basis of autoimmune thyroiditis, which requires replacement with levothyroxine (T$_4$).[10] Supplementation should occur as soon as the diagnosis of hypothyroidism is made. How and when to treat subclinical hypothyroidism (high level of TSH and normal level of free T$_4$) during pregnancy are unknown. However, the preponderance of data suggesting neurologic damage to the fetus with overt hypothyroxinemia warrants prevention of hypothyroidism during pregnancy.[11] For this reason, supplementation for subclinical hypothyroidism is recommended during pregnancy, despite the lack of clinical trials demonstrating a benefit with this approach.[4,6] The dosage should be titrated to achieve normal levels of TSH and free T$_4$ levels, usually 1.6 to 1.7 µg/kg body weight.

Of special note is the management of the patient with previously identified hypothyroidism. Most women will require an increase in dosage over the course of gestation.[12] Levels of TSH and free T$_4$ should be assessed every 8 to 12 weeks if no recent dose adjustment has been made. These measurements can be done conveniently every trimester. If the dose requires alteration, levels of TSH and free T$_4$ should be checked 4 to 6 weeks after adjustment for adequacy of replacement. The postpartum period is another period of rapid, dynamic alteration of thyroid function. A TSH level should be obtained at 6 weeks postpartum unless the patient is symptomatic or a recent dose adjustment was made. As with many autoimmune diseases, women with antithyroidal antibodies may have a flare postpartum, with previously subclinical disease becoming clinically evident.[13] Because new mothers have symptoms that are similar to those of clinical hypothyroidism, clinicians should have a low threshold for testing thyroid functions in the postpartum period.

KEY POINT

Most women with stable thyroxine replacement before pregnancy will require an increase in thyroxine dosage during pregnancy as a result of increased TBG.

What is the Evidence?

There are no randomized clinical trials demonstrating the benefit of achieving and maintaining a euthyroid state during pregnancy in the absence of iodine dietary deficiency.[2] There is good evidence or consensus for the following recommendations.

1. Treatment of overt hypothyroidism is required for maternal health irrespective of pregnancy.[10] Reports of impaired neurodevelopmental outcome in women with thyroid dysfunction are derived from preliminary population-based data and

will require clinical trials before universal screening and treatment of subclinical disease is warranted.

2. Women with a family history of thyroid disease or autoimmune disease should be screened for thyroid disease during pregnancy. Women with slight enlargement of the thyroid gland do not require testing if no other risk factors apply.[9]

3. Clinicians should inquire about iodine intake and consider testing and/or supplementation if low intake is suspected.[2,4]

4. Levels of TSH and/or free T_4 should be monitored in women with thyroid disease during pregnancy. Dosage for adequate replacement may increase early in gestation.[12]

5. The pediatrician should be made aware of the presence of maternal thyroid disease to ensure appropriate follow-up of neonatal thyroid function.[7,9]

Guiding Questions in Approaching the Patient

1. Has the patient been diagnosed or tested previously for thyroid disease?
2. Is there a family history of thyroid disease?
3. Does the patient come from an area in which iodide dietary deficiency is common? (In most European countries, iodine intake is marginal; in some African countries, it is severely depleted.)
4. Is there a history of goiter?
5. Is there a history of recurrent miscarriages?

Conclusion

Hypothyroidism is common in pregnancy. In fact, women with subclinical hypothyroidism may develop overt hypothyroidism during pregnancy. While a modest decrease in IQ is associated with untreated hypothyroidism, universal screening for subclinical hypothyroidism is not currently warranted. Testing may be indicated by the patient's history and physical examination and by strong family history of thyroid disease or autoimmune disease. Thyroid function tests need to be followed during pregnancy since many women will need a greater amount of replacement thyroid hormone. Patients should also be assessed in the postpartum period.

Discussion of Cases

CASE 1: PRIMIGRAVIDA WITH A FAMILY HISTORY OF THYROID DISEASE

A new obstetric patient has arrived for routine prenatal care. She is a 24-year-old gravida 1, para 1. Her pregnancy is approximately 8 weeks. She is on no medications. She states that all four of her sisters have "thyroid problems." Her current examination indicates normal weight and height. Her skin is slightly dry. Uterine size is consistent with 8 weeks of gestation.

What tests should be ordered in addition to prenatal laboratory tests?

Levels of TSH and free T$_4$ should be determined.

Laboratory results indicated a borderline high level of TSH and a normal level of free T$_4$.

How should these laboratory results be interpreted?

At this gestational stage, the TSH level should be suppressed by hCG. The high level of TSH and normal level of free T$_4$ suggest subclinical hypothyroidism.

How should this patient be treated?

Because there are no data demonstrating a benefit from treatment of subclinical hypothyroidism during pregnancy, there are two acceptable approaches. One is to repeat the measurement of levels of TSH and free T$_4$ in the midtrimester after hCG-induced suppression has abated. If TSH level is high, therapy should proceed even if the level of free T$_4$ is normal. An alternative is to start treatment at this time to avoid any possibility of transient hypothyroxinemia. In either event, T$_4$ should be started at a dose of 0.05–0.10 mg/day.

When should adequate replacement levels be rechecked and what laboratory tests should be ordered?

Levels of TSH and free T$_4$ should be rechecked 4 weeks after starting medication or changing the dose.

Four weeks later, the patient's levels of TSH and free T$_4$ are normal.

When should these levels be rechecked?

Laboratory tests should be rechecked every 8 to 12 weeks. In this case, because pregnancy can increase requirements, especially early in gestation, it is prudent to check at 8 weeks and then every 12 weeks if results are stable.

The patient has delivered her infant. On physical examination, she feels well and has no goiter.

How will this observation alter her treatment?

It is likely she will need a decreased dose or, in this case, she may not need any replacement postpartum. She is at increased risk for development of hypothyroidism over the next 5 years (as high as 50%), so she should have her thyroid functions checked intermittently. In addition, some recommend assessment for antithyroid antibodies. This increases her risk for overt hypothyroidism within the next year.[13] She should have levels of TSH and free T$_4$ evaluated early in her next pregnancy (or, optimally, as she plans her next pregnancy). Long-term planning is best done with an endocrinologist.

CASE 2: AFRICAN IMMIGRANT WITH A GOITER

A woman presents at 18 weeks of gestation after a recent moved to the United States from Africa. Her pregnancy history is significant for occasional irregular cycles and one miscarriage. In her town, most women develop a "big neck" when pregnant and she has noticed some enlargement since the beginning of the pregnancy. On examination, she has a smooth, symmetric, slightly enlarged thyroid gland that is nontender. The initial laboratory results include a normal TSH level, a normal free T_4 level, and a slightly increased level of free T_3.

What is the likely etiology of her goiter and what laboratory tests will help answer this question?

Examination results may be consistent with pregnancy, but because the patient is from an area where iodine deficiency is common, testing is prudent. This laboratory profile of normal values but a slight increase in T_3 may indicate iodine dietary deficiency. Diagnosis is made by assessment of urinary iodine excretion. When obtained, her excretion level is 10 μg/L.

How should this result be interpreted and what treatment should be ordered?

Laboratory work suggests iodine deficiency. It is prudent to advise consuming iodized salt, but she may need a more extensive workup to determine her thyroid volume, including ultrasound and assessment of thyroid antibody status. Additional iodine replacement can be considered but should be under the direction of an endocrinologist to prevent hyperthyroidism from oversupplementation.

The patient is evaluated by an endocrinologist who diagnoses a simple goiter and no antithyroid antibodies and determines that no further medications are required. How should the patient be followed throughout gestation?

She should have an examination and TSH and free T_4 measurements every 8 weeks to ensure euthyroid status. In some cases, T_4 may be considered to prevent worsening of the goiter.

REFERENCES

1 Ayala A, Wartofsky L. The case for more aggressive screening and treatment for thyroid failure. *Cleve Clinic J Med* 2002;69:313–320.

2 Wu T, Liu GJ, Li P, Clar C. Iodised salt for preventing iodine deficiency disorders. *Cochrane Database Syst Rev* 2003;(1).

3 Haddow JE, Palomaki GE, Allan WC, et al. Maternal thyroid deficiency during pregnancy and subsequent neuropsychological development of the child. *N Eng J Med* 1999;341:549–555.

4 Glinoer D. The regulation of thyroid function in pregnancy: pathways of endocrine adaptation from physiology to pathology. *Endocrinol Rev* 1997;18:404–433.

5 Lazarus JH, Kokandi A. Thyroid disease in relation to pregnancy: a decade of change. *Clin Endocrinol* 2000;53:265–278.

6 Cooper DS. Subclinical hypothyroidism. *N Engl J Med* 2001;345: 260–265.

7 Smallridge RC, Ladenson PW. Hypothyroidism in pregnancy: consequences to neonatal health. *J Clin Endocrinol Metab* 2001;86: 2349–2353.

8 Hollowell JG, Staehling NW, Hannon WH, et al. Iodine nutrition in the United States: trends and public health implications: iodine excretion data from National Health and Nutrition Examination Surveys I and III (1971–1974 and 1988–1994). *J Clin Endocrinol Metab* 1998;83:3401–3408.

9 Thyroid disease in pregnancy. *Obstet Gynecol* 2002;100:389–396.

10 Toft AD. Thyroxine therapy. *N Engl J Med* 1994;331:174–180.

11 de Escobar GM, Obregon MJ, del Rey FE. Is neuropsychological development related to maternal hypothyroidism or to maternal hypothyroxinemia? *J Clin Endocrinol Metab* 2000;85:3975–3987.

12 Mandel SJ, Larsen PR, Seely EW, Brent GA. Increased need for thyroxine during pregnancy in women with primary hypothyroidism. *N Engl J Med* 1990;323:91–96.

13 Amino N, Tada H, Hidaka Y, Izumi Y. Postpartum autoimmune thyroid syndrome. *Endocrinol J* 2000;47:645–655.

Evaluation for Suspected Hyperthyroidism

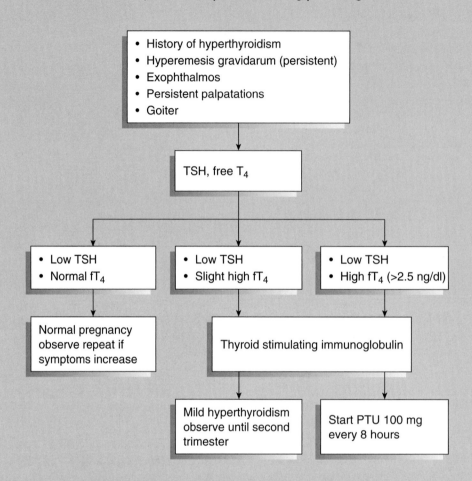

3 Hyperthyroidism

Marjorie C. Meyer

Introduction

Hyperthyroidism is the second most common endocrine disease in pregnancy, with only diabetes seen more frequently. The physiologic increase in thyroid gland activity during early pregnancy, as noted in Chap. 2 (Hypothyroidism), can make the diagnosis difficult to establish. Hyperthyroid symptoms overlap with symptoms of other diseases that complicate pregnancy, i.e., hyperemesis gravidarum in the first trimester and preeclampsia in the third trimester. Thus, clinicians must consider the possibility of hyperthyroidism when evaluating patients throughout gestation.

Pathophysiology of Hyperthyroidism

KEY POINT

Ninety percent of hyperthyroidism during pregnancy is due to Graves' disease.

Although Graves' disease accounts for only 60–80% of hyperthyroidism in the general population, during pregnancy 90% of women with hyperthyroidism will have a thyroid stimulating immunoglobulin (TSI) as the etiology of disease.[1] As with other autoimmune diseases during pregnancy, patients with preexisting disease can see worsening of disease in the puerperium. TSIs directly stimulate the thyroid gland by binding to thyroid stimulating hormone (TSH) receptors.

FIRST AND SECOND TRIMESTERS

As discussed in Chap. 2, early pregnancy is characterized by suppression of TSH by human chorionic gonadotropin (hCG), largely related to thyrotropic activity of hCG on the thyroid gland, mediated by the TSH receptor. Given the pathophysiology of Graves' disease, it is not surprising that women may initially manifest or have an

31

exacerbation of hyperthyroidism during the first trimester. To complicate matters further, the hypermetabolic state of pregnancy, with increased heart rate, fatigue, and heat intolerance, mimics symptomatic hyperthyroidism. There is no sensitive or specific clinical symptom to differentiate normal pregnancy from mild hyperthyroidism. The best diagnostic tool is evaluation of laboratory data when hyperthyroidism is part of the differential diagnosis. If the level of free T_4 is slightly high and symptoms are not severe, hyperthyroidism may be transient and repeating the laboratory work in 4–6 weeks is indicated.[2] Overzealous treatment with antithyroid medications at this stage may result in hypothyroidism later in gestation, a complication to be avoided (see Chap. 2). Treatment with antithyroid medications is indicated for severe symptoms with a high level of free T_4. All women with high levels of free T_4 should be tested for TSI, although the presence of this antibody alone is not an indication for antithyroid treatment. Although there are reports of triiodothyronine (T_3) hyperthyroidism, this disease is rare during pregnancy. The diagnosis of T_3 hyperthyroidism can be considered in the patient with severe symptoms, decreased TSH, and normal levels of free T_4. A high level of free T_3 is indicative of T_3 thyrotoxicosis.

A common indication for testing for hyperthyroidism is hyperemesis gravidarum. Decreased levels of TSH, hCG, and free T_4 have been correlated with hyperemesis. However, antithyroid drugs do not decrease vomiting in these patients, even when thyroid function tests have been normalized. In the absence of a clear diagnosis of hyperthyroidism, medications to block thyroid function are not indicated for hyperemesis. It is important to note that most women with hyperthyroidism in early pregnancy have had symptoms before pregnancy. A careful history for symptoms preceding pregnancy will help clinicians recognize these patients.

SECOND AND THIRD TRIMESTERS

After the first trimester, the hCG suppression of TSH is decreased and TSH often normalizes. Thyroid function tests should be performed if nausea and vomiting of pregnancy persist without abatement into the second trimester. Severe hyperthyroidism or thyroid storm can precipitate severe hypertension, congestive heart failure, and altered mental status, findings that mimic severe preeclampsia. Thus, hyperthyroidism should be considered in any patient who had severe preeclampsia with atypical features

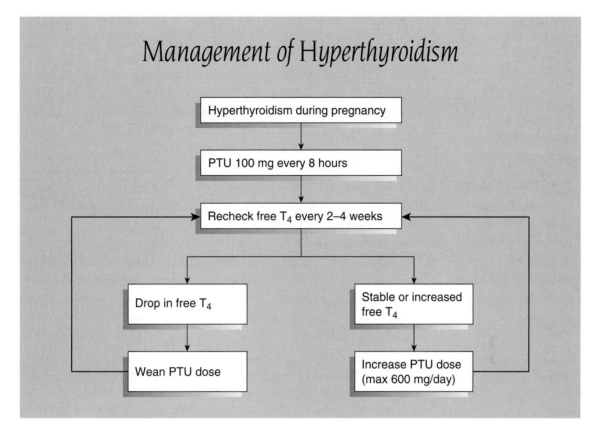

Management of Hyperthyroidism

Hyperthyroidism during pregnancy

↓

PTU 100 mg every 8 hours

↓

Recheck free T_4 every 2–4 weeks

Drop in free T_4

Wean PTU dose

Stable or increased free T_4

Increase PTU dose (max 600 mg/day)

such as early gestational age, fever, diarrhea, or tachycardia out of range of other symptoms. Prompt recognition is essential because antithyroid medication should be administered for good maternal and fetal outcome.

Fetal effects of maternal disease range from hypothyroidism from the transplacental passage of antithyroid drugs to hyperthyroidism from stimulation of the fetal thyroid gland by maternal TSI. Fetal effects are not correlated with maternal disease, but fetal hyperthyroidism is increased in women with high levels of TSI.[3] Fetal symptoms can include growth restriction, fetal tachycardia, hydrops, or fetal goiter. Fetal goiter can be seen with ultrasound in the antenatal period. It is important to identify a goiter before delivery because hyperextension of the neck can create difficulty with delivery or airway problems at birth. Fetal thyroid abnormalities can be treated in utero, but the exact diagnosis requires fetal blood sampling.[4] This invasive test is indicated only if severe, treatable fetal disease is suspected.

KEY POINT

Severe hyperthyroidism can mimic severe preeclampsia and should be suspected with atypical preeclampsia.

Treatment of Hyperthyroidism

The mainstay of treatment for hyperthyroidism is blockade of production of thyroid hormone. In general, women with a free T_4 levels higher than 2.5 ng/dL should be treated.[5] In the United States, the most commonly used drugs are propylthiouracil (PTU) and methimazole (MMU). PTU has been the drug of choice in the United States because it was initially felt that the high level of protein binding decreased transfer to the fetus. Resolution of symptoms may be more rapid with PTU because this drug can also decrease extrathyroidal conversion of T_4 to T_3 in the periphery. Moreover, MMU has been associated with increased risk for aplasia cutis in the neonate, a rare finding characterized by congenital absence of the skin. A typical lesion is 0.5–3 cm and located on the scalp at the parietal hair whorl. Although there are reports refuting this association, there was a threefold increase in aplasia cutis in regions of Spain where MMU was used illegally as a fattening agent in animal feed.[5] Because there has been no demonstrable benefit of MMU over PTU aside from dosing convenience, the risk-benefit ratio favors PTU as the initial drug of choice. MMU should be reserved for those who cannot tolerate PTU.

PTU is started at a dose of 100 mg every 8 hours, with repeat free T_4 level assessed at 2 weeks. Because PTU works by inhibiting the production of thyroid hormone, the thyroid must exhaust the existing supply of stored hormone before the effect of PTU can be assessed. TSH suppression can persist for weeks or months and therefore cannot be used to assess therapy. Atenolol can be added for a few days (25–50 mg/day orally) for symptom control, if needed. The dose of PTU should be increased if there is no response, with doses as large as 600 mg/day occasionally necessary. Treatment failure due to noncompliance should be considered if there is no effect after using larger doses of PTU. When levels of free T_4 begin to decrease, the dose should be decreased by half and free T_4 concentrations evaluated again in 2 weeks. PTU dose can be weaned in this manner every 2–4 weeks. The goal of therapy is to have a stable level of free T_4 at approximately the upper third of the normal range. TSH will normalize at approximately 8 weeks. Most women will need less PTU in the third trimester, with many women completely weaned from PTU by 32–36 weeks. If hyperthyroidism recurs, medication can be restarted.

New treatment paradigms, such as "block-replace" regimens, which administer large doses of PTU with thyroxine replacement, have not been studied during pregnancy. Because of possible fetal thyroid effects, use of these protocols should be restricted to research protocols.[1] Radioactive iodine is contraindicated during pregnancy because the iodine is taken up by the fetal thyroid gland and can destroy the developing gland. Surgery on the thyroid gland during pregnancy is reserved for only extreme cases that are unresponsive to medical therapy because severe maternal morbidity and mortality have been reported.

Evaluation of Maternal and Fetal Status During Treatment

KEY POINT

Ultrasound for fetal growth and assessment for goiter should be performed in the third trimester.

In addition to thyroid function testing, mother and fetus require assessment for complications of treatment or disease. Because PTU is associated with agranulocytosis or hepatic dysfunction, a complete blood cell count and liver function tests should be performed before treatment and periodically during therapy. Assessment of the fetus includes routine assessment of fetal growth, including careful evaluation of the fetal neck for goiter during the third trimester.

Postpartum Care

KEY POINT

Thyroid function of the neonate should be evaluated periodically because of the influence of transplacental maternal TSIs.

Hyperthyroidism may become evident for the first time with exacerbation postpartum, as is common with autoimmune diseases. Recurrence of disease in women treated earlier in pregnancy is very high, at greater than 75%.[6] Treatment is similar to that of pregnancy. PTU is compatible with breast feeding, with little drug transferred in breast milk. As with hypothyroidism, neonatal thyroid function should be monitored closely because of the effects of maternal thyroid antibodies on neonatal thyroid function. Radioactive iodine treatment can be considered after cessation of breast feeding but may require separation of mother from infant for a short time depending on the dose of iodine administered.

What is the Evidence?

There are no randomized clinical trials demonstrating the benefit of achieving and maintaining a euthyroid state during pregnancy in the absence of iodine dietary deficiency, but overt hyperthyroidism should be treated for maternal and fetal wellbeing. There is good evidence or consensus for the following recommendations: Women with a family history of thyroid disease or autoimmune disease should be screened for thyroid disease during pregnancy. Women with slight enlargement of the thyroid gland do not require testing if no other risk factors apply. Levels of TSH and/or free T4 or free thyroid index should be monitored in women with hyperthyroidism but are not warranted in women with hyperemesis. The pediatrician should be made aware of the presence of maternal thyroid disease to ensure appropriate follow-up of neonatal thyroid function.

Guiding Questions in Approaching the Patient

1. Is this hyperthyroidism from Graves' disease or is this transient gestational hyperthyroidism?
2. Should treatment be initiated and how?
3. How should the fetus be monitored?

Conclusion

Hyperthyroidism remains a common medical complication of pregnancy. It usually is caused by Grave's disease which poses a risk for fetal and neonatal hyperthyroidism. While thyroid test abnormalities are often seen with hyperemesis gravidarum, neither routine thyroid function tests nor medical treatment are indicated. Hyperthyroidism should be considered in cases of atypical severe preeclampsia. If medical therapy is indicated, propylthiouricil is preferred over methimazole. Ultrasound examination in the third trimester is indicated for surveillance for fetal growth restriction.

Discussion of Cases

CASE 1: PRIMIGRAVIDA IN FIRST TRIMESTER WITH NAUSEA AND VOMITING

A 27-year-old gravida 1 presents at 9 weeks of gestation with persistent nausea and vomiting of 1 week in duration. She denies fever, chills, or abdominal pain. Physical examination shows mild, diffuse thyromegaly without tenderness. The abdomen is soft and nontender. Pelvic examination is consistent with menstrual dating. Vital signs show normal blood pressure (90/60 mm Hg), slighty increased heart rate (95 beats/min), and normal respirations. There is a weight loss of 5 lbs from the previous week.

What testing is needed for evaluation?

Ultrasound for viability and to rule out twins or gestational trophoblastic disease, electrolytes and urinalysis to check for ketones, and determination of TSH and free T$_4$ levels.

Ultrasound shows a viable twin pregnancy, electrolytes are normal, urinalysis demonstrates large ketones but is otherwise normal, TSH is undetectable, and free T$_4$ is 1.0 ng/dL.

Does the patient require further testing or management?

Although she requires treatment for hyperemesis, the low level of TSH in the face of a high but normal level of free T$_4$ are expected in the setting of very high levels of β-hCG associated with twin gestation. Her symptoms are related to pregnancy and antithyroid medication is not indicated.

CASE 2: MULTIPARA WITH WEIGHT LOSS AND FATIGUE

A 30-year-old gravida 2, para 1001 with an uncomplicated previous pregnancy presents at 23 weeks with complaints of weakness and extreme fatigue. Her first pregnancy was uneventful, with the term delivery of a 3500-g male infant. The current pregnancy has been complicated by first-trimester nausea without vomiting, but the patient lost 8 lbs during the first trimester and has not regained any weight. She states that her appetite is not good, but she is able to keep food down. She admits to mild anxiety and has had difficulty sleeping, which are new symptoms that she cannot explain. On examination, she appears tired but otherwise normal. The thyroid is mildly enlarged but not tender. Fundal examination shows 24 cm from the symphysis pubis. Vital signs include a blood pressure of 130/80 mm Hg and a heart rate of 120.

What evaluation is indicated?

Ultrasound for multiple gestation or gestational trophoblastic disease if it had not already performed; determination of TSH and free T$_4$ concentrations; and determination of thyroid stimulating antibody if the free T$_4$ level is high.

This case illustrates the vague symptoms that should raise a suspicion of hyperthyroidism but that it may not be related to a somatic disease. It would be reasonable to consider a serum creatinine measurement and liver function tests because chronic renal disease and liver disease can present with vague symptoms. Previous ultrasound demonstrated a single viable pregnancy at 9 weeks of gestation. TSH was undetectable and free T$_4$ was 3.0 ng/dL.

What treatment, if any, is indicated?

Start PTU 100 mg orally every 8 hours; perform ultrasound to assess the fetal neck for goiter.

Because the patient's level of free T$_4$ is high and she is symptomatic, she should be started on PTU 100 mg orally every 8 hours. Because she is symptomatic with fatigue, a β-blocker can be added for 2 weeks until the effects of thyroid inhibition become apparent.

What follow-up test should be ordered?

Check levels of free T$_4$ every 2 weeks; check complete blood cell counts at 2 weeks and repeat as indicated; PTU should be decreased when free T$_4$ levels begin to decrease; and perform ultrasound every 4–6 weeks to monitor fetal growth and fetal goiter.

The goal is to have the patient on the smallest possible dose of PTU for management of disease, including discontinuation when possible. Agranulocytosis is a rare complication of PTU therapy; therefore, a complete blood cell count should be checked after initiation of therapy. The fetus has an increased risk of growth restriction and development of goiter. Thyroid stimulating antibodies can cross the placenta and create fetal hyperthyroidism and goiter; likewise, PTU can cross the placenta and inhibit fetal thyroid hormone production, which can also cause fetal goiter.

What should be done postpartum?

Notify the infant's pediatrician and measure levels of TSH and free T$_4$.

Because many women do not require medication late in pregnancy, it is important to inform the pediatrician about the mother's disease state. The neonate is at risk for hyperthyroidism due to transplacental passage of thyroid stimulating antibody. Any patient with an autoimmune disease may develop a flare-up postpartum. The patient should be followed carefully for relapse, especially during the first year postpartum.

REFERENCES

1 Weetman AP. Graves disease. *N Engl J Med* 2000;343:1236–1248.

2 Goodwin TM, Hershman JM. Hyperthyroidism due to inappropriate production of human chorionic gonadotropin. *Clin Obstet Gynecol* 1997;40:32–44.

3 Peleg D, Cada S, Peleg A, Ben-Ami M. The relationship between maternal serum thyroid stimulating immunoglobulin and fetal and neonatal thyrotoxicosis. *Obstet Gynecol* 2002;99:1040–1043.

4 Wenstrom KD, Weiner CP, Williamson RA, Grant SS. Prenatal diagnosis of fetal hyperthyroidism using funipuncture. *Obstet Gynecol* 1990;76;513–517.

5 Mandel SJ, Cooper DS. The use of anti-thyroid drugs in pregnancy and lactation. *J Clin Endocrinol Metab* 2001;86:2354–2359.

6 Mestman JH. Hyperthyroidism in pregnancy. *Endocrinol Metab Clin North Am* 1998;27:127–149.

Detection and Management of Gestational Diabetes

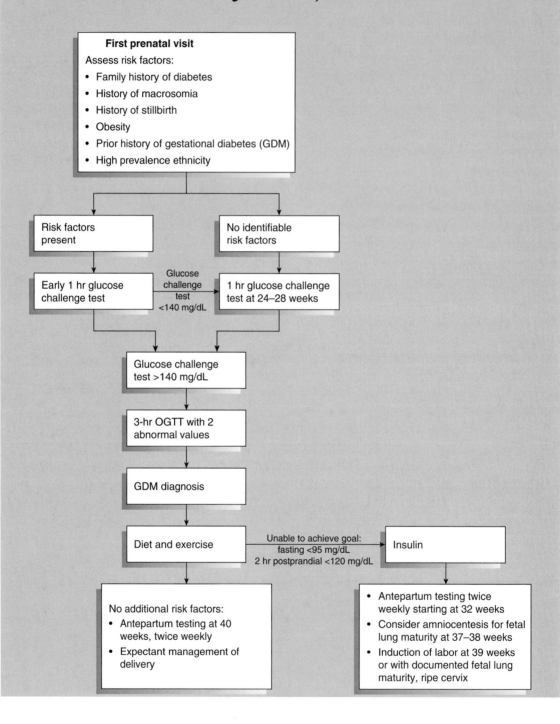

4 Gestational Diabetes

Jennifer T. Ahn
Judith U. Hibbard

Introduction

Diabetes is one of the most common metabolic disorders encountered during pregnancy and occurs in 2–5% of gravidas.[1] Gestational diabetes mellitus (GDM), which accounts for 90% of diabetic cases during pregnancy, is defined as carbohydrate intolerance with its initial onset or recognition during pregnancy.[2] In long-term follow-up studies, more than 50% of patients with GDM will develop diabetes later in life.[3]

Physiology of Gestational Diabetes

Changes in maternal metabolism provide a constant source of glucose by facilitated transport across the placenta to the growing fetus. Changes in the latter half of pregnancy heighten the diabetogenic state with increasing levels of human placental lactogen and insulin growth factors, which are promoters of insulin resistance. The resultant hyperinsulinemic state mobilizes maternal hepatic glycogen stores and potentiates gluconeogenesis. GDM is the consequence of inadequate maternal insulin production in the face of pregnancy-induced insulin resistance. The fetal response to maternal hyperglycemia is increased insulin production that can act as a growth hormone and result in macrosomia.[4]

Screening and Diagnosis

National organizations have not agreed on screening recommendations for GDM. The American College of Obstetricians and

41

***Table 4-1.*   CHARACTERISTICS OF WOMEN AT LOW RISK
               FOR GESTATIONAL DIABETES**

Must meet all following criteria

Age <25 years

Member of an ethnic group with a low prevalence of gestational
  diabetes mellitus

Weight normal before pregnancy

No known diabetes in a first-degree relative

No history of abnormal glucose tolerance

No history of poor obstetric outcome

Gynecologists (ACOG) advocates universal screening.[2] Risk-based
screening is recommended by the World Health Organization and
the American Diabetes Association (ADA).[1] Women who meet all
the criteria for being at low risk (Table 4-1) may not need screening. A subpopulation of gravidas at increased risk for developing
GDM has been identified (marked obesity, personal history of GDM
or delivery of a macrosomic infant, glycosuria, or a strong family
history of diabetes).[1] The ADA recommends that these individuals undergo screening at the first prenatal visit. For these women,
if GDM is not diagnosed during initial screening, testing should be
repeated at 24–28 weeks of gestation. Although outcomes with
early identification have not been adequately investigated, early
testing may identify individuals with previously undiagnosed type
2 diabetes. The remainder of women should have screening at
24–28 weeks. If screening is normal at 24–28 weeks and the patient
develops findings potentially consistent with GDM (macrosomia,
hydramnios), then repeat screening is indicated.

KEY POINT

*Early screening
should be done in
women with
identified risk
factors.*

Customarily, screening consists of a 50-g, 1-hour glucose challenge test administered at 24–28 weeks. This recommendation is
based on testing at the time of peaked insulin resistance and at an
early enough gestational age to allow intervention. The threshold
for an abnormal value is arbitrary and seeks to maximize sensitivity with acceptable specificity. Some data suggest that a threshold of 130 mg/dL has 90% sensitivity, with 23% of the population
requiring testing, and that a threshold of 140 mg/dL has 80% sensitivity and requires testing 14% of the population. Either threshold is considered acceptable by the ACOG, although using the
140-mg/dL cutoff is most cost effective.[2]

After an abnormal result on a glucose challenge test, a diagnostic 100-g, 3-hour oral glucose tolerance test (OGTT) should be performed. Before testing, patients should be instructed to fast overnight for 8–14 hours and ingest at least 150 g/day of carbohydrates for 3 consecutive days. This should avoid carbohydrate depletion, which could cause falsely high test results. Conditions should allow patients to be seated, and women should refrain from smoking during the testing period.[2]

Currently, three sets of diagnostic criteria for an OGTT are recognized[1,2] (Table 4-2). In the United States, the Carpenter-Coustan and National Diabetes Data Group criteria are used primarily. The diagnosis of GDM is made when a high glucose level is measured in at least two of the four parameters. Much debate surrounds which criteria are preferred. Some data suggest that the Carpenter-Coustan criteria are associated with improved outcomes including decreased incidence of fetal macrosomia. This approach also increases the number of women meeting the diagnosis of GDM and is associated with an increase in the rate of cesarean section. The ADA has adopted the stricter Carpenter-Coustan criteria, whereas the ACOG accepts either approach as long as consistency is practiced.

Current guidelines use two abnormal values for the diagnosis of GDM. However, those gravidas with one abnormal value should have close follow-up because the incidence of macrosomia was significantly higher in this subgroup than in the normal and treated GDM groups.[5] Another study showed a higher rate of cesarean section in this group.[6] If other risk factors are present (e.g., ultrasonographic evidence of large for gestational age), one

Table 4-2. **DIAGNOSTIC CRITERIA FOR GESTATIONAL DIABETES[a]**

	CARPENTER-COUSTAN (100-G GLUCOSE LOAD)	**NDDG** (100-G GLUCOSE LOAD)	**WHO** (75-G GLUCOSE LOAD)
Fasting	95 mg/dL, 5.3 mmol/L	105 mg/dL, 5.8 mmol/L	95 mg/dL, 5.3 mmol/L
1 h	180 mg/dL, 10.0 mmol/L	190 mg/dL, 10.6 mmol/L	180 mg/dL, 10.0 mmol/L
2 h	155 mg/dL, 8.6 mmol/L	165 mg/dL, 9.2 mmol/L	155 mg/dL, 7.8 mmol/L
3 h	140 mg/dL, 7.8 mmol/L	145 mg/dL, 9.0 mmol/L	N/A

[a] Diagnosis of gestational diabetes mellitus is made when a high value is seen in two parameters.
N/A = not available; NDDG = National Diabetes Data Group; WHO = World Health Organization.

may consider initiation of a diabetic diet. Re-evaluation with the OGTT should be done at 32 weeks.

Maternal and Neonatal Complications

The incidence of congenital anomalies noted in GDM is no greater than that in the general population. In GDM, hyperglycemia occurs after organogenesis. GDM is associated with excess fetal growth that is attributed to accelerated metabolism. Fetal macrosomia, the most common morbidity, occurs 10 times more frequently in women with GDM than in women without GDM.[7] As a consequence, the fetus is at increased risk for shoulder dystocia, clavicle fracture, birth trauma, and even fetal death. Polyhydramnios can result from GDM, but the mechanism of this is unclear. In addition, the neonate may face metabolic disturbances such as hypoglycemia, hyper-bilirubinemia, hypocalcemia, and polycythemia, which may require care in a neonatal intensive care unit. GDM is associated with a greater prevalence of chronic and gestational hypertension. Rates of cesarean delivery and operative vaginal delivery are increased.

Treatment

KEY POINT

The goal of therapy is maintaining euglycemia and preventing macrosomia.

The goal for management of GDM is to maintain euglycemia. Once a patient is diagnosed with GDM and appropriate therapy has been initiated, home blood glucose monitoring is initiated. Most clinicians follow monitoring protocols with daily fasting and post-prandial measurements. Current therapeutic recommendations aim toward 2-hour postprandial values lower than 120 mg/dL and fasting blood sugar levels below 95 mg/dL. A direct correlation between postprandial hyperglycemia and fetal weight has been observed.[8] There is a lack of consensus as to whether postprandial glycemic goals should reflect 1-hour values lower than 130–140 mg/dL or the more standard 2-hour value below 120 mg/dL.

DIET

Dietary modification is first-line therapy for GDM. There is incomplete evidence on the optimal nutritional elements. Consultation with a registered dietician should be encouraged. Decreasing the carbohydrate intake to 35–40% and maintaining a weight-specific caloric regimen improve postprandial glycemic control, with fewer patients needing insulin therapy.[4,9] Specifically, the caloric recommendations are 30 kcal/kg for normal-weight individuals and

20–25 kcal/kg for obese (body mass index >30 kg/m^2) women. Because limiting caloric intake may enhance ketosis, a complication weakly associated with diminished intelligence quotients in offspring, intermittent monitoring for ketonuria is reasonable.

EXERCISE

In the nonpregnant diabetic population, studies have documented that exercise can decrease glucose intolerance by targeting insulin resistance, thus obviating insulin therapy.[10] For all women, exercise during pregnancy is recommended. Programs of moderate physical exercise have been shown to decrease maternal glucose levels. Incorporating exercise into a therapy program for GDM appears to be not only safe but also prudent. Although the effect of exercise on neonatal complications associated with GDM awaits rigorous clinical trials, the beneficial glucose-lowering effects warrant a recommendation that women without medical or obstetric contraindications be encouraged to start or continue a program of moderate exercise as a part of therapy for GDM.

INSULIN

When euglycemia is not achieved by diet and exercise, insulin therapy, required by 10–15% of gravidas with GDM, is recommended. Insulin should be initiated when several postprandial blood sugar levels remain high despite appropriate dietary modifications. Insulin use in GDM has been documented to decrease the incidence of macrosomia. Types of insulin preparations and pharmacokinetics are listed in Table 4-3, with regular insulin and

Table 4-3. **INSULIN PREPARATIONS**

TYPE OF INSULIN	ONSET	PEAK	EFFECTIVE DURATION
Rapid acting Insulin lisPro (Humalog) Insulin aspart (NovoRapid)	<15 min	1 h	3 h
Short acting Regular	0.5–1 h	2–3 h	3–6 h
Intermediate acting NPH/lente	2–4 h	7–8 h	10–12 h
Long acting Ultralente Insulin glargine (Lantus)	4 h 1–2 h	Variable Flat/ predictable	18–20 h 24 h

NPH = neutral protamine hagedorn.

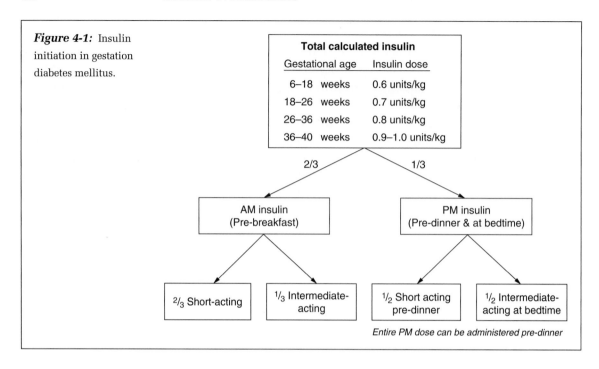

Figure 4-1: Insulin initiation in gestation diabetes mellitus.

neutral protamine hagedorn (NPH) being the most commonly used varieties. A combined split-dose subcutaneous injection of short-acting and intermediate-acting insulin is the usual route of administration. Anticipated insulin requirements can be calculated by maternal weight and gestational age (Figure 4-1), with refinements of doses after noting an individual patient's response.

Several new insulin analogs have been introduced, with a paucity of reported use during pregnancy. The short-acting analogs, insulin lispro and insulin aspart, more accurately mimic the first-phase pancreatic secretions of insulin after meals, potentially improving postprandial glycemia. Unfortunately, these analogs may accelerate maternal retinopathy. The long-acting insulin analog, insulin glargine, provides a continuous, steady release of insulin over 24 hours, a desirable quality that simulates basal insulin requirements. However, there are no studies to date that have evaluated glargine use during pregnancy. Insulin lispro and insulin aspart are listed as category C medications. Caution would urge that insulin analogs have limited use in pregnancy until data from more clinical trials are available.

ORAL AGENTS   Before recent studies, use of oral hypoglycemic agents during pregnancy was considered inappropriate due to concerns about placental transfer and neonatal outcome. Several nonrandomized reports evaluated glyburide and other oral hypoglycemics, including metformin, during pregnancy.[11–13] All but one study[12] demonstrated no adverse effects. After several pharmacokinetic studies demonstrated negligible placental transfer of the drug, 404 women with GDM were randomized to therapy with insulin or glyburide.[14] Nearly normal glucose levels were achieved by both groups, with no detected neonatal complications present in the pregnancies managed with glyburide. Although the results are promising, use of oral hypoglycemic drugs during pregnancy is not current standard of care.

Antepartum Management

Diabetic counseling is crucial for the gravida with GDM because this may be the first encounter with dietary restrictions and a need to self-monitor glucose levels. A diabetic educator can help counsel, educate, and support the diabetic gravida. Frequent office visits are necessary to assess adequacy of glycemic control. Some physicians use glycosylated hemoglobin A1C levels as another assessment of effectiveness of therapy. This test evaluates an average blood glucose concentration over the lifespan of the red blood cell, i.e., 120 days. Due to enhanced erythropoiesis during pregnancy, these values may be obtained as often as every 6 weeks.

There is consensus that antepartum testing to decrease the risk of fetal death is indicated for women with GDM who require insulin, are poorly compliant with therapy and home blood glucose monitoring, have hypertension, or have a history of fetal death. There is no consensus regarding antepartum testing for women who achieve euglycemia on diet and exercise and who are compliant with home blood glucose monitoring. If euglycemia is achieved, the risk for intrauterine demise in GDM is similar to that in the general population. Therefore, routine antepartum testing may not be warranted for uncomplicated diet-controlled GDM in the absence of risk factors, but initiating testing at 40 weeks of gestation seems prudent.[15] Some clinicians routinely initiate testing in this group.

Different antepartum testing regimens are available (nonstress tests, oxytocin challenge tests, and biophysical profiles).

One common regimen is twice-weekly nonstress testing with a weekly amniotic fluid index or weekly biophysical profiles initiated at 32 weeks of gestation. Such surveillance has decreased the rate of stillbirth from 6.1 to 1.9 in 1000 in an investigation that compared once-weekly with twice-weekly testing.[16] Instructions for fetal kick counting should also be reviewed with the patient who should detect at least 10 movements in a 2-hour period.

Ultrasonography to determine fetal weight is widely employed despite conflicting reports of reliability. Several biometric measurements been evaluated to ascertain the macrosomic fetus at risk for shoulder dystocia or other associated birth traumas. Clinical estimation by Leopold evaluation and maternal estimate of fetal weight have been shown to predict birth weight more accurately than ultrasound examination.[17] Thus, fetal weight estimations may be highly dependent on the skills of the sonographer, the potential for inaccuracy of estimated fetal weight at the higher ranges of estimated fetal weight, and the clinician's clinical acumen.

Delivery

KEY POINT

Induction of labor should be considered by 39 weeks of gestation in insulin-requiring GDM.

Timing of delivery should be carefully balanced between increased fetal morbidity and lung maturation. To decrease the risk of fetal morbidity in insulin-requiring GDM, a prospective, randomized trial compared induction of labor at 38–39 weeks of gestation with expectant management.[18] There was no apparent difference in rates of cesarean section between the two groups, but a larger number of macrosomic infants was born to the latter group. Additional investigators confirmed these results by demonstrating a greater incidence of shoulder dystocia in the expectantly managed groups.[19,20]

To prevent injury from shoulder dystocia, prophylactic cesarean delivery has been suggested for GDM patients with a range of estimated fetal weights. The American College of Obstetricians and Gynecologists recommends consideration of a cesarean section with an estimated fetal weight of at least 4500 g.[2,21] Fetal lung maturation by amniocentesis should be assessed in elective deliveries before 39 weeks of gestation. Delivery before 39 weeks is considered for women with poor glucose control, poor compliance, or comorbidities such as hypertension. Rigorous glycemic control should be maintained during the intrapartum period to prevent immediate neonatal metabolic disturbances including hypoglycemia. For well-controlled GDM on diet only, this may entail measuring blood glucose levels every 2–4 hours, with more intensified therapy needed for those maintained on insulin or in poor control.

Postpartum Follow-up

More than 50% of women with GDM will eventually develop diabetes during their lifetime. Therefore, the ACOG and ADA recommend a postpartum 75-g OGTT at least 6 weeks after delivery. Some clinicians forgo the 75-g OGTT in women who were diet controlled and had a normal result from random fingerstick blood glucose postpartum. Because some women with GDM will have had unrecognized glucose intolerance before pregnancy, the ADA suggests the following postpartum reclassification based on a 75-g OGTT: diabetes, impaired fasting glucose, impaired glucose tolerance (IGT), or normoglycemia.[22] There are no universally recognized diagnostic criteria for diabetes but the following criteria are often accepted: symptoms of diabetes with a random glucose level of at least 200 mg/dL, or a fasting (>8 hours) glucose level of at least 126 mg/dL, or a 2-hour postprandial (or after 75-g OGTT) glucose level of at least 200 mg/dL (Table 4-4).[22] Impaired fasting glucose is defined as a fasting blood sugar level higher than 110 mg/dL but lower than 140 mg/dL. Individuals who have IGT are usually euglycemic with nearly normal or normal levels of hemoglobin A1c but demonstrate hyperglycemia when challenged with an OGTT. Recent studies have clearly documented the role of diet and exercise in preventing or delaying the conversion of IGT or insulin growth factors to diabetes in adults at increased risk for type 2 diabetes.[23] Therefore, all women identified with a risk for diabetes should be advised of this, counseled, and a diet and

Table 4-4. **POSTPARTUM FOLLOW-UP USING 75-G OGTT**

	IMPAIRED FASTING GLUCOSE	*IMPAIRED GLUCOSE TOLERANCE*	*DIABETES*[a]
Fasting	≥110 mg/dL, <126 mg/dL *and*	<110 mg/dL *and*	≥126 mg/dL *or*
2 h	<140 mg/dL	≥140 mg/dL, <200 mg/dL	≥200 mg/dL

[a] Diagnosis requires two abnormal challenge tests.
OGTT = oral glucose tolerance test.

exercise program initiated. They should be advised to notify their primary care provider about the results of the OGTT.

Guiding Questions in Approaching the Patient

Assessing a patient at the first prenatal visit

- Does the patient have any identifiable risk factors associated with diabetes?
- Is there a history of poor pregnancy outcome?

Assessing plans for antenatal testing and delivery

- How well has the GDM been controlled?
- Is the patient on insulin?
- Will she need an amniocentesis to assess fetal lung maturity?
- Is there evidence of macrosomia?
- Is there a history of shoulder dystocia or cesarean section in a previous delivery?

What's the Evidence?

The majority of evidence about GDM has been retrospective and descriptive. Few studies have been controlled. There are numerous places in this text that point out controversy about data and lack of high quality data. There have been a few randomized trials. One recent prospective, randomized trial evaluated the use of oral hypoglycemic medications as opposed to insulin.[14] Research trials of timing of delivery also have been performed.[18,20]

Conclusion

Gestational diabetes will be encountered by every obstetrical care provider. A standardized approach will allow prompt therapy to improve glycemic control which will mitigate the adverse consequences of gestational diabetes. A key feature is selecting a strategy for screening whether selective or universal and performing early screening for high risk women. Therapy may include diet, exercise, insulin, or oral hypoglycemic agents. The goal of therapy is to decrease the likelihood of macrosomia and neonatal hypoglycemia. All women with gestational diabetes have an increased risk of diabetes. They should have formal screening done in the postpartum period and periodic screening for the rest of their lives.

Discussion of Cases

CASE 1: OBESE MULTIPARA WITH A HISTORY OF FETAL MACROSOMIA

A 26-year-old gravida 2, para 1001 Hispanic female presents for her initial prenatal visit. According to her last menstrual period, she is at approximately 16 weeks of gestation. She discloses her obstetric history of a previous uncomplicated vaginal delivery of a 4560-g infant at 40 weeks of gestation. She denies any personal history of diabetes, but her father has insulin-dependent diabetes. Physical examination demonstrates a moderately obese woman, with a weight of 195 lb and a height of 62 inches.

You advised a 50-g glucose challenge test that shows a high glucose level of 164 mg/dL. Follow-up 3-hour OGTT results were a fasting level of 110 mg/dL, a 1-hour level of 172 mg/dL, a 2-hour level of 151 mg/dL, and a 3-hour level of 120 mg/dL.

What risk factors does she have for diabetes?

Previous delivery of a macrosomic infant, obesity with a calculated body mass index of 35.7 kg/m^2, Hispanic ethnicity, and a family history of diabetes.

What are your recommendations for future management?

Currently, the patient does not meet the diagnostic criteria for GDM. However, she does have one abnormal value on her OGTT, which may be suggestive of impaired glucose tolerance. She should repeat the 3-hour OGTT at 24–28 weeks. Because she has demonstrated a high level on the 1-hour screening test, this test does not need to precede the repeat OGTT.

She asks you if she should be placed on a special diet to prevent her from becoming diabetic. What would you recommend?

Although few studies have demonstrated no difference in preventative measures for GDM, this patient has a multitude of risk factors, and her obesity carries an increased risk for morbidity. Caloric restriction with 35% carbohydrates may be advised. Regular exercise may be helpful.

She returns to your office at 22 weeks, now with 4+ glucosuria. A random fingerstick blood sugar level is 246 mg/dL. What do you recommend?

A random blood sugar level above 200 mg/dL is highly suggestive of diabetes and is diagnostic in a nonpregnant patient. Therefore, it is not necessary for her to undergo further diagnostic testing. Counseling for a diet appropriate for diabetics and home glucose monitoring should be initiated. She should be encouraged to exercise moderately. If her blood glucose levels remain above therapeutic goals, insulin should be initiated.

CASE 2: INSULIN REQUIRING GDM AND FETAL MACROSOMIA

A 28-year-old gravida 2, para 2002 with GDM who has been on insulin since 32 weeks presents at 34 weeks of gestation for a follow-up growth ultrasound study due to the suggestion of fetal macrosomia by fundal height and 30-week ultrasound, with growth in the 85th percentile. She states her glycemic control has been adequate. Her current insulin regimen consists of regular insulin 14 U with NPH 30 U in the morning, regular insulin 10 U at dinner, and NPH 12 U at bedtime. This week's blood sugar levels (mg/dL) are listed below:

FBS* (MG/DL)	2 H AFTER BREAKFAST	2 H AFTER LUNCH	2 H AFTER DINNER
74	119	122	124
98	132	118	108
122	157	126	113
105	98	112	96
99	125	105	123
118	141	97	106

*Fasting blood sugar.

Today's growth scan shows a fetus that measures 3900 g and higher than the 95th percentile.

What changes should be made to her insulin regimen?

Most of her fasting blood sugar levels are above 95 mg/dL. Her levels after breakfast are also high, with four of six values above 120 mg/dL. Some of her blood sugar levels after lunch and dinner are high but for the most part are within target ranges. She should increase her NPH insulin at bedtime to help decrease her fasting blood sugars. In addition, her regular insulin dosage should be increased in the morning.

What complications may arise during delivery?

She is at risk for macrosomia with consequent risks for shoulder dystocia, clavicle fracture, and operative delivery.

She reports that her previous delivery of a 4120-g infant was done with forceps. She is fearful that this pregnancy will have the same outcome. What do you recommend?

She should be advised that this infant is excessively grown and is at risk for complications. Due to her inadequate glucose control, induction of labor is indicated at 37–38 weeks after an amniocentesis to assess lung maturity. At this time, growth should be reassessed. If the estimated weight is above 4500 g, a cesarean delivery may be indicated. Twice-weekly antepartum fetal testing and daily fetal kick counts should be continued in the interim period.

REFERENCES

1 American Diabetes Association. Gestational diabetes mellitus. *Diabetes Care* 2003;26(suppl 1):S103–S105.

2 Gestational diabetes. *ACOG Pract Bull* Number 30, September 2001.

3 Damm P, Kuhl C, Bertelsen A, et al. Predictive factors for the development of diabetes in women with previous gestational diabetes mellitus. *Am J Obstet Gynecol* 1992;167:607–616.

4 Persson B, Hanson U. Neonatal morbidities in gestational diabetes mellitus. *Diabetes Care* 1998;21(suppl 2):79B–84B.

5 Langer O, Brustman L, Anyaegbunam A, Mazze R. The significance of one abnormal glucose tolerance test value on adverse outcome in pregnancy. *Am J Obstet Gynecol* 1987;15:758–763.

6 Gruendhammer M, Brezinka C, Lechleitner M. The number of abnormal plasma glucose values in the oral glucose tolerance test and the feto-maternal outcome of pregnancy. *Eur J Obstet Gynecol* 2003;108: 131–136.

7 Spellacy WN, Miller S, Winegar A, et al. Macrosomia—maternal characteristics and infant complications. *Obstet Gynecol* 1985;66:158– 161.

8 Jovanovic-Peterson L, Oetersib CM, Reed GF, et al. Maternal postprandial glucose levels and infant birth weight: the Diabetes in Early Pregnancy Study. The National Institute of Child Health and Human Development–Diabetes in Early Pregnancy Study. *Am J Obstet Gynecol* 1991;164:103–111.

9 Langer O. Management of gestational diabetes. *Clin Obstet Gynecol* 2000;43:106–115.

10 Jovanovic-Peterson L, Peterson CM. Is exercise safe or useful for gestational diabetic women? *Diabetes* 1991;40(suppl 2):179–181.

11 Elliot B, Schenker S, Langer O, et al. Oral hypoglycemic agents: profound variation exists in their rate of human placenta transfer. *Am J Obstet Gynecol* 1994;171:653–160.

12 Hellmuth E, Damm P, Molsted-Pederson L. Oral hypoglycaemic agents in 118 diabetic patients. *Diabet Med* 2000;17:507–511.

13 Gluek CJ, Phillips H, Cameron D, et al. Metformin therapy throughout pregnancy reduces the development of gestational diabetes in women with polycystic ovary syndrome. *Fertil Steril* 2002;77:520– 525.

14 Langer O, Conway DL, Berkus MD, et al. A comparison of glyburide and insulin in women with gestational diabetes mellitus. *N Engl J Med* 2000;343:1134–1138.

15 Landon MB, Gabbe SG. Fetal surveillance in the pregnancy complicated by diabetes mellitus. *Clin Perinatol* 1993;20:549–560.

16 Boehm FH, Salyer S, Shah DM, et al. Improved outcome of twice weekly nonstress testing. *Obstet Gynecol* 1986;67:566–568.

17 Sherman DJ, Arieli S, Tovbin J, et al. A comparison of clinical and ultrasonic estimation of fetal weight. *Obstet Gynecol* 1998;91:212– 217.

18 Kjos SL, Henry OA, Montoro M, et al. Insulin-requiring diabetes in pregnancy: a randomized trial of active induction of labor and expectant management. *Am J Obstet Gynecol* 1993;169:611–615.

19 Lurie S, Insler V, Hagay ZJ. Induction of labor at 38 to 39 weeks of gestation reduces the incidence of shoulder dystocia in gestational diabetic patients class A2. *Am J Perinatol* 1996;13:293–296.

20 Gonen O, Rosen DJ, Dolfin Z, et al. Induction of labor versus expectant management in macrosomia: a randomized study. *Obstet Gynecol* 1997;89:913–917.

21 Conway DL, Langer O. Elective delivery of infants with macrosomia in diabetic women: reduced shoulder dystocia versus increased cesarean deliveries. *Am J Obstet Gynecol* 1998;178:922–925.

22 Expert Committee on the Diagnosis and Classification of Diabetes Mellitus. Report of the Expert Committees on the Diagnosis and Classification of Diabetes Mellitus. *Diabetes Care* 2003;26(suppl 1): S5–S20.

23 Tuomilehto J, Lindstrom J, Eriksson JG, et al. Prevention of type 2 diabetes mellitus by changes in lifestyle among subjects with impaired glucose tolerance. *N Engl J Med* 2001;344:1343–1350.

Suggested Management of Pregestational Diabetes Preconception or in Early Pregnancy

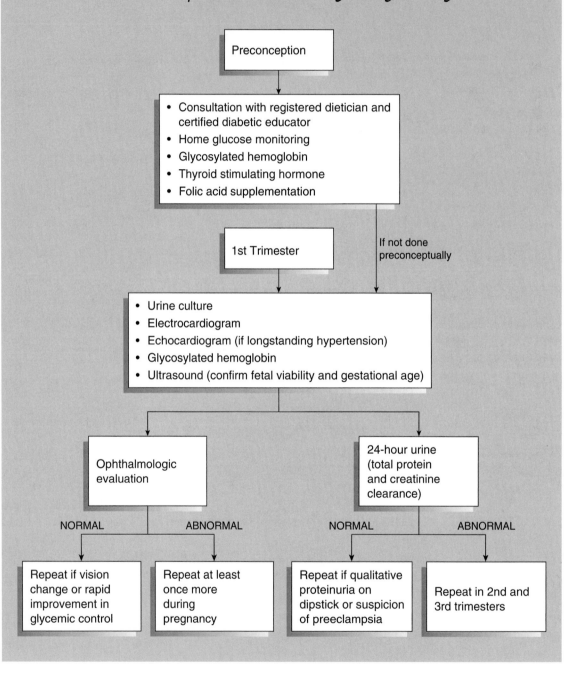

5 Pregestational Diabetes

Patricia C. Devine

Introduction

Diabetes mellitus is a chronic metabolic disorder that is characterized by an absolute or relative insulin deficiency that results in hyperglycemia. The prevalence of diabetes in pregnancy greatly depends on the population studied. As many as 3–10% of all pregnancies are complicated by some degree of insulin resistance or deficiency. In more than 80% of these pregnancies the insulin resistance is due to gestational diabetes (diabetes that is first recognized during pregnancy). Because glucose is freely transported across the placenta throughout pregnancy, the fetus is at risk for in utero hyperglycemia and increased perinatal morbidity and mortality. This chapter reviews the basic pathophysiology of pregestational diabetes, the complications that may arise with diabetes in pregnancy, and the interventions that may optimize pregnancy outcome.

Pathophysiology

Euglycemia is maintained through a series of interactions of nutrient transfer, hormones, and counter-regulatory hormones that occur in response to food intake. Hemodynamic changes of pregnancy, metabolic demands of the fetus, and function of the placenta affect glucose balance is such a way that pregnancy is often referred to as a diabetogenic state. In addition, changes that occur vary in response to gestational age and different patient characteristics such as maternal weight.

The first half of pregnancy is associated with an increased tendency toward hypoglycemia. Increased levels of estrogen and

KEY POINT

The first trimester is marked by a tendency toward decreased insulin requirements.

57

progesterone cause a decrease in hepatic glucose production and an increase in peripheral glucose utilization. Maternal glucose levels are also decreased by the uninhibited transfer of glucose from the mother to the fetus across the placenta by facilitated transport and by diminished food intake secondary to nausea and vomiting.

The second half of pregnancy is associated with increasing insulin requirements. During this period, increased levels of prolactin, cortisol, glucagons, and placental hormones combine to produce increased insulin resistance. Insulin resistance is more marked in the obese population. As a consequence, it is not uncommon for insulin requirements to increase by twofold throughout pregnancy.

After delivery, hormone levels are markedly decreased, and insulin requirements will usually decrease to prepregnancy levels or less. Many patients may not require any insulin in the first several days after delivery. Insulin requirements will generally return to prepregnancy levels by 4–6 weeks postpartum.

KEY POINT

Larger insulin doses are needed during the second and third trimesters.

Classification of Diabetes

Different classification schemes have been used to describe patients with diabetes. Traditionally, women with diabetes in pregnancy have been grouped according to White's classification. This classification system, first proposed by Priscilla White in 1940, attempted to identify women with longstanding or severe disease by grouping women according to duration of disease and presence of end-organ involvement (Table 5-1). In the 1970s, the National Diabetes Data Group proposed a different classification scheme based on pathophysiology. This scheme includes type I, type II, and gestational diabetes. Diabetes is classified as type I or type II according to whether or not the patient requires insulin to avoid diabetic ketoacidosis. Each can be subcategorized as presence or absence of vascular disease. Type I diabetes refers to patients who have an absolute insulin deficiency and require lifelong insulin supplementation. Women with type I diabetes who have a successful insulin regimen to maintain euglycemia before pregnancy are at significant risk to develop hypoglycemia in the first trimester when levels of glucose are lower.

Most pregnant patients with pregestational diabetes have type II diabetes. These patients are generally older and heavier than are patients with type I diabetes, although variations in presentation

KEY POINT

Patients at greatest risk of complications are women with type 1, insulin-deficient diabetes who have vascular disease or hypertension.

Table 5-1. **WHITE'S CLASSIFICATION OF DIABETES**
           IN PREGNANCY

White's Class	*Age at Onset (years)*	*Duration of Disease (years)*	*Systemic Complications*
Gestational diabetes			
A1			
A2			Insulin requiring
Pregestational diabetes			
B	≥20	≤10	No vascular disease
C	10–19	10–19	No vascular disease
D	<10	≥20	Background retinopathy or hypertension
F			Nephropathy (>500 mg/d proteinuria)
H			Arteriosclerotic heart disease
R			Proliferative retinopathy or hemorrhage
T			After renal transplantation

are seen. The pathogenesis of type II diabetes is very different from that of type I diabetes, with hyperglycemia occurring as a result of insulin resistance and β-cell dysfunction, with an inadequate insulin response to a given glucose load. The pathophysiology of gestational diabetes is similar to that of type II diabetes. Although these patients are not always insulin dependent and are not at risk for ketoacidosis, they may eventually require insulin to maintain euglycemia.

Effect of Pregnancy on Diabetes

Pregnancy may have a significant effect on glucose metabolism and, hence, glycemic control and insulin requirements as soon as the first few weeks of pregnancy. This section reviews the effect of pregnancy on preexisting diabetic retinopathy, nephropathy, and cardiovascular disease.

DIABETIC RETINOPATHY

Retinopathy is the most common chronic complication of diabetes and is the leading cause of blindness between ages 24 and 64 years.

The prevalence of retinopathy is directly related to duration of disease and degree of glycemic control. Changes consistent with the earliest stage of retinopathy, "background retinopathy," are seen in approximately 98% of patients who have had type I diabetes longer than 15 years. Virtually all patients who have type II diabetes longer than 25 years will have some degree of retinopathy.

Much attention has been given to the possibility that pregnancy is a risk factor for progression of diabetic retinopathy. Recent studies have provided a favorable prognosis, indicating that the degree of baseline retinopathy is a more significant risk factor for progression of disease than the occurrence of pregnancy.[1] Overall, pregnancy is associated with an approximately twofold increased risk for progression of preexisting retinopathy.[2] However, this risk is very low for patients with background retinopathy or no changes on baseline eye examination. The Diabetes in Early Pregnancy study also confirmed that patients with minimal or no changes on baseline eye examination are at a lower risk for progression of disease than are patients with more advanced baseline findings.[3]

Several studies have suggested that rapid induction of glycemic control in early pregnancy can result in increased retinal vascular proliferation and, therefore, progression of disease. There is controversy about the particular risk associated with insulin lispro.[4] The risk of progression is greatest for patients with longstanding significant hyperglycemia (glycosylated hemoglobin >10%) who achieve rapid improvement in glycemic control. However, when the total effect of pregnancy on the status of retinopathy is considered, women who are pregnant demonstrate a slower progression of disease than does the non-pregnant population. Therefore, deterioration of retinal status that is seen with rapid improvement of control early in pregnancy is offset by the benefits of excellent control that are maintained during and after pregnancy. Hypertension and nephropathy may be additional risk factors for progression of retinopathy in pregnancy.

Ideally, all women should have a comprehensive eye examination and therapy, if indicated, before conception. All women with pregestational diabetes should have an eye examination by an ophthalmologist early in pregnancy. Many patients may need to have serial examinations in pregnancy, and all patients will require evaluation

KEY POINT

Women with a history of retinopathy or a drastic improvement in control in the first trimester need close ophthalmologic evaluation for proliferative retinopathy.

after delivery.[5] Some controversy exists as to whether women with background retinopathy need more than an initial ophthalmologic examination. Fortunately, most changes related to retinopathy are temporary and reversible, with most patients demonstrating a return to their baseline status by 6 months after delivery. If necessary, laser photocoagulation may be completed in pregnancy. A minority of women with severe disease and no response to photocoagulation may be at risk for further progression of their disease and loss of vision. Early delivery could be considered for this group, although there is no literature to confirm that this will improve a patient's outcome.

DIABETIC NEPHROPATHY

As with diabetic retinopathy, the risk of nephropathy is directly related to the duration of disease and degree of control. A diagnosis of nephropathy is associated with a decrease in life expectancy, with a significant percentage of these patients developing overt renal failure within 10–20 years. Baseline renal function is the single most important predictor of pregnancy outcome in any patient with underlying renal disease.[6] The two factors most predictive of outcome are proteinuria higher than 3.0 g/24 hours or serum creatinine concentrations higher than 1.5 mg/dL before 20 weeks of gestation. Patients with decreased renal function are at increased risk for preeclampsia (up to 55%), low birth weight (up to 20%), and preterm delivery (up to 75%).[7]

Most women will have an iprovement in renal function in the first half of pregnancy secondary to increases in plasma volume, renal blood flow, and glomerular filtration that occur with pregnancy. However, most studies have demonstrated that pregnancy is not associated with an increased risk of developing nephropathy or permanent worsening of preexisting renal disease.[1,8,9] Patients who develop proteinuria in pregnancy will usually see a return to baseline after delivery. Patients who have a decrease in creatinine clearance are at significant risk to develop preeclampsia. The bulk of the information available suggests that, for most women, pregnancy does not cause permanent deterioration in kidney function. There is some evidence that women who have severe renal disease during pregnancy may develop accelerated progression to end-stage renal disease.[1]

Recommendations for the treatment of patients with diabetic nephropathy in pregnancy include serial assessment of renal function, good glycemic control, and aggressive blood pressure

KEY POINT

Women with diabetic nephropathy can have a significant increase in the amount of proteinuria during pregnancy. Most will return to baseline after pregnancy.

The comorbidity of diabetic nephropathy increases risks of preeclampsia, premature delivery, and fetal growth restriction. The diagnosis of superimposed preeclampsia can be difficult.

management. The drug of choice for the management of hypertension in these patients is not certain. The use of angiotensin-converting enzyme inhibitors is contraindicated in pregnancy. These drugs can have an adverse effect on fetal renal function and have been associated with fetal death.

Patients with longstanding type I diabetes and nephropathy are at risk for progression to end-stage renal failure and the need for hemodialysis. Advances in the care of these patients have resulted in an improved overall state of health, with many of these patients becoming pregnant. The prognosis for a successful pregnancy in patients who require hemodialysis remains poor. However, there is a very high likelihood of good outcome after successful renal transplantation.[10]

CARDIOVASCULAR DISEASE

Cardiovascular diseases seen in the pregnant diabetic patient include chronic hypertension, preeclampsia, and ischemic myocardial disease. Hypertensive disorders are estimated to complicate up to 30% of all diabetic pregnancies and are a risk factor for preterm delivery, fetal growth restriction, and abruption. Chronic hypertension is estimated to complicate approximately 10% of all diabetic pregnancies, but this risk is doubled for patients with preexisting nephropathy. Preeclampsia is more likely in pregnant patients with diabetes. Patients with diabetes complicated by nephropathy or chronic hypertension are at increased risk for preeclampsia.[11]

Although uncommon, a small number of women with longstanding diabetes may have coronary artery disease. Patients with this complication have a mean age of 34 years and nearly always exhibit evidence of retinopathy or nephropathy. Studies published before 1980 reported maternal mortality rates on the order of 70%. Series and reports since then have been more optimistic, with mortality rates up to 10%.[1] Pregnancy remains a significant risk due to obligatory physiologic changes and the increased demands required by delivery. Successful outcome is dependent on a team approach with goals of good glucose control without hypoglycemia, surveillance for maternal and fetal statuses, and delivery planning that considers cardiac function.

Effect of Diabetes on Pregnancy Outcome

Because glucose can freely cross the placenta, maternal hyperglycemia is associated with fetal hyperglycemia and subsequent fetal hyperinsulinemia. Fetal hyperinsulinemia has a negative effect on the developing fetus that results in increased storage of nutrients and subsequent macrosomia. The fetus responds to the increased level of nutrients with an increase in catabolism that requires energy and can result in depletion of fetal oxygen stores. Chronic hypoxia can have significant effects on the developing fetus that result in multiple hematologic and cardiovascular adaptations with subsequent morbidity.

FETAL AND NEONATAL DEMISE

In the past, a large number of pregnancies in diabetic women resulted in unexplained fetal demise. Although improvements in care have resulted in a significant decrease in the incidence of fetal demise, the risk remains approximately twice that of the general population. Risk factors for fetal demise include history of poor glycemic control, vasculopathy, preterm delivery, macrosomia, and preeclampsia. The ability to assess gestational age and fetal lung maturity before delivery has made delivery before 39 weeks of gestation much safer. The use of antenatal testing and ultrasound surveillance has been instrumental in decreasing the risk of fetal death. With the decrease in incidence of intrauterine fetal demise and neonatal demise secondary to hyaline membrane disease, the most common current cause of perinatal loss in this population is congenital anomalies.

FETAL MALFORMATIONS

Among the general population, the risk of having a major birth defect in approximately 1–2%. This risk is increased by two- to sixfold in women with diabetes before conception.[12,13] The Diabetes in Early Pregnancy study has confirmed these numbers, with a 9% incidence of major anomaly among 279 women with diabetes compared with a 2.1% incidence in a nondiabetic control population.[14,15] No single malformation is specific to diabetes, but malformations tend to be more severe and commonly involve the central nervous or cardiovascular system.

The etiology of malformations is not certain but is felt to be directly related to the degree of glycemic control early in pregnancy. Lucas and colleagues reported an overall risk of 13% for malformation in a series of 105 diabetic patients. In this series, the risk of delivering a malformed infant was not increased above that of the general population if hemoglobin A1c values were lower than 7%, and increased directly with hemoglobin A1c to a risk of 25% for values higher than 11.2%.[16] Although hyperglycemia is a significant risk factor for fetal malformation, the etiology is felt to be multifactorial, with increased levels of ketones, somatomedin inhibitors, and free oxygen radicals proposed as possible factors related to teratogenesis in this population.

MACROSOMIA

Multiple definitions have been used to describe macrosomia and include birth weight greater than 4000 or 4500 g or greater than the 90th percentile for a given gestational age. Macrosomia is estimated to occur in up to 40% of pregnancies in women with pregestational diabetes, with the risk of delivering a baby weighing greater than 4500 g increased 10-fold over that of the nondiabetic population.[17]

Fetal macrosomia remains a significant clinical issue because it is associated with increases in maternal and neonatal morbidities. Macrosomia is associated with an increased need for cesarean section delivery and increased risks of shoulder dystocia, neonatal acidosis, hypoglycemia, and hyperbilirubinemia. Neonatal morphometric measurements indicate that infants born to patients with diabetes have a greater proportion of fat deposition in the abdominal and intrascapular areas. The disproportionate growth within the abdomen can be detected prenatally, with accelerated growth of the abdominal circumference seen after 24 weeks. There remains no reliable way to make an accurate estimate of fetal weight.

Data from the Diabetes in Early Pregnancy trial have indicated that birth weight correlates best with second and third trimester postprandial levels and not with fasting levels. In addition, strict glycemic control that improves postprandial levels can decrease the risk of macrosomia. When postprandial glucose levels were maintained within the normal range (<120 mg/dL), the incidence of macrosomia was 20% compared with 35% when the average postprandial value was 160 mg/dL.[18]

FETAL GROWTH RESTRICTION

Although pregnancies of women with diabetes are most often complicated by excessive fetal growth, a small number of these pregnancies will result in fetal growth restriction, especially in those with underling vascular disease. Additional risk factors for poor fetal growth include longstanding diabetes (>10 years), baseline nephropathy, vascular disease, maternal hypertension, and the presence of a fetal anomaly.

NEONATAL MORBIDITY

Maternal hyperglycemia can result in fetal hyperglycemia and hyperinsulinemia. Longstanding fetal hyperglycemia and hyperinsulinemia have a significant effect on the uterine environment and can result in increased neonatal morbidity. Neonates of women with diabetes are at risk for multiple metabolic abnormalities in the neonatal period, including hypoglycemia, polycythemia, hyperbilirubinemia, and hypocalcemia.

Hypoglycemia is defined as a glucose level lower than 35–40 mg/dL within the first 12 hours of life. It is commonly seen in macrosomic neonates and affects up to 50% of these babies. The risk and severity of hypoglycemia is increased in patients with poorly controlled diabetes in the third trimester or during labor and delivery. Prolonged fetal hyperglycemia results in β-cell hyperplasia and hyperinsulinemia. Delivery interrupts the excessive supply of glucose; however, the exaggerated insulin response persists with subsequent hypoglycemia. If unrecognized, significant hypoglycemia may result in seizures, coma, and brain damage.

In utero hyperglycemia and hyperinsulinemia can also result in depletion of oxygen stores. The subsequent hypoxia is a powerful stimulant of fetal erythropoietin, resulting in polycythemia. Excessive red cell production can cause hyperviscosity, with subsequent vascular sludging and ischemia or hyperbilirubinemia secondary to destruction of the increased levels of red blood cells. Decreased serum levels of calcium and magnesium are detected more commonly in neonates of mothers with diabetes, even when additional risk factors such as prematurity and birth asphyxia are controlled.

Prolonged in utero hyperglycemia may also have an adverse affect on fetal cardiac development. Fetuses exposed to prolonged hyperglycemia may develop hypertrophic cardiomegaly, with asymmetric septal hypertrophy (ASH).[19] The risk of developing ASH is related to the degree of antenatal glycemic control, with the neonatal diagnosis associated with increased birth weight (4009 vs. 3475 g) and maternal glycosylated hemoglobin levels (6.7% vs. 5.7%).[20] However, excellent control does not exclude the possibility of ASH.[19]

RESPIRATORY DISTRESS SYNDROME

Before the 1970s, respiratory distress syndrome was the most common complication seen in newborns born to mothers with diabetes, and planned preterm delivery was often used as a means to avoid fetal demise. Management of late pregnancy evolved with the implementation of ultrasound and antenatal surveillance. Preterm delivery could be avoided more often, and ultrasound and fetal lung maturity testing allowed preterm delivery to be completed more safely. The incidence of respiratory distress syndrome has decreased from 31% to 3%.

Maternal diabetes is known to have a negative effect on fetal lung maturation. Early studies assessing amniotic fluid samples reported a delay in normal timing of pulmonary maturation in diabetic pregnancies, with phosphatidylglycerol (PG) detected later in diabetic pregnancies. Some studies indicate that pulmonary maturation may be adversely affected only in pregnancies with poor glycemic control.[21] Therefore, in diabetic women with less than ideal control, it is not safe to assume that there is no risk for respiratory distress syndrome until at least a gestational age of 39 weeks. Any delivery planned before this time for other than the most urgent maternal or fetal indication should be preceded by documentation of fetal lung maturity.[22] The gold standard for fetal lung maturity studies is documentation of the presence of PG. A lecithin/sphingomyelin ratio higher than 2.0 alone is considered to be insufficient. Currently, many physicians use other amniotic fluid assays for assessment of lung maturity. An obstetrician should be aware of the performance ability of the specific assay used to assess lung maturity.

KEY POINT

If delivery is considered before 39 weeks without a clearly compelling indication, an amniocentesis for lung maturity is necessary.

Management of Pregnancy Complicated by Pregestational Diabetes

The goal of management of diabetes is to achieve euglycemia to limit maternal and neonatal mortality and morbidity and limit the hypoglycemia that may be associated with intensive insulin therapy. Euglycemia is usually achieved through a combination of diet modifications, insulin therapy, and exercise.

Dietary management is critical to the successful control of diabetes. Optimally, the patient should also receive dietary instruction from a registered dietician and a certified diabetic educator. The goal is for patients to avoid a single large meal that will cause a significant increase in glucose levels. Three meals with several small intervening snacks are recommended to limit the glucose load to the body at any given time and limit the risk of interprandial hypoglycemia. The current dietary recommendations are for a total caloric intake of 35 kcal/(kg · d) that is based on prepregnancy weight and composed of 50–60% carbohydrates, 20% protein, and 25–30% fat. Dietary education should also include carbohydrate counting. Weight reduction by dieting in pregnancy is not advised.

Frequent blood glucose monitoring is a fundamental part of achieving good glycemic control. It involves the patient in her own care and provides immediate feedback on the effectiveness of the diet or current insulin dosage. The frequency of home glucose monitoring should be individualized for each patient but should include postprandial levels because they have the strongest correlation with fetal growth. The typical regimen involves the patient assessing the glucose level immediately after rising in the morning (fasting) and 2 hours after each meal. Studies have demonstrated that glycemic control can be further improved if preprandial glucose levels are assessed. Preprandial values allow the insulin to be adjusted based on the current glucose state and the composition of the meal through a method of carbohydrate counting.

The target glucose levels for each of these checks are higher 65 mg/dL but lower than 95 mg/dL in the fasting state and lower than 120 mg/dL 2 hours postprandial. Significant hypoglycemia should be avoided. The patient should maintain a log that tracks dietary intake, insulin dosage, and glucose level to allow immediate feedback.

Insulin can be provided through several different regimens that vary in the type of insulin used and the mode and time of delivery. Insulin levels usually need to be decreased by as much as 10–15% in the first trimester and then are gradually increased beginning in the second trimester as insulin resistance develops in response to placental hormones.

Most patients are managed with a regimen of multiple subcutaneous injections of a combination of short- and intermediate-acting insulin. Table 5-2 lists the types of insulin most commonly used in pregnancy. Although neutral protamine hagedorn (NPH) and regular insulin is the combination used most often in pregnancy, lispro is a short-acting insulin that is being used more often in pregnancy in place of regular insulin.[23] Its use has been addressed by a randomized trial demonstrating it to be at least as effective as regimens with regular insulin.[24] When compared with regular insulin, the peak serum concentration of lispro is higher and achieved more rapidly and the duration of action is half as long. Hence, lispro is very effective in preventing postprandial hyperglycemia and prevents the interprandial hypoglycemia that can be seen with increasing doses of insulin that has a longer duration of action. It can be substituted for regular insulin in a 1:1 ratio.

Table 5-2. **INSULIN PREPARATIONS FREQUENTLY UTILIZED IN PREGNANCY**

TYPE OF INSULIN	TIME TO PEAK ACTION (H)	DURATION OF ACTION (H)	COMMENTS
Humalog (lispro)	1	2	Given immediately before meals Decreased incidence of interprandial hypoglycemia
Regular	2	4	Given 20–30 min before meals Risk for interprandial hypoglycemia when large doses are required
NPH	4	8	Usually given before breakfast and in the evening before bedtime Risk of 3 AM hypoglycemia
Lantus (glargine)	Flat/predictable	24	Onset in 1–2 h Commonly given at bedtime

A common calculation for the initial 24-hour dose requirement of insulin is 0.5 U/day in the first trimester, 0.75 U/day in the second trimester, and 1.0 U/day in the third trimester. Two-thirds of the dose is given in the morning before breakfast distributed as two-thirds intermediate-acting insulin and one-third short-acting insulin. The remaining third of the dose is given before dinner with half as short-acting insulin and half as intermediate-acting insulin. Many people take the intermediate-acting component at bedtime.

Patients who use carbohydrate counting generally administer short-acting insulin before each meal, with the dose based on the amount of carbohydrate to be ingested. These calculations can be simple such as short-acting insulin 1 U for each 10 g of carbohydrate to be ingested or can be quite complex. They also take scheduled intermediate- or long-acting insulin. A long-acting insulin is commonly given at bedtime.

Women with diabetes are being managed with a continuous subcutaneous infusion of insulin with increasing frequency. The insulin pump allows for a constant infusion of a low dose of short-acting insulin, with boluses administered before meals. Although only limited data are available describing use of the insulin pump in pregnancy, several studies suggest that it is a safe and effective management tool in pregnancy.[25] Pump use is currently limited to a small number of highly motivated patients.

ANTEPARTUM FETAL EVALUATION

The surveillance and anteparum testing algorithm lists the various elements of fetal and maternal surveillance that should be used throughout pregnancy. Ultrasound evaluation is critical to assess viability, confirm gestational age early in pregnancy, and then assess for fetal anomalies and appropriate fetal growth in the second and third trimesters. Antenatal testing is generally initiated at 32–34 weeks of gestation for all patients with pregestational diabetes but should be initiated sooner in patients with fetal growth restriction, poorly controlled hypertension, or persistent hyperglycemia. Antenatal fetal testing can be completed with the biophysical profile or nonstress test but should include daily fetal kick counting.

TIMING AND MODE OF DELIVERY

The goal for delivery is to await spontaneous labor, if possible, until 39 weeks, when the risk of pulmonary immaturity is extremely low. In general, delivery should be accomplished by 40 weeks, after which time the risk of fetal demise is known to increase. Induction should be avoided, if possible, because it places the patient at risk for a prolonged hospitalization and cesarean section delivery. Expectant management until term is an appropriate option for patients with good glycemic control, normal fetal growth, and reassuring fetal testing. Early delivery should be considered for patients with evidence of maternal or fetal compromise (e.g., hypertension, preeclampsia, fetal growth restriction, or nonreassuring fetal testing). Fetal lung maturity testing is not usually indicated in these patients. Patients with hyperglycemia may need to be delivered before 39 weeks, but assessment of fetal lung maturity should be considered.

Delivery of the macrosomic infant at term is more complicated. Diabetes and macrosomia are the risk factors most strongly associated with shoulder dystocia, with women with diabetes having significantly greater rates of shoulder dystocia at any given fetal weight. The American College of Obstetricians and Gynecologists (ACOG)

Surveillance and Antepartum Testing for Pregestational Diabetes in Pregnancy

Second trimester

- Urine culture
- Thyroid stimulating hormone level
- Glycosylated hemoglobin

Prentatal diagnosis:

- Maternal serum screening (15 to 18 weeks' gestation)
- Level II ultrasound evaluation (16 to 20 weeks' gestation)
- Fetal echocardiography (20 to 22 weeks' gestation)
- 24-hour urine or ophthalmologic examinations if needed

Third trimester

- Urine culture
- Glycosylated hemoglobin
- 24-hour urine or ophthalmologic examinations if needed
- Ultrasound evaluation to assess fetal growth
  (26, 30, 34, and 38 weeks and as indicated)

- Antenatal testing
- Twice weekly BPP or NST

Hypertension, fetal growth restriction, oligohydramnios

NO

YES

Start at 32–34 weeks

Start at 28 weeks or when diagnosed

currently recommends that cesarean section be considered for all diabetic patients with an estimated fetal weight (EFW) greater than 4500 g.[26] Because of the increased risk of shoulder dystocia in the diabetic population at any given birth weight, caution should also be used when considering operative vaginal delivery or continued expectant management in patients with a prolonged second stage.

The role of induction of labor to prevent macrosomia and limit the risk of shoulder dystocia is uncertain. This option is limited by the inability to assess accurately fetal weight at term and the increased risk of cesarean section that is associated with induction. Several studies that compared expectant management with induction of labor in patients with diabetes have indicated that induction of labor may result in decreased birth weight and incidence of shoulder dystocia without increasing the cesarean section rate. However, these studies did not include fetuses with suspected macrosomia, and these results have not been replicated in the non-diabetic population.[27,28] One randomized study in the nondiabetic population reported similar rates for cesarean section and shoulder dystocia when comparing induction with expectant management in patients with an EFW of 4000–4500 g.[29]

KEY POINT

Diabetic mothers with macrosomic fetuses are at risk for shoulder dystocia. ACOG recommends cesarean birth if the EFW is greater than 4500 g.

INTRAPARTUM GLYCEMIC CONTROL

Because the neonatal status can be affected by intrapartum hyperglycemia, especially in patients with prolonged labors, it is important to maintain euglycemia (range 80–100 mg/dL) throughout labor. Many patients will require little or no insulin in labor. Frequent fingerstick blood sugar testing must be done and intermittent urine analysis should be assessed for ketones. If delivery is planned by induction or cesarean section, the patient should be counseled to follow her usual dietary and insulin regimen of insulin the evening before delivery, have nothing to eat or drink after midnight, and take no additional insulin the morning of delivery. Some physicians ask the patient to take one-third of her usual intermediate-acting insulin dose that morning. Patients undergoing elective cesarean section should be scheduled as the first case of the day to avoid long periods without food intake or insulin. Although there are many ways to manage insulin therapy in labor, Table 5-3 lists general guidelines for intrapartum glucose management.

Table 5-3.   GLUCOSE MANAGEMENT IN LABOR

Usual dietary and insulin regimen the evening before delivery;
  morning insulin is held
Glucose assessment every hour (may be decreased to every 2 h in
  early labor if stable)
Intravenous infusion of saline is initiated
Once active labor begins or glucose level decreases <70 mg/dL,
  infusion is changed from saline to 5% dextrose and delivered
  at rate of 2.5 mL/(kg · min)
Short-acting insulin (regular) is administered by intravenous
  infusion rate, as needed as follows:

Glucose Level (mg/dL)	Insulin Infusion Rate (U/h)
<80	Insulin off
80–100	0.5
101–140	1.0
141–180	1.5
181–220	2.0

Patients who use an insulin pump may continue with the pump in labor
  after adjusting the basal dose as required

Guiding Questions in Approaching the Patient

- What type of diabetes does the patient have: type I or type II?
- How many years has the patient had diabetes?
- Is the diabetes well controlled? What is the baseline glycosylated hemoglobin level? What are the most recent glucose
  levels?
- Is the patient currently taking insulin? What is her insulin
  regimen? Does it need to be adjusted?
- Does the patient have a history of systemic complications:
  retinopathy, nephropathy, or cardiovascular disease? What
  are the baseline values for renal function, ophthalmologic
  evaluation, and blood pressure?
- What is the gestational age of the pregnancy? Has the pregnancy dating been confirmed with ultrasound evaluation?
- Has fetal evaluation been initiated to include maternal
  serum screening, level 2 ultrasound evaluation, and fetal
  echocardiography?

What's the Evidence?

Most of the information about maternal and perinatal outcomes relies on multiple population-based observational studies, some with cohort controls. Limited study has addressed therapeutic options, but there have been some recent controlled studies of different insulin management regimens that may help guide clinical care.[23,24] Clinical trials have addressed the issue of timing of delivery.[27,28] Several issues impair studying these issues. One is the difficulty in any research trial studying pregnant women. In addition, many of the outcomes of interest with regard to maternal health will not be determined for many years and are difficult to study. In all likelihood there will be some new knowledge derived from basic embryology research that will provide tools to prevent birth defects and improve glucose control.

Conclusion

Although pregestational diabetes is relatively common, it has the potential to complicate pregnancy significantly from patient and pregnancy outcome standpoints. Depending on maternal comorbidities and compliance, with compulsive management, a good outcome is highly likely.

Discussion of Cases

CASE 1: PRENATAL CARE FOR DIABETIC PATIENT

A 26-year-old women with a 16-year history of diabetes at 10 weeks of gestation presents for her initial obstetric evaluation. The patient reports good glycemic control with an insulin regimen of multiple injections of short- and intermediate-acting insulin. She has had some nausea in the mornings over the past several weeks.

Her initial evaluation in the office is significant for a singleton pregnancy, with ultrasound confirming the pregnancy dating. Blood pressure is 120/60 mm Hg with 2+ protein on urine analysis. The glucose level in the office, approx-

imately 2 hours after the patient ate breakfast, is 75 mg/dL, and the glycosylated hemoglobin level is 5.4%. Review of the glucose log shows 2-hour postprandial levels of 55–70 mg/dL. The remaining fingersticks are normal.

What additional tests would you recommend at this time?

Urine culture, 24-hour urine for protein and creatinine clearance, electrocardiogram, and ophthalmologic evaluation.

Does the patient require any changes in her insulin regimen?

The morning postprandial values are lower than the recommended target levels. Patients with pregestational diabetes are at risk for hypoglycemia early in the pregnancy due to metabolic changes related to pregnancy and decreased intake secondary to nausea. The morning dose of short-acting insulin should be decreased, and nutritional consultation should be obtained to ensure proper dietary intake. If nausea and vomiting are severe, antiemetics may be recommended.

What is your recommendation for evaluation of the fetus during the pregnancy?

The normal glycosylated hemoglobin suggests that the patient is not at an increased risk for fetal anomalies due to her history of diabetes. However, ultrasound evaluation to assess for fetal anomalies should be completed at 18–20 weeks of gestation. Fetal echocardiography at 20–22 weeks of gestation should also be considered, especially if level 2 ultrasound evaluation is unable to fully evaluate the cardiac anatomy. Maternal serum screening should also be completed at 15–18 weeks of gestation to screen for neural tube and abdominal wall defects. Ultrasound evaluation and fetal testing should be completed in the third trimester to assess fetal growth and fetal well-being.

CASE 2: MANAGEMENT OF DIABETES NEAR TERM

A 38-year-old women with pregestational diabetes for 2 years is currently at 37 weeks of gestation. She had two previous pregnancies that were complicated by gestational diabetes and fetal macrosomia, resulting in vaginal delivery of 9-lb babies. The current pregnancy has been complicated by persistent hyperglycemia, with postprandial glucose levels persistently above 200 mg/dL. The current insulin regimen consists of multiple injections of short- and long-acting insulin. Ultrasound examination demonstrates excessive fetal growth with an EFW of 3800 g and polyhydramnios. Fetal testing is reassuring.

What intervention should be considered at this time?

Because of persistent hyperglycemia at this gestational age, delivery should be considered at this time. If delivery is not initiated immediately, the insulin dose should be adjusted and fetal testing should be maintained at a frequency of twice weekly.

Should any special procedures be completed before delivery?

Because the gestational age is only 37 weeks and there is no evidence of fetal or maternal distress requiring urgent delivery, assessment of fetal lung maturity should be completed.

What mode of delivery do you recommend?

Induction of labor with vaginal delivery is recommended for this patient with an EFW of 3800 g. Patients with diabetes and macrosomia are at significant risk for shoulder dystocia, with the risk directly related to the birth weight.

REFERENCES

1 Rosenn BM, Miodovnik M. Medical complications of diabetes mellitus in pregnancy. *Clin Obstet Gynecol* 2000;43:17–31.

2 Diabetes and Control and Complications Trial Research Group. Effect of pregnancy on microvascular complications in the Diabetes Control and Complications Trial. *Diabetes Care* 2000;23:1084–1091.

3 Chew EY, Mills JL, Metzger BE, et al. Metabolic control and progression of retinopathy. The Diabetes in Early Pregnancy Study. *Diabetes Care* 1995;18:631–637.

4 Kitzmiller JL. Insulin lispro and the development of proliferative diabetic retinopathy during pregnancy. *Am J Obstet Gynecol* 2001; 185:775–775.

5 American Diabetes Association. Diabetic retinopathy. *Diabetes Care* 2000;suppl 1:S73–S76.

6 Biesenbach G, Grafinger P, Stoger H, Zazgornik J. How pregnancy influences renal function in nephropathic type 1 diabetic women depends on their pre-conceptional creatinine clearance. *J Nephrol* 1999;12:41–46.

7 Rosenn BM, Miodovnik MM, Khoury JC, et al. Outcome of pregnancy in women with diabetic nephropathy. *Am J Obstet Gynecol* 1997;176: S631.

8 Rissing K, Jacobsen P, Hommel E, et al. Pregnancy and progression of diabetic nephropathy. *Diabetologia* 2002;45:36–41.

9 Leguizamon G, Reece EA. Effect of medical therapy in progressive nethropathy: influence of pregnancy, diabetes and hypertension. *J Matern Fetal Med* 20009:70–78.

10 Lessen-Pezeshki M. Pregnancy after renal transplantation: points to consider. *Nephrol Dial Transpl* 2002;17:703–707.

11 Hiilesmaa V, Suhonen L, Teramo K. Glycaemic control is associated with pre-eclampsia but not with pregnancy-induced hypertension in women with type 1 diabetes mellitus. *Diabetologia* 2000;43:1534–1539.

12 Kitzmiller JL, Buchanan TA, Kjos S, et al. Pre-conception care of diabetes, congenital malformations, and spontaneous abortions. *Diabetes Care* 1996;19:514–541.

13 Greene MF. Spontaneous abortions and major malformations in women with diabetes mellitus. *Semin Reprod Endocrinol* 1999;17: 127–136.

14 Mills JL, Knopf RH, Simpson JP, et al. Lack of relations of increased relations increased malformation rates in infants of diabetic mothers to glycemic control during organogenesis. *N Engl J Med* 1988;318: 671–676.

15 Mills JL, Knopp RH, Simpson JL, et al. Lack of relation of increased malformation rates in infants of diabetic mothers to glycemic control during organogenesis. *N Engl J Med* 1988;318:671–676.

16 Lucas MJ, Leveno KJ, Williams ML, et al. Early pregnancy glycosylated hemoglobin, severity of diabetes and fetal malformations. *Am J Obstet Gynecol* 1989;161:426–431.

17 Jaffe R. Identification of fetal growth abnormalities in diabetes mellitus. *Semin Perinatol* 2002;26:190–195.

18 Jovanovic-Peterson L, Peterson CM, Reed GF, et al. Maternal postprandial glucose levels and birthweight. The National Institute of Child Health and Human Development–Diabetes in Early Pregnancy Study. *Am J Obstet Gynecol* 1991;164:103–111.

19 Rizzo G, Arduini D, Romanini C. Accelerated cardiac growth and abnormal cardiac flow in fetuses of type I diabetic mothers. *Obstet Gynecol* 1992;80(3 pt 1):369–376.

20 Cooper MJ, Enderlein MA, Tarnoff H, Roge CL. Assymetric septal hypertrophy in infants of diabetic mothers. Fetal echocardiography and the impact of maternal diabetic control. *Am J Dis Child* 1992; 146:226–229.

21 Piper JM. Lung maturation in diabetes in pregnancy: if and when to test. *Semin Perinatol* 2002;26:206–209.

22 Landon MB. Obstetric management of pregnancies complicated by diabetes mellitus. *Clin Obstet Gynecol* 2000;43:65–74.

23 Masson EA, Patmore JE, Brash PD, et al. Pregnancy outcome in type 1 diabetes mellitus treated with insulin lispro (Humalog). *Diab Med* 2003;20:46–50.

24 Persson B, Swahn ML, Hjertberg R, et al. Insulin lispro therapy in pregnancies complicated by type 1 diabetes mellitus. *Diabetes Res Clin Pract* 2002;58:115–121.

25 Gabbe S. New concepts and applications in the use of insulin pump during pregnancy *J Matern Fetal Med* 2000;9:42–45.

26 Fetal macrosomia. *ACOG Pract Bull* 2000;22.

27 Kjos SL, Henry OA, Montoro M, et al. Insulin-requiring diabetes in pregnancy: a randomized trial of induction of labor and expectant management. *Am J Obstet Gynecol* 1993;169:611–615.

28 Lurie S, Insler V, Hagay ZJ. Induction of labor at 38 to 39 weeks of gestation reduces the incidence of shoulder dystocia in gestational diabetic patients Class A2. *Am J Perinatol* 1996;13:293–296.

29 Gonen O, Rosen DJ, Dolfin Z, et al. Induction of labor versus expectant management in macrosomia: a randomized study. *Obstet Gynecol* 1997;89:913–917.

PCOS *with Insulin Resistance*

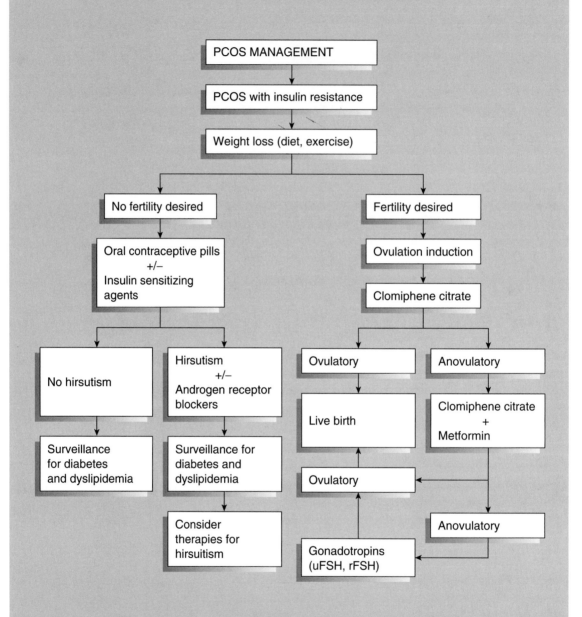

6 Polycystic Ovary Syndrome

Kelly Pagidas

Introduction

Polycystic ovarian syndrome (PCOS) is the most common cause of hyperandrogenic anovulatory infertility. The syndrome affects up to 6% of women of reproductive age.[1] The underlying cause of this syndrome remains uncertain, but it involves an array of neuroendocrine and metabolic abnormalities. The features of PCOS include a combination of clinical or biochemical hyperandrogenism, ovulatory dysfunction, and a unique form of insulin resistance. Insulin resistance leads to compensatory hyperinsulinemia and dyslipidemia.

Obesity is a common feature of PCOS, although 50% of women with PCOS are not obese. Obesity is also associated with insulin resistance and hyperinsulinemia. The presence of obesity in women with PCOS amplifies the degree of insulin resistance associated with PCOS, resulting in overt hyperinsulinemia, dyslipidemia, and fibrinolytic defects. Neuroendocrine and metabolic disturbances between obese and nonobese women with PCOS are quite distinct. This disturbance is key to understanding and evaluating the clinical and laboratory manifestations of the disease and, more importantly, the long-term sequelae and antenatal complications in pregnancy (Figure 6-1).

KEY POINT

PCOS is the most common cause of hyperandrogenic anovulation and infertility.

Diagnosis of PCOS

In 1990, the National Institute of Child Health and Human Development sponsored the first consensus conference on the diagnostic criteria for PCOS.[2] Considerable discussions led to the current diagnostic criteria for PCOS. PCOS is a diagnosis of exclusion in the

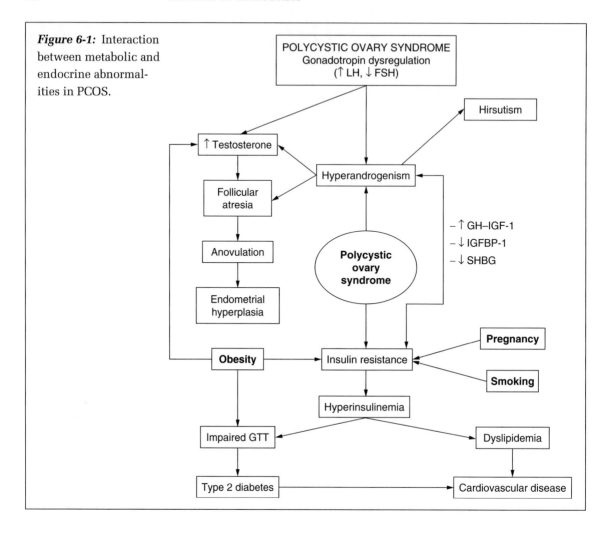

Figure 6-1: Interaction between metabolic and endocrine abnormalities in PCOS.

presence of clinical or biochemical evidence of hyperandrogenism and ovulatory dysfunction. The current definition of PCOS is:

- Chronic anovulation
- Hyperandrogenism (biochemical and clinical)
- Exclusion of other disorders (thyroid, pituitary, adrenal)

Since the 1990 conference on PCOS sponsored by the National Institute of Child Health and Human Development, there has been an increasing awareness that the clinical manifestations of PCOS are broader than originally defined. The 2003 Rotterdam consensus workshop reviewed the definition of PCOS and recommended

KEY POINT

PCOS is a diagnosis of exclusion in women with hyperandrogenism and ovulatory dysfunction.

that PCOS requires only two of the following criteria to make the diagnosis[3]:

- Oligo- and/or anovulation
- Clinical and/or biochemical hyperandrogenism
- Polycystic ovaries on ultrasound (specific criteria were established)

Pathophysiology of PCOS

KEY POINT

> *Obesity is commonly seen in PCOS but is not required for its development. Obesity amplifies the insulin-resistant state and hyperandrogenism.*

The cause of PCOS remains to be elucidated. The emphasis has been on the metabolic and endocrine disorders categorized by the syndrome, all of which may play an active role in the pathogenesis of the syndrome, including gonadotropin releasing hormone (GnRH) pulse generator dysregulation, insulin resistance, obesity, and lipoprotein lipid profile abnormalities.

The classic syndrome is characterized by inherent defects of gonadotropic inputs by intraovarian and paracrine regulators and co-gonadotropic inputs such as insulin and growth hormone. In addition, PCOS in combination with obesity may be a modified version of the syndrome.

GNRH PULSE GENERATOR DYSREGULATION

A unique feature in PCOS is the disproportionately high level of luteinizing hormone (LH) and relatively low level of follicle stimulating hormone (FSH). The underlying cause is linked to an accelerated GnRH pulse generator activity and heightened pituitary responses to GnRH. An increased LH pulse frequency is a feature specific for PCOS independent of obesity.[4] As a consequence, there is a low and constant FSH level in women with PCOS that likely is the key mechanism that causes follicular arrest in this syndrome and therefore can be restored by exogenous administration of small doses of FSH.

INSULIN RESISTANCE IN PCOS

Insulin resistance is a common finding in PCOS independent of obesity. Obesity contributes an additive effect to insulin resistance in women with PCOS, with a corresponding increase in the extent of compensatory hyperinsulinemia. The degree of peripheral insulin resistance in PCOS is similar in magnitude to that seen with non–insulin-dependent diabetes (NIDDM). Approximately 30–50% of women with PCOS are insulin resistant. Prevalence estimates for insulin resistance in non-obese women with PCOS and obese women with PCOS are 30% and 70–80%, respectively. The insulin signaling pathways involved in PCOS are for glucose transport stimulation and antilipolysis.

CLINICAL DIAGNOSIS OF INSULIN RESISTANCE

Determining insulin resistance in a clinical setting is not clear cut or required for the diagnosis of PCOS as recommended by the 2003 consensus workshop.[3] Different methods are available to assess insulin sensitivity, such as a fasting glucose:insulin ratio lower than 4.5 or a peak insulin level higher than 100 mU/L during an oral glucose tolerance test.[5] The insulin-resistant syndrome in women with PCOS is vital to detect because its presence is the basis for development of cardiovascular disease, dyslipidemia, fibrinolytic abnormalities, and NIDDM. The recommendation is to measure fasting lipid and lipoprotein profiles in all women with PCOS, including high-density lipoprotein (HDL), low-density lipoprotein (LDL), and triglycerides. In obese women with PCOS, plasma glucose levels should also be measured during fasting and 2 hours after a 75-g glucose load as a screen for glucose intolerance, in accordance with criteria of the World Health Organization and the American Diabetes Association:

KEY POINT

Women with PCOS and insulin resistance are at increased risk for impaired glucose tolerance and diabetes. Diabetes screening is recommended.

- Fasting glucose levels lower than 110 mg/dL are normal, levels of 110–126 mg/dL indicate impaired glucose tolerance, and levels of at least 126 mg/dL indicate NIDDM.
- A 2-hour glucose value lower than 140 mg/dL is normal, a value of 140–199 mg/dL indicates impaired glucose tolerance, and a value of at least 200 mg/dL indicates NIDDM.

In one study the prevalence of NIDDM in obese women with PCOS was 7.5%. The prevalence of impaired glucose tolerance was 31%.[6]

OBESITY

Obesity (body mass index [BMI] ≥ 30 kg/m^2) is present in approximately 50% of women with PCOS, which is greater than the incidence of obesity in the general population. Body fat distribution also has significant effect on long-term sequelae of PCOS. Central distribution of body fat is associated with higher rates of morbidity and mortality than is peripheral fat distribution. Insulin is a known stimulator of a critical transcription factor in the regulation of adipogenesis found in adipose tissue called peroxisome proliferator-activated receptor.[7] A new class of insulin-sensitizing compounds, thiazolidinediones, consists of specific ligands for peroxisome proliferator-activated receptor. They enhance insulin action and improve insulin resistance states in patients with NIDDM and PCOS, as evident by recent clinical trials.[8]

LIPOPROTEIN LIPID PROFILE ABNORMALITIES

In women with PCOS, peripheral insulin resistance leads to defects of glucose metabolism and activation of antilipolytic activity, with the end result being abnormal lipoprotein lipid profile. The degree of abnormality has been related to the extent of insulin resistance and independent of androgen levels and BMI.[9]

Abnormalities in lipid profile compared with that in BMI-matched control subjects are as follows:

- Increased levels of triglycerides, LDL, very LDL cholesterol, apolipoproteins A1 and B, and free fatty acids
- Decreased levels of HDL cholesterol

In addition, plasminogen activator inhibitor (PAI) is increased in women with PCOS. All of these abnormalities result in an increased incidence of hypertension, coronary heart disease, and thrombosis in women with PCOS. The key factors that lead to these increased risks are insulin resistance, hyperinsulinemia, and altered lipoprotein lipase activity.[9] The extent of the defects in lipids in women with PCOS can be influenced by diet, exercise, and lifestyle. Weight reduction is an effective means in obese women with PCOS due to decreased hyperinsulinemia.

Long-Term Sequelae and Risks of PCOS

Endocrine and metabolic abnormalities associated with PCOS place women with this syndrome at risk for the development of NIDDM, hypertension, coronary artery disease, intravascular thrombosis, and endometrial cancer.

NON–INSULIN-DEPENDENT DIABETES

Women with PCOS and insulin resistance are at increased risk for impaired glucose tolerance or diabetes. Up to 40% of obese PCOS women have impaired glucose tolerance or NIDDM by the fourth decade of life. Classically, fasting glucose levels are typically in the normal range, and impairments are detected only by glucose tolerance testing. Because pregnancy is associated with insulin resistance, it is anticipated that there will be an increase in the incidence of gestational diabetes in women with PCOS during pregnancy.[10] Evidence to date suggests that the main predictor of the development of gestational diabetes in women with PCOS is a BMI greater than 25 kg/m^2 before pregnancy, although the presence of PCOS itself may exert a small contribution. Therefore, the recommendation for women with PCOS and obesity is to have a glucose tolerance test early in pregnancy and then at 26–28 weeks of gestation.

CARDIOVASCULAR DISEASE

The insulin resistance and hyperlipidemia found in PCOS and the exacerbating influences of obesity constitute the basis for an increase in cardiovascular risk. An added independent cardiovascular risk factor is an increased level of PAI related to insulin resistance that increases the incidence of intravascular thrombosis.[11] Improved insulin resistance is accompanied by a decrease in PAI levels. Hence, women with PCOS have an increased risk of cardiovascular disease that includes myocardial infarction and atherosclerosis. The relative risk of myocardial infarction in women with PCOS is estimated to be 7.4 times that of women without PCOS.[12,13]

Theoretically, high PAI levels in pregnant women with PCOS could increase the thrombotic risk of pregnancy. No increased prevalence of inherited thrombophilias has been reported in women with PCOS compared with controls with the exception of a trend toward a higher prevalence of 5-10 methylenetetrahydrofolate reductase gene mutation and higher homocysteine levels.[14] This abnormality has not been associated with an increase in adverse pregnancy outcome in the general population.

PREGNANCY

KEY POINT

Long-term sequelae of PCOS include development of endometrial cancer, type 2 diabetes, and cardiovascular abnormalities.

In multiple studies using logistic regression analysis to control for parity, multiple gestations, and maternal age, pregnancy outcomes for women with PCOS did not exhibit increased perinatal morbidity and mortality rates nor was PCOS a predictor for hypertension or preeclampsia.[15] Controversy exists as to whether women with PCOS are at increased risk for recurrent pregnancy loss. In a cohort of women with recurrent pregnancy loss, PCOS was seen in 40% of patients; women with PCOS and recurrent pregnancy loss had a live birth rate similar to that in women with no PCOS (61% vs. 59%, respectively).[16]

Management of PCOS

The goal of PCOS management is to decrease long-term consequences of metabolic sequelae and the chronic anovulatory state. It is particularly important to try to ameliorate the abnormal metabolic state including insulin resistance before pregnancy. Achieving pregnancy likely will require medical therapy for ovulation induction.

DIET AND EXERCISE

Obesity is associated with a negative effect on the effectiveness of all medical and surgical therapies for PCOS. Weight reduction in women with PCOS by dietary restriction decreases insulin resistance and hyperinsulinemia. Exercise is an important adjunct to dietary restriction. Moderate exercise increases fuel expenditure and is associated with an improved hormonal profile. Only a modest amount of weight loss, 5–10%, can be sufficient to produce these changes. Thus, weight loss is recommended to all women with PCOS to improve the odds of spontaneous ovulation and pregnancy and for the overall benefit on the metabolic manifestations of the syndrome. Continued exercise regimens during pregnancy have clear maternal and fetal benefits. Further weight loss during pregnancy is disadvantageous. Even obese women need to gain 15 lb during pregnancy to avoid fetal growth restriction.

OVARIAN SUPPRESSION

For women who do not desire fertility, the use of oral contraceptive pills is the treatment of choice to alleviate risk of endometrial hyperplasia or cancer with or without the use of androgen blocking agents in the presence of significant hirsutism. The use of androgen-receptor blocking agents in women attempting conception is contraindicated.

OVULATION INDUCTION

Ovulation induction is the mainstay of treatment for women with PCOS who desire fertility. Clomiphene citrate is first-line therapy to induce ovulation in women with PCOS. It is a selective estrogen receptor modulator that exerts its effects on the hypothalamus and pituitary, acting as an antagonist to the estrogen receptor, with the end result being an increase in the production and release of FSH. Approximately 15% of women with PCOS will be resistant to clomiphene.

Administration of exogenous gonadotropin is reserved for women whose conventional clomiphene treatment fails with or without the use of metformin because of the particularly high incidence of hyperstimulation and multiple gestations. The goal of treatment is monofollicular development that limits hyperstimulation and multiple pregnancies. Using in vitro fertilization also controls the risk of multiple pregnancies. Among the risks of a multiple gestation is increasing insulin resistance.

INSULIN-SENSITIZING AGENTS Women with PCOS, whether or not they desire fertility, benefit from decreasing the insulin-resistant state and hyperandrogenemia. Recent advances in the availability of insulin-sensitizing agents have afforded a new option with targeted therapeutic goals of decreasing insulin resistance and hyperinsulinemia and their associated sequelae of dyslipidemia, glucose intolerance, and hyperandrogenemia. A new class of antidiabetic insulin-sensitizing agents has been developed. The insulin-sensitizing agents most studied in women with PCOS are metformin, a biguanide, and rosiglitazone, a thiazolidinedione. However, use of insulin-sensitizing agents in nondiabetic women has not been approved by the U.S. Food and Drug Administration, and its use in women with PCOS is off-label. No data exist regarding the effect of long-term use of these drugs for PCOS.

METFORMIN Metformin decreases insulin resistance and hyperinsulinemia. Its major action is on glucose homeostasis by suppression of hepatic glucose output by activating glucose transporters that allow passage of glucose into hepatic and muscle cells. The drug has been approved by the U.S. Food and Drug Administration to control NIDDM and is a category B drug. Metformin has been used in women with PCOS to treat insulin resistance and promote ovulation. In a recent meta-analysis, metformin monotherapy was found to have an odds ratio of 3.9 to induce ovulation compared with placebo.[17] This meta-analysis also found beneficial effects of decreasing fasting insulin levels, blood pressure, and LDL cholesterol.

Longitudinal studies have been done on prevention of diabetes with the use of metformin. The Diabetes Prevention Program reported that the use of metformin decreased the rate conversion of impaired glucose tolerance to type 2 diabetes by 31% in the study population of women without PCOS.[18] To date, evidence of long-term benefit of metformin in minimizing metabolic risks associated with PCOS is unproved. Randomized, prospective trials sponsored by the National Institutes of Health are currently in progress to assess metformin as monotherapy and in combination with clomiphene in women with PCOS women with end points to include pregnancy outcomes.

ROSIGLITAZONE Rosiglitazone is an insulin-sensitizing agent and a member of the thiazolidinedione family of compounds. These drugs have been shown to increase oral glucose tolerance and decrease insulin resistance and defects in β-cell function in obese patients with impaired glucose tolerance. Rosiglitazone currently is under active investigation for management of PCOS. Rosiglitazone is a category C drug. It has been shown to improve total body insulin action, resulting in lower circulating levels of insulin and androgen and induction of ovulation in women with PCOS.[8] Currently, in women with PCOS and insulin resistance, rosiglitazone is second-line therapy to metformin and prospective, randomized trials are needed.

METFORMIN USE IN PREGNANCY There is no evidence of a benefit with metformin before pregnancy with regard to the development of gestational diabetes. No teratogenic effects have been documented from animal data. Several small case series have found no adverse fetal effect from metformin. An abstract report documented a series of 82 women with NIDDM and treated with metformin or glyburide and found no increased rates of abnormalities.[19] A retrospective cohort study published in 2000 that spanned 1966–1991 investigated pregnancy outcomes of 118 women with diabetes, 50 of whom were treated with metformin.[20] Findings included an increased prevalence of preeclampsia and increased perinatal mortality rates in women treated with metformin in the third trimester. No difference was seen in numbers of congenital abnormalities.

A single group of investigators has produced three reports on the use of metformin in pregnancy. The first report is a consecutive case series that described an apparent decrease in the spontaneous abortion rate in women with PCOS who took metformin compared with patients' previous pregnancy outcomes, which

KEY POINT

Alleviation of insulin resistance and hyperinsulinemia can be achieved with diet, exercise, and insulin-sensitizing agents, resulting in amelioration of hormonal and metabolic aberrations of the syndrome.

had a high prevalence of miscarriage.[21] The investigators postulated a theoretic role for the effect of metformin decreasing PAI levels, which they found to be correlated with the risk of miscarriage. In a second study they reported that gestational diabetes occurred in 1 of 33 (3%) women with PCOS who took metformin throughout pregnancy.[22] There was no traditional control group. The outcomes of the study patients were compared with combined outcomes of previous pregnancy outcomes of subjects and outcomes of a separate group of 39 women with PCOS. The composite group had a rate of 31% for gestational diabetes. The third publication documented similar findings with further accumulation of subjects into their trial.[23]

Until more rigorously studied data are available, it is currently common practice to stop metformin once pregnancy is achieved. Fortunately, the data are reasonably clear that there is no associated teratogenic syndrome. Once pregnancy is achieved, monitoring needs to be implemented for early detection of gestational diabetes. For women with diabetes, aggressive glucose management is indicated from the very beginning of pregnancy. A regimen of diet and exercise is vital in optimizing outcome in pregnant women, and a calorie-restricted, low-carbohydrate, high-protein diet should be encouraged in women with PCOS and insulin resistance.

What's the Evidence?

After the 1990 conference on PCOS sponsored by the National Institutes of Health, the revised 2003 Rotterdam consensus workshop concluded that PCOS is a syndrome of ovarian dysfunction with cardinal features of hyperandrogensim and polycystic morphology. Insulin resistance and high LH levels are common features of the syndrome. Obese women with PCOS need to be screened for the metabolic syndrome, including glucose intolerance with an oral glucose tolerance test. Criteria for the metabolic syndrome include centripetal obesity, hypertension, fasting hyperglycemia, and dyslipidemia. Identification of the metabolic syndrome in women with PCOS is associated with an increased risk of type 2 diabetes and cardiovascular events. Lifestyle changes (diet and exercise) should be a vital part of treatment because such changes have been shown to decrease the risks of type 2 diabetes and cardiovascular disease. The need to select additional therapy for PCOS is based on a woman's desire to conceive in the presence or absence of impaired glucose tolerance or type 2 diabetes. Further research studies need to address the potential effect of insulin-sensitizing agents on pregnancy outcome.

Guiding Questions in Approaching the Patient

Women who desire fertility

- Is the metabolic syndrome present (abdominal obesity, hypertriglyceridemia, low HDL cholesterol, hypertension, high level of fasting blood glucose)?
- Has type 2 diabetes been ruled out?
- Has a program of diet and exercise been initiated?
- Have conventional ovulation induction regimens failed to achieve ovulatory cycles?
- Would metformin be beneficial to this patient?

Women who do not desire fertility

- Is the metabolic syndrome present?
- Has type 2 diabetes been ruled out?
- Has a program of diet and exercise been initiated?
- Would the patient benefit from metformin or other insulin-sensitizing agent?
- Are there any contraindications to the use of oral contraceptive pills for cycle regulation?
- Is there any significant hirsutism that requires management?

Conclusion

Polycystic Ovary Syndrome is the most common cause of hyperandrogenic anovulation and infertility. Insulin resistance is present and increases the likelihood of pregestational and gestational diabetes. Obesity is commonly present and increases the risk of adverse maternal and neonatal outcomes. Without co-morbidities, PCOS does not increase the risk of adverse pregnancy outcome. Further research is needed regarding potential benefits of use of metformin in the first trimester.

Discussion of Cases

CASE 1: INFERTILITY EVALUATION OF A WOMAN WITH OLIGOMENORRHEA AND HIRSUTISM

A 32-year-old woman presents for evaluation and management of oligomenorrhea and infertility. She has been off oral contraceptives for the past year and is attempting pregnancy but has not had any menses. Her current physical examination is significant for a blood pressure of 120/70 mm Hg, weight of 220 lb and height of 5 ft 3 in., facial hirsutism, and acne.

What testing would you recommend at this point?

Endocrine profile (LH, FSH, thyroid stimulating hormone, and prolactin), androgen profile (testosterone, dehydroepiandrosterone sulfate, 17-OH progesterone), and metabolic profile (fasting lipid levels and glucose and insulin level during fasting and 2 hours after 75-g oral glucose tolerance testing).

The patient's endocrine profile is normal, her androgen profile is normal, but her metabolic profile shows a high fasting level of LDL cholesterol and glucose 190 mg/dL and insulin 130 mU/L 2 hours after a 75-g glucose load.

What is your first-line therapy for this patient?

Ovulation induction is indicated. The working diagnosis in this patient is PCOS with insulin resistance in the presence of obesity. The recommendation would be that she initiates a regimen of diet and exercise to decrease her weight by 5–10% concurrent with the initiation of clomiphene citrate to induce ovulation. Clomiphene citrate is started at 50 mg daily for 5 days and increased to 150 mg with no ovulatory cycles documented.

What would you do next?

Given her obesity and the presence of impaired glucose tolerance, it would be useful to add metformin to the treatment regimen.

After two cycles of clomiphene and metformin, a positive pregnancy test is detected.

What should be recommended?

The recommendation would be to stop the metformin and initiate early antennal evaluation and management of diabetes.

CASE 2: YOUNG WOMAN WITH METRORRHAGIA AND HIRSUTISM

You are asked to evaluate an 18-year-old girl with irregular cycles and hirsutism. Thus far, she has not been evaluated for her complaints. Physical examination shows mild facial hirsutism, weight of 130 lb and height of 5 ft 7 in., normal breast development, and an unremarkable pelvic examination.

What testing would you recommend at this point?

Endocrine profile, androgen profile, and metabolic profile.

The patient's endocrine profile shows high levels of LH and low levels of FSH (LH:FSH ratio 3.5), her androgen profile shows high levels of total testosterone, and her metabolic profile is normal.

What is your diagnosis and recommendation for future management?

The working diagnosis is PCOS without evidence of insulin resistance, or "lean PCOS." Treatment can simply be instituted with oral contraceptive pills to allow regularization of her menstrual cycles and protection of the endometrium from unopposed estrogen stimulation.

What is the next step?

She needs to be seen annually and monitored due to the diagnosis of PCOS. If no sequelae manifest, she is to remain on oral contraceptive pills until fertility is desired.

REFERENCES

1 Knochenhauer ES, Key TJ, Kahsar-Miller M, et al. Prevalence of the polycystic ovary syndrome in unselected black and white women of the southeastern Unites Sates: a prospective study. *J Clin Endocrinol Metab* 1998;83:3078–3082.

2 Zawadaki JK, Dunaif A. Diagnostic criteria for polycystic ovary syndrome: towards a rationale approach. In: Dunaif A, Given JR, Haseltine F, Merriam GR, eds. *Polycystic Ovary Syndrome.* Boston: Blackwell, 1992; p. 377–384.

3 Fauser B. Revised 2003 consensus on diagnostic criteria and long-term health risks related to polycystic ovary syndrome. *Hum Reprod* 2004;19:41–47.

4 Morales AJ, Laughlin GA, Butzow T, et al. Insulin, somatotropic and LH axes in lean and obese women with polycystic ovary syndrome: common and distinct features. *J Clin Endocrinol Metab* 1996;81:2854–2864.

5 Legro RS, Finegood D, Dunaif A. A fasting glucose to insulin ratio is a useful measure of insulin sensitivity in women with polycystic ovary syndrome. *J Clin Endocrinol Metab* 1998;83:2694–2698.

6 Legro RS, Kunselman AR, Dodson WC, Dunaif, A. Prevalence and predictors of the risk for type 2 diabetes mellitus and impaired glucose tolerance in polycystic ovary syndrome: a prospective, controlled study in 254 affected women. *J Clin Endrocrinol Metab* 1999;84:165–169.

7 Shalev A, Siegrist-Kaiser CA, Yen PM, et al. The peroxisome proliferator-activated receptor is a phosphoprotein: regulation by insulin. *Endocrinology* 1996;137:4499–4502.

8 Dunaif A, Scott D, Finegood D, et al. The insulin-sensitizing agent troglitazone improves metabolic and reproductive abnormalities in the polycystic ovary syndrome. *J Clin Endocrinol Metab* 1996;81: 3299–3306.

9 Norman RJ, Hague WM, Masters SC, et al. Subjects with polycystic ovaries without hyperandrogenemia exhibit similar disturbances in insulin and lipid profiles as those with polycystic ovary syndrome. *Hum Reprod* 1995;10:2258–2261.

10 Lanzone A, Caruso A, DiSimone N, et al. Polycystic ovary disease. A risk factor for gestational diabetes? *J Reprod Med* 1995;40:312–316.

11 Sampson M, Kong C, Patel A, et al. Ambulatory blood pressure profiles and plasminogen activator inhibitor (PA-1) activity in lean women with and without the polycystic ovary syndrome. *Clin Endocrinol* 1996;45:623–629.

12 Dahlgren E, Jansen PO, Johansson S, et al. Polycystic ovary syndrome and risk for myocardial infarction. Evaluated from a risk based on a prospective population study. *Acta Obstet Gynaecol Scand* 1992; 71:599–604.

13 Talbott E, Guzick D, Clerici A, et al. Coronary heart disease risk factors in women with polycystic ovarian syndrome. *Arterioscler Thromb Vasc Biol* 1995;15:821–826.

14 Schachterr M, Raziel A, Friedler S, et al. Insulin resistance in patients with polycystic ovary syndrome is associated with elevated plasma homocysteine. *Hum Reprod* 2003;18:721–727.

15 Mikola M, Hiilesemma V, Halttunen M, et al. Obstetric outcome in women with polycystic syndrome. *Hum Reprod* 2001;16:226–229.

16 Rai R, Backos M, Rushworth F, Regan L. Polycystic ovaries and recurrent miscarriage—a reappraisal. *Hum Reprod* 2000;15:612–615.

17 Lord JM, Flight IHK, Norman RJ. Insulin-sensitizing drugs (metformin, troglitazone, rosiglitazone, pioglitazone, D-chiro-inositol) for polycystic ovary syndrome. *Cochrane Database Syst Rev* 2003;2.

18 The Diabetes Prevention Program Research Group. Effects of withdrawal from metformin on the development of diabetes in the diabetes prevention program. *Diabetes Care* 2003;26:977–980.

19 Langer O, Conway D, Berkus M, Xenakis EM. There is no association between oral hypoglycemic use and fetal anomalies. *Am J Obstet Gynecol* 1999;180:S38.

20 Hellmuth E, Damm P, Molsted-Pedersen L. Oral hypoglycemic agents in 118 diabetic pregnancies. *Diabet Med* 2000;17:507–511.

21 Glueck CJ, Phillips H, Cameron D, et al. Continuing metformin throughout pregnancy in women with polycystic ovary syndrome

appears to safely reduce first-trimester spontaneous abortion: a pilot study. *Fertil Steril* 2001;75:46–52.

22 Glueck CJ, Wang P, Kobayashi S, et al. Metformin therapy through-out pregnancy reduces the development of gestational diabetes in women with polycystic ovary syndrome. *Fertil Steril* 2001;77: 520–525.

23 Glueck CJ, Wang P, Goldenberg N, Sieve-Smith L. Pregnancy out-comes among women with polycystic ovary syndrome treated with metformin. *Hum Reprod* 2002;17:2858–2864.

Approach to the Patient with Anemia

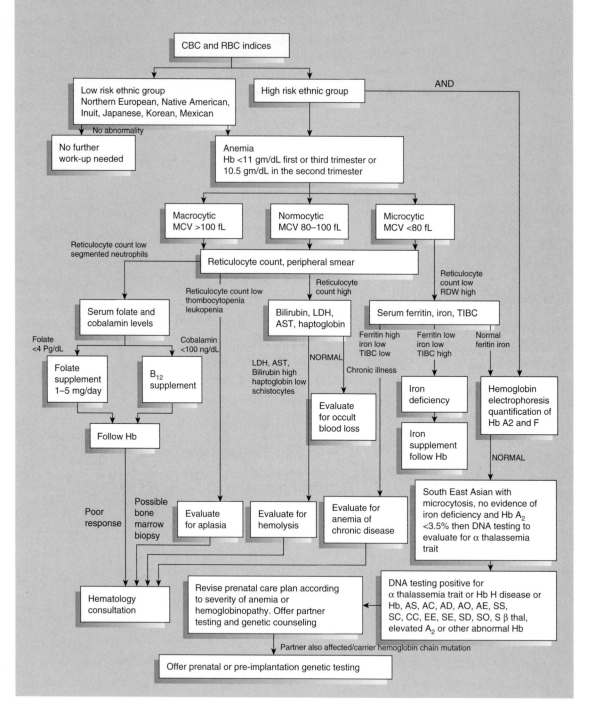

7 Anemia

Michelle Russell
Lisa Dunn-Albanese

Introduction

Anemia is a disorder characterized by a decrease in the number of circulating erythrocytes or the amount of functional hemoglobin that can result in tissue hypoxia. Anemia may be acquired or hereditary in origin. It is commonly encountered in women of childbearing age and during pregnancy. The effects of anemia on pregnancy depend on the etiology. The causes of acquired anemia include iron deficiency, acute or occult blood loss, chronic disease states, vitamin deficiency, aplasia or hypoplasia of erythroid cells, and hemolysis. The hereditary anemias are a result of genetic mutations that affect the production of or shorten the life span of the circulating erythrocytes. The group of hereditary anemias is large and includes the sickle cell disorders, thalassemias, unstable hemoglobin variants, and other hemoglobinopathies. This chapter reviews the acquired causes of anemia and the diagnosis and management of these disorders during pregnancy.

Acquired Anemia

In the United States anemia affects up to 5% of individuals and 29% of pregnant women. Clinically, it manifests as pallor of the skin and mucous membranes, dyspnea on exertion, dizziness, headaches, palpitations, syncope, lethargy, fatigability, sleep and mood disturbances, and, rarely, congestive heart failure. The underlying causes of anemia can be divided into those that lead to decreased erythroid cell production, increased red blood cell (RBC) destruction, or loss of blood from the circulatory system.

The normal circulating life span of an erythrocyte is approximately 120 days. For nonpregnant women a hemoglobin value between 12 and 15 g/dL is normal, but a hemoglobin value of 7 g/dL can meet oxygen-carrying requirements if tissue perfusion is maintained. In the second trimester the plasma component expansion is greater than the increase in the cellular components of blood leading to a dilutional or "physiologic anemia." Because of the physiologic anemia of pregnancy, normal values of hemoglobin are lower. In 1998, the Centers for Disease Control (CDC) defined anemia in pregnancy as hemoglobin values less than 11 g/dL, 10.5 g/dL, and 11g/dL in the first, second, and third trimesters, respectively.[1] A hemoglobin level less than 6 g/dL has been associated with significant maternal morbidity.[2]

EVALUATION

The initial laboratory evaluation of anemia includes a complete blood count (CBC) with platelets, leukocyte differential, and RBC indices. An absolute reticulocyte count, peripheral smear, serum ferritin, serum iron, or a hemoglobin electrophoresis may aid in the diagnosis of anemia. Additional laboratory studies may be indicated. Blood tests to evaluate the etiology of an anemia must be drawn before blood transfusion and, ideally, before therapy. The etiology of an individual's anemia at times is difficult to determine because acquired and hereditary anemia often have similar characteristics.

The initial laboratory evaluation is an important tool in differentiating the anemias. Using the RBC indices, the common types of anemia can be categorized by the size of the erythrocytes, which is measured by the mean corpuscular volume (MCV). In a normocytic anemia the mean corpuscular volume (MCV) is 80–100 fL. In a microcytic anemia the MCV is smaller than 80 fL, and in a macrocytic anemia the MCV is larger than 100 fL. Information can also be gained from evaluation of the other RBC indices. For instance, the RBC distribution width (RDW) is a measurement of variability of erythrocyte size. A high RDW indicates increased variability in cell size, and a normal RDW indicates a homogeneous population of RBCs. The RDW is high in iron deficiency anemia but is normal in thalassemia. Iron deficiency anemia decreases the total RBC

KEY POINT

During pregnancy, iron deficiency is the most common nutritional deficiency and is responsible for up to 75% of cases of anemia.

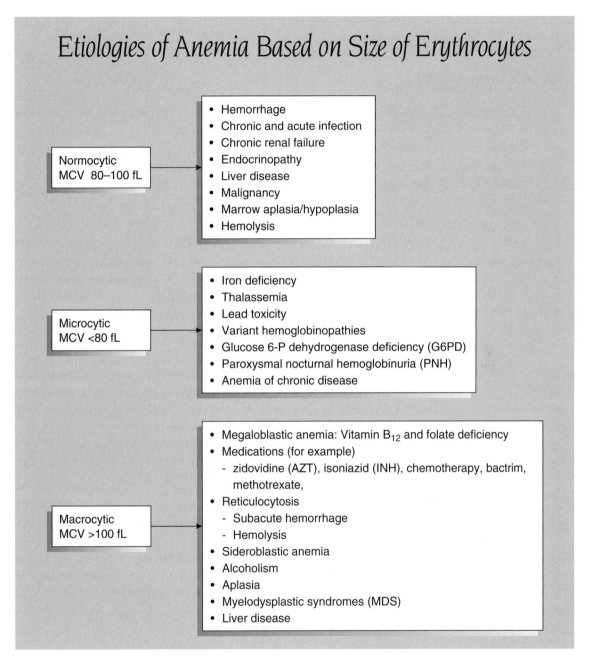

Etiologies of Anemia Based on Size of Erythrocytes

Normocytic
MCV 80–100 fL

- Hemorrhage
- Chronic and acute infection
- Chronic renal failure
- Endocrinopathy
- Liver disease
- Malignancy
- Marrow aplasia/hypoplasia
- Hemolysis

Microcytic
MCV <80 fL

- Iron deficiency
- Thalassemia
- Lead toxicity
- Variant hemoglobinopathies
- Glucose 6-P dehydrogenase deficiency (G6PD)
- Paroxysmal nocturnal hemoglobinuria (PNH)
- Anemia of chronic disease

Macrocytic
MCV >100 fL

- Megaloblastic anemia: Vitamin B_{12} and folate deficiency
- Medications (for example)
  - zidovidine (AZT), isoniazid (INH), chemotherapy, bactrim, methotrexate,
- Reticulocytosis
  - Subacute hemorrhage
  - Hemolysis
- Sideroblastic anemia
- Alcoholism
- Aplasia
- Myelodysplastic syndromes (MDS)
- Liver disease

count but thalassemia is associated with an increase in the RBC count. The mean cell hemoglobin is decreased in iron deficiency anemia but not in thalassemia.

The peripheral smear is another tool useful in the diagnosis and differentiation of the cause of anemia. There are numerous erythrocyte shapes and characteristics that can help to determine the etiology of an anemia.

Iron Deficiency Anemia

The CDC estimates that iron deficiency affects 8 million American women of childbearing age. The prevalence of iron insufficiency in women living in the United States varies by age, race, parity, and socioeconomic status. African and Mexican American women have the highest prevalence rates, with up to 22% affected by iron deficiency outside pregnancy. Menstrual blood loss, poor nutritional status, and inadequate dietary intake of sources of iron contribute to this frequent disorder.[3] Fewer than 50% of non-pregnant women have iron stores adequate to meet their requirements during pregnancy. Further, dietary sources of iron are inadequate to meet the approximate iron requirement of normal pregnancy and supplements are often needed. The recommended daily allowance of iron for reproductive age women is 12–18 mg/day. Up to 80% of women who do not receive iron supplements during pregnancy will develop iron deficiency by the third trimester. Iron deficiency anemia during the first and second trimesters of pregnancy has been associated with poor maternal weight gain, preterm birth, and low-birth-weight infants.[3] Infants born to mothers with iron deficiency anemia are at increased risk of developing anemia during the first year of life.[4] Although a correlation has been identified through epidemiologic studies, a direct cause-and-effect relation has not been established. Iron supplementation has not been shown to alter the obstetric outcome in pregnancies affected by iron deficiency anemia.[5]

DIAGNOSIS

KEY POINT

A serum ferritin value less than 15 µg/dL confirms iron deficiency anemia and is the best parameter to judge the degree of iron deficiency.

The diagnosis of iron deficiency anemia is made by identifying the characteristic changes that occur and by excluding other causes of anemia. In iron deficiency anemia, there is a depletion of iron stores from the liver, spleen, and bone marrow, a decrease in serum iron and ferritin levels, a decrease in saturation of transferrin receptors, an increase in total iron binding capacity (TIBC), a decrease in hemoglobin and hematocrit, and production of microcytic, hypochromic erythrocytes. The CBC may demonstrate a normocytic, normochromic anemia in the early stages of deficiency, with a microcytic, hypochromic anemia developing as the condition worsens. A measured serum iron level lower than 30–60 mg/dL or a serum ferritin level lower than 15–30 µg/L suggests iron deficiency.

Management of Iron Deficiency Anemia in Pregnancy

- Oral iron supplementation 200–300 mg QD and continue 3 months postpartum
- Consider IV or IM iron supplementation if unresponsive, poorly compliant or unable to absorb

↓

Follow hemoglobin every month until corrected then each trimester

↓

- If poorly responsive to therapy, evaluate for and exclude other causes of anemia and chronic blood loss
- Consider hematology consult

↓

Reserve transfusion for symptomatic anemia unresponsive to treatment or hemoglobin ≤6–7 gm/dL

↓

Consider monitoring fetal growth in cases of severe anemia

↓

- Minimize acute blood loss at delivery
- Assure blood products available at delivery

A TIBC higher than 360 µg/dL and a transferrin receptor saturation of less than 15–20% are additional indicators of iron deficiency.

THERAPY

Therapy for iron deficiency anemia during gestation can be accomplished by oral iron supplementation. Oral supplements are effective and show a dose-dependent increase in hemoglobin in iron-deficient pregnant women.[6] The goal of therapy is to administer elemental iron 60–120 mg/day and continue treatment for at least 3 months after resolution of the anemia. Ascorbic acid can enhance iron absorption. Women taking therapeutic doses of iron should also be supplemented with zinc and copper. The common oral iron preparations vary in the amount of absorbable elemental iron, and noncompliance with prescription is frequently due to gastrointestinal disturbances. Oral preparations containing sustained-release capsules, slow absorbable compounds, or syrups may decrease side effects and improve compliance. The amount of elemental iron varies in the commonly prescribed oral iron preparations (Table 7-1). Anecdotally, the preparations containing ferrous gluconate produce fewer gastrointestinal side effects. Rarely, iron deficiency anemia is controlled by intramuscular or intravenous iron administration. The hematologic response to parenteral preparations is no more rapid than when supplementation by the oral route is accomplished. Parenteral routes of administration are associated with a higher risk of adverse reactions such as venous thrombosis, anaphylaxis, and pain. There is little evidence to support the use of administration routes other than oral except in rare circumstances when oral therapy is not tolerated, anemia is refractory to therapy, or gastrointestinal absorption is impaired.[7] Conditions such as subtotal gastrectomy, malabsorption syndromes, short bowel syndrome, chronic bowel obstruction, protein-calorie malnutrition, and hemodialysis may warrant parenteral therapy.

KEY POINT

Although management of iron deficiency anemia during pregnancy has not been shown consistently to improve obstetric outcome, neonatal iron stores have been shown to correlate with maternal iron status.

PREVENTION

Populations at risk of iron deficiency should have annual screening of hemoglobin levels during routine health maintenance visits and preconception evaluations. Supplementation can be administered if a deficiency is detected. Prevention of iron deficiency anemia during pregnancy can be accomplished by selective or routine administration of elemental iron 65–80 mg/day or its equivalent throughout gestation and for 3 months postpartum.

Table 7-1. **COMMON ORAL IRON COMPOUNDS**

Preparation	*Dose (mg)*	*Elemental Iron (%)*	*Elemental Iron (mg)*
Ferrous sulfate	325	20	65
Ferrous fumarate	325	33	107
Ferrous gluconate	325	11.6	38

What's the Evidence?

PREGNANCY OUTCOME In an exhaustive recent literature review, Rasmussen[5] concluded that there was ample evidence of an association between maternal anemia and size at birth, duration of gestation, and neonatal and perinatal mortality. However, supplementation with iron, folic acid, or both did not appear to increase birth weight or length of gestation.

Megaloblastic Anemia

This group of anemias is associated with macrocytic erythrocytes where the MCV is larger than 100 fL and often larger than 110 fL. Megaloblastic anemia arises from a disorder that results in impaired DNA synthesis and abnormal erythroid cell division. Macrocytic, megaloblastic erythroid cells are destroyed in the bone marrow, leading to a decrease in production of circulating erythrocytes. Neutrophil hypersegmentation is often seen on the peripheral smear. Megaloblastic anemias are less common than iron deficiency anemias during pregnancy but can occur and require evaluation and management. Causes of megaloblastic anemia include folate deficiency, cobalamin deficiency, medications, and hereditary metabolic disorders. Not all macrocytic anemias are due to megaloblastic changes. Rapid reticulocytosis in response to acute blood loss or recently treated deficiency can also increase the MCV.

Folate Deficiency

Folate deficiency is the most common cause of acquired megaloblastic anemia during pregnancy, but folate deficiency in general is uncommon in the United States due to government-mandated fortification of foods with this nutrient since 1997. Natural dietary folate is derived from fruits and vegetables or meats such as liver and kidney. Many grains and cereals have been fortified with folate. The nonpregnant daily folate requirement is 0.05–0.1 mg and increases to 0.8–1.0 mg during pregnancy. Folate deficiency can occur during states of high folate requirement and in conditions in which dietary intake does not meet the increased need, such as during pregnancy and with the chronic hemolytic anemias. A short interval between gestations and multiple gestation pregnancies may increase the risk of folate deficiency. Certain populations such as teenagers are prone to folate deficiency due to the rapid linear growth phase and diets poor in sources of folate. Other causes that contribute to folate deficiency are the use of antiepileptic medications, alcoholism, malignancy, chronic hemodialysis, intestinal malabsorption syndromes, and parasitosis.

DIAGNOSIS

The diagnosis of folate deficiency can be made by measuring serum folate levels. RBC folate or serum homocysteine levels can be used to support the diagnosis. Normal serum folate levels are 6–20 ng/mL, and values lower than 4 ng/mL suggest folate deficiency. Serum folate levels reflect recent folate consumption, whereas RBC folate levels are representative of folate stores in the tissues. A measurement of serum homocysteine level is occasionally used because levels may be high early in folate-deficient states before hematologic changes.

THERAPY

Megaloblastic anemia due to folate deficiency responds quickly to therapy with supplementation of oral folate 1–5 mg/day. Concurrent cobalamin deficiency should be excluded in individuals on prolonged courses of folate supplementation or in individuals whose anemia does not respond to folate therapy.

PREVENTION

Prevention of folate-induced megaloblastic anemia in the healthy individual can be accomplished by appropriate dietary practices or by administration of a daily multivitamin that contains folate. Individuals with conditions that increase utilization, alter metabolism, or decrease absorption of folate may need higher daily preventative doses in the range of 1–5 mg/day. In addition to megaloblastic anemia, folate deficiency has been implicated as a factor in congenital anomalies such as neural tube defects, cleft lip/palate, and some cardiac defects.[8,9] The CDC recommends that all healthy women of reproductive age who are at risk of an unplanned pregnancy or who are planning to conceive should be advised to consume in their diets or take a daily supplement containing the recommended daily allowance of folate 400 µg to decrease the risk of birth defects.

Cobalamin Deficiency

Cobalamin (vitamin B_{12}) deficiency during pregnancy is a rare cause of megaloblastic anemia, but deficiency can occur in healthy women who consume a strict vegetarian diet and in women with medical conditions. Cobalamin is necessary for the metabolism of folic acid; hence, when deficiency of cobalamin occurs, the anemia pattern is similar to that of the macrocytic, megaloblastic anemia associated with folate deficiency. Additional causes include pernicious anemia, gastrectomy, intestinal resection, intestinal absorptive disorders, intrinsic factor deficiency, parasitosis, and medications.

In contrast to folate deficiency, there are irreversible neurologic abnormalities that can occur with a deficiency of cobalamin. Vitamin B_{12} is an important component in the process of neuronal myelination, and a deficiency can lead to peripheral neuropathy, central nervous system abnormalities, psychiatric disturbances, and gastrointestinal symptoms. To avoid irreversible neurologic deficits, a concurrent vitamin B_{12} deficiency must be excluded when prescribing prolonged courses of folate supplementation or when anemia is refractory to therapy. In addition to anemia and neurologic complications, a deficiency of vitamin B_{12} during early gestation, similar to a deficiency of folate, may be associated with an increased risk of congenital anomalies such as neural tube defects.[10]

DIAGNOSIS

The diagnosis of cobalamin deficiency can be made by measuring serum cobalamin levels. Occasionally, serum methylmalonic acid (MMA) levels may be helpful. Normal serum B_{12} levels are 200–900 pg/mL and values lower than 100 pg/mL indicate deficiency. Normal serum MMA levels are lower than 0.4 µmol/L and values above this level are considered increased. MMA and homocysteine levels are high in individuals deficient in vitamin B_{12} and are reflective of decreased tissue stores. Evaluation for autoantibodies associated with pernicious anemia may be indicated.

THERAPY

Mild cobalamin deficiency due to dietary practices can be managed with oral supplements of cobalamin 300–1000 µg/day, but severe deficiency or deficiency attributed to malabsorption is better managed by parenteral administration of cyanocobalamin. One regimen for vitamin B_{12} deficiency is cyanocobalamin 100 µg/day given intramuscularly for 1 week and then 100 µg weekly until a goal of 2000 µg over the first 6 weeks is reached. Maintenance doses of cyanocobalamin 100 µg are administered intramuscularly every month. The anemia responds quickly to therapy. Hematology and gastroenterology consultations may be helpful when managing severe cases of megaloblastic anemia due to vitamin B_{12} deficiency.

Anemia of Chronic Disease

Acquired anemia associated with chronic disease is the result of a decrease in erythroid cell proliferation. It is uncommon during pregnancy because the severity of the underlying disease often impairs fertility. Anemia of chronic disease arises from disease states such as end-stage renal disease, severe hypothyroidism, liver disease, starvation, chronic infections, malignancy, human immunodeficiency virus, chronic inflammatory bowel disease, and rheumatologic disorders.

DIAGNOSIS

Anemia of chronic disease is diagnosed after other frequently encountered causes of anemia are excluded. Diagnostic tests include a CBC, absolute reticulocyte count, serum iron, serum ferritin, and TIBC. Occasionally, erythropoietin levels are helpful. The diagnosis of anemia of chronic disease is suspected when iron and hemoglobin electrophoresis studies are undemonstrative in an individual with a hypochromic, microcytic anemia arising in the setting of chronic inflammation or a chronic disease condition. Typically, there is normal or decreased serum iron, normal or low TIBC, and a high serum ferritin level. In addition, serum erythropoietin levels may be decreased, particularly in anemia associated with chronic renal failure.

THERAPY

Successful management of most cases of anemia of chronic disease relies on resolution of the chronic inflammatory state. Administration of recombinant erythropoietin is effective in ameliorating anemia in cases attributed to insufficient erythropoietin production and renal impairment.

Aplastic Anemia

Aplastic anemia is a rare but serious hematologic disorder characterized by pancytopenia and bone marrow hypocellularity in the absence of underlying malignancy. Anemia arises because of decreased or absent of erythroid cell proliferation. Presenting clinical manifestations of acquired aplastic anemia are symptoms of severe anemia and thrombocytopenia. Uncommonly, infection due to neutropenia is a presenting symptom.

ETIOLOGY

Most cases of aplastic anemia are acquired but rare forms may be inherited. One of the inherited conditions associated with aplasia is Fanconi's anemia. It should be excluded in all patients with acquired aplastic anemia.[11] There are many causes of acquired aplastic anemia including medications, viral infection, connective tissue disorders, organic compound exposures, recreational drug use, and radiation.

Numerous medications have been associated with anemia, but many are uncommonly used during pregnancy. Classes of medications used during pregnancy that have been linked with aplastic anemia include certain antimicrobials, anti-inflammatory agents, anticonvulsants, antithyroid drugs, sulfonamides, antihypertensive agents, and antihistamines. Viral agents associated with acquired aplastic anemia include the viral hepatitides A, B, and C, Epstein-Barr virus (EBV), human immunodeficiency virus, and parvovirus B_{19}. More recently, the recreational drug Ecstasy has been associated with acute acquired aplastic anemia, and as such, a history of drug use should be sought. One-half to two-thirds of cases of acquired aplastic anemia have no causative agent identified and are therefore idiopathic.

Pregnancy may be coincidental to aplastic anemia, but it has also been implicated as an etiologic factor in some recurrent relapsing cases. Aplastic anemia is associated with significant risk of morbidity and mortality. In cases of aplastic anemia complicating pregnancy, maternal mortality attributable to hemorrhage and infection is increased to 20–60%.[12] Successful pregnancy outcome has been documented in women previously treated for aplastic anemia with immunosuppressive therapy. Up to 19% of these successfully treated cases may relapse during pregnancy or may require repetitive transfusion therapy.[13] Management of women with aplastic anemia should be done in consultation with a hematologist.

DIAGNOSIS

The CBC with leukocyte differential and RBC indices generally show pancytopenia with a normochromic, normocytic anemia. Reticulocyte count is low, platelets are normal in size, and there are no abnormal cells in the differential diagnosis. Evaluation of a bone marrow aspirate or biopsy can confirm the diagnosis and exclude an infiltrative malignant or premalignant condition.

THERAPY   Management of aplastic anemia during pregnancy involves withdrawal of the inciting agent, if it is known, supportive transfusion of blood components, and immunosuppressive therapy. Recombinant hematopoietic growth factors are sometimes indicated and may be particularly useful in cases of severe neutropenia after immunosuppressive therapy. Autologous peripheral blood stem cell transplantation or related donor human leukocyte antigen matched bone marrow transplantation can be curative but is not performed during pregnancy. Irradiated, leuco-depleted, cytomegalovirus-negative blood components should be used during pregnancy and in patients who may be candidates for bone marrow transplantation.[11] As with any transfusion-dependent anemia, iron overload toxicity is a risk and should be monitored with serum ferritin levels. Special precautions should be taken in neutropenic gravidas. Control of infections in neutropenic patients requires broad-spectrum antibiotic therapy until a specific organism can be identified.

Hemolytic Anemia

Hemolytic anemia arises because of increased destruction of erythroid cells. Hemolytic anemias are a heterogeneous collection of acquired anemias that more frequently affect women than men. Chronic inheritable forms exist and are often a result of structural abnormalities of the erythroid cells or variant unstable hemoglobins. The hallmark of hemolytic anemia is a normal or increased erythroid cell production but a shortened RBC survival in the peripheral circulation. There is evidence of cellular destruction including antibodies, abnormal RBC morphology, and increased RBC enzymes. Common presenting symptoms of hemolytic anemia are symptoms of severe anemia and of jaundice. Splenomegaly may occur and contribute to symptoms.

ETIOLOGY   Numerous etiologies of hemolytic anemia include autoimmune, collagen vascular disease, infection, microangiopathy, paroxysmal nocturnal hemoglobinuria (PNH), transfusion-related, medications, structural abnormalities of RBCs, and hemoglobin variants.

DIAGNOSIS The diagnosis of hemolytic anemia is made by evaluation of a CBC with RBC indices, total reticulocyte count, and peripheral smear. A hemoglobin electrophoresis should be completed to exclude a hemoglobinopathy. Serum bilirubin, lactate dehydrogenase, serum aspartate aminotransferase, and serum haptoglobin can support the diagnosis. The CBC generally shows a normocytic anemia and the peripheral smear shows anisocytosis, schistocytes, helmet cells, and nucleated RBCs. Total and indirect serum bilirubin levels, the breakdown products of hemoglobin, are high. Haptoglobin binds free hemoglobin and as a result is decreased in cases of hemolytic anemia. The coagulation profile is helpful when evaluating microangiopathic hemolytic anemias. Direct and indirect Coombs' tests are at times revealing in cases of autoimmune and transfusion-related hemolytic anemias, respectively.

Autoimmune Hemolytic Anemia

In autoimmune hemolytic anemia, direct Coombs' test is often positive and the antibody-bound erythrocytes are destroyed after passage through the spleen and the liver. Warm active antibodies may be found in 80–90% of cases. Autoimmune hemolytic anemia may be associated with an underlying disease state in half of cases. Associated disease entities include malignancy or collagen vascular disorders such as systemic lupus erythematosus. Recurrent pregnancy-induced hemolytic anemia has been reported in successive pregnancies and may have an autoimmune basis.[14]

Management of autoimmune hemolytic anemia generally involves glucocorticoid therapy and occasionally intravenous immunoglobulin (Ig) therapy or plasmapheresis.[15] In refractory cases, plasma exchange transfusion, splenectomy, cytotoxic agents, cyclosporin, azathioprine, or, rarely, thymectomy can be beneficial. Transfusion therapy may be necessary in severe cases but should be approached with caution due to the presence of anti-RBC antibodies and increased risk of transfusion reactions. Premedication therapy before blood component transfusions in this setting is indicated.

Infectious Hemolytic Anemia

Infectious causes of hemolytic anemia include *Mycoplasma pneumoniae*, EBV, cytomegalovirus, hepatitis C virus, and, occasionally, hepatitis B virus. Hemolytic anemia due to *M. pneumoniae* or EBV is due to cold agglutinin disease or cold active antibodies of the IgM class. Testing for viral serology or cold agglutinins can occasionally be demonstrative if an infectious etiology is suspected. Transient hemolytic anemia associated with gram-negative endotoxins can also be observed in cases of severe pyelonephritis complicating pregnancy.

Microangiopathic Hemolytic Anemia

Hemolytic anemia during pregnancy is commonly associated with microangiopathic changes. A common cause of microangiopathic hemolytic anemia arising during pregnancy is severe preeclampsia or the syndrome of hemolysis, elevated liver enzymes, and low platelets (HELLP). Disseminated intravascular coagulation (DIC) may be encountered during pregnancy. Management of DIC depends on the underlying cause. DIC associated with sepsis is controlled with antibiotics and supportive blood component transfusions, whereas DIC related to retained products of conception requires uterine evacuation. Placental abruption is associated with DIC and may require pregnancy termination or delivery. Other microangiopathic causes of anemia are known as thrombotic microangiopathies. Thrombotic microangiopathies are often in the differential diagnosis of hemolytic anemia occurring during pregnancy and include hemolytic uremic syndrome (HUS) and thrombotic thrombocytopenia purpura (TTP).

Hemolytic Uremic Syndrome

HUS is more common in children but it can affect young adults of reproductive age. It can be triggered by bacterial cytotoxins that are associated with diarrheal and respiratory illnesses. HUS is a cytokine-mediated prothrombotic process involving microvascular thrombosis, hemolysis, hypocomplementemia, cardiac injury, uremia, and proteinuria. There are familial forms of HUS that are of unknown pathogenesis and are associated with poor prognosis. HUS is controlled with supportive therapy, plasma component transfusion, or plasma exchange transfusion, which have been shown to improve survival in nonpregnant patients.[16] The uremia generally resolves, but severe cases may require temporary or long-term hemodialysis.

Thrombotic Thrombocytopenic Purpura

TTP arises from an abnormality in von Willebrand factor (vWF) cleaving protease. In TTP there is microvascular thrombosis, hemolysis, fever, thrombocytopenia, central nervous system dysfunction, cardiac dysfunction, and paradoxical bleeding. TTP has been reported during pregnancy and in the postpartum period and should be considered in the differential diagnosis of acquired acute anemia and thrombocytopenia.[17]

The diagnosis of TTP requires a high index of suspicion because the presentation may resemble HELLP or HUS. Serum vWF protease activity and inhibitor studies have been used as diagnostic tools. In TTP the vWF protease activity is decreased or absent and the presence of an inhibitor is detected.

Similar to HUS, therapy consists of plasma and blood component transfusions, plasma exchange, and glucocorticoids. Platelet transfusions should be avoided. For HUS and TTP, therapy with intravenous Igs and antibiotics has been used with limited success.

Paroxysmal Nocturnal Hemoglobinuria

Hemolytic anemia due to PNH is the result of an acquired mutation of a cell surface protein that results in complement-mediated hemolysis. Primary manifestations of PNH are marrow aplasia, intravascular hemolysis, and thrombophilia. PNH can be differentiated from other forms of hemolytic anemia by the absence of specific cell surface proteins in flow cytometric analysis. Exacerbations of hemolysis can occur in response to infection, menses, transfusions, surgery, and iron therapy. Pregnancy in women with acquired PNH is associated with a 75% risk of maternal morbidity and up to a 10% risk of mortality that is attributed to a 10–40% risk of venous thrombosis. Transfusions, antiplatelet therapy, and anticoagulation are necessary in pregnancies complicated by PNH.[18] Corticosteroids are sometimes used to manage PNH during pregnancy. Outside pregnancy donor-related human leukocyte antigen, matched bone marrow transplant may be the only potential for cure.

Transfusion Reaction

Transfusion-induced hemolytic anemia should be suspected when there is an acute onset of anemia consistent with hemolysis after blood component therapy. It can be confirmed by a positive indirect Coombs' test. Antibodies of the IgM or IgG type can cause transfusion-related hemolysis. IgG antibodies can cross the placenta and potentially cause neonatal hydrops fetalis.

Medication

Medications commonly used during pregnancy that have been implicated in hemolytic events include α-methyldopa, penicillin, cephalosporins, hydralazine, quinidine, and procainamide.

Hereditary Hemolytic Anemia

Rare forms of chronic hemolytic anemia include abnormalities of RBC structure such as spherocytosis and ovalocytosis. Inherited unstable hemoglobin variants result in chronic hemolytic anemia. Splenectomy is often the therapy used in these cases. Women who have previously undergone a splenectomy have a more favorable outcome during pregnancy than do those who have not.[19] X-linked inherited erythrocyte enzyme defects such as complete or partial glucose-6-phosphate dehydrogenase deficiency can be found in approximately 2–15% of African American women. It can result in recurrent hemolytic anemia when the individual is exposed to oxidation medications or compounds.

Consultation with hematology is indicated when managing cases of hemolytic anemia during pregnancy with the exception of obstetric cases arising as a result of HELLP syndrome or DIC.

Guiding Questions in Approaching the Patient

- What is the morphology of the anemia (MCV)?
- What is the mechanism of anemia—decreased production, increased destruction of RBCs, or blood loss?
- Is the patient in an ethnic group that has an increased risk of hemoglobinopathy or enzymopathy?
- Does the patient have risk factors for folate or vitamin B_{12} deficiency?

Conclusion

Anemia is common in pregnancy. Mild anemia has minimal consequences on pregnancy, but severe anemia has been associated with adverse maternal, fetal, and newborn outcomes. The most frequently encountered cause of acquired anemia in pregnancy is iron deficiency. The obstetrician needs to be aware of the numerous causes of anemia that can coincide with pregnancy and must have a familiarity with the evaluation and management of various acquired anemias. In addition, the obstetrician has a responsibility to identify inheritable forms of anemia and to offer appropriate prenatal counseling and testing. Diagnosis and therapy of aplastic anemia, hemolytic anemia, and anemia refractory to therapy should be done with hematology consultation.

Discussion of Cases

CASE 1: MULTIPATA WITH ANEMIA AND A HISTORY OF AN EATING DISORDER

A 37-year-old gravida 2, para 1 presents for prenatal care at 23 weeks of gestation and is found to have a hemoglobin level of 9.0 g/dL. Her medical history is significant for an eating disorder and alcoholism. Her MCV is 85.4 fL (normal 82–99 fL), platelet count is 457 K/µL, and white blood cell count is 15.3 K/µL.

Are there any other tests you would order at this time?

Peripheral smear and reticulocyte count, ferritin level, and, because of her history of nutritional deficiency, folate and vitamin B_{12} levels.

The absolute reticulocyte count is 65×10^9/L (normal $48–152 \times 10^9$/L). The peripheral smear shows normochromic/normocytic red blood cells with some poikilocytosis. The ferritin level is 13 µg/dL, B_{12} is 497 pg/mL (normal 211–911 pg/mL), and folate is 1296 ng/mL (normal >95 ng/mL).

What is your initial management plan?

Ferrous sulfate 325 mg three times daily.

Follow-up testing in 3 weeks shows a hemoglobin level of 11.8 g/dL. How long should therapy be continued?

It will take approximately 3 months for restitution of iron stores after correction of anemia. For optimal absorption, iron should be taken 30 minutes before a meal and preferably with vitamin C.

If the initial laboratory assessment had not included folate and B_{12} levels, then the absolute reticulocyte count could have been rechecked. One would have expected an increase in 7 to 10 days after therapy initiation. If this was not observed, then the folate and B_{12} levels could have been assessed at that time.

CASE 2: GRAND MULTIPARA WITH SEVERE ANEMIA

A 25-year-old African American gravida 8, para 6 presents at 31 weeks of gestation in preterm labor. She has had no prenatal care thus far this pregnancy. She has a history of five full-term deliveries and one spontaneous preterm birth at 32 weeks. Her hemoglobin is 4.3 g/dL, and platelet and white blood cell counts are within normal limits. The peripheral smear shows 3+ microcytosis and 2+ hypochromasia. The absolute reticulocyte count is 0.0720 M/μL (within normal limits).

What other laboratory tests are indicated at this time?

Hemoglobin electrophoresis is indicated. Because of microcytic cells and inappropriately low reticulocyte count, a serum ferritin level should also be performed to rule out iron deficiency. An assessment for hemolysis is also indicated.

Hemoglobin electrophoresis demonstrates a sickle cell trait. Serum ferritin level is 5 ng/mL. Haptoglobin level is also low at below 8 mg/dL. Serum folate and B_{12} levels are also checked and are normal. Because of the patient's ethnicity and low haptoglobin level, a glucose-6-phosphate dehydrogenase qualitative assessment was done, and activity was present.

After further assessment with ultrasound, the patient was noted to have a twin pregnancy. How do you interpret the findings?

The patient's anemia is a result of severe iron deficiency. She has had her iron stores depleted by multiple pregnancies separated by short intervals. Hemodilution of the current pregnancy is exacerbated by the twin gestation. Her sickle cell status may have contributed to the mild hemolysis.

What are options for treatment?

Offering the patient a transfusion is appropriate, but she refused. She was also unwilling to take oral iron therapy three times per day, so she was given parenteral iron therapy. Before her delivery 5 weeks later, she had a hemoglobin level of 8.9 g/dL.

REFERENCES

1 Yip R. Iron deficiency. *Bull World Health Organ* 1998;76(suppl 2):121–123.

2 Williams M, Wheby M. Anemia and pregnancy. *Med Clin North Am* 1992;76:631–647.

3 Scholl T. High third trimester ferritin concentration: associations with very preterm delivery, infection, and maternal nutritional status. *Obstet Gynecol* 1998;92:161–166.

4 Savoie N, Rioux F. Impact of maternal anemia of the infant's iron status at 9 months of age. *Can J Public Health* 2002;93:203–207.

5 Rasmussen K. Is there a causal relationship between iron deficiency or iron-deficiency anemia and weight at birth, length of gestation and perinatal mortality? *J Nutr* 2001;131(suppl 2):590S–601S.

6 Sloan N, Jordan E, Winikoff B. Effects of iron supplementation on maternal hematologic status in pregnancy. *Am J Public Health* 2002; 92:288–293.

7 Cuervo L, Mahomed K. Treatments for iron deficiency anemia in pregnancy. *Cochrane Database Syst Rev* 2001;2:CD003094.

8 Hartridge T, Illing H, Sandy J. The role of folic acid in oral clefting. *Br J Orthod* 1999;26:115–120.

9 Hernandez-Diaz S, Werler M, Walker A, et al. Folic acid antagonists during pregnancy and the risk of birth defects. *N Engl J Med* 2000;343:1608–1614.

10 Suarez L, Hendricks K, Felkner M. Maternal serum B_{12} levels and risk for neural tube defects in a Texas-Mexican border population. *Ann Epidemiol* 2003;13:81–88.

11 Ball S, The modern management of severe aplastic anemia. *Br J Haematol* 2000;110:41–53.

12 Aitchison R, Marsh J, Hows J, et al. Pregnancy associated with aplastic anemia: a report of five cases and review of current management. *Br J Haematol* 1989;73:541–545.

13 Tichelli A, Socie G, Marsh J, et al. Outcome of pregnancy and disease course among women with aplastic anemia treated with immunosuppression. *Ann Intern Med* 2002;137:164–172.

14 Kumar R, Advani A, Sharan J, et al. Pregnancy induced hemolytic anemia: an unexplained entity. *Ann Hematol* 2001;80:623–626.

15 Benraad C, Scheerder H, Overbeeke M. Autoimmune haemolytic anaemia during pregnancy. *Eur J Obstet Gynecol Reprod Biol* 1994; 55:209–211.

16 Ruggenenti P, Remuzzi G. Pathophysiology and management of thrombotic microangiopathies. *J Nephrol* 1998;11:300–310.

17 McMinn J, George J. Evaluation of women with clinically suspected thrombotic thrombocytopenia purpura-hemolytic uremic syndrome during pregnancy. *J Clin Apheresis* 2001;16:202–209.

18 Meyers G, Parker C. Management issues in paroxysmal nocturnal hemoglobinuria. *Int J Hematol* 2003;77:125–132.

19 Pajor A, Lehoczky D, Szakacs Z. Pregnancy and hereditary spherocytosis. Report of 8 patients and a review. *Arch Gynecol Obstet* 1993;253:37–42.

Approach to the Patient with a Possible Hemoglobinopathy

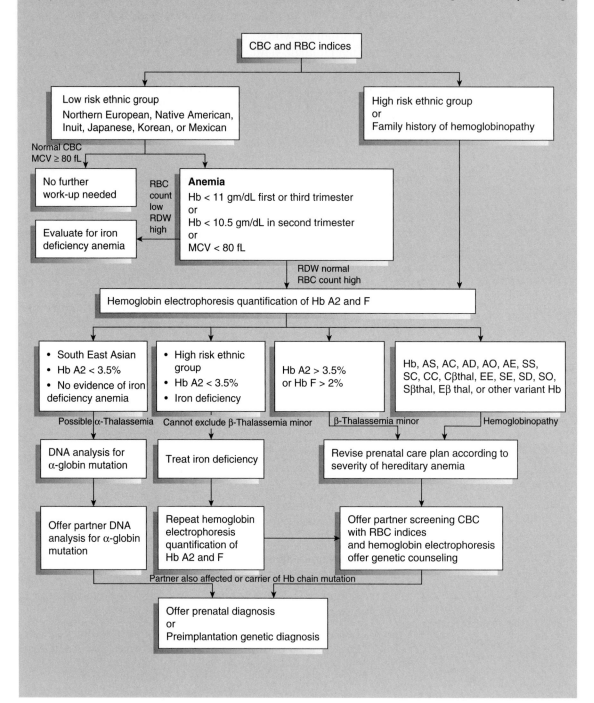

8 Hemoglobinopathy

Michelle Russell

Introduction

KEY POINT

Hemoglobinopathies occur in many ethnic groups.

Hemoglobinopathies are the most common genetic diseases of humans. According to the World Health Organization, the worldwide carrier frequency is 4.5%, and the affected birth rate is 2 in 1000 live births. Hemoglobin disorders are present in many ethnic groups. The prevalence of disease depends on the carrier frequency of hemoglobin mutations in the population.

Disease can result from a change in the structure, quantity, function, or stability of the hemoglobin protein. This chapter on hemoglobinopathies reviews the pathophysiology, diagnosis, and management of thalassemia, altered oxygen affinity, variant hemoglobin, unstable hemoglobin, and methemoglobinemia disorders. Considerations of sickle cell anemia are excluded because this subject is addressed in Chap. 9.

Normal Hemoglobin

KEY POINT

All prenatal patients from ethnic groups other than those identified as having low risk, including those with unexplained anemia or microcytosis, or a family history of hemoglobinopathy should be offered screening.

One needs to understand the structure and function of normal hemoglobin to understand the pathologic effects of abnormal hemoglobin. Normal hemoglobin is comprised of a tetramer of globin chains and an iron-containing heme group that is covalently linked to each of the globin chains. The iron of the heme group binds, carries, and delivers oxygen to the tissues. The normal individual has four copies of the α-globin–like genes and two copies of the β-globin–like genes. A normal tetramer of globin chains consists of two α-globin–like chains and two β-globin–like chains. The variation in globin tetramers determines the type of hemoglobin and its function.

115

Hemoglobin A is the predominant hemoglobin found in erythrocytes of the adult, comprising 95–98% of the hemoglobin. A small amount of hemoglobin A_2, normally less than 3.5%, is also present in the adult erythrocyte. Adult hemoglobin is generally comprised of less than 0.5–2% hemoglobin F (fetal hemoglobin). Genetic mutations that alter the globin chain or quantity of globin chains produced will yield a variant hemoglobin with abnormal properties.

Hemoglobinopathies

Hundreds of genetic mutations in hemoglobin have been described and occur in many populations.[1] When these mutations alter globin chain production, structure, or function, they shorten the life span of the erythrocyte and produce clinical symptoms. The spectrum of disease state ranges from asymptomatic to severe anemia incompatible with life. Pregnancies in women with hemoglobinopathies are at higher risk of obstetric and nonobstetric complications that can be minimized with modification in prenatal care. Carriers of globin chain mutations are at increased risk of producing offspring with a similar or a clinically more significant hemoglobin abnormality. Women with a family history of hemoglobinopathy, unexplained anemia, or microcytosis on routine prenatal testing should be offered screening. The widening ethnic and geographic distributions of human hemoglobinopathies have made identification of individuals at increased risk by ethnic or racial origin less reliable. Hence, it may be easier to identify low-risk groups. All couples of ethnic groups other than northern European, Japanese, Inuit, Native American, Mexican, and Korean should routinely be offered screening for hemoglobinopathy carrier status.

SCREENING AND DIAGNOSIS

KEY POINT

Screening tests include CBC with RBC indices and hemoglobin electrophoresis with quantification of hemoglobins A_2 and F.

Diagnostic tests must be completed before blood product transfusion. The complete blood count (CBC) with red blood cell (RBC) indices and hemoglobin electrophoresis with quantification of hemoglobins A_2 and F are the initial screening tools. Hemoglobin electrophoresis identifies variant hemoglobins by the electrophoretic migration pattern (Table 8-1). A peripheral smear may be helpful because it can show characteristic changes such as target cells, fragmented cells, or sickle cells in the presence of a hemoglobin abnormality. Evaluation for iron deficiency is occasionally indicated and, if present, requires therapy and repeat screening to exclude

Table 8-1. **INTERPRETATION OF HEMOGLOBIN ELECTROPHORESIS AND COMPLETE BLOOD CELL COUNT**

DISORDER	HB (G/DL)	MCV (FL)	HB A (%)	HB A$_2$ (%)	HB F (%)	OTHER HB	PERIPHERAL SMEAR	DISEASE STATE
Normal	13	85	95–98	<3.5	<2	None	Normal	None
β-Thalassemia trait	12.5	70	90	>3.5	<8	None	Target	Mild anemia
β-Thalassemia major	6	65	<40	>5	>60	None	Nucleated RBCs	Severe anemia
S trait	13	85	60	<3.5	<2	Hb S 40	Sickle	Asymptomatic
S trait/α-thalassemia trait	13	80	70	<3.5	<2	Hb S 30	Sickle	Asymptomatic
S/β$^+$-thalassemia	10	65	25	>3.5	<20	Hb S 70	Sickle	Severe anemia
S/β^0-thalassemia	8	65	0	>3.5	<30	Hb S 90	Sickle	Severe anemia
SS disease	7	65	0	<3.5	<30	Hb S 90	Sickle	Severe anemia
SS/α-thalassemia	8	75	0	<3.5	<35	Hb S 90	Sickle	Moderate/severe anemia
SC disease	10	80	0	<3.5	<2	Hb S 50 Hb C 50	Sickle, target	Moderate/severe anemia
C trait	13	80	50	<3.5	<2	Hb C 50	Target	Asymptomatic
CC disease	12	80	0	<3.5	<2	Hb C 95	Target	Mild anemia
α-Thalassemia silent carrier	13	85	95	<3.5	<2	None	Normal	Asymptomatic
α-Thalassemia trait	10	80	95	<3.5	<2	None	Rare target	Asymptomatic
α-Thalassemia intermedia	10	70	90	<3.5	<5	None	Hb H inclusions	Mild/moderate anemia
E trait	13	70	70	<3.5	<2	Hb E 30	Targets	Asymptomatic
E trait/α-thalassemia	13	65	80	<3.5	<2	Hb E 20	Targets	Asymptomatic
EE disease	11	60	0	<3.5	<8	Hb E 90	Targets	Mild anemia
E/β-thalassemia	8	60	0	>3.5	<8	Hb E 80	Targets, nucleated RBCs	Severe anemia

Hb = hemoglobin; MCV = mean corpuscular volume; RBCs = red blood cells.

117

concurrent hemoglobinopathy. DNA analysis is the only diagnostic tool that can exclude or confirm the presence of α-thalassemia silent carrier, α-thalassemia trait, uncommon types of β-thalassemia, and complex compound heterozygous states. When a hemoglobin abnormality is identified during preconception or prenatal evaluation, the partner should be offered similar screening and diagnostic testing.

Thalassemia

Thalassemia disorders are a diverse group of microcytic, hemolytic anemias that have defective synthesis of α-globin or β-globin chains. They occur in individuals of Mediterranean, Middle Eastern, South East Asian, African, and Asian Indian descent. Clinically significant thalassemia disorders include homozygous α-thalassemia, α-thalassemia intermedia, β-thalassemia major, β-thalassemia intermedia, and compound heterozygous thalassemia states such as hemoglobin E/β-thalassemia and α-thalassemia coinherited with hemoglobin Constant Spring. Thalassemia is becoming an increasingly significant world health problem, and recent immigration trends are affecting certain regions of the United States.

α-Thalassemia

α-Thalassemia is a genetic disorder that results in deletions of α-globin genes. The severity of the disorder is directly related to the number of genes affected by mutations (Table 8-2). Thalassemia can arise from nondeletion mutations. More than 30 such mutations affecting the α-globin gene have been identified. Hemoglobin Constant Spring is an abnormally long-chain α-globin. It occurs in South East Asian populations and can result in a severe thalassemia syndrome if compound heterozygosity occurs with an α-globin chain mutation. Up to 40% of cases of α-thalassemia intermedia in the United States are a result of coinheritance of α-thalassemia trait and hemoglobin Constant Spring.

HOMOZYGOUS α-THALASSEMIA

Homozygous $α^0$-thalassemia is a mutation that deletes all four α-globin chains. When α-globin chains are absent, abnormal β-globin such as homotetramers $γ^4$ and $β^4$, hemoglobin Bart, and hemoglobin H are formed.[2] These have a high affinity for oxygen, poorly oxygenate

Table 8-2. GENE DELETIONS IN α-THALASSEMIA

Deletions (No. of Genes)	Disorder	Diagnostic Tests	Disease	Ethnic Group	Reproductive Transmission Risk
αα/αα (none)	Normal	None	None	Any	No
αα/α–(1)	Silent carrier, α-thalassemia 2, minima	DNA analysis	None	South East Asian, African American	Yes; risk of α-thalassemia intermedia
αα/—(2) Cis	α⁰-thalassemia trait, α-thalassemia 1, minor	DNA analysis	None to mild, microcytic anemia	South East Asian	Yes; risk of homozygous α-thalassemia
α–/α– (2) Trans	α⁺-thalassemia trait, α-thalassemia 1	DNA analysis	None to mild microcytic anemia	African American	Yes; risk of α-thalassemia intermedia
α–/—(3)	Intermedia, hemoglobin H disease	Hemoglobin electrophoresis, peripheral smear, DNA analysis	Variable anemia	South East Asian	Yes; risk of homozygous α-thalassemia
—/—(4)	Major, hemoglobin Bart's disease	Hemoglobin electrophoresis, DNA analysis	In utero hydrops fetalis	South East Asian	No

tissues, and cause erythrocyte hemolysis. Homozygous α-thalassemia (hemoglobin Bart's disease) is generally incompatible with life. It occurs in South East Asian populations and in certain other high-risk groups.

Hemoglobin Bart constitutes up to 98% of the hemoglobin in affected fetuses and produces severe anemia and intrauterine hypoxia. The result is high-output cardiac failure and hydrops fetalis in the second or third trimester of pregnancy. Intrauterine or neonatal demise is the most common outcome for homozygous α^0-thalassemia. Ultrasound findings that have some value in predicting homozygous α^0-thalassemia include cardiothoracic ratios, placental thickness, and middle cerebral artery Doppler.[3,4] Definitive diagnosis can be made by chorionic villous sampling, amniocentesis, and cordocentesis, which have been done as early at 12 weeks of gestation.[5]

There have been a few case reports of intrauterine transfusion in α-thalassemia homozygous fetuses. Fetal therapy has allowed some fetuses to survive what is usually a lethal condition. Structural abnormalities including limb reduction defects have been reported.[6] However, the outcome can involve neurologic impairment. Limited experience with intrauterine stem cell transplantation has been reported and may be the future therapy for selected fetuses.[7]

Pregnancies complicated by hydrops fetalis impose risks on the mother. Preeclampsia occurs in up to 61% of pregnancies. Retained placenta requiring manual extraction and postpartum hemorrhage necessitating transfusion occur in up to 50% of patients. Fetal malpresentation and dystocia due to hydrops fetalis contribute to a higher rate of cesarean section delivery.

α-THALASSEMIA INTERMEDIA

In contrast to homozygous α-thalassemia, α-thalassemia intermedia is compatible with extrauterine life, but a spectrum of clinical severity occurs.[2] Some affected individuals develop mild anemia, others require transfusions, and still others succumb to in utero hydrops fetalis. Genetic factors are responsible for the variable presentation. Deletion of three of the four α-globin genes (—α–) leads to hemoglobin H disease. This causes a decrease in α-globin chains and a disproportion in the quantity of β-globin–like chains. The excess β-globin–like chains form homotetramers β_4 (hemoglobin H) that comprise 16–30% of adult hemoglobin.[8] It delivers oxygen ineffectively, is unstable, and precipitates in the erythrocyte. Precipitation of hemoglobin H leads to ineffective erythropoiesis and erythrocyte hemolysis.[2]

Many pregnancies have been reported in women with α-thalassemia intermedia. Most women with α-thalassemia intermedia do not require modification in routine prenatal care beyond management of the chronic hemolytic anemia, but pregnancies in severely affected women should be managed similar to pregnancies in women with β-thalassemia major.

Preconceptual or prenatal assessment for liver, endocrine, and cardiac diseases from iron overload is important. Initial laboratory evaluation includes CBC, platelets, fasting glucose, calcium, liver function tests, albumin, partial thromboplastin time, and thyroid function tests. Repeat laboratory testing may be indicated as gestation advances. Multiply transfused women should have screening for RBC antibodies, hepatitis B surface antigen, hepatitis C virus antibodies, and human immunodeficiency virus. Ferritin levels should be obtained during preconception testing or early in prenatal care.

A detailed late second-trimester ultrasound examination is advisable because there is a proposed risk for fetal abnormalities due to folate deficiency, iron overload, and linked chromosome abnormalities. Because of the increased risk of intrauterine growth restriction with severe anemia, fetal growth evaluation by serial ultrasonography is indicated. Weekly or twice weekly fetal antenatal testing should be initiated at 28–32 weeks depending on the condition of the patient and the fetus.

In general, anemia worsens during pregnancy. Acute worsening of anemia can occur due to increased erythrocyte hemolysis induced by bacterial infections, fever, parvovirus B_{19} infections, oxidative medications, secondary hypersplenism, and pregnancy. Transfusion support may be required. Iatrogenic exacerbations can be diminished by the avoidance of oxidating medications such as Pyridium (phenazopyridine), sulfonamides, and nitrofurantoin.

Gravidas with hemoglobin H disease should receive folate supplementation 1–5 mg/day. Prolonged administration of large doses of folate may warrant periodic evaluation of serum vitamin B_{12} levels to exclude an underlying deficiency. Oral iron supplements should be prescribed only if laboratory studies indicate iron deficiency.

Women with hemoglobin H disease may have iron overload toxicity unrelated to transfusion and supplementation history.[8] The enhanced erythropoietic state leads to an increase in gastrointestinal absorption. Chronic iron toxicity can affect the endocrine system, leading to diabetes mellitus, hypothyroidism, hypoparathyroidism, and gonadal dysfunction. It can also affect the liver, leading to fibrosis and cirrhosis, and the heart, leading to ventricular dysfunction and dysrhythmias. Congestive heart failure has been observed in up to 9% of pregnant women with hemoglobin H disease.[2] Cardiac evaluation and surveillance with an electrocardiogram and echocardiogram during pregnancy are warranted if there is evidence of iron overload. Chelation therapy should be considered for ferritin levels above 1000–1300 ng/dL or if cardiac or hepatic iron toxicity is present.

Hepatosplenomegaly and symptomatic cholelithiasis are common in patients with α-thalassemia intermedia.[2] Evaluation and management of cholelithiasis before pregnancy should be considered. Outside pregnancy, splenectomy is performed in severe thalassemia cases. Women who have had a splenectomy are at higher risk of thromboembolism, and prophylactic anticoagulation should be considered if prolonged bedrest is prescribed.

Delivery should be accomplished when there is evidence of fetal lung maturity or sooner if there is evidence of maternal or fetal compromise. Regional anesthesia is preferred. An obstetric anesthesia consultation before delivery can be advantageous.

A multidiscipline approach to care with maternal fetal medicine, hematology, cardiology, and anesthesiology should be considered for treatment of pregnant women with α-thalassemia intermedia.

α-THALASSEMIA TRAIT AND SILENT CARRIER STATE

Individuals with the carrier states of α-thalassemia, α-thalassemia trait, and silent carrier are asymptomatic. α-Thalassemia trait (α-thalassemia minor) occurs when two of four α-globin genes are deleted. It has little clinical significance in an individual beyond mild, microcytic anemia. The α^+-thalassemia trait (α–α–) is a trans-type mutation that deletes one of the two α-globin genes on each chromosome. It is more common in African Americans. The α^0-thalassemia trait (αα/—) is a cis-type mutation that deletes both α-globin genes on one chromosome. It occurs in South East Asian populations. Populations with cis-type mutations are at risk of producing offspring with homozygous α^0-thalassemia. Offspring with α-thalassemia intermedia can result if a pregnancy occurs in an individual who has an_α-globin gene mutation such as hemoglobin Constant Spring.

KEY POINT

Severe hemoglobinopathies require modifications in prenatal management that is best provided by a multidiscipline approach.

Silent carrier α-thalassemia, or α-thalassemia minima, arises when one of four α-globin genes is deleted (αα/α–) It can affect reproduction similar to $α^+$-thalassemia trait.

Pregnancy in women with α-thalassemia trait and silent carrier α-thalassemia is uncomplicated, and the hemoglobin abnormality is often unrecognized. Routine obstetric care is appropriate for these conditions.

β-Thalassemia

β-Thalassemia is a heterogeneous genetic disorder of the β-globin gene. The type and carrier frequency of β-globin gene mutations vary across populations. Populations with a high prevalence include Mediterraneans, South East Asians, Middle Easterners, Asian Indians, and African Americans. Most cases are autosomal recessive, but dominant patterns of inheritance exist. Coinheritance of a β-globin chain mutation such as hemoglobins Lepore, E, and C can result in severe disease.

β-THALASSEMIA MAJOR

β-Thalassemia major is also known as Cooley's anemia. In this disorder there is an absence of β-globin chain production, but α-globin chain synthesis is maintained. The excess α-globin chains are incapable of forming globin homotetramers and precipitate in erythrocytes. The precipitation of α-globin chains leads to erythrocyte hemolysis and to ineffective erythropoiesis. Fetal hemoglobin production is increased, but it delivers oxygen poorly. This leads to bone marrow expansion, skeletal deformity, hypermetabolism, wasting, gout, folate deficiency, iron toxicity, and death. Onset of severe hemolytic anemia occurs in infancy and blood transfusions are required. If untreated, the life expectancy of an individual is approximately 6 years. Transfusion therapy extends the lives of individuals with this disease but leads to iron overload. Iron toxicities include cardiac and hepatic dysfunctions and endocrinopathies such as diabetes mellitus, hypothyroidism, and hypoparathyroidism. Hypertransfusion protocols to suppress ineffective erythropoiesis combined with intensive iron chelation therapy decreases morbidity related to this disease and iron overload.

Previously, women with β-thalassemia major were infertile as a result of gonadal dysfunction. Improvement in the care of individuals with β-thalassemia major has extended life expectancies into the third decade and decreased morbidity. As a result, many of these women are reaching childbearing age with reproductive capabilities intact. There are an increasing number of case reports of pregnancy in women with β-thalassemia major.[9] These pregnancies are often complicated by preeclampsia, preterm delivery, and fetal growth restriction.

Preconceptual or early prenatal care should include a thorough physical assessment for cardiac, liver, and splenic abnormalities. Laboratory studies including evaluation of CBC, platelets, ferritin, electrolytes, calcium, partial thromboplastin time, total protein, albumin, liver function, renal function, thyroid function, and fasting glucose levels should be completed. A screen for RBC antibodies and blood-borne viral infections by testing for hepatitis B surface antigen, hepatitis C virus antibodies, and human immunodeficiency virus is indicated in patients previously exposed to blood transfusions. Hepatitis B vaccination should be given, if indicated. Repeat evaluation of the CBC every 2 weeks and ferritin monthly is suggested. Evaluation of liver function, thyroid function, and electrolytes should be repeated each trimester. Glucose tolerance testing should be performed early and repeated if initially normal. Gravidas with β-thalassemia major are at risk of folate depletion and should receive supplementation of up to 5 mg/day. Iron supplementation should be avoided.

A detailed evaluation of fetal anatomy should be offered because of the association of open neural tube defects with folate deficiency. Fetal growth should be monitored. Once- or twice-weekly antepartum testing can be initiated at 28–32 weeks of gestation depending on maternal and fetal statuses.

Worsening of anemia occurs during gestation and requires intensification of the transfusion and surveillance regimen. Similar to the nonpregnant state, a blood hypertransfusion protocol to maintain the hemoglobin level near 10 g/dL is recommended to avoid increased erythropoiesis and lessen the risks of fetal compromise such as intrauterine growth restriction.[9]

Secondary hypersplenism may occur in nonsplenectomized women, leading to thrombocytopenia, leukopenia, and profound anemia. The risk of thromboembolism is increased in patients who have predisposing risk factors such as postsplenectomy thrombocytosis, cardiomyopathy, diabetes, liver abnormalities, or hypothyroidism.[10] Prophylactic anticoagulation should be considered, particularly if immobilization occurs. Symptomatic cholelithiasis is common, and evaluation and management of cholelithiasis before conception is indicated.[9]

Iron-related cardiac toxicity has been demonstrated by echocardiography in 38% of asymptomatic chelated patients with β-thalassemia major.[11] Pulmonary hypertension and right-side heart failure can occur. Cardiac decompensation is the most common cause of death in transfused patients with thalassemia. Cardiac evaluation by electrocardiogram and echocardiogram should be completed during preconception or in early pregnancy. Pregnancy is discouraged if the resting left ventricular ejection fraction is less than 55% or if there is evidence of pulmonary hypertension. A normal measured resting left ventricular ejection fraction does not predict normal cardiac function with stress.[9] Pregnancy, anemia, preeclampsia, intercurrent infection, labor, and delivery may compromise cardiac function and are associated with cardiac decompensation. Cardiac surveillance should be repeated in the second and third trimesters of pregnancy.

Before pregnancy, most patients with transfusion-dependent β-thalassemia major are on a regimen of iron chelation therapy with a goal of maintaining serum ferritin levels below 1000–1300 ng/mL. In unchelated pregnant patients, serum ferritin levels increase only 10%, but in others it may increase significantly.[12] Chelation therapy is often discontinued before or during early pregnancy due to unknown teratogenic risks in human pregnancy. Animal studies indicate an increased risk of skeletal dysplasia at large doses. There are several case reports involving at least 40 pregnancies in which continued chelation therapy with deferoxamine showed no evidence of adverse fetal effects.[12] The risks of iron chelation therapy during breast feeding are also unknown, but the agent is poorly absorbed by the oral route and unlikely to attain levels in the neonate. Breast-fed infants should be monitored closely for evidence of iron deficiency. If iron chelation therapy is terminated, it is advisable to discontinue ascorbic acid to avoid an undesired increase in intestinal absorption of iron.

Women with β-thalassemia major often have skeletal abnormalities and small stature due to marrow expansion and hypermetabolism. They are at increased risk of cephalopelvic disproportion during delivery. Most reported deliveries have been by scheduled cesarean section. As transfusion and chelation therapy improve the physical condition of these women, vaginal delivery will be more likely to be successful. With a few exceptions, cesarean delivery can be reserved for the usual obstetric indications.

Anesthesia for labor and delivery is an important component of prenatal care. The pain response and hemodynamic changes of labor can place intolerable stresses on the cardiovascular system. Regional epidural is the preferred anesthesia technique, but each case must be individualized depending on the presence of comorbidities. Predelivery consultation with an obstetric anesthesiologist may facilitate provision of adequate labor and delivery analgesia.

Birth control needs should be addressed, and unplanned pregnancies should be discouraged. Estrogen-containing oral contraceptives may increase the risk of thromboembolic disease in women who have undergone a splenectomy.

Although not performed during pregnancy, human leukocyte antigen matched bone marrow transplantation is the only cure for severe transfusion-dependent thalassemia and has a 90–95% disease-free survival rate in low-risk patients.[13] Successful pregnancies are reported in women after bone marrow transplantation. Stem cells derived from fetal cord blood or fetal liver have been successfully used for transplantation.

β-THALASSEMIA INTERMEDIA

β-Thalassemia intermedia occurs when there is decreased β-globin chain synthesis and an excess of α-globin chains. β^+-Thalassemia intermedia results from compound heterozygosity or coinheritance of a genetic mutation that modifies the ratio of β-globin chains to α-globin chains. Many of the earlier reports of pregnancies in women with β-thalassemia were cases of β-thalassemia intermedia. Women with β-thalassemia intermedia have a moderate hemolytic anemia but are not transfusion dependent as children.[14] The spectrum of disease ranges from asymptomatic, mild anemia to transfusion dependency during stress including pregnancy, infection, and surgery. Iron overload toxicity can occur without an antecedent history of transfusion. Serum ferritin levels should be monitored. An evaluation of the cardiac, endocrine, and hepatic systems is performed if there is evidence of iron overload.

Iron supplementation can be given if iron deficiency is present by laboratory evaluation. Folate supplementation 1–5 mg/day is recommended. Complications arising due to severe β-thalassemia intermedia are similar to the complications of β-thalassemia major, and management during pregnancy is similar.

β-THALASSEMIA MINOR

Women with β-thalassemia minor are generally asymptomatic before pregnancy. During pregnancy these women may develop moderate worsening of anemia, but this usually has no significant effect on pregnancy outcome. Rarely, they require transfusion support during pregnancy. Folate supplementation 1–5 mg/day should be advised, and iron supplementation can be given, if needed.

Hemoglobin E

Hemoglobin E results from a point mutation in the β-globin gene. It is the second most common β-globin chain mutation worldwide, occurring in more than 30 million people mostly from South East Asia. In at-risk populations, the carrier frequency is as high as 36%. The homozygous state causes an asymptomatic, mild microcytic anemia. Anemia can worsen with physiologic stressors. Oxidating medications should be avoided. Hemoglobin E trait and homozygous hemoglobin E have little effect on pregnancy.

When hemoglobin E is coinherited with a β-thalassemia gene, it can manifest as a severe form of transfusion-dependent thalassemia. There are reported cases of compound heterozygous hemoglobin E and β-thalassemia in the obstetric literature. Complications include severe maternal anemia, extramedullary hematopoiesis, and intrauterine growth restriction. Management of pregnancies in women with compound heterozygous thalassemia should be similar to management of those with β-thalassemia major or sickle cell disease.

Hemoglobin C

Hemoglobin C arises from a point mutation in the β-globin gene. It is seen predominantly in persons of West African descent. Hemoglobin C trait is asymptomatic, and homozygous hemoglobin C manifests as a mild microcytic anemia, splenomegaly, and hemolysis. Neither condition has a significant effect on pregnancy outcome.[15]

Compound heterozygous individuals who inherit hemoglobin C with hemoglobin S or β-thalassemia can have a clinically significant sickle cell anemia or thalassemic disorder, respectively. In contrast to SC disease, hemoglobin C/β-thalassemia has minimal effect on pregnancy.

Unstable Hemoglobin

Unstable hemoglobin mutants other than the thalassemias are uncommon. There are more than 100 rare variants described that are dominantly inherited. They are not specific to an ethnic group. Point mutations in the globin gene result in altered globin structure and increased susceptibility of hemoglobin to oxidation or insolubility. The abnormal hemoglobin precipitates in the erythrocyte. The screening hemoglobin electrophoresis may be normal, and the diagnosis may require isopropanol precipitation testing or DNA analysis. The clinical picture is of chronic hemolytic anemia of varying severity, jaundice, and splenomegaly. It is generally diagnosed in infancy but occasionally can be first evident in adults after oxidative stress such as exposure to oxidative medications. Transfusion support and splenectomy may be required in severe cases. Thromboembolic events and infections with encapsulated microorganisms are increased after splenectomy. Supplementation with folic acid 1–5 mg/day should be considered. Close maternal and fetal surveillance is important. Fetal growth surveillance and fetal nonstress testing may be warranted if anemia is severe. Pregnancy outcome may be affected by severe hemolytic anemia.[16]

Hemoglobin with Altered Oxygen Affinity

More than 80 mutations exist that increase or decrease the oxygen affinity of hemoglobin. Mutations that increase the oxygen affinity of hemoglobin result in tissue hypoxia and erythrocytosis. Symptoms of hyperviscosity can occur, and the risk of thromboembolism is increased. Hemoglobin electrophoresis may be normal, and the diagnosis is made by clinical evaluation. Erythropoietin levels are high in the high oxygen affinity disorders. Rare cases of poor pregnancy outcome have been reported. No special therapy is routinely recommended for these conditions, but fetal growth assessment and nonstress testing should be considered.

Hemoglobin M

Hereditary methemoglobinemia due to hemoglobin M disease is found in Japanese populations. It has an autosomal dominant transmission pattern, and homozygosity is not compatible with survival. It arises from a point mutation in the α- or β-globin chain that maintains the iron molecule in the ferric state and is incapable of carrying oxygen. Cyanosis is evident in early childhood. The diagnosis can be confirmed by DNA analysis. Pregnancy is unaffected, and there is no treatment available or needed for this condition.[16] Fetal growth assessment and nonstress testing are prudent if maternal cyanosis is evident.

Prenatal Testing

Couples that are found to be carriers of mutations in the α- or β-globin chains should be offered prenatal testing. Prenatal screening programs in high-prevalence populations are effective and have decreased the incidence of homozygous β-thalassemia from 1 in 250 to 1 in 4000 live births. Prenatal diagnosis has been performed with DNA-based methods such as polymerase chain reaction and Southern blotting techniques on trophoblastic tissue obtained by chorionic villous sampling and on amniocytes obtained by amniocentesis. Using a combination of tests may avoid misdiagnosis.

Preimplantation genetic diagnosis is an alternative to prenatal testing. Similar DNA-based techniques have been used successfully to diagnose sickle cell disease, homozygous β-thalassemia, and homozygous α-thalassemia in blastocyst stage embryos, thus avoiding the transfer of an affected embryo.[17]

What's the Evidence?

There are only case reports of pregnancy management and outcome in women with hemoglobinopathies. Management protocols are based on case reports or extrapolated from studies performed in nonpregnant patients.

Guiding Questions in Approaching the Patient

- Is the patient at risk of having a hemoglobinopathy?
- How do I screen for hemoglobinopathy?

- How does the hemoglobinopathy affect pregnancy?
- How do I need to modify the prenatal management?
- Can the hemoglobinopathy be genetically transmitted to the fetus?
- Does the father also have a hemoglobinopathy that can be transmitted to the fetus?
- How can the patient find out if the fetus is affected?
- How can the couple prevent giving birth to an affected infant if both are carriers of a hemoglobin mutation?

Conclusion

Obstetricians need to be familiar with the diagnosis and complications of hereditary anemias. Management of pregnancies in women with transfusion-dependent hemoglobinopathies should be undertaken in a multidisciplinary approach that involves maternal fetal medicine, hematology, anesthesiology, and cardiology. Homozygous α-thalassemia is generally incompatible with extrauterine life, and pregnancy carries maternal risks. Management of asymptomatic non–transfusion-requiring hemoglobinopathies does not differ significantly from routine prenatal care with the exception of monitoring anemia. When a β- or α-globin chain mutation is identified in a patient, the prenatal care provider should offer partner testing, genetic counseling, and prenatal testing.

Discussion of Cases

CASE 1: FILIPINO COUPLE WITH PRIOR PREGNANCY COMPLICATED BY HYDROPS

A 25-year-old Filipino woman and her Filipino partner present to your office at 16 weeks of gestation for their first prenatal visit. The couple's pregnancy history is significant for a previous pregnancy complicated by fetal hydrops and an intrauterine fetal demise at 28 weeks of gestation. Autopsy findings and DNA testing found that the fetus had homozygous α-thalassemia.

What do you do next?

You offer the couple genetic counseling and prenatal testing. They are counseled that both are carriers of a cis-type α-globin chain mutation. This mutation gives the couple a 25% risk of producing an offspring with homozygous α-thalassemia. The couple chooses prenatal diagnosis.

How do you test for this condition?

An amniocentesis is performed. Amniotic fluid is sent for a DNA analysis that fails to detect α-globin chain sequences and makes the diagnosis of homozygous α-thalassemia. If the couple had presented earlier in gestation, chorionic villous sampling could have been offered and sent for similar testing.

How do you counsel the couple?

The couple is informed that the fetus is affected by homozygous α-thalassemia. They are counseled that homozygous α-thalassemia nearly always is incompatible with survival and frequently leads to intrauterine hydrops and fetal death. The mother is at increased risk for preeclampsia, preterm labor, placenta previa, cesarean section, and postpartum hemorrhage.

How do you propose to manage this pregnancy and what referrals do you make?

They are offered pregnancy termination, but they elect expectant management. You refer the couple to a tertiary care center where there are maternal fetal medicine specialists and neonatologists.

How do you think this case turned out?

At 25 weeks, a surveillance ultrasound showed fetal ascites. Subsequently, the patient developed severe preeclampsia, and fetal death occurred at 27 weeks. She was delivered of the stillborn and had moderate postpartum hemorrhage.

CASE 2: WEST AFRICAN PRIMIGRAVIDA WITH LIFE-LONG ANEMIA

A 17-year-old West African primigravida presents to your office at 15 weeks of gestation for first her prenatal visit. She reports a history of chronic anemia and needing transfusions on a few occasions as a child. Her mother and sister also have chronic anemia. She underwent a splenectomy for splenomegaly, thrombocytopenia, severe chronic anemia, and nonhealing leg ulcers in the previous year. She has cholelithiasis, but she has not had a cholecystectomy.

What tests do you want to order?

CBC, hemoglobin electrophoresis, reticulocyte count, low-density lipoprotein, iron studies, haptoglobin, folate, and vitamin B_{12}.

The CBC shows a white blood cell count of 13.0 K/μL, hemoglobin of 8.2 g/dL, hematocrit of 27.5%, platelet count of 797 K/μL, mean

corpuscular volume of 71.4 fL, RBC distribution width of 25.1, and mean cell hemoglobin of 21.3 pg. Hemoglobin electrophoresis shows 34.5% hemoglobin A, 3.2% hemoglobin A_2, and 62.3% hemoglobin F. Peripheral smear demonstrates multiple cell abnormalities including target cells, schistocytes, spherocytes, and others. The reticulocyte count is 22%, lactate hydrogenase is 210 μ/L, haptoglobin is lower than 14 mg/dL, and serum ferritin is 1000 ng/mL. Folate and B_{12} levels are normal. These tests are consistent with a hereditary hemolytic anemia. The patient is diagnosed with β-thalassemia intermedia.

She has had a splenectomy. How does that affect her risk of infection and complications?

After a splenectomy, there is increased risk of infection with encapsulated microorganisms. You inquire about immunizations and she confirms that she received immunizations for *Pneumococcus* and *Heliobacter influenzae* 1 year previously, before the splenectomy. She has thrombocytosis and is at increased risk of thromboembolic disease. You advise her to continue her current small dose of aspirin. You advise her that she may need additional thromboembolism prophylaxis if other risk factors arise during her pregnancy.

How do you counsel this patient?

She is offered genetic counseling, prenatal testing, and partner testing (CBC and hemoglobin electrophoresis). This would have determined the risk of an affected fetus. She declined testing including amniocentesis.

How do you plan to modify her prenatal care?

You plan to follow her hematologic studies and transfuse blood products if her anemia significantly worsens. Due to her high levels of ferritin, electrocardiogram and echocardiogram are indicated. She also needs evaluation for endocrinopathies and referral for possible chelation.

Her CBC is followed closely and remains stable. At 28 weeks, it shows a hemoglobin level of 7.7 gm/dL, hematocrit of 28.6%, and a platelet count of 877,000. You recommend serial fetal growth ultrasounds and advised antepartum testing twice weekly starting at 32 weeks. You perform an ultrasound for fetal growth at 34 weeks and the estimated fetal weight is 2235 g.

Are there any pregnancy complications for which she is at risk?

Women with β-thalassemia intermedia are at risk for preeclampsia, preterm labor, and fetal intrauterine growth restriction.

At her 37-week visit her blood pressure is 152/106 mm Hg and urine analysis shows 3+ protein. She is admitted for labor induction with a diagnosis of preeclampsia. The patient is delivered of a small-for-gestational-age male infant that weighs 2375 g.

Is she at risk of other complications after her cesarean section delivery and postpartum?

Her postpartum course is uncomplicated. Her postoperative hemoglobin level is 6.6 gm/dL. She is maintained on her daily regimen of baby aspirin and lower extremity compression boots until full ambulation is resumed. She is discharged home on folic acid 2 mg and progesterone-only oral contraceptives. You advise her that her partner can be tested for the presence of hemoglobin mutations before her next pregnancy. You advise her to seek surgical consultation for her cholelithiasis before her next planned pregnancy. Her hemoglobin level returns to 8.7 m/dL by her 6-week postpartum evaluation.

How should the newborn be followed?

A newborn screen is performed and shows the presence of hemoglobin S. On follow-up evaluation, the infant's hemoglobin level is 10.2 gm/dL, and mean corpuscular volume is 65 fL. Hemoglobin electrophoresis shows 3.2% hemoglobin A_2, 26% hemoglobin F, and 70% hemoglobin S. The infant is diagnosed with compound heterozygous sickle/β⁺-thalassemia.

REFERENCES

1 Clarke G, Higgins T. Laboratory investigation of hemoglobinopathies and thalassemias: review and update. *Clin Chem* 2000;46(8 pt 2): 1284–1290.

2 Chui D, Fucharoen S, Chan V. Hemoglobin H disease: not necessarily a benign disorder. *Blood* 2003;101:791–800.

3 Sohan K, Billington M, Pamphilon D, et al. Normal growth and development following in utero diagnosis and treatment of homozygous alpha-thalassemia. *BJOG* 2002;109:1308–1310.

4 Lam Y, Tang M, Lee C. Prenatal ultrasonographic prediction of homozygous type-1 α-thalassemia at 12-13 weeks of gestation. *Am J Obstet Gynecol* 1999;180:148–150.

5 Lam Y, Tang M. Prenatal Diagnosis of hemoglobin Bart's disease by cordocentesis at 12–13 weeks—experience with the first 59 cases. *Prenat Diagn* 2000;20:900–904.

6 Lam Y, Tang M, Sin S, et al. Limb reduction defects in fetuses with homozygous alpha-thalassemia-1. *Prenat Diagn* 1997;17:1143–1146.

7 Flake A, Zanjani E. In utero transplantation for thalassemia. *Ann N Y Acad Sci* 1998;850:300–311.

8 Chen F, Ooi C, Ha S, et al. Genetic and clinical features of hemoglobin H disease in Chinese patients. *N Engl J Med* 2000;343:544–550.

9 Aessopos A, Karabatsos F, Farmakis D, et al. Pregnancy in patients with well treated beta-thalassemia: outcome for mothers and newborn infants. *Am J Obstet Gynecol* 1999;180:360–365.

10 Borgna P, Carnelli V, Caruso V, et al. Thromboembolic events in beta-thalassemia major: an Italian multicenter study. *Acta Haematol* 1998;99:76–79.

11 Spirito P, Lupi G, Melevendi C, et al. Restrictive diastolic abnormalities identified by Doppler echocardiography in patients with thalassemia major. *Circulation* 1990;82:88–94.

12 Singer S, Vichinsky E. Deferoxamine treatment during pregnancy: is it harmful? *Am J Hematol* 1999;60:24–26.

13 Giardini C, Lucarelli G. Bone marrow transplantation for beta-thalassemia. *Hematol Oncol Clin North Am* 1999;13:1059–1064.

14 Weatherall D. The thalassemias. In: Buetler E, ed. *Williams Hematology,* 6th ed. New York: McGraw-Hill, 2001; p. 547–579.

15 Maberry M, Mason R, Cunningham F, et al. Pregnancy complicated by hemoglobin CC and C-beta-thalassemia disease. *Obstet Gynecol* 1990;76:324–327.

16 Rust O, Perry K. Disorders of hemoglobin structure, function, and synthesis. In: Gleicher N, Buttino L, Elkayam U, eds. *Principles and Practice of Medical Therapy in Pregnancy,* 3rd ed. Norwalk: Appleton & Lange, 1998; p. 1168–1173.

17 De Rycke M, Van V, Sermon K. Preimplantation genetic diagnosis for sickle cell anemia and beta-thalassemia. *Prenat Diagn* 2001;21: 214–222.

Management of Sickle Cell Disease in Pregnancy

First trimester

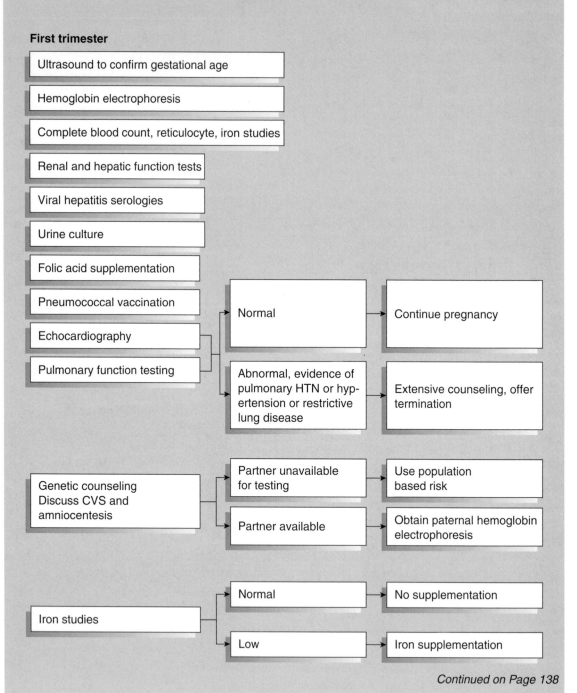

Ultrasound to confirm gestational age

Hemoglobin electrophoresis

Complete blood count, reticulocyte, iron studies

Renal and hepatic function tests

Viral hepatitis serologies

Urine culture

Folic acid supplementation

Pneumococcal vaccination

Echocardiography

Pulmonary function testing

- Normal → Continue pregnancy
- Abnormal, evidence of pulmonary HTN or hypertension or restrictive lung disease → Extensive counseling, offer termination

Genetic counseling Discuss CVS and amniocentesis

- Partner unavailable for testing → Use population based risk
- Partner available → Obtain paternal hemoglobin electrophoresis

Iron studies

- Normal → No supplementation
- Low → Iron supplementation

Continued on Page 138

9 Sickle Cell Disease and Pregnancy

Jeff B. Chapa
Judith U. Hibbard

Introduction

Sickle cell disease refers to a group of autosomal recessive disorders resulting from production of hemoglobin (Hb) S. With advances in our understanding of the pathophysiology of these diseases, medical care of afflicted individuals has improved immensely. Life expectancy for those with sickle cell disease now extends well into the fifth decade. Increasing numbers of women are reaching childbearing age and achieving pregnancy; thus, obstetricians need to be aware of the associated implications for mother and fetus. In this chapter we review the underlying pathophysiology of sickle hemoglobinopathies, discuss the clinical manifestations and available therapies with an emphasis on aspects relevant to the gravida, and outline a strategy for pregnancy management.

Molecular Basis and Epidemiology

Hb S is due to the alteration of a single nucleotide in the β-globin gene that leads to substitution of the neutral amino acid, valine, for the negatively charged glutamine at the sixth position from the N-terminus of the β-globin molecule. Homozygosity (SS or sickle cell anemia) and the combination of Hb S with other abnormalities in hemoglobin synthesis manifest in a pathologic state of chronic hemolytic anemia and vasoocclusion, often precipitating severe pain.

In the African American population, nearly 8%, or 1 in 12 individuals, are heterozygous for the sickle cell gene.[1] Most are asymptomatic and exhibit abnormalities of minimal clinical significance. Because of the relatively low percentage of Hb S in

137

Management of Sickle Cell Disease in Pregnancy (Cont.)

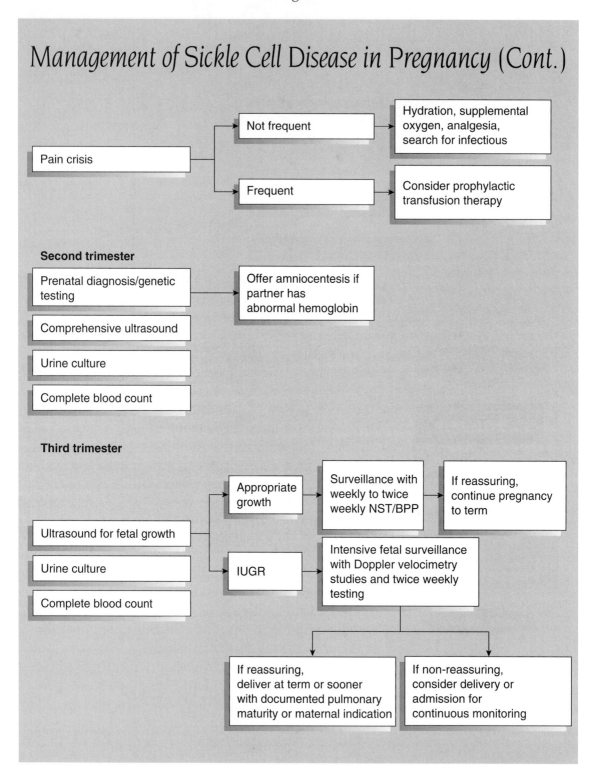

Pain crisis

Not frequent → Hydration, supplemental oxygen, analgesia, search for infectious

Frequent → Consider prophylactic transfusion therapy

Second trimester

Prenatal diagnosis/genetic testing → Offer amniocentesis if partner has abnormal hemoglobin

Comprehensive ultrasound

Urine culture

Complete blood count

Third trimester

Ultrasound for fetal growth

Urine culture

Complete blood count

Appropriate growth → Surveillance with weekly to twice weekly NST/BPP → If reassuring, continue pregnancy to term

IUGR → Intensive fetal surveillance with Doppler velocimetry studies and twice weekly testing

If reassuring, deliver at term or sooner with documented pulmonary maturity or maternal indication

If non-reassuring, consider delivery or admission for continuous monitoring these individuals, sickling episodes occur only with extreme oxygen desaturation. Based on the frequency of sickle cell trait, one would expect the incidence of sickle cell anemia in the black population to be 1 in 576; however, due to childhood mortality, the disease is noted less frequently in adulthood and pregnancy. Sickle hemoglobinopathies are also more prevalent in those of Middle Eastern and South Asian descent. In addition, up to 1 in 1000 African Americans are afflicted with sickle cell Hb C (SC) disease or sickle cell β-thalassemia. The molecular basis and epidemiology of Hb C and the thalassemias are discussed in detail in Chap. 8, but their heterozygous state in combination with Hb S may result in morbidities similar to those seen in sickle cell anemia. For example, sickle cell β-thalassemia is often clinically similar to sickle cell anemia, but some patients produce detectable amounts of Hb A and are less severely affected. In pregnancy, these patients are also at risk for sickling complications and adverse outcomes.

Experience with Sickle Cell Disease in Pregnancy—What's the Evidence?

Although sickle cell disease was once considered by some to be a contraindication to pregnancy, advances in the understanding and management of the disease have greatly improved pregnancy outcome. The Cooperative Study of Sickle Cell Disease reported on 445 pregnancies in 297 women with sickle hemoglobinopathies.[2] Although 28.8% of these pregnancies ended in voluntary termination and another 6.3% resulted in spontaneous abortion, those pregnancies that proceeded to 28 weeks of gestation or beyond resulted in a 99% live birth rate. The most frequent pregnancy complications were hypertensive disease (15%), preterm labor (9%), and preterm premature rupture of the membranes (6%). Women with SS anemia were nearly twice as likely (27% vs. 14%) to deliver a preterm infant than were women with SC disease. Intrauterine growth restriction was more common, particularly in women with SS genotype, in whom 21% of infants were small for gestational age at birth. The two most significant risk factors for poor fetal growth were preeclampsia and a history of acute anemic episodes. Two maternal deaths, both in SS gravidas, were reported in this series, one resulting from pulmonary embolism and the other from acute chest syndrome and renal failure.

Sun and associates[3] reported their experience with sickle cell disease in pregnancy at a single inner city medical center over a 20-year period in patients with SS and SC disease compared with normal (AA) race-matched controls. Maternal mortality rate was not reported in this series, but perinatal mortality was increased only in SS patients (RR 3.0, 95% CI 1.0–8.9). In patients with SS and with SC, antepartum admission was required more frequently, primarily due to pain crises, pyelonephritis, and acute anemia. SS patients were more likely to receive blood transfusions than were SC individuals. Preterm labor and preterm premature rupture of the membranes were also increased in SS patients but not in SC patients. Interestingly, the risk of preeclampsia was not significantly increased in either group. In the postpartum period, SS and SC patients had higher rates of infectious morbidity, chiefly endometritis, despite not having a significantly higher cesarean section rate than the control group.

One specific management issue that has received research attention is the utility of transfusion. The role of prophylactic transfusion of red blood cells to prevent complications associated with sickle cell disease in pregnancy is controversial but offers the advantage of replacing the patient's sickle cells with normal red blood cells, thus greatly improving oxygen carrying capacity and suppressing synthesis of sickle hemoglobin. Disadvantages of transfusion therapy include risks of transfusion reactions, transmission of infection, and development of maternal alloantibodies. With current blood banking techniques, the former morbidities are relatively uncommon, and experience to date suggests that the risk of neonatal isoimmunization and hemolytic disease is not increased significantly. However, if immunoglobulin G alloantibodies are present, the patient must be managed is the same way as any other gravida with alloimmunization.

Booster and exchange methods of transfusion are performed, but the latter is preferred because it places less stress on the cardiovascular system and results in a more significant increase in Hb A concentration. Exchange transfusion during pregnancy requires close monitoring because uterine blood flow is particularly sensitive to changes in maternal hemodynamic status. Lee and colleagues[4] demonstrated that, despite substantial hematologic alterations resulting from exchange transfusion, the procedure could be performed in minimally symptomatic gravidas with sickle cell disease without significantly altering the hemodynamic and metabolic profile of these women. If booster transfusions are given, careful monitoring of maternal volume status is required, and diuretics should be administered as needed to prevent and treat fluid overload.

Studies from longer than 20 years ago suggested that prophylactic red cell transfusions decrease rates of maternal morbidity and perinatal mortality.[5] Although these studies seemed to demonstrate improvement in outcome with transfusion therapy, they were limited because their subjects were not randomized but were compared with historical cohorts that did not have transfusion therapy available to them. In a well-designed protocol, Koshy and associates[6] randomized 72 pregnant women with sickle cell disease to prophylactic transfusions or exchange transfusion, only if indicated. These investigators reported a significant decrease in painful sickle cell crises with prophylactic therapy, but perinatal outcomes were not markedly improved. More recently, Mahomed[7] reviewed the Cochrane Database and determined that there is not enough evidence currently available to draw conclusions on the use of prophylactic transfusions in pregnant women with sickle cell disease. A large multicenter randomized clinical trial is needed to resolve these unanswered questions. At present, an individualized approach to this issue is reasonable, reserving transfusion for those patients who are repeatedly symptomatic with painful crises. Prophylactic transfusion for fetal indications is not indicated.

Pathophysiology and Clinical Manifestations

The key feature in the pathophysiology of sickle cell disease is the tendency for Hb S to polymerize in response to deoxygenation and other physiologic stresses. Polymerization of hemoglobin results in a conformational change or "sickling" of the red blood cell membrane. These sickle cells have difficulty traversing capillaries, leading to ischemia and infarction in many organs. Pain and organ dysfunction are the hallmarks of sickle crisis. Chronic cycles of infarction from sickling lead to a multitude of pathologic changes, including osteonecrosis, particularly of the femoral and humeral heads, renal medullary damage, hepatomegaly, ventricular hypertrophy, cardiac failure, pulmonary infarction, cerebrovascular accidents, seizure disorder, and leg ulcers. Infarction of the bone marrow and splenic atrophy results in decreased immunity and a propensity toward infection and sepsis due to encapsulated organisms. The repetitive conformational change associated with sickling episodes damages the red blood cell membrane and significantly shortens its life span, predisposing to hemolysis and anemia.

Pain Crises

Pain in sickle cell disease may be acute, chronic, or a combination. Acute pain, typically sudden in onset and quite intense, results from infarction of bone or soft tissue, whereas chronic pain is usually due to avascular necrosis of bone that typically affects joints and the spine. Pain crises are often triggered by infection, dehydration, acidosis, and hypoxia. Pregnancy-associated physiologic changes including hemodilution, circulatory stasis, increased metabolic demand, and greater susceptibility to infection may predispose to sickling. Approximately 50% of gravidas with sickle cell anemia and 19–25% of those with SC disease will require hospitalization during pregnancy for acute pain crisis.[5,6] It is important in the evaluation of these women to differentiate between pain due to sickling and that due to obstetric causes such as uterine contractions, placental abruption, and pyelonephritis.

Management of an acute sickle cell pain crisis involves providing appropriate analgesia and supportive care. Intravenous fluids and supplemental oxygen must be given to improve hydration and oxygen saturation. A search for underlying infection as the inciting event, particularly in the urinary and respiratory systems, must be undertaken. Laboratory studies including complete blood count, reticulocyte count, and hemoglobin electrophoresis may help in determining the severity of the crisis. Pain should be treated, as it would be in the nonpregnant state, with administration of intravenous narcotics. Patient-controlled analgesia is safe and effective in this setting and preferred by many patients. Constipation, nausea, vomiting, and pruritus are common side effects of narcotics and should be controlled appropriately. As symptoms improve, the dosage should be weaned and the patient switched to equivalent doses of oral medications. Chronic pain can also be managed with oral analgesics; however, additional modes of therapy, including nerve block, physiotherapy, and cognitive behavior therapy, may also be beneficial.

Unfortunately, prolonged narcotic therapy may lead to dependence and addiction in the patient with sickle cell disease. Caregivers need to be wary of signs of addiction such as a patient's insistence on determining the dose and timing of drug administration, objection to dose reduction, and demand for increase in dosage. These patients, although small in number, can consume a great deal of time and resources and become a source of frustration for the physician caring for them. Consultation with those familiar in managing drug dependence and chronic pain may be helpful in tailoring an approach to this difficult problem.

ACUTE CHEST SYNDROME

In addition to episodes of pain, patients with sickle cell disease may present with more serious sequelae, including the acute chest syndrome, a form of acute lung injury characterized by fever, respiratory compromise, and a new pulmonary infiltrate on chest radiograph. Recent estimates of the incidence of acute chest syndrome in pregnant women are 7% with the SS genotype and 3% in those with Hb SC. Acute chest syndrome is the leading cause of death in sickle cell disease[8] because it can quickly progress to acute respiratory distress syndrome and multisystem organ failure. Most commonly, the causes underlying these findings are infection, pulmonary fat embolus, and pulmonary infarction.[9] Treatment should be supportive and includes transfusion to improve oxygenation, mechanical ventilation, broad-spectrum antibiotic therapy, and bronchodilator therapy. Any respiratory compromise in the gravida with sickle cell disease must be taken seriously and warrants thorough evaluation for infectious and embolic etiologies. Worsening respiratory status calls for prompt consultation with a critical care team; delivery may be indicated with advanced gestation or deterioration of maternal condition.

ACUTE ANEMIA

Another potential complication for the gravida with sickle cell disease is that of acute anemia. Although the disproportionate increase in plasma volume associated with gestation results in a dilutional anemia, more severe forms of anemia can result from splenic sequestration and aplastic crisis due to bone marrow failure. The former is not usually a problem in the patient with SS disease during pregnancy because most individuals with this genotype will have had splenic infarction during multiple previous sickle crises in childhood; however, patients with SC disease typically still have splenic function. A sickle crisis in these individuals may result in massive sequestration of red blood cells in the spleen. These patients typically present with left upper quadrant pain due to an extremely enlarged spleen and severe anemia. This is a life-threatening complication. Medical therapy, with aggressive volume replacement and blood transfusion, and splenectomy have been employed successfully. In contrast, aplastic crisis results from a transient arrest of erythropoiesis in the bone marrow and is characterized by an abrupt decrease in hemoglobin and reticulocyte count. These crises may be precipitated by infection, particularly with parvovirus B_{19}, and are temporary. Transfusion therapy is the mainstay of treatment.

NEW THERAPIES

Advances in the management of sickle cell disease have been made with the implementation of new treatments. Nitric oxide has shown promise in preventing injury due to ischemia induced by sickle cell disease through regulation of vascular tone, endothelial adhesion, and platelet activity.[10] Because of its relaxant effect on smooth muscle, nitric oxide may benefit the gravida by improving uterine blood flow and maintaining uterine quiescence; a trial in pregnancy is warranted. Hydroxyurea is another agent used with increasing frequency in young patients with sickle cell disease. By increasing fetal hemoglobin (Hb F) production, this antineoplastic drug suppresses Hb S synthesis in erythroid precursors and has been shown to decrease hospitalizations, pulmonary sequelae, and pain episodes in patients with sickle cell disease. Despite theoretical concerns and teratogenic effects reported in animal studies, the drug has been used in pregnancy without adverse fetal effects.[11]

SICKLE CELL TRAIT

Hb SC, a milder variant of sickle cell anemia with nearly normal levels of hemoglobin, can be relatively asymptomatic in nonpregnant women and may not have been recognized previously. During pregnancy these patients are susceptible to sickle crises; thus, it is helpful to make the diagnosis before pregnancy. Patients with sickle cell trait (AS) have traditionally not been thought to be at increased risk for pregnancy complications; however, a recent report indicates that these women may be at increased risk for preeclampsia, preterm birth, and low birth weight.[12] These individuals are also at a increased risk for urinary tract infections[13] and should be screened periodically with urine culture. Iron deficiency anemia may also occur and should be screened for in each trimester. During labor, oxygenation should be maintained because sickling can occur if PaO_2 falls too low. Davies[14] reported intraoperative maternal death from extensive sickling in this setting.

Management of Pregnancy Complicated by Sickle Cell Disease

PRECONCEPTIONAL
Ideally, before attempting pregnancy, women with sickle cell disease, particularly those with significant comorbidities, should have a preconception evaluation to assess risk for adverse outcomes and make plans for optimal prenatal care. Because most pregnancies are not planned, this assessment and planning most often occur at a first prenatal visit. For women with more severe disease and preexisting end-organ pathology, planning a multidisciplinary approach, including consultation with subspecialists in hematology, pulmonary medicine, anesthesiology, and critical care, may be helpful. These patients may also benefit from care at a medical center familiar with controlling sickle cell disease and its complications. Patients who are severely ill need to be counseled about the risks to their heath. Women who have developed pulmonary hypertension due to restrictive lung disease have high rates of maternal mortality during pregnancy.[15] The option of termination of pregnancy should be addressed with these women.

Genetic counseling, education, and testing are best started before pregnancy. Each patient needs a clear explanation of inheritance, possibility of paternal genotype testing, and options for prenatal diagnosis. Early preparation gives the patient an opportunity to make an informed decision regarding prenatal diagnosis. If the patient's partner has a hemoglobinopathy and the couple anticipates additional pregnancies, they should be informed about the possibility of cord blood banking. Cord stem cells from a fetus with normal hemoglobin or only heterozygous status for sickle cell could be helpful for an affected sibling.

EARLY AND MID GESTATION
For the patient with sickle hemoglobinopathy, prenatal care should be initiated upon recognition of pregnancy. Because of the increased metabolic demands of pregnancy and the associated increase in red blood cell mass, supplementation with folic acid 1 mg/day or

higher is recommended. Levels of hematocrit and hemoglobin are typically decreased, but iron supplements should not be routinely given unless serum iron and ferritin levels are low. Routine administration of iron in patients who may have undergone multiple previous transfusions may lead to iron overload and hemochromatosis. Serum ferritin and iron levels should be obtained to assess the need for supplementation. An early first-trimester ultrasound for confirmation of gestational age should be performed. Women with sickle cell disease are at risk for complications later in pregnancy, and firm establishment of gestational age will be extremely valuable in making management decisions regarding timing of delivery.

The obstetrician must not overlook the fact that sickle cell disease results in chronic damage to many organs. In addition to standard laboratory testing normally performed in pregnancy, prenatal evaluation of renal, hepatic, and cardiopulmonary functions is warranted, especially among those patients who have been symptomatic or have evidence of preexisting disease. Appropriate tests include a 24-hour urine study for creatinine clearance and protein, liver function tests, and viral hepatitis serology. Consideration should be given for pulmonary function tests and echocardiography. Cardiopulmonary disease, particularly restrictive lung disease and pulmonary hypertension, can be seen in these patients and is a significant risk factor for adverse maternal outcome. Sickle cell disease is considered to a hypercoagulable state, and pregnancy may add further risk for thrombosis. Although it is not standard practice, prophylactic heparin therapy could be considered in women with sickle hemoglobinopathies who have additional risk factors for thrombosis, including morbid obesity, prolonged bedrest, and history of thromboembolic disease.

Patients with sickle cell disease have a significant degree of immunosuppression and have developed a propensity for infection with encapsulated bacteria. This risk increases in pregnancy, when immune function is further suppressed. Infection in addition to emotional and physical stresses may trigger the onset of pain crisis in these women. It is reasonable to perform urine cultures every 4–6 weeks antenatally and control bacteriuria with antibiotics. If not managed promptly, cystitis can rapidly progress to pyelonephritis and sepsis. These patients are also at greater risk for pneumonia from *Streptococcus pneumoniae* and *Haemophilus influenza.* Vaccination for these organisms is recommended and can be administered safely in pregnancy if not already given. During influenza season vaccination is indicated. Osteomyelitis due to *Staphylococcus aureus* and *Salmonella* species occurs more frequently, and a high clinical suspicion for this complication in the presence of unexplained fever and bone pain should be maintained.

Genetic counseling should also be initiated early to provide the patient with optimal time to make decisions regarding prenatal diagnosis. Hemoglobin electrophoresis should be performed on the father of the fetus. If the father is unavailable for screening or unwilling to be tested, counseling should still be provided based on carrier frequencies for the father's ethnic group. A mother with sickle cell anemia with an untested African American partner has a risk of 4% (1 in 24) for a fetus with sickle cell disease. In addition, there is a risk for other sickle cell syndromes, including Hb SC disease and sickle cell β-thalassemia. Prenatal diagnosis is available for sickle cell disorders and can be performed on cultured cells obtained by chorionic villus sampling or amniocentesis. Recently, an oligonucleotide ligation assay coupled with laser-induced capillary fluorescence detection has been introduced and enables diagnosis of Hb S and Hb C within a matter of hours.[16] Preimplantation diagnosis has been described with single-blastomere DNA analysis.[17]

LATE GESTATION

KEY POINT

Close surveillance of the pregnancy is particularly important in the third trimester to detect potential maternofetal complications.

As pregnancy progresses, evaluation of hemoglobin and hematocrit should be performed routinely, with the idea of maintaining adequate oxygen delivery to the fetus. The role of transfusion therapy has previously been addressed. Patients with sickle cell disease are at increased risk for adverse obstetric outcomes, including intrauterine growth restriction, intrauterine fetal demise, and preeclampsia. Placental ischemia and thrombosis appear to be a common finding in these cases. As pregnancy progresses, fetal growth should be assessed with serial sonographic examinations. Evidence of fetal growth restriction warrants more intensive surveillance with nonstress testing and biophysical profile. There is some evidence that third-trimester uterine and umbilical artery Doppler studies demonstrate changes in flow patterns that precede abnormal antenatal testing by several weeks.[18]

PERIPARTUM

Delivery should be performed at term but may be achieved sooner with documentation of fetal pulmonary maturity and a favorable cervical examination. In the gravida who has frequent crises, timing of delivery during a crisis-free period is desirable. Nonreassuring antepartum testing or compromised maternal status, such as that which occurs with preeclampsia, may necessitate premature delivery. In these cases, if gestational age is less than 34 weeks, corticosteroids should be administered to promote fetal lung maturity. Vaginal delivery is preferred because maternal morbidity is significantly decreased compared with cesarean section. Gravidas with sickle cell disease may be at increased risk for postoperative complications including thromboembolic disease, infection, and poor wound healing.[19] Throughout the course of labor and delivery, the parturient must remain well oxygenated and hydrated at all times, and continuous fetal monitoring should be performed. Cesarean section should be reserved for standard obstetric indications.

Analgesia is an important aspect of labor management in the parturient with sickle cell disease. Labor, with its increased metabolic demands, may predispose to sickling and pain crisis. Moreover, pain associated with labor leads to an increase in circulating catecholamine levels, further aggravating the problem. Epidural and spinal analgesia can be used effectively in this setting. Achieving good pain control decreases catecholamine levels. Alternatively, narcotics, administered intermittently or by a patient-controlled infusion system, may be used in those parturients unable to receive a regional block.

In those women requiring cesarean delivery, care must be taken to avoid conditions that could precipitate sickling in the perioperative period. The patient must be kept warm, well oxygenated, and well hydrated at all times, particularly in the operating room. Danzer and associates[20] recommended keeping the room temperature at 78°F and liberal use of warming blankets. Regional anesthesia can be safely used for cesarean delivery and is the preferred method. This requires adequate prehydration and a rapid means of infusing fluids or blood products, if needed, because the associated sympathetic block and surgical blood loss may lead to profound hypotension. In patients with associated cardiopulmonary disease, the threshold to use more invasive forms of hemodynamic monitoring including pulmonary artery catheterization should be low. Prophylactic antibiotics are essential. Postoperatively, sequential compression devices or prophylactic heparin should be administered, with early ambulation to decrease the risk of thromboembolic events. Good pulmonary toilet and incentive spirometry are also beneficial.

Ideally, the pediatrician or neonatologist caring for the child should be familiar with sickle cell disease and potential complications. Prolonged intrauterine exposure to large doses of narcotics can lead to an abstinence syndrome in the neonate, which is characterized by irritability, hypertonia, jitteriness, seizures, sneezing, tachycardia, diarrhea, and feeding difficulty. The pediatrician evaluating the infant at birth should be made aware of the mother's medication history including time and amount of most recent narcotic dose, because neonatal respiratory depression can occur. If prenatal testing was not performed, the infant should be screened for sickle hemoglobinopathies.

Contraception is essential for women with sickle cell diseases, especially in those complex patients in whom pregnancy should be avoided. Concerns regarding combined oral contraceptive preparations resulting in increased risk for thromboembolic disease are based on theoretical concerns regarding the estrogen component of these formulations and anecdotal case reports. In truth, there is little evidence to suggest that a woman with sickle cell disease is more likely to sustain a thromboembolic insult compared with the general population when using these agents. Pregnancy may carry greater risks, particularly in those women with significant comorbidities. Recent in vitro studies suggest that red cell deformability in patients with sickle cell disease is not altered by oral contraceptive formulations.[21] The current very low-dose oral contraceptive formulations are a safe and effective means of contraception for women with sickle cell disease. If other contraindications exist, particularly a history of thromboembolic disease or hepatic dysfunction, nonhormonal forms of contraception should be prescribed. Very effective alternatives include injectable progestins, progesterone-only oral contraceptives, and intrauterine devices. In particular, depot medroxyprogesterone acetate injections may be recommended because they may decrease the incidence of painful crises.[22] Sterilization should be encouraged in women who have sickle cell disease and have completed childbearing.

Conclusion

With improvements in medical management, more women with sickle cell disease are not only surviving to reproductive age but also desiring and achieving pregnancy. However, sickle hemoglobinopathies remain a significant cause of maternal and perinatal morbidity and mortality. Care of the gravida with sickle cell disease requires not only an understanding of the underlying pathophysiology but also anticipation and prompt management of potential complications. With close supervision and adherence to the principles outlined in this chapter, the chance for favorable pregnancy outcomes in women with sickle cell disease will be maximized.

Discussion of Cases

CASE 1: NULLIPARA WITH SC DISEASE

A 24-year-old gravida 1, para 0, African American woman at 14 weeks of gestation presents after results of her hemoglobin electrophoresis screen showed that she has Hb SC disease. She has never had any symptoms related to this diagnosis and her hematocrit was 31% at the initial screen. She is concerned about the chances for her unborn child of having SS or SC disease.

What further testing at this point would you recommend to assist in determining fetal risk?

Hemoglobin electrophoresis performed on the father of this fetus.

The results of the father's hemoglobin electrophoresis are consistent with sickle cell trait (AS).

Based on these results, what would the risk be for the fetus having SC disease or SS disease?

The fetus has a 25% chance of being affected with SC disease and a 25% chance of being affected with SS disease. There is also a 25%
chance that the fetus will be a carrier of Hb C trait and a 25% chance that the fetus will have sickle cell trait.

The patient was counseled as to these risks, and she declined to have prenatal diagnosis. At this point, she is concerned regarding the risk for adverse outcome with the pregnancy.

Based on her benign history, is it safe to assume the patient will have an uneventful pregnancy?

No. Although patients with Hb SC disease generally have a milder course through pregnancy than their counterparts with Hb SS disease, they are still at increased risk for adverse maternal and perinatal outcomes. In addition, the physiologic changes associated with pregnancy may predispose to exacerbation of her underlying hemoglobinopathy, which until this point has not been a problem. The patient will require close supervision throughout the remainder of this and subsequent pregnancies.

CASE 2: SICKLE CELL CRISIS AT 24 WEEKS

A 26-year-old gravida 1, para 0, African American woman with known sickle cell disease presents at 24 weeks of gestation with complaints of severe back and lower extremity pain. She has a history of frequent pain crises and has managed her pain at home with oral narcotics. Her temperature is 37.3°C, blood pressure is 130/80 mm Hg, respiratory rate is 24 breaths/min, and pulse is 110 beats/min. Fetal heart tones are approximately 150 beats/min with good variability; no contractions are noted on the tocometer. On physical examination, the patient demonstrates exquisite tenderness over the lower lumbar vertebrae and the pretibial areas in the lower extremities. Laboratory data include a white blood cell count of 17.8, hematocrit of 21%, and reticulocyte count of 2.4%. Hemoglobin electrophoresis demonstrates 91% Hb S, 2% Hb A_2, and 7% Hb F. Urinalysis was significant for large white blood cell counts and many bacteria.

What therapy would you prescribe for this patient?

It appears that the patient most likely has a sickle cell pain crisis that was possibly triggered by a concurrent urinary tract infection. A urine culture should be performed and antibiotic therapy initiated. For relief of the patient's symptoms, adequate intravenous hydration and supplemental oxygenation should be given in addition to parenteral narcotics. If pain is severe enough, patient-controlled analgesia may be useful.

How would you manage her anemia?

Patients with sickle cell anemia should receive folic acid supplementation. Iron studies should be performed; only if iron stores are depleted should supplementation with oral ferrous sulfate be initiated. Because this patient has had frequent pain crises, she may benefit from exchange transfusions to improve her fraction of Hb A.

At 32 weeks the patient presents for an ultrasound examination, which shows an estimated fetal weight of 900 g and appears to be consistent with intrauterine growth restriction.

What fetal surveillance would you recommend at this point?

Weekly to twice-weekly nonstress tests should be performed. In addition, umbilical artery Doppler studies may be useful in determining fetal risk for adverse outcomes. Abnormal testing warrants administration of corticosteroids for fetal lung maturity if done before 34 weeks of gestation and potential delivery. Fetal growth should be followed with serial ultrasounds.

REFERENCES

1 Motulsky AG. Frequency of sickling disorders in US blacks. *N Engl J Med* 1973;288:31.

2 Smith JA, Espeland M, Bellevue R, et al. Pregnancy in sickle cell disease: experience of the cooperative study of sickle cell disease. *Obstet Gynecol* 1996;87:199–204.

3 Sun PM, Wilburn W, Raynor BD, et al. Sickle cell disease in pregnancy: twenty years of experience at Grady Memorial Hospital, Atlanta, Georgia. *Am J Obstet Gynecol* 2001;184:1127–1130.

4 Lee W, Werch J, Rokey R, et al. Physiologic observations of pregnant women undergoing prophylactic erythrocytapheresis for sickle cell disease. *Transfusion* 1991;31:59–62.

5 Cunningham FG, Pritchard JA, Mason R. Pregnancy and sickle cell hemoglobinopathies: results with and without prophylactic transfusions. *Obstet Gynecol* 1983;62:419–424.

6 Koshy M, Burd L, Wallace D, et al. Prophylactic red-cell transfusions in pregnant patients with sickle cell disease: a randomized cooperative study. *N Engl J Med* 1988;319:1447–1452.

7 Mahomed K. Prophylactic versus selective blood transfusion for sickle cell anemia during pregnancy. *Cochrane Database Syst Rev* 2000;2: CD000040.

8 Castro O, Brambilla DJ, Thorington B, et al. The acute chest syndrome in sickle cell disease: incidence and risk factors: the Cooperative Study of Sickle Cell Disease. *Blood* 1994;84:643–649.

9 Vichinsky EP, Neumayr LD, Earles AN, et al. Causes and outcomes of the acute chest syndrome in sickle cell disease. *N Engl J Med* 2000; 342:1855–1865.

10 Morris CR, Kuypers FA, Larkin S, et al. Arginine therapy: a novel strategy to induce nitric oxide production in sickle cell disease. *Br J Haematol* 2000;111:498–500.

11 Diav-Citrin O, Hunnisett L, Sher GD, et al. Hydroxyurea use during pregnancy: a case report in sickle cell disease and review of the literature. *Am J Hematol* 1999;60:148–150.

12 Larrabee KD, Monga M. Women with sickle cell trait are at increased risk for preeclampsia. *Am J Obstet Gynecol* 1997;177:425–428.

13 Baill IC, Witter FR. Sickle cell trait and its association with birthweight and urinary tract infections in pregnancy. *Int J Gynaecol Obstet* 1990;33:19–21.

14 Davies SC. Intraoperative death during cesarean section in a patient with sickle-cell trait. The Anaesthesia Advisory Committee to the Chief Coroner of Ontario. *Can J Anaesth* 1987;34:67–70.

15 Pope CS, Boley TJ. Successful pregnancy outcome with cardiac and severe restrictive lung disease requiring mechanical ventilation: a case report and literature review. *J Matern Fetal Med* 2001;10:64–67.

16 Day NS, Tadin M, Christiano AM, et al. Rapid prenatal diagnosis of sickle cell diseases using oligonucleotide ligation assay coupled with laser-induced capillary fluorescence detection. *Prenat Diagn* 2002;22: 686–691.

17 Xu K, Shi ZM, Veeck LL, et al. First unaffected pregnancy using preimplantation genetic diagnosis of sickle cell anemia. *JAMA* 1999; 281:1701.

18 Anyaegbunam A, Langer O, Brustman L, et al. The application of uterine and umbilical artery velocimetry to the antenatal supervision of pregnancies complicated by maternal sickle hemoglobinopathies. *Am J Obstet Gynecol* 1988;159:544–547.

19 Scott-Connor CEH, Brunson CD. Surgery and anesthesia. In: Embury SH, Hebbel RP, Mohandas N, Steinberg MH, eds. *Sickle Cell Disease: Basic Principles and Clinical Practice.* New York: Raven Press, 1994; p. 809–827.

20 Danzer BI, Birnbach DJ, Thys DM. Anesthesia for the parturient with sickle cell disease. *J Clin Anesth* 1996;8:598–602.

21 Yoong WC, Tuck SM, Yardumian A. Red cell deformability in oral contraceptive pill users with sickle cell anemia. *Br J Haematol* 1999; 104:868–870.

22 De Abood M, de Castillo Z, Guerrero F, et al. Effect of depo-Provera or microgynon on the painful crises of sickle cell anemia patients. *Contraception* 1997;56:313–316.

Workup of Thrombocytopenia in Pregnancy

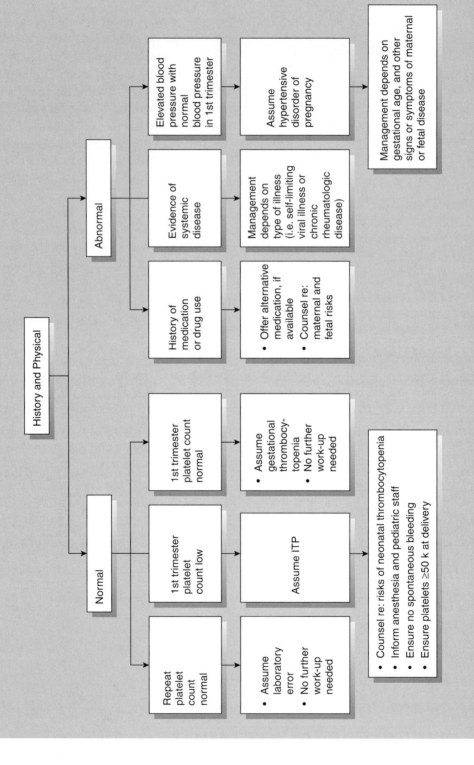

Thrombocytopenia in Pregnancy

Sara H. Garmel

Introduction

Thrombocytopenia often affects pregnant women and is sometimes diagnosed before pregnancy or discovered during pregnancy when a complete blood count is obtained during routine prenatal screening. Thrombocytopenia can be caused by medical conditions that have serious implications for the pregnancy or by benign self-limiting conditions that pose no risk to mother or fetus. This chapter will review the most common etiologies of thrombocytopenia seen in pregnancy, discuss the evaluation of thrombocytopenia, and review maternal and fetal risks.

Definition of Thrombocytopenia

The normal range for platelets in nonpregnant women is 150,000–400,000. Thrombocytopenia is defined as mild if the platelet count is 100,000–150,000, moderate if the platelet count is 50,000–100,000, and severe if the platelet count is lower than 50,000. Bleeding with trauma or surgery may occur if the platelet count is lower than 50,000 and spontaneous bleeding can occur if the platelet count is lower than 10,000. Figure 10-1 shows a normal peripheral smear, and Figure 10-2 shows a peripheral smear from a pregnant patient with thrombocytopenia (platelet count 30,000). Platelets are normal in size and red blood cells and white blood cells are normal in appearance.

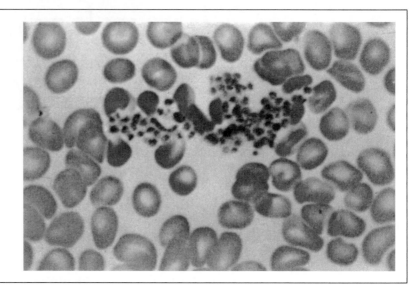

Figure 10-1: Platelets are non-nucleated cells approximately 2–3 µm in diameter. In blood smears, they are often clumped together, as in this micrograph. (Printed with permission from Wheater PR, Burkitt HG, Daniels VG. Blood. In: *Functional Histology.* New York: Churchill Livingstone, 1979; p. 32.)

Workup of Thrombocytopenia in Pregnancy

Thrombocytopenia can occur due to increased consumption or decreased production of platelets, depending on the etiology (Table 10-1). Table 10-2 lists the many causes of thrombocytopenia, some of which are seen only in pregnancy. Those encountered

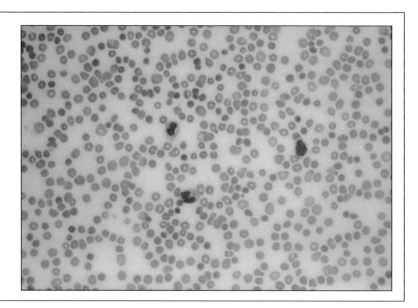

Figure 10-2: Peripheral smear of pregnant patient with thrombocytopenia (platelet count of 30,000). Platelets are normal in size, and red blood cells and white blood cells are normal in appearance. (Courtesy M. F. Schaldenbrand, MD.)

Table 10-1. **PATHOGENESIS OF THROMBOCYTOPENIA**

Consumption > production	
Dilutional	Massive transfusion
Sequestration	Splenomegaly
Immune destruction	Immune thrombocytopenic purpura
	Drug induced
	Systemic lupus erythematosus
Nonimmune destruction	Inflammation
	Leukemia
	Intravascular coagulopathy
	Trauma
	Arterial or venous thrombosis
	Neoplasia
	Hemangioma
Pregnancy specific	Gestational thrombocytopenia
	Preeclampsia-associated thrombocytopenia
Decreased production	
Congenital disorders	Fanconi's anemia
	Wiskott-Aldrich syndrome
Infection	Rubella
	Hepatitis
	Cytomegalovirus
Drugs and toxins	Cytotoxic drugs
	Drug reactions
	Hydrocarbons
	Alcohol
	Radiation
Vitamin deficiency	B_{12}
	Folate
Marrow replacement	Leukemia
	Myeloproliferative disorder
	Tumor

Source: Modified with permission from Pathogenesis of thrombocytopenia. In: Harvey AM, Johns RJ, McKusick VA, et al, eds. *The Principles and Practice of Medicine.* Norwalk, Connecticut: Appleton & Lange, 1988.[1]

KEY POINT

History and physical examination are usually adequate to determine the etiology of thrombocytopenia.

most often are discussed in detail below. (From ACOG Practice Bulletin #6, September 1999, with permission).

Important elements of a history should include questions about bleeding or bruising or about bleeding with previous surgeries, systemic symptoms such as fever, headache, rash, or arthralgias; or flu-like symptoms. Medication or drug use should be assessed, as should risk factors for infectious disease such as

Table 10-2. **CAUSES OF THROMBOCYTOPENIA IN PREGNANCY**[2]

Gestational thrombocytopenia
Pregnancy-induced hypertension
HELLP syndrome
Pseudothrombocytopenia (laboratory artifact)
HIV infection
Immune thrombocytopenic purpura
Systemic lupus erythematosus
Antiphospholipid syndrome
Hypersplenism
Disseminated intravascular coagulation
Thrombotic thrombocytopenic purpura
Hemolytic uremic syndrome
Congenital thrombocytopenias
Medications (heparin, quinine, quinidine, zidovudine, sulfonamides)

HELLP = hemolysis, elevated liver enzymes, low platelets; HIV = human immunodeficiency virus.

human immunodeficiency virus (HIV). A family history of thrombocytopenia should also be ascertained.

Important components of a physical examination include signs of bleeding, jaundice or other evidence of liver disease, evidence of autoimmune disease such as rash or goiter, evidence of infection such as lymph node enlargement, or evidence of thrombosis. A consensus panel for the American Society of Hematology developed practice guidelines for the diagnosis of patients with immune thrombocytopenic purpura (ITP) (Table 10-3) that are helpful in evaluating patients with thrombocytopenia from any cause and should be part of any complete history and physical examination.

What's the Evidence?

There are few evidence-based guidelines for clinicians to rely on when evaluating and counseling patients with thrombocytopenia. All physicians would agree that a careful history and physical examination are warranted, and these recommendations for initial evaluation of thrombocytopenia are based on clinical experience and are standard practice for most clinicians. There are several reports documenting the lack of fetal risk in women with gestational thrombocytopenia, but the conclusions are based on limited or inconsistent evidence. Most of the questions regarding thrombocytopenia in

***Table 10-3.* PRINCIPAL ELEMENTS OF THE HISTORY AND PHYSICAL EXAMINATION IN AN ADULT WITH THROMBOCYTOPENIA**

History

Bleeding symptoms
  Type of bleeding
  Severity of bleeding
Duration of bleeding
Hemostasis with prior surgeries, pregnancies
Systemic symptoms, including weight loss, fever, headache, and
  symptoms of autoimmune disorders such as arthralgias,
  skin rash, alopecia, and venous thrombosis
Risk factors for HIV infection
Medications
Transfusion history
Family history of thrombocytopenia, including bleeding symptoms
  and symptoms of autoimmune disorders

Physical examination

Bleeding signs
  Type of bleeding
  Severity of bleeding
Liver, spleen, and lymph nodes; jaundice and other stigmata of liver
  disease
Evidence for infection, particularly bacteremia or HIV
Evidence for autoimmune disease, such as arthritis, goiter, nephritis, or
  cutaneous vasculitis
Evidence for thrombosis
Neurologic function
Skeletal anomalies

HIV = human immunodeficiency virus.
Source: Modified with permission from George JN, Woolf SH, Raskob GE, et al. Idiopathic thrombocytopenic purpura: a practice guideline developed by explicit methods for the American Society of Hematology. *Blood* 1996;88:3–40.[3]

pregnancy involve patients with a history of ITP or possible new-onset ITP in pregnancy and concerns for fetal thrombocytopenia. Proponents of fetal blood sampling before delivery cite case reports and theoretical risks of intracranial hemorrhage secondary to trauma with fetal thrombocytopenia, but there are no randomized clinical trials of optimal management. A decision analysis compared the three common strategies for managing term pregnancies complicated by ITP and found percutaneous umbilical blood sampling (PUBS) preferable to scalp sampling when testing was performed but did not recommend no testing over PUBS.[4]

Etiology of Thrombocytopenia

GESTATIONAL
THROMBOCYTOPENIA

Gestational thrombocytopenia is the most common cause of thrombocytopenia during pregnancy. It complicates 5–10% of term pregnancies and accounts for most (approximately 75%) cases of thrombocytopenia in pregnancy.[5] Patients do not have a history of thrombocytopenia, except perhaps in previous pregnancies. Usually the thrombocytopenia is mild ($\geq$100,000, and typically not <70,000). However, there is no value below which gestational thrombocytopenia may be excluded and new-onset ITP can be diagnosed with certainty.[6] It is difficult to distinguish from new-onset ITP because there is no test available to differentiate the two and the diagnosis of both is based on the finding of thrombocytopenia without another cause. When late pregnancy platelet counts are lower than 100,000, the distinction between gestational thrombocytopenia and ITP is very difficult to make. Platelet counts in patients with gestational thrombocytopenia typically return to normal within 2–12 weeks postpartum. This may make the diagnosis easier to make retrospectively. It poses no risk to mother or fetus.

KEY POINT

Most pregnant women with a low platelet count have gestational thrombocytopenia.

IMMUNE
THROMBOCYTOPENIC
PURPURA

ITP occurs in 1 in 1000 to 10,000 gestations, making it one of the most common autoimmune disorders that complicates pregnancy. Antibodies are produced against one's own platelets, and these platelets are prematurely destroyed in the spleen, resulting in thrombocytopenia. The course of ITP is not affected by pregnancy. Fetal thrombocytopenia results from destruction of fetal platelets by maternal immunoglobulin G (IgG) antiplatelet antibodies that cross the placenta. It is a diagnosis of exclusion because there is no definitive diagnostic test for this disorder. Because the presence of antiplatelet antibody is nonspecific, it should not routinely be assessed.

KEY POINT

Patients with ITP need to be informed of the risk of thrombocytopenia in the fetus.

   The reported incidence of severe neonatal thrombocytopenia in infants born to mothers with ITP, defined as a platelet count lower than 50,000, is 0–25%.[7] The management of ITP in labor varies because the data do not clearly support an advantage of cesarean section over vaginal delivery for women carrying severely thrombocytopenic fetuses. There are a handful of reported cases of intracranial hemorrhage in severely thrombocytopenic fetuses, presumably from labor-related trauma. These reports suggest a possible association between vaginal delivery and adverse outcome in severely thrombocytopenic fetuses. Some investigators believe that the risk of intracranial hemorrhage is low enough to obviate cesarean section, even for patients carrying fetuses with severe thrombocytopenia. Others are of the opinion that, although the risk of intracranial hemorrhage is low, the sequelae are serious enough to warrant cesarean section in all patients with ITP or at least in those patients carrying severely thrombocytopenic fetuses (Box 10-1).[8]

Maternal platelet counts do not correlate with fetal platelet counts. Fetal platelet counts can be directly determined by scalp sampling during labor or by PUBS before labor. Scalp sampling procedures carry a negligible risk of morbidity, whereas PUBS carries a small but real risk of fetal complication. PUBS, however, offers certain advantages. It is more reliable than scalp sampling for determination of the true platelet count because scalp sampling is more likely to show an artificially low count from platelet clumping, dilution from amniotic fluid, or scalp edema. Moreover, PUBS may be performed before labor; scalp sampling must be performed during labor with ruptured membranes. The timing of intracranial hemorrhage in cases of severe thrombocytopenia is unclear; it may occur early in labor, before scalp sampling is feasible. Most important to referral patients, a normal fetal platelet count after PUBS allows most patients (those carrying fetuses with normal platelet counts) to deliver vaginally at their community hospitals without specialized neonatal care. Those patients carrying severely thrombocytopenic fetuses can deliver by cesarean section at a tertiary care facility and can receive immediate neonatal therapy in the form of platelet transfusions, steroid administration, or intravenous gamma IgG (IVIgG).

Occasionally, therapy is needed to increase the maternal platelet count in women with signs of bleeding or dangerously low platelet counts (<30,000–50,000) (Box 10-2). Prednisone 1 mg/(kg · day) but no higher may be given in divided doses over 2–3 weeks, with a response in approximately 70% of patients within 3 days to 3 weeks. The dose is then tapered to the lowest dosage needed to maintain a platelet count of at least 50,000. IVIgG 0.4–2 g/(kg · day) in divided doses over 2–5 days may effect a response in more than 80% of patients, typically within a week.[9] IVIgG may be especially useful in term patients to ensure hemostasis at delivery or in patients with acute bleeding complications. The effect of steroids and IVIgG on the fetal platelet count is unclear, and maternal therapy should not be given solely in the hope of increasing the fetal

Box 10-1.   *CONTROVERSIES IN THE MANAGEMENT OF ITP IN PREGNANCY*

- What is the risk of severe fetal thrombocytopenia?
- Should the fetal platelet count determine mode of delivery?
- Is intracranial hemorrhage decreased by cesarean section?

- Is the risk of intracranial hemorrhage low enough to obviate cesarean section, even in severely thrombocytopenic fetuses? Or are sequelae serious enough to warrant cesarean section in all patients with severely thrombocytopenic fetuses?

platelet count. Platelet transfusion should be used only as a temporizing measure before cesarean section or in the face of life-threatening maternal hemorrhage. Splenectomy during pregnancy is almost never needed.

Most anesthesiologists agree that regional anesthesia is safe in patients with platelet counts higher than 100,000. Many will not administer regional anesthesia if the platelet count is lower than 100,000, and most will not administer regional block if the platelet count is lower than 50,000. Patients with thrombocytopenia should be offered consultation with an anesthesiologist before delivery to discuss these issues, if possible.

Box 10-2.   *MANAGEMENT OF ITP*

Maternal management
- A normal platelet count is not necessary.
- No maternal treatment is needed if the platelet count is higher than 50,000 and the patient is asymptomatic.
- Medical therapy is indicated (prednisone or IgG) if the platelet count is lower than 50,000 and the patient is approaching third trimester.
- Anesthesia consultation should occur before labor.

- Counsel regarding risk of fetal thrombocytopenia and options for testing.
- Avoid operative vaginal delivery if fetal platelet count unknown.

Neonatal management
- Inform pediatric staff.
- Measure platelet count at birth and repeat during first few days of life.
- Confirm normal count before circumcision.

HYPERTENSIVE DISORDERS IN PREGNANCY

Approximately 5% of pregnancies are complicated by hypertensive disorders, and patients with gestational hypertension or preeclampsia-associated thrombocytopenia account for approximately 20% of thrombocytopenias in pregnancy. Therefore, this bears some discussion at this point, although a full discussion of hypertensive disorders in pregnancy is beyond the scope of this chapter because it is a complex and controversial area (see Chap. 25).

Hypertensive disorders in pregnancy include gestational hypertension, preeclampsia, eclampsia, superimposed preeclampsia, and chronic hypertension. There are well-defined risk factors for this spectrum of disease including nulliparity, adolescence, or advanced maternal age, underlying chronic hypertension, renal disease, diabetes, multiple gestation, and previous preeclampsia. Thrombocytopenia can be seen in patients with gestational hypertension, preeclampsia, eclampsia, or superimposed preeclampsia. The syndrome of hemolysis, elevated liver enzymes, and low platelets is one end of the spectrum of preeclampsia and by definition includes thrombocytopenia. Most likely, thrombocytopenia associated with gestational hypertension or preeclampsia is due to platelet activation and consumption. Any patient with thrombocytopenia (defined as <100,000/μL) associated with preeclampsia has clinically significant disease, with potential maternal and fetal risks. For example, thrombocytopenia may be severe and life-threatening for the mother, although it has no direct risks to the fetus aside from prematurity related issues due to the need for delivery secondary to maternal disease.

KEY POINT

Preeclampsia must be ruled out in all pregnant patients with thrombocytopenia.

DRUGS OR MEDICATIONS

Many drugs commonly used in pregnancy may result in thrombocytopenia by suppressing bone marrow, accelerating platelet destruction, or by some unknown mechanism of antiplatelet action. Heparin, for example, is associated with thrombocytopenia in fewer than 5% of patients. Its onset occurs 3–15 days after beginning treatment. Although most cases of heparin-induced thrombocytopenia are mild, some can result in serious thrombotic complications. Acetaminophen (Tylenol) and penicillin, two of the most commonly used medications in pregnancy, have also been associated with thrombocytopenia. See Table 10-4 for a more complete list of drugs that can produce thrombocytopenia.[10] If a medication is identified as a cause of thrombocytopenia, it should be discontinued.

Table 10-4.   DRUGS THAT MAY CAUSE THROMBOCYTOPENIA

Drugs that suppress the marrow
Cytotoxic agents such as those used in cancer chemotherapy
  (nitrogen mustard, cyclophosphamide, 5-fluorouracil,
  methotrexate, and many others)

Drugs that by immune mechanisms accelerate platelet destruction
Chlorothiazides
Chlorpropamide
Diazepam
Diphenylhydantoin
Gold salts
Quinidine
Quinine
Sulfisoxazole

Drugs whose mechanism of antiplatelet activity is unknown
Acetaminophen
Aminopyrine
Chlorpromazine
Cimetidine
Furosemide
Heparin
Heroin
Penicillamine
Penicillin
Phenylbutazone
Various sulfonamides
Tolbutamide

SOURCE: Printed with permission from Anderson HM. Maternal hematologic disorders. In: Creasy RK, Resnik R, eds. *Maternal–Fetal Medicine: Principles and Practice.* Philadelphia: WB Saunders, 1989; p. 908.[10]

Recreational drugs such as alcohol, cocaine, or heroin may also result in thrombocytopenia. Therefore, any patient with newly diagnosed thrombocytopenia should have urine and serum drug screening obtained as warranted.

SYSTEMIC DISEASE   *VIRAL INFECTION*   Many viral infections can cause thrombocytopenia due to decreased platelet production or increased platelet destruction. Any patient with newly diagnosed thrombocytopenia should be evaluated for viral disease, including a thorough history and physical examination and HIV screening, as recommended for all pregnant women.

SYSTEMIC LUPUS ERYTHEMATOSUS (SEE CHAP. 34) Systemic lupus erythematosus (SLE) is a chronic autoimmune disease that usually affects many organ systems. The American College of Rheumatology's classification criteria for SLE includes hematologic disorders as one of 11 criteria seen with SLE, and thrombocytopenia may be the only hematologic manifestation of lupus seen. Thrombocytopenia may be severe enough to be life-threatening. Patients with lupus require high-risk obstetric care and long-term follow-up after delivery because of a possible increase in disease activity.

Patients newly diagnosed with thrombocytopenia should be questioned regarding any signs or symptoms of SLE, and it would be reasonable to obtain an antinuclear antibody to screen for SLE. Although the test is nonspecific, 95% of patients with SLE will have a positive result. A positive screen would prompt further testing for SLE as a cause of the thrombocytopenia.

ANTIPHOSPHOLIPID SYNDROME Antiphospholipid syndrome (APS) is another autoimmune condition that is associated with thrombocytopenia in approximately 40% of cases. Other features include thromboses, fetal loss, and, less likely, amaurosis fugax or transient ischemic attacks, chorea, hemolytic anemia, and livedo reticularis. High levels of IgG anticardiolipin antibodies and/or lupus anticoagulant are also present. Typically, patients must have one clinical feature plus laboratory evidence of APS before the diagnosis is made. As with patients with SLE, those with APS require close observation during their pregnancy, with careful follow-up after delivery because of risks of significant medical problems. Any history suggestive of this disorder should prompt further testing in a patient with newly diagnosed thrombocytopenia.

THROMBOTIC THROMBOCYTOPENIC PURPURA Thrombotic thrombocytopenic purpura (TTP) usually occurs in previously healthy patients who present with severe thrombocytopenia, microangiopathic hemolytic anemia, fever, central nervous system abnormalities, and renal disease. Pregnancy may predispose patients to TTP, and, when associated with pregnancy, the disease typically occurs near term or in the peripartum period. The pathophysiology of this disease is thought to be a deficiency of von Willebrand factor cleaving protease. TTP should be suspected in patients with severe thrombocytopenia, especially when it persists for more than several days postpartum and in combination with other signs or symptoms described above.

DISSEMINATED INTRAVASCULAR COAGULATION   Disseminated intravascular coagulation is not a specific disease process but rather one encountered in many different scenarios, such as infection, cancer, and trauma, in addition to obstetric complications such as abruption, hemorrhage, amniotic fluid embolism, abortion, or retention of a dead fetus. Clotting factors are consumed, which results in bleeding and ischemia. Thrombocytopenia is seen, as are hypofibrinogenemia and prolonged prothrombin time and partial thromboplastin time.

OTHER ETIOLOGIES   Von Willebrand's disease, rare inherited thrombocytopenias such as Bernard-Soulier and May-Hegglin, certain anemias such as aplastic anemia or megaloblastic anemia, and sepsis may also be associated with thrombocytopenia; in most cases a thorough history will point to the etiology.

PSEUDOTHROMBO-CYTOPENIA

Pseudothrombocytopenia is seen in fewer than 1% of adults and is usually due to clinically insignificant platelet agglutinins that cause platelet clumping when mixed with the anticoagulant ethylene-diamine-tetra-acetic acid. The peripheral smear should then be reviewed to rule out platelet clumping to confirm thrombocytopenia.

NEONATAL ALLOIMMUNE THROMBOCYTOPENIA

Another platelet disorder with significant pregnancy implications is neonatal alloimmune thrombocytopenia. The mother is healthy with a normal platelet count and no history of thrombocytopenia, so a detailed review is not covered in this chapter. This fetal or neonatal disorder is often called the platelet equivalent of Rh disease, although previous exposure for sensitization is not necessary and first-born babies may be affected. Neonatal alloimmune thrombocytopenia occurs in 1 in 2000 to 5000 births; the HPA-1a antigen is the most common antigen responsible for sensitization. Neonates are born with severe thrombocytopenia or develop symptoms within hours after birth. Between 10% and 20% have intracranial hemorrhage. Treatment strategies require perinatology consultation and often necessitate invasive testing.

Guiding Questions in Approaching the Patient

If the patient does not have a history of thrombocytopenia

- Did she have a normal first-trimester platelet count?
- Is she on any medications or taking any drugs that might cause thrombocytopenia?
- Does she have any preexisting medical problems that might cause thrombocytopenia?
- Is her blood pressure normal?
- How low is her platelet count?

If the patient has a history of thrombocytopenia or has a very low platelet count

- Have you discussed the risk of fetal and neonatal thrombocytopenia?
- Have you discussed the option of determining the platelet count before delivery?
- Have you discussed the possibility that a regional anesthetic may not be available?
- Have you discussed the need for neonatal follow-up?

Conclusion

Thrombocytopenia is a relatively common finding during pregnancy. Etiologies are varied and range from clinically nonsignificant gestational thrombocytopenia to ITP, which poses risks to mother and fetus. When thrombocytopenia is a new finding during pregnancy, attention should be given to determining an underlying cause. Given the implications for delivery, pregnancy-associated hypertensive disorders should always be ruled out. Gestational thrombocytopenia and ITP are diagnoses of exclusion. Therapy is determined by the underlying cause.

Discussion of Cases

CASE 1: MULTIPAROUS PATIENT WITH ITP

You are evaluating a 36-year-old gravida 3, para 2 (two previous vaginal deliveries) with a known history of ITP. Her platelet count at her initial visit was 17,000. She is on prednisone 20 mg/day. She reports no spontaneous bleeding or easy bruisability. She has no other medical problems and is on no medications. Her examination shows a viable fetus with the fundus at the umbilicus. There is no evidence of bruising or petechiae.

Does she require any further testing or evaluation at this point?

No. With a known history of ITP and no current complaints or medications, the thrombocytopenia is most likely caused by ITP. At this early gestation, neither preeclampsia nor gestational thrombocytopenia is a concern.

Are you concerned about the degree of thrombocytopenia?

Yes. A platelet count this low can result in spontaneous bleeding (certainly seen with a platelet count <10,000 and sometimes seen with a count <20,000 or <30,000). Further, any trauma or emergency surgery can put this patient in life-threatening danger. Her medication regimen should be adjusted to bring her platelet count up to at least 50,000. A larger dose of steroids should be tried (up to 1–2 mg/[kg · day]), and frequent platelet counts should be obtained. If the patient were closer to term, then IVIgG would be administered to increase the platelet more quickly in the event that labor were to ensue.

How would you counsel this patient regarding risks to her baby?

In the presence of known ITP, the risk of fetal thrombocytopenia is approximately 15%. Only a small percentage of these thrombocytopenic babies will have thrombocytopenia severe enough to warrant admission to the intensive care unit, medical treatment, or blood transfusion. Fetal sampling by scalp sampling in labor or cordocentesis before labor should be discussed because of a possible risk of intracranial hemorrhage in babies with thrombocytopenia who are delivered vaginally. Cesarean section can be offered to those women whose fetuses have documented severe thrombocytopenia to prevent potential trauma during labor.

If fetal sampling is not performed, care should be taken to ensure that appropriate pediatric care is available in the event that the baby is born severely thrombocytopenic; in some cases this may require delivery at a tertiary center. Consultation with an anesthesiologist should be offered because many will not offer regional anesthesia if a platelet count is lower than 100,000, even if counts have been stable. Most physicians would not deliver this patient by vacuum or forceps, unless the fetal platelet count was known to be normal. If this patient delivers a baby boy, he should not be circumcised until his platelet count is known.

CASE 2: INCIDENTAL FINDING OF THROMBOCYTOPENIA

You are evaluating a healthy 36-year-old gravida 1, para 0 at 28 weeks of gestation. You order a complete blood cell count with a 1-hour glucose screen. The glucose screen is normal, but the platelet count is 100,000. Her first-trimester platelet count was 215,000. The remainder of her pregnancy has been uncomplicated thus far.

What testing, if any, would you recommend at this point?

Because this patient is at risk for developing preeclampsia, that should be ruled out. Values for blood pressure, weight, and urine dipstick should be obtained and compared with previous recordings. The patient should be queried about symptoms of preeclampsia such as headache, vision change, or epigastric pain. A thorough history should be obtained regarding evidence of other illnesses, such as a recent viral infection or recent medication or drug use.

What would you recommend for the remainder of the pregnancy?

If preeclampsia is ruled out, no extraordinary obstetric care is needed. This patient most likely has gestational thrombocytopenia, which does not put her or her baby at any increased risk. It may make sense to recheck a platelet count later in the pregnancy and on admission to labor and delivery to make sure it does not decrease significantly; however, with gestational thrombocytopenia, the platelet count typically does not decrease lower than 70,000 or 100,000. If the platelet count decreases, further evaluation of an etiology would include questioning the patient about signs or symptoms of SLE and testing for antinuclear antibody and HIV.

If the diagnosis appears to be gestational thrombocytopenia, there is no need to inform the pediatric staff of the diagnosis; the baby's platelet count will not be affected and therefore does not need to be assessed after birth.

REFERENCES

1 Harvey AM, Johns RJ, McKusick VA, et al, editors. *The Principles and Practice of Medicine.* Norwalk, Connecticut: Appleton & Lange, 1988.

2 American College of Obstetricians and Gynecologists Practice Bulletin #6, September 1999, Thrombocytopenia in pregnancy.

3 George JN, Woolf SH, Raskob GE, et al. Idiopathic thrombocytopenic purpura: a practice guideline developed by explicit methods for the American Society of Hematology. *Blood* 1996;88:3–40.

4 Stamilio DM, Macones GA. Selection of delivery method in pregnancies complicated by autoimmune thrombocytopenia: a decision analysis. *Obstet Gynecol* 1999;94:41–47.

5 Burrows RF, Kelton JG. Incidentally detected thrombocytopenia in healthy mothers and their infants. *N Engl J Med* 1988;319:142–145.

6 McCrae KR, Samuels P, Schreiber AD. Pregnancy-associated thrombocytopenia: pathogenesis and management. *Blood* 1992;80:2697–2714.

7 Garmel SH, D'Alton ME. Immune thrombocytopenia in pregnancy. *The Female Patient.* 1996;21:77–80.

8 Peleg D, Hunter SK. Prenatal management of women with immune thrombocytopenic purpura: survey of US perinatologists. *Am J Obstet Gynecol* 1999;180:645–649.

9 Cines DB, Blanchette VS. Immune thrombocytopenia. *N Engl J Med* 2002;346:995–1008.

10 Anderson HM. Maternal hematologic disorder. In: Creasy RK, Resnik R, eds. *Maternal Fetal Medicine: Principles and Practice.* Philadelphia: Saunders, 1989; p. 908.

Chronic Renal Insufficiency

- Control hypertension
- Symptomatic care for edema
- Treat anemia (iron or erythropoietin as indicated)
- Baseline laboratory studies:
  - Electrolytes, BUN, creatinine, uric acid, albumin, total protein, AST, ALT, CBC, 24-hour urine for protein and creatinine
- Repeat laboratory studies:
  - Monthly electrolytes, BUN, creatinine, CBC
- First trimester ultrasound examination for pregnancy dating
- 18-week ultrasound examination for fetal growth and morphology
- Third trimester ultrasounds for fetal growth (monthly or more frequently as indicated)
- Surveillance for preeclampsia:
  - Consider diagnosis if significantly worsening hypertension or proteinuria
- Antenatal testing:
  - Ultrasound examination, nonstress tests, Doppler, biophysical profile

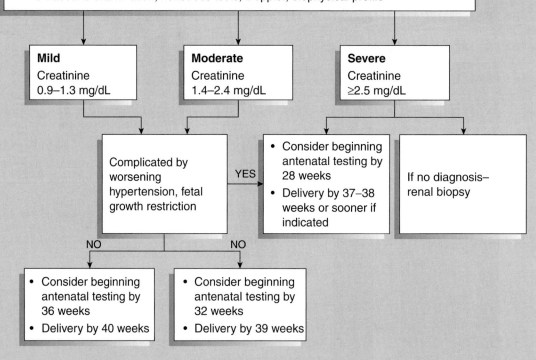

Mild
Creatinine
0.9–1.3 mg/dL

Moderate
Creatinine
1.4–2.4 mg/dL

Severe
Creatinine
≥2.5 mg/dL

Complicated by worsening hypertension, fetal growth restriction

YES

- Consider beginning antenatal testing by 28 weeks
- Delivery by 37–38 weeks or sooner if indicated

If no diagnosis–renal biopsy

NO   NO

- Consider beginning antenatal testing by 36 weeks
- Delivery by 40 weeks

- Consider beginning antenatal testing by 32 weeks
- Delivery by 39 weeks

11 *Chronic Renal Disease and Pregnancy*

Jeanine A. Carlson

Introduction

When a woman with chronic renal disease is contemplating pregnancy, many issues need to be considered including the effects of the pregnancy on the underlying kidney disease and effects of the underlying kidney disease on pregnancy outcomes. One needs to identify how the clinical manifestations and laboratory parameters of kidney disease are affected by pregnancy. The likelihood of maternal morbidity and perinatal morbidity and mortality depends on the degree of renal impairment, the presence or absence of hypertension and proteinuria, and the underlying renal histology.

Evaluation of Renal Function

In the nonpregnant patient, serum creatinine should not exceed 1.4 mg/dL, and the 24-hour urine protein excretion should be less than 150 mg. Levels that exceed these limits are suggestive of renal disease and warrant an evaluation. In the pregnant patient, renal plasma flow and glomerular filtration rate increase in the first trimester and reach levels 30–50% above those in the nonpregnant state by the second trimester.[1,2] This results in a decrease in the serum creatinine concentration to 0.4–0.8 mg/dL, and a level higher than this in pregnancy is consistent with impaired renal function.[3] The pregnancy-associated increase in glomerular filtration rate also results in an increase in proteinuria from

171

150 mg per 24 hours in the normal nonpregnant woman to as much as 300 mg per 24 hours in the normal pregnant woman.

In prenatal clinics, urine protein is usually measured by semi-quantitative dipstick analysis. If the measurement on a clean-catch specimen is at least 2+ (100 mg/dL) or if there is persistent 1+ proteinuria (30 mg/dL), a 24-hour urine specimen should be obtained to quantify the protein excretion.[3] In the absence of preeclampsia, when the 24-hour urine protein excretion exceeds 500 mg per 24 hours, it is unequivocally abnormal, and the patient should be evaluated for underlying renal disease.

The urine sediment should also be examined. There should be fewer than 5 red blood cells per high-power field (RBC/HPF) and fewer than 3 white blood cells per high-power filed (WBC/HPF), and neither RBC casts nor WBC casts should be seen. An abnormality in the urine sediment should prompt further evaluation. Although isolated hematuria or pyuria may reflect only an uncomplicated urinary tract infection or an asymptomatic renal stone, the presence of casts is indicative of a parenchymal renal disease.

On occasion, abnormalities in these parameters will be first noted at a prenatal visit, and a more thorough evaluation for renal disease will need to be undertaken at that time. Reversible causes of renal insufficiency should be identified and treated. Examples of reversible causes include intravascular volume depletion due to dehydration, blood loss or gastrointestinal losses, cardiac or vascular disorders, and nephrotoxic medications. A renal ultrasound should be obtained to document the presence of two kidneys and their size and to eliminate obstruction as a cause of impaired renal function.

If a reversible cause of the abnormality is not identified, a renal biopsy should be considered, especially if there is a sudden deterioration in renal function, if nephrotic syndrome occurs before 30–32 weeks of gestation, or if an active urine sediment (RBC or WBC casts) is present in a patient not previously evaluated. In 1987, Packham and Fairley reported on 111 percutaneous renal biopsies in pregnant women and noted that the complication rate was equivalent to that in the nonpregnant patient.[4] Chen and associates reported similar findings in 2001 and concluded that renal biopsy performed during pregnancy is not contraindicated, and that the histopathologic studies may be very useful when counseling the patient regarding continuation of the pregnancy, potential maternal and fetal outcomes, and treatment options.[5]

BASELINE STUDIES The following baseline data should be obtained at the earliest possible prenatal appointment in all pregnant women with kidney disease, whether they were first identified as having kidney disease during the pregnancy or diagnosed and evaluated before conception.

- Serum electrolytes, blood urea nitrogen, creatinine, uric acid
- Serum albumin, aspartate aminotransferase, alanine amino-transferase
- Complete blood cell count, platelet count
- 24-hour urine levels for protein and creatinine
- Blood pressure
- Renal biopsy results, if available

These parameters are frequently abnormal in patients with chronic kidney disease. These values, obtained at the beginning of the pregnancy, are then used as a patient-specific baseline for comparison with values obtained later in the pregnancy, resulting in an improved ability to interpret the later diagnostic tests. These baseline data may also permit the clinician to define better the risks of the pregnancy for that particular patient, and this will enable the patient to make a more informed decision regarding continuation of the pregnancy.

Effect of Pregnancy on Underlying Renal Disease

RENAL DISEASE WITH NORMAL RENAL FUNCTION Jungers and colleagues reported on 360 women of childbearing age with biopsy-proved primary chronic glomerulonephritis (GN) and normal renal function.[6] One hundred seventy-one patients became pregnant at least once after the clinical onset of GN, and the remaining 189 did not. The investigators found no difference between the group that became pregnant after clinical onset of GN and the group that did not. The average period of follow-up was 15 years.[6] Other investigators have reported similar findings.[7–9]

RENAL DISEASE WITH MILD RENAL INSUFFICIENCY In pregnant women with mild renal insufficiency (serum creatinine >0.8 mg/dL and <1.4 mg/dL), the underlying renal disease does not appear to be adversely affected by the pregnancy. A mild to

KEY POINT

The major risk factor for pregnancy-induced deterioration in renal function is the degree of renal impairment at conception.

moderate decrease in renal function was seen in 16% of these pregnancies, but renal function returned to baseline after delivery.[7] Significant hypertension occurred in 20–23% of patients, but in 50% of these patients hypertension was present before conception, and it resolved after delivery.[7,10] Increased proteinuria was the most common complication, occurring in 47% of pregnancies. In two thirds of these patients, 24-hour protein excretion exceeded 3 g. This also resolved postpartum, with the incidence of persistent proteinuria decreasing to prepregnancy levels.[7]

RENAL DISEASE WITH MODERATE RENAL INSUFFICIENCY

Forty-three percent of women with moderate renal insufficiency (serum creatinine 1.4–2.4 mg/dL) at the first antepartum visit will develop a pregnancy-related decline in renal function of as much as 50%, occurring during gestation (20%) or immediately after delivery (23%). However, recovery of renal function occurred by 6 months postpartum in all but 1 of 49 patients whose registration creatinine was lower than 2.0 mg/dL. In women with registration creatinine between 2 and 2.4 mg/dL, three of nine sustained an accelerated and irreversible loss of renal function.[11]

The frequency of hypertension, defined as a mean arterial pressure higher than 105 mm Hg, increased from 28% at baseline to 48% in the third trimester.[11] High-grade proteinuria (urine protein excretion >3000 mg/day) present in 23% of these pregnancies at baseline ultimately occurred in 41% of the pregnancies.[11]

RENAL DISEASE WITH SEVERE RENAL INSUFFICIENCY

Pregnancy is a rare occurrence in women with severe renal insufficiency, usually defined as a serum creatinine level higher than 2.5 mg/dL, because these women have difficulty conceiving. One study reported an accelerated decline in renal function in 33% of these women.[11] Another study reported that 100% of these pregnancies were complicated by anemia (hematocrit <30%) and 65% by preeclampsia.[12]

RENAL DISEASE BY SPECIFIC HISTOLOGIC TYPE

Pregnancy may not be the sole culprit when renal function deteriorates during pregnancy. The deterioration may reflect the natural history of the underlying disease. Earlier studies, which were retrospective, generally reported on small numbers of patients and grouped all renal diseases together irrespective of histology. They did not take into consideration the time course of the deterioration of renal function before, during, and after the pregnancy.

KEY POINT

*Deterioration in
renal function may
be due to the
natural history of
the underlying
disease.*

In addition, they did not compare women who did have a pregnancy with a control population matched for renal disease, degree of renal impairment, and rate of progression before pregnancy.

Given this information it would not be possible to determine whether a pregnancy-associated decline in renal function was due to the pregnancy per se or if the natural history of the underlying renal disease would be expected to result in a comparable decline in renal function over the course of 12 months. Likewise, it would not be possible to detect a small incremental decline in renal function due to pregnancy.

Abe combined data from eight separate studies that evaluated the effect of pregnancy on the course of various types of GN and found that the effect of pregnancy was not uniform among the histologic types of GN studied.[13] More recently, two case-controlled studies were performed to address these issues and found that pregnancy after the onset of GN does not increase the likelihood of progression to end-stage renal disease (ESRD).[6,9] The histologic form of GN, however, is a predictive factor for the development of ESRD, but this is independent of pregnancy status. The odds ratios for progression to ESRD for immunoglobulin A (IgA) GN, membranoproliferative GN, and focal-segmental glomerulosclerosis were two to seven times higher than that for membranous GN, the reference group.[6]

Effect of Underlying Renal Disease on Pregnancy

CLINICAL AND
DIAGNOSTIC
PARAMETERS

Women with chronic kidney disease frequently will have one or more of the following abnormalities predating the pregnancy: hypertension, proteinuria, high levels of creatinine, high levels of uric acid, and anemia. During pregnancies that will ultimately prove to be uncomplicated, it is common for these women to develop an increase in blood pressure (20–100% of these patients) or an increase in proteinuria (39–100% of these patients).

KEY POINT

*Chronic
hypertension and
anemia are
common
comorbidities in
women with
chronic renal
disease.*

Women with chronic kidney disease and chronic hypertension are also at increased risk for preeclampsia. It may develop earlier in their pregnancies, occasionally occurring in the second trimester. Increasing hypertension and proteinuria are two parameters that clinicians typically monitor for the development of preeclampsia. The diagnosis of preeclampsia is difficult in women with chronic kidney disease due to abnormalities in clinical parameters at baseline, but it should be suspected if there is a significant increase in blood pressure or proteinuria after 20 weeks of gestation and certainly if there is evidence of other manifestations of severe preeclampsia such as HELLP syndrome (hemolysis, elevated liver enzymes, and low platelets).

MATERNAL
COMPLICATIONS

In women with chronic kidney disease who become pregnant, the maternal complications most frequently reported are worsening hypertension, increasing proteinuria, and development of preeclampsia. The incidence and severity of these complications are correlated with the degree of preexisting renal insufficiency and the presence or absence of hypertension before conception.

When renal function is preserved or renal insufficiency is mild (creatinine <1.4 mg/dL), the complications, if they occur, tend to be mild and usually reversible. In one study, preconception hypertension was present in 20% of patients. During the pregnancies, it was noted in 23%. Renal function decreased during pregnancy in 16% of these patients. Pregnancy-associated changes in renal function and hypertension resolved postpartum. Proteinuria was present in 33% of these women before gestation but exceeded 1 g per 24 hours in fewer than 50% of them. The incidence of proteinuria increased in 47% during pregnancy, and two thirds had proteinuria higher than 3 g per 24 hours. After delivery, proteinuria higher than 3 g per 24 hours persisted in 4%.[7]

Maternal complications of pregnancy in women with moderate renal insufficiency (creatinine 1.4–2.5 mg/dL) appear to correlate with the presence or absence of hypertension. For the 63%

KEY POINT

Women with chronic hypertension have an increased risk of adverse maternal and fetal outcomes.

of the women who had moderate renal insufficiency and chronic hypertension, there was an 80% chance they would develop preeclampsia and a 20% chance that their serum creatinine would increase by more than 50%. Only 30% of the women who were normotensive before conception developed preeclampsia, and none of them had an accelerated decline in their renal function.[12]

When renal insufficiency is severe (creatinine >2.5 mg/dL), anemia with a hematocrit value lower than 30% appears to be the norm, occurring in 100% of women in one series; 80% were hypertensive and 65% developed preeclampsia.[12]

Women with isolated chronic proteinuria (>500 mg/24 hours) have as much as a threefold greater risk of preeclampsia during gestation but a relatively unchanged incidence of growth-retarded infants or preterm delivery when compared with the general obstetric population.[3]

FETAL EFFECTS AND
PREGNANCY OUTCOME

KEY POINT

Fetal complications of maternal renal disease include intrauterine growth retardation (IUGR), preterm delivery, and decreased perinatal survival.

KEY POINT

There is a clear correlation between the incidence of fetal complications and the degree of maternal renal impairment.

Successful pregnancy outcomes in this population have become significantly more common. One study reported that the pregnancy success rate improved from 65% in the decade between 1975 and 1984 to 91% between 1985 and 1994.[14] This most likely reflects improvements in maternal blood pressure management, intrauterine fetal monitoring, and postnatal care for the neonate.[15] This is of particular importance and should be kept in mind when reviewing the outcomes data from earlier studies.

When renal function is preserved or renal insufficiency is mild (maternal creatinine <1.4 mg/dL), the pregnancy outcome is fairly good. IUGR is seen in 11–24% of pregnancies, and preterm delivery occurs in 16–20%. There is a 95% chance of a live birth, and perinatal survival is reported to be 89–92%.[7–9,13]

Moderate maternal renal insufficiency (creatinine 1.4–2.4 mg/dL) is associated with overt fetal growth retardation (birth weight <10th percentile) in 31% of infants, preterm delivery in 55% of pregnancies, and an overall fetal survival rate of 93%.[11]

For pregnancies in which there is severe maternal renal insufficiency (creatinine ≥2.5 mg/dL), the frequency of IUGR is 43–57%, that of preterm delivery is 73–86%, and those of fetal and neonatal survival are 64–100%.[11,12]

For every level of renal dysfunction, there is an additional increase in adverse pregnancy outcomes when chronic hypertension is also present.[3]

The relative risk of fetal loss is reported to be 10.6 times greater when hypertension is present at conception than when the blood pressure is normal.[14] Pregnancies complicated by chronic isolated proteinuria appear to have an equivalent incidence of IUGR and preterm delivery as the general obstetric population.[11]

Management Considerations

PRECONCEPTUAL
COUNSELING

Women who have underlying renal disease, preserved renal function, do not have hypertension, and whose proteinuria is at most moderate at conception usually have uncomplicated and successful pregnancies. Maternal complications, including accelerated deterioration in renal function, are more frequent, and fetal prognosis more compromised when renal function is impaired. The greater the degree of renal insufficiency, the greater the risks to the mother and her fetus.

Some investigators have recommended that women with known renal disease not delay childbearing and have counseled them to complete their childbearing while their renal function is still well preserved (creatinine <1.2 mg/dL).[16]

When moderate renal insufficiency is present, approximately 30% of women will develop more than the expected decline in their renal function (based on the underlying renal disease alone). Unfortunately, we are unable to predict which of these women will be in the 30% whose renal disease progresses at an accelerated rate. The experience of women with IgA nephropathy suggests that the severity of the changes seen on renal biopsy may prove to be an indicator.

However, even in these patients, fetal outcome is generally good. If the long-term outlook for maternal renal disease is poor in any event, some of these women may decide to conceive anyway. This may be the only chance for a woman with renal disease to bear a child.

Although successful pregnancies have been reported after renal transplantation, the average waiting time on the transplant list for a cadaveric renal transplant is 3 years, and fertility rates decline with advancing maternal age. In addition, although renal transplantation does improve the metabolic milieu, by definition these women have renal insufficiency because they have only one functioning kidney.

There is increasing experience with management of pregnant women who have had kidney transplantation. In general, good outcomes are likely and depend on prepregnancy renal function and evidence of rejection. Most immunosuppressive agents are acceptable in pregnancy. A common recommendation to women is to wait 2 years after transplantation to achieve a pregnancy.

There is also modest experience with need for dialysis for pregnant women with ESRD. Hemodialysis and peritoneal dialysis have been used successfully. Details of this management are beyond the scope of this chapter. Management of these women requires a team approach with maternal fetal medicine specialists and nephrologists.

HYPERTENSION Meticulous control of maternal blood pressure is crucial because, for every renal disease and all levels of renal function, the presence of hypertension likely increases the incidence of maternal and fetal complications. Hypertension has an independent adverse effect on kidney function, thus prompting an additional reason for control of hypertension in pregnancy. Specific management recommendations for hypertension are well reviewed elsewhere in this textbook. In counseling a woman about choosing an antihypertensive medication before pregnancy, one issue is that there is evidence that fetal exposure to angiotensin-converting enzyme inhibitors in the first trimester does not result in significant fetal morbidity as compared with exposure in the second and third trimesters, during which time fetal oliguria, skull defects, and death have been found. Depending on the circumstance, one might choose not to use them in women seeking pregnancy. It is important to discontinue angiotensin-converting enzyme inhibitors when a pregnancy is diagnosed.

PROTEINURIA Worsening proteinuria during pregnancy is common in women with renal disease. Women with proteinuria higher than 3 g per 24 hours may develop significant and disabling edema during pregnancy. Salt restriction alone usually does not provide appreciable improvement in symptoms. When applied judiciously, diuretics have been safely used. They should be introduced at a very small dose, and the dose should be increased gradually as necessary but avoid hypotension and rapid fluid shifts that could impair placental perfusion. The goal of therapy is diminution, not elimination, of edema. Serum electrolytes should be monitored carefully for hypokalemia or hyponatremia.

ANEMIA Anemia, which is caused by decreased production of erythropoietin, is common in patients with chronic renal disease. The decrement in hematocrit tends to parallel the decrease in renal function. As a result, anemia usually does not become severe enough to require specific management until renal disease is quite advanced. A hematocrit of 34% is considered normal in pregnancy. This "physiologic anemia of pregnancy" is caused by a 40–50% increase in plasma volume but only a 30% increase in RBC mass.

Some women with severe renal insufficiency may develop profound anemia during pregnancy. If the hematocrit value is lower than 25% and no other cause of the anemia is identified (iron, folate, B_{12} deficiency, or blood loss), erythropoietin 150 U/kg per week subcutaneously has been shown to be effective in correcting the anemia.[17,18] Erythropoietin does not cross the placenta to the fetus and is considered a risk factor "C" in pregnancy.[19]

OBSTETRIC MANAGEMENT

The goal of the first trimester is to assess preexisting maternal condition with regard to renal function, hypertension, and anemia. Even in the presence of confident menstrual dates, it is reasonable to confirm dating with a first- or early second-trimester ultrasound examination. Baseline laboratory studies should be obtained as noted above. An ultrasound examination at 18–20 weeks is indicated for surveillance for early onset growth restriction and for morphologic survey especially in the setting of medication exposures.

In the third trimester, ultrasound examinations should be obtained every 4 weeks or more frequently if there is evidence of developing growth restriction or oligohydramnios. Antenatal testing including assessment of amniotic fluid volume should be initiated by 32 weeks of gestation or sooner if there is evidence of uteroplacental insufficiency by findings of growth restriction, abnormal Doppler velocimetry, or oligohydramnios.

Clinic visits should be frequent in the third trimester for surveillance for preeclampsia. Although mild to modest increases in the amount of proteinuria is to be expected, repeating a 24-hour urine collection should be considered if there is an increase in the amount of protein detected on dipstick. A substantial increase would significantly increase the likelihood of superimposed preeclampsia.

Detecting the development of superimposed preeclampsia in the woman with chronic hypertension and renal disease with proteinuria can be quite difficult. One needs to rely on presence or absence of symptoms and the rate of change of hypertension and proteinuria. The presence of abnormal liver enzymes (transaminases) and thrombocytopenia clearly favors the diagnosis of superimposed preeclampsia. Expectant management of severe preeclampsia should be undertaken with extraordinary caution, if at all.

Delivery needs to be considered if there is evidence of severe growth restriction, superimposed preeclampsia, or rapidly worsening renal failure. For women with mild renal insufficiency, in the absence of evidence of hypertension, uteroplacental insufficiency, or nonreassuring fetal testing, it is reasonable to allow avoidance of induction of labor until 40 weeks of gestation with continued close surveillance. For women with moderate or severe renal insufficiency and no other indication for delivery, delivery should be accomplished as soon as lung maturity is demonstrated and no later than 39 weeks.

What's the Evidence

Similar to many medical problems in pregnancy, there is a paucity of good quality data regarding renal disease. Most of the information available consists of descriptions of outcomes of populations of women with renal disease. Several features hamper interpretation of the literature. The studies generally report outcomes of relatively small numbers of women and can span a number of years during which the overall outcomes for mother and babies have generally improved. A few studies have attempted to form control groups but are nevertheless retrospective. None of the interventions has been subjected to a randomized trial.

Guiding Questions in Approaching the Patient

- What is the degree of the renal insufficiency?
- Does the woman have preexisting hypertension?
- Will the pregnancy result in deterioration of renal function?
- What is the likelihood of adverse fetal outcome?
- What are the potential maternal complications?
- What are the effects on fetal and infant survival?

Conclusion

When a woman with chronic renal disease is contemplating pregnancy, we can stratify the risk of the pregnancy to her residual renal function based on her creatinine level at conception, the presence or absence of chronic hypertension, and the histologic type of renal disease that she has. The incidence of maternal and fetal complications during pregnancy correlates with the degree of renal insufficiency and the presence of chronic hypertension.

Although the likelihood of a successful pregnancy outcome appears to correlate inversely with preconception level of serum creatinine, fetal and neonatal survival rates have improved over the past two decades. This suggests that the correlation is not absolute, and that as we develop a more complete understanding of the metabolic complications chronic renal disease and continue to make improvements in prenatal and neonatal management, we can improve outcome.

Discussion of Cases

CASE 1: NEW DIAGNOSIS OF RENAL DISEASE DURING PREGNANCY

A 25-year-old gravida 3, para 2 presents at 16 weeks of gestation with a blood pressure of 140/100 mm Hg. Although she has been feeling well during this pregnancy, she has noted some dependent edema. Her medical history is significant for preeclampsia during her second pregnancy that resulted in early delivery at 32 weeks of gestation. Otherwise, she has had no medical illnesses, including hypertension. She has no family history of hypertension.

Physical examination shows a blood pressure of 140/100 mmg Hg, a heart rate of 80 beats/min, a height of 5 ft 5 in., and a weight of 151 lb. Funduscopic examination shows arteriolar narrowing, no atrioventricular nicking, hemorrhages, or exudates. Chest sounds are clear. Heart rate, rhythm, and S1S2 are normal. The abdomen is gravid. Examination of the extremities show 2+ pitting edema to the knees. Neurologic examination is normal.

Laboratory data show a BUN of level 20 mg/dL, a creatinine level of 0.9 mg/dL, a chloride level of 106 mmol/L, and a HCO₃ level of 21 mmol/L.

What is your differential diagnosis at this time?

This is unlikely to represent preeclampsia. Although preeclampsia can occur at an earlier gestational age, it is rare for it to present before 20 weeks. Second-trimester preeclampsia can occur in a molar pregnancy, but this can be excluded by ultrasound.

Essential hypertension is unlikely in this patient who previously had a normal blood pressure and no family history of hypertension. Further evaluation is indicated for other causes such as thyroid disease, renal disease, hyperparathyroidism, and renal artery stenosis.

What do the values of creatinine 0.9 mg/dL and BUN 20 mg/dL suggest?

In pregnancy renal plasma flow and glomerular filtration rate increase in the first trimester and reach levels 30–50% above those in the nonpregnant state by the second trimester. This results in a decrease in the serum creatinine concentration to 0.4–0.8 mg/dL. This patient's value of 0.9 mg/dL most likely represents mildly impaired renal function.

What other testing would you recommend at this point?

Urinalysis, serum albumin, and 24-hour urine for total protein and creatinine.

Urinalysis shows a specific gravity of 1.018, 3+ protein, negative glucose, and negative blood values. Microscopy demonstrates 0–1 RBC/HPF, 1 WBC/HPF, and no casts.

Serum albumin is 1.7 g/dL, total protein is 2.9 g/dL, and 24-hour urine is 800 mg protein (normal in pregnancy is ≤300 mg/24 hours).

Renal ultrasound shows two normal-size kidneys, and fetal ultrasound shows a normally grown fetus.

These findings suggest primary glomerular disease with nephritic syndrome causing decreased glomerular filtration, hypoalbuminemia, edema, hypertension, and proteinuria.

Further evaluation for specific diagnosis with serology studies includes serum complements (C3, C4, CH50), antinuclear antibody, and hepatitis B surface antigen and antibody. If a diagnosis can not be made with blood tests, a renal biopsy should be considered, especially if renal function is deteriorating. Hypertension should be controlled. Common medications include methyldopa and labetalol. Edema can be decreased with salt restriction and bedrest.

She had induction of labor at 37 weeks for severe hypertension that required multiple medications for control. Proteinuria did not resolve in the 6 months after delivery. Renal biopsy performed 6 months postpartum demonstrated focal segmental glomerulosclerosis. She continued to require medication for hypertension and has a serum creatinine of 1.4 mg/dL.

How do you counsel this patient and her husband regarding future pregnancies?

She has moderate renal insufficiency (creatinine 1.4–2.5 mg/dL), hypertension, and proteinuria. There is at least an 80% likelihood that she will develop accelerated hypertension or preeclampsia in future pregnancies, and at least a 20% chance that her renal function will decrease by more than 50%. In terms of the fetus, moderate renal insufficiency is associated with overt fetal growth restriction in 30% of pregnancies and preterm delivery in 55%.

CASE 2: PRIMIGRAVIDA WITH CHRONIC GLOMEROLONEPHRITIS

A 30-year-old primigravida presents at 8 weeks of gestation for initial prenatal care. She reports that she has had brown urine in the past but has not had medical evaluation. She has no back, flank, or abdominal pain. She has no history of chronic illness including hypertension. Her blood pressure is 120/70 mm Hg and her physical examination is normal.

Laboratory data show a BUN level of 20 mg/dL, creatinine level of 0.7 mg/dL, and 24-hour urine protein level of 500 mg/dL. Hematocrit is 30%. Urinalysis demonstrates large blood and RBC casts. Renal ultrasound examination is normal.

What is your differential diagnosis at this time?

Chronic Glomerolonephritis is likely.

What other testing would you recommend at this point?

A consultation with a nephrologist is indicated for further evaluation for a specific diagnosis with serology studies including serum complements (C3, C4, CH50), antinuclear antibody, and hepatitis B surface antigen and antibody.

Her pregnancy was uncomplicated until 26 weeks, when her creatinine level increased to 2.0 mg/dL. Renal biopsy diagnosed IgA nephropathy. At 37 weeks, another increase in creatinine was noted, and she was delivered of a 2500-g baby.

How do you counsel this patient and her husband regarding future pregnancies?

At present she has moderate renal insufficiency that, if it persists, is associated with preeclampsia, fetal growth restriction, worsening of renal function, and prematurity. She is at risk for developing hypertension, proteinuria, and progressively decreased renal function.

REFERENCES

1 Davison JM, Dunlop W. Renal hemodynamics and tubular function in normal human pregnancy. *Kidney Int* 1980;18:152.

2 Myers SA, Gleicher N. Physiologic changes in normal pregnancy. In: Gleicher N, ed. *Principles and Practice of Medical Therapy in Pregnancy,* 2nd ed. New York: Appleton & Lange, 1992; p. 43.

3 Stettler RW, Cunningham FG. Natural history of chronic proteinuria complicating pregnancy. *Am J Obstet Gynecol* 1992;167:1219.

4 Packham D, Fairley KF. Renal biopsy: indications and complications in pregnancy. *Brit J Obstet Gynecol* 1987;94:935.

5 Chen HH, Lin HC, Yeh JC, et al. Renal biopsy in pregnancies complicated by undetermined renal disease. *Acta Obstet Gynecol Scand* 2001;80:888.

6 Jungers P, Houillier P, Forget D, et al. Influence of pregnancy on the course of primary chronic glomerulonephritis. *Lancet* 1995;346:1122.

7 Katz AI, Davison JM, Hayslett JP, et al. Pregnancy in women with kidney disease. *Kidney Int* 1980;18:192.

8 Barcelo P, Lopez-Lillo J, Cabero L, et al. Successful pregnancy in primary glomerular disease. *Kidney Int* 1986;30:914.

9 Abe S. The influence of pregnancy on the long-term renal prognosis of IgA nephropathy. *Clin Nephrol* 1994;41:61.

10 Surian M, Imbasciati E, Cosci P, et al. Glomerular disease and pregnancy: a study of 123 pregnancies in patients with primary and secondary glomerular disease. *Nephron* 1984;36:101.

11 Jones DC, Hayslett JP. Outcome of pregnancy in women with moderate or severe renal insufficiency. *N Engl J Med* 1996;335:226.

12 Cunningham FG, Cox SM, Harstad TW, et al. Chronic renal disease and pregnancy outcome. *Am J Obstet Gynecol* 1990;163:453.

13 Abe S. An overview of pregnancy in women with underlying renal disease. *Am J Kidney Dis* 1991;17:112.

14 Jungers P, Chauveau D, Choukroun G, et al. Pregnancy in women with impaired renal function. *Clin Nephrol* 1997;47:281.

15 Jones DC. Pregnancy complicated by chronic renal disease. *Clin Perinatol* 1997;24:483.

16 Jungers P, Houillier P, Chaveau D, et al. Pregnancy in women with reflux nephropathy. *Kidney Int* 1996;50:593.

17 Yankowitx J, Piraino B, Laifer SA, et al. Erythropoietin in pregnancies complicated by severe anemia of renal failure. *Obstet Gynecol* 1992;80:485.

18 Scott LL, Ramin SM, Richey M, et al. Erythropoietin use in pregnancy: two cases and a review of the literature. *Am J Perinatol* 1995;12:22.

19 Briggs GG, Freeman RK, Yaffe SJ. *Drugs in Pregnancy and Lactation,* 5th ed. Baltimore: Williams and Wilkins, 1998; p. 384.

Algorithm for the Investigation of Symptomatic Kidney Stones in Pregnancy

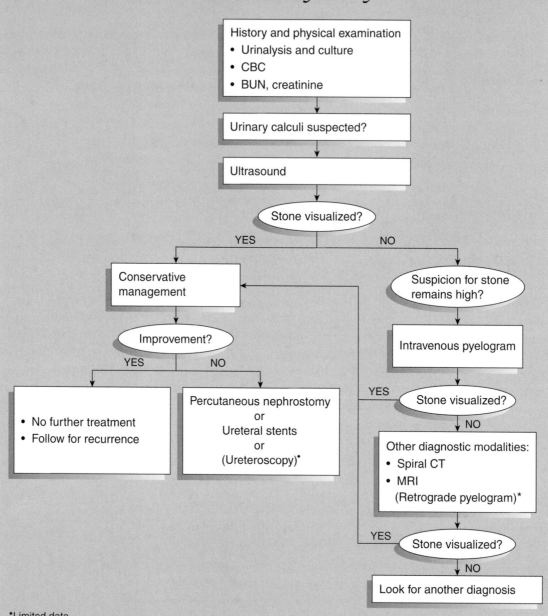

History and physical examination
- Urinalysis and culture
- CBC
- BUN, creatinine

Urinary calculi suspected?

Ultrasound

Stone visualized?

YES → Conservative management

NO → Suspicion for stone remains high?

Conservative management → Improvement?

YES →
- No further treatment
- Follow for recurrence

NO → Percutaneous nephrostomy
or
Ureteral stents
or
(Ureteroscopy)*

Suspicion for stone remains high? → Intravenous pyelogram

Intravenous pyelogram → Stone visualized?

YES → (Conservative management)

NO → Other diagnostic modalities:
- Spiral CT
- MRI
(Retrograde pyelogram)*

Stone visualized?

YES → (Conservative management)

NO → Look for another diagnosis

*Limited data
*Shield utenis, limit fluoroscopy, and do not perform if infection present

12 Nephrolithiasis

Garfield A. Clunie

Introduction

Nephrolithiasis is an uncommon condition in pregnancy, with an estimated incidence of 0.03–0.5%.[1,2] The actual incidence is unknown because small kidney stones can be asymptomatic and can pass through the renal tract undetected. Ureteral dilatation that normally occurs in pregnancy can also permit easier passage of small calculi.[3] The incidence of nephrolithiasis is reportedly increasing.[4] Nephrolithiasis occurs more commonly in whites than in blacks,[5] affects multiparous women three times more often than nulliparous women,[6] and occurs more often with an increasing number of pregnancies.[7] Women with a history of kidney stones are at higher risk of forming subsequent stones, but there has been no evidence that pregnancy is an independent risk factor for kidney stone formation.[1,8] Calcium-containing stones are the most common cause of nephrolithiasis, followed by struvite stones, uric acid stones, and cystine stones.[9,10] Most kidney stones present during the second and third trimesters of pregnancy,[11] with only 20% presenting in the first trimester.[12] Pain is the most common presenting sign of kidney stones, and pain secondary to kidney stones is one of the most common nonobstetric conditions that require hospitalization in pregnancy.[1,2,13]

Diagnosis of renal stones in pregnancy can be difficult due to the anatomic and physiologic changes that occur within the urinary tract during pregnancy. Physiologic hydronephrosis, which occurs in up to 90% of pregnancies by the third trimester,[1,7] can sometimes be difficult to differentiate from pathologic obstruction caused by a kidney stone. The fetal skeleton and the enlarged gravid uterus also distort the pelvic anatomy, making detection of urinary stones by conventional techniques a challenge. Once the diagnosis is confirmed, the clinician must determine whether conservative or surgical management is appropriate. Fortunately, up to 80% of symptomatic renal stones will pass spontaneously with conservative management.[6,11,14]

Pregnancy-Related Changes in the Renal System

There are various changes that occur within the urinary tract during normal pregnancy that may promote stone formation. Pregnancy itself does not appear to be an independent risk factor for nephrolithiasis, but physiologic hydronephrosis of pregnancy is the only known predisposing factor to the development of stones.[7]

Physiologic hydronephrosis generally begins as early as 6 weeks and is caused by hormonal and mechanical effects. This phenomenon can persist up to 6 weeks postpartum.[1,13] Progesterone affects the urinary smooth muscle during early pregnancy, causing decreased peristalsis and dilation of the ureter above the pelvic brim.[1] The right ureter is far more commonly affected than the left, 85% versus 15%, because of compression from the right ovarian vein and uterine dextrorotation.[1,13] However, kidney stones occur on each side with equal frequency.[6,13] Beyond the pelvic brim, the ureter appears normal unless a pathologic obstruction is present. Studies have shown that ureteral dilation does not occur when the ureter does not cross the pelvic brim, as observed in patients with a pelvic kidney or an ileal conduit.[1,7] Physiologic hydronephrosis, in combination with the decreased peristalsis and ureteral compression resulting in stasis, is thought to increase the risk of nephrolithiasis.[7] However, for a stone to form in the urinary tract, a crystal must form, be retained, aggregate, and grow.[15] Calcium, usually with oxalate or phosphate, is the most common constituent of stones and is present in some form in almost 90% of all kidney stones.[9]

Calcium homeostasis is regulated by parathyroid hormone (PTH), vitamin D, and calcitonin. Normally, when calcium levels in the blood are low, the parathyroid gland is stimulated to secrete PTH. PTH has three major effects in the kidney. It increases calcium reabsorption, acts on osteoblasts in bone, which in turn stimulates osteoclasts to cause bone breakdown, and activates vitamin D. Active vitamin D acts on the kidney to increase calcium reabsorption, stimulate osteoblast activity, and stimulate absorption of active calcium and phosphate in the duodenum and jejunum. Calcitonin is secreted by the parafollicular cells of the parathyroid gland and is secreted in response to increased blood calcium. Calcitonin inhibits reabsorption of calcium and phosphate in the kidney, and in bone calcitonin inhibits osteoclast activity to decrease erosion of bone, thereby preventing calcium and phosphate release into blood.

In pregnancy, calcium homeostasis is altered in several ways. Renal plasma flow steadily increases to 60–80% more than preconception values and then decreases in the third trimester but remains 50% above the prepregnancy rate.[16] This in turn causes the glomerular filtration rate to increase by 30–50%, peaking by 11 weeks of gestation.[1,16] The filtered load of calcium, sodium, and uric acid is subsequently increased, resulting in increased excretion.[4,15,16] Despite an increase in these solutes in urine, there is no resultant increase in the rate of stone formation over the nonpregnancy rate for the following reasons. The increased urinary excretion of citrate and magnesium that occurs in pregnancy inhibits calcium stone formation, and the increased excretion of glycosaminoglycans and acidic glycoproteins inhibits the formation of oxalate stones. In addition, respiratory alkalosis of pregnancy results in alkaline urine, which inhibits uric acid stone formation.[16] Low urine pH is a critical factor in producing uric acid stones.[9] Therefore it is likely that stasis and decreased peristalsis are the factors that promote formation of these types of stones.

KEY POINT

Hormonal and mechanical factors that occur in normal pregnancy predispose women to nephrolithiasis.

Another possible cause of calcium-containing kidney stone formation in pregnancy is the placental secretion of 1,25-dihydroxyvitamin D_3 to ensure that enough calcium is available for fetal skeletal formation. Fetal skeletal formation is greatest in the second and third trimesters,[11] which is also the time when kidney stones present. More calcium is absorbed than is required for the fetal skeleton. Thus the excess calcium is collected by the kidneys for excretion, where it can promote kidney stone formation. There is no overall increase in the incidence of calcium-containing stones over the nonpregnant rate.

Clinical Presentation

The most common presenting signs and symptoms of nephrolithiasis are flank pain, gross or microscopic hematuria, and urinary
tract infection. Of these, flank pain is the most common, occurring
in 90% of patients with nephrolithiasis.[4,12,13] Flank pain often radiates to the groin or lower abdomen. Microscopic hematuria occurs
in 75–100% of cases and gross hematuria occurs in up to 20% of
cases.[1,7] Other reported signs of kidney stones include irritative
voiding, chills, nausea, and vomiting. This nonspecific nature of
the presentation leads to a wide differential diagnosis including
appendicitis, pyelonephritis, diverticulitis, preterm labor, renal
calyx rupture, renal vein rupture, cholecystitis, abruption, and
liver involvement from preeclampsia[13,14] (Table 12-1). Because the
differential is so varied, the diagnosis of urolithiasis must be firmly

Table 12-1.   **DIFFERENTIAL DIAGNOSIS OF RENAL COLIC**

Abdominal aortic aneurysm
Renal artery thrombosis, embolism, or dissection
Appendicitis
Pyelonephritis
Ectopic pregnancy
Ovarian torsion
Diverticulitis
Musculoskeletal pain
Peritonitis
Ischemic bowel
Acute myocardial infarction
Bowel obstruction
Henoch-Schönlein purpura
Renal papillary necrosis
Ovarian cyst
Endometriosis
Psoas abscess or hematoma
Retroperitoneal mass
Biliary colic
Urinary retention
Fitz-Hugh-Curtis syndrome
Superior mesenteric artery occlusion
Internal hernia
Malingering

SOURCE: Manthey DE, Teichman J. Nephrolithiasis. *Emerg Med Clin North Am* 2001;19:633.

established to institute appropriate therapy. Treatment for the presumptive diagnosis of urolithiasis may be inadequate for the actual underlying pathology and can result in further morbidity. Marlow also reported that the persistence of fever after 48 hours of parental antibiotics for pyelonephritis is strongly suggestive of a calculus.[2] Stothers and Lee reported an incorrect diagnosis of appendicitis, diverticulitis, and placental abruption in 28% of patients in whom a stone was subsequently confirmed.[17] Therefore, a thorough history and careful physical examination are warranted.

On physical examination, flank tenderness is almost always present, but the patient may exhibit costovertebral angle (CVA) tenderness and abdominal muscle guarding. Renal stones may be discovered in any portion of the urinary tract but are most likely to be symptomatic when in the ureter. Renal colic may occur episodically over several hours to days until the stone has passed into the bladder. Auscultation of the abdomen is not particularly helpful because bowel sounds can range from hyper- to hypoactive.[2] Frank peritonitis is uncommon and should prompt a search for another diagnosis.

KEY POINT

Flank pain and microscopic hematuria are the most common presenting signs and symptoms of nephrolithiasis.

Diagnostic Evaluation

Diagnosis of nephrolithiasis in pregnancy can be problematic. The gravid uterus, fetal skeleton, and physiologic hydronephrosis can make detection of small kidney stones quite difficult. There is also an inherent reluctance on the part of clinicians to perform radiography or invasive diagnostic procedures in pregnant women because they often involve exposing the fetus to radiation and contrast material. Fetuses exposed to less than 5 rad of radiation are not at increased risk of anomaly, growth restriction, or spontaneous abortion.[18] Table 12-2 lists the approximate radiation doses to a fetus from various radiographic studies. Exact dosages will vary according to the size of the patient, gestational age of the fetus, anatomic location of the fetus, and radiographic technology and equipment used.[7,15] Techniques used to minimize the amount of radiation to which a fetus is exposed include irradiating only the side suspected to have a stone, shielding the maternal pelvis, and limiting the number of films taken.[4] A medical physicist can be consulted if knowledge of exact dosages is required.

Table 12-2. **APPROXIMATE RADIATION DOSAGES TO FETUS FROM RADIOGRAPHIC STUDIES**

Radiographic Study	*Dosage to Fetus (rad)*
Radiography of kidneys, ureter, and bladder	0.023–0.055
Intravenous pyelogram (5 films)	0.686–1.398
Abdominal computed tomography	1.7–2.6
Retrograde pyelogram	0.109–0.220
Ultrasound	0
Magnetic resonance imaging	0

Source: Cunningham FG, MacDonald PC, Gant NF, et al. *Williams Obstetrics*, 20th ed. Stanford CT: Appleton & Lange, 1997.

ULTRASOUND

Traditionally, diagnosing kidney stones involved performing plain abdominal radiographs of the kidney, ureters, and bladder and an intravenous pyelogram (IVP). Although safe, these tools expose the fetus to small amounts of radiation and/or intravenous contrast materials. Because of the concern for potential risks to the fetus from these agents, ultrasound has become the current standard first-line investigation.[1] Evaluation of the entire ureter must be performed to obtain the greatest benefit from the ultrasound examination. A dilated ureter that tapers to a normal caliber at the level of the pelvic brim without associated calculi is likely the result of physiologic hydronephrosis of pregnancy. In contrast, a dilated ureter extending to the level of a calculus results from pathologic obstruction.[1,7] Ellenbogen and colleagues in 1978 reported that sonography had a sensitivity of 98% for the detection of hydronephrosis when obstruction was present.[19] However, when differentiating pathologic obstruction due to kidney stones from physiologic hydronephrosis, ultrasound was much less effective. More recently reported sensitivities for transabdominal ultrasound in detecting kidney stones range from 24% to 74%.[1,6,14,20] Although the sensitivity varies greatly, ultrasound is commonly used because it is a noninvasive diagnostic tool. The *combination* of a plain abdominal radiograph and transabdominal ultrasound can increase the sensitivity to 95%.[6] The addition of transvaginal ultrasound improves the detection rate of kidney stones over transabdominal ultrasound alone, especially for stones in the distal ureter.[1]

KEY POINT

The combination of plain abdominal radiograph and ultrasound has a 95% sensitivity for detecting kidney stones.

COLOR DOPPLER ULTRASOUND

In recent years, color Doppler ultrasound has been proposed as an alternative to simple ultrasound as a method for detecting kidney stones. It is attractive because it does not require radiation and is noninvasive. Color Doppler ultrasound has also been reported to improve the detection rate of kidney stones by enabling calculation of the resistive index (RI), identifying ureteral jets, and showing the relation of a dilated ureter to iliac vessels. An RI of less than 0.70 is reportedly normal in nonpregnant women, but it increases within 6 hours after an acute renal obstruction and returns to normal when the obstruction is relieved.[13] Hertzberg and associates found that the RI values in the kidneys of pregnant women were not significantly different from those in nonpregnant patients, in each case measuring less than 0.70 in all pregnant patients whether or not physiologic hydronephrosis of pregnancy was present.[21] These findings suggest that normal pregnancy does not affect the intrarenal RI and that a high RI during pregnancy should not be attributed to normal physiologic changes of pregnancy.[13] Therefore, color Doppler ultrasound can be used to calculate the mean intrarenal RI, which can be used to help differentiate upper tract dilatation from functional obstruction.[11]

Color Doppler ultrasound has also been used to identify ureteral jets. The presence of ureteral jets is thought to indicate a free-flowing, nonobstructed ureter. An undetectable ureteral jet on the side where obstruction is suspected has been reported to have a diagnostic sensitivity of 100% and a specificity of 91% for ureteral obstruction.[13] In contrast, a subsequent study noted complete unilateral absence of ureteral jets in four asymptomatic pregnant patients.[1] Further, Burge and coworkers reported that patients with incomplete ureteral obstruction or urinary calculi not causing ureteral obstruction may have ureteral jets that appear normal.[4] Therefore, the absence of ureteral jets as an adjunct procedure for the diagnosis of ureteral calculus obstruction remains controversial.

Color Doppler ultrasound has been used to identify the relation of the dilated ureter to the iliac vessels. Ureteral calculi should be suspected when a dilated ureter extends into the pelvis, past the common iliac artery. If the ureter tapers to normal when crossing the pelvic brim, physiologic hydronephrosis rather than a pathologic process is the most likely cause.[13]

INTRAVENOUS PYELOGRAM

When sonography is nondiagnostic for kidney stones and there is still a high index of suspicion, an IVP should be performed. The sensitivity of an IVP after a nondiagnostic ultrasound is 93%.[20]

An IVP enables the radiologists to readily locate and measure ureteral calculi, establish the presence of obstruction, estimate renal function, detect altered renal physiology caused by acute ureteral obstruction, and identify anatomic abnormalities that would affect management.[13] The major drawback of the IVP is that it requires intravenous contrast and radiation. The intravenous contrast places the mother at increased risk for adverse reactions due to allergy. Fortunately, no adverse effects on fetal development have been reported from contrast material.[13] The amount of radiation that the fetus is exposed to during a limited IVP is much less than 5 rad (see Table 12-2). One problem that limits the usefulness of IVP in the diagnosis of obstructing ureteral calculi during pregnancy is the difficulty in differentiating delayed excretion of contrast material associated with physiologic hydronephrosis of pregnancy from the delayed excretion that is associated with an obstructing kidney stone. Delayed films up to several hours may be needed to differentiate the two entities.

There is consensus that a limited number of exposures during IVP is recommended over a standard protocol to minimize the radiation dose delivered to the fetus. However, there is some debate regarding the definition of a "limited" IVP.[13] There is no set protocol for the use of IVP for the diagnosis of kidney stones in pregnancy. Table 12-3 lists IVP protocols using limited exposures, with

Table 12-3.   **REPORTED LIMITED OR "ONE-SHOT" INTRAVENOUS PYELOGRAPHIC PROTOCOLS**

REFERENCE	*PROTOCOL*
Butler et al.[3]	Single film at 30 min[a]
Stothers and Lee[17]	Plain film; second film at 20–30 min; delayed film at 60 min[b]
Drago et al.[22]	Plain film; second film at 30–60 min[b]
Klein[23]	Plain film; second film at 20 min; delayed films as needed[b]
Waltzer[24]	Plain film; second film at 15 min; if obstruction, then film at 60 min[b]
Boridy et al.[13]	Plain film; second film at 1 min; third film at 15 min; delayed film at 45–120 min[b]

[a] Thirty minutes after administering intravenous contrast material.
[b] Subsequent films are made after administering intravenous contrast material.

delayed films as needed. Aside from the "one-shot" IVP, the first film in an IVP is the scout film or plain abdominal radiograph of the kidney, ureters, and bladder. When done as an initial test, it alone has a sensitivity of 57%.[20] If the first set of radiographs shows evidence of obstruction but the point of obstruction is not shown, delayed films are generally needed to differentiate physiologic hydronephrosis from pathologic obstruction.[13] As with ultrasound, ureteral dilation that tapers to normal caliber above or below the pelvic brim is highly suggestive of a stone.[7]

COMPUTED TOMOGRAPHY

When sonography and IVP are inconclusive and expectant management is not appropriate, additional diagnostic studies may be considered. Unenhanced helical computer tomography (spiral CT) is an excellent tool for differentiating kidney stones from blood clots and tumors.[13,15] It appears to have greater sensitivity than IVP for the diagnosis of kidney stones,[13,25] but studies did not involve pregnant patients. The radiation dose to the fetus from CT of the pelvis, although still below 5 rads, is significantly higher than other methods including a limited IVP and therefore is a less desirable method in pregnancy.[6,13,26]

MAGNETIC RESONANCE IMAGING

Magnetic resonance excretory urography (MRU) is a technique that has been recently investigated as an alternative to IVP when ultrasound is inconclusive. It provides useful information regarding urinary obstruction without the need for ionizing radiation or intravenous contrast. Kidney stones do not elicit a characteristic magnetic resonance signal, but they can be detected as a signal void superimposed on the high-intensity signal of urine on heavily T_2-weighted images.[13,15] MRU holds a promise of becoming an important imaging modality in diagnosing obstruction of the urinary system in pregnancy because, like IVP, it will show hydronephrosis and can be used to assess urinary tract function. Therefore, it can potentially differentiate between physiologic hydronephrosis and pathologic obstruction.[6] The technique will show where the level of compression is in relation to the iliac vessels. The drawbacks of MRU are that it is expensive and is not universally available, and the procedure can be somewhat uncomfortable for some patients who experience claustrophobia. In the future, MRU may be an alternative to unenhanced helical CT or IVP but is currently considered investigational.

RETROGRADE PYELOGRAM

KEY POINT

Minimizing the radiation exposure to the fetus is the most important factor when choosing a diagnostic test.

Retrograde pyelogram can be useful when ultrasound and IVP are inconclusive for ureteral stones. During this procedure, a stent can be placed, if required. Retrograde pyelogram has been reported to increase the risk of sepsis.[1] This procedure also requires radiation and cystoscopy but does not provide any information regarding urinary tract function. For the pregnant population, the general consensus is that retrograde pyelogram should be avoided, if possible, because of the high levels of radiation associated with fluoroscopy. When this procedure is deemed necessary, the uterus must be shielded and pulsed fluoroscopy should be used to decrease the amount of radiation exposure to the fetus.[6]

Management

CONSERVATIVE MANAGEMENT

KEY POINT

Conservative management of nephrolithiasis in pregnancy most often results in spontaneous resolution.

The smaller the stone, the more likely it is to pass spontaneously, Thus, management of nephrolithiasis in pregnancy is in most cases initially conservative. Conservative management includes increasing oral hydration to achieve a urine output of 2–3 L/day and using oral narcotic analgesics, antiemetics, and antibiotics, if infection is present.[6,14,15] Swanson and colleagues reported that stones with a diameter of 4 mm or smaller will pass 80% of the time in nonpregnant patients versus stones that are larger than 8 mm, which will pass only 20% of the time.[15] This may not be exactly the same for pregnant women because the physiologic hydronephrosis may make it easier to pass larger stones. However, spontaneous passage of symptomatic renal calculi reportedly occurs in up to 80% of pregnant women who are treated conservatively.[6,11,14] The remaining patients require surgical intervention. Surgical intervention is indicated when the following occur: sepsis, obstruction of a solitary kidney, bilateral ureteric obstruction, or failure of conservative management.[6]

Treatment with medications that are used to prevent various types of kidney stones are not recommended in pregnancy, with the exception of antibiotics. When a kidney stone can be obtained, mineral analysis should be performed, but drug therapy to prevent stone formation should be delayed until the postpartum period. Likewise, serologic and urinary tests to confirm the suspected etiology of kidney stones should also be deferred until 6 weeks postpartum.

SURGICAL MANAGEMENT

Surgical management for symptomatic kidney stones includes ureteral stent placement, percutaneous nephrostomy tube placement, and ureteroscopic lithotripsy with stone extraction. The first two procedures are done with the intention of temporizing until definitive treatment can be performed in the postpartum period. Ureteroscopic lithotripsy enables definitive treatment to occur during pregnancy. Although there have been reports of patients delivering normal babies after inadvertently having extracorporeal shock wave lithotripsy while unknowingly pregnant, this procedure is currently considered contraindicated during pregnancy.[11]

URETERAL STENT

Ureteral stent placement is the most common technique used to relieve obstruction due to nephrolithiasis.[7] It involves the placement of a double-J stent or pigtail catheter within the ureter cystoscopically or under ultrasound guidance to relieve an obstruction until definitive therapy can be scheduled in the postpartum period. Advantages of this procedure are that it does not require radiation and it can be done under local anesthesia or with intravenous sedation, thus avoiding general anesthesia and its related complications. It also requires less care than a percutaneous nephrostomy tube. A major disadvantage of this procedure is encrusting of the indwelling catheter, which makes it necessary to change the catheter as frequently as every 4–6 weeks.[6] The cause of the encrusting is unknown but is most likely related to the causative factors that initially lead to the formation of the kidney stone. Other disadvantages include irritative voiding symptoms, pain from the catheter itself, and urinary tract infection. Houshiar and associates recommended urine cultures every 2–4 weeks with treatment for asymptomatic bacteriuria but also reported that prophylactic antibiotics can be given in lieu of serial urine cultures.[14]

PERCUTANEOUS NEPHROSTOMY TUBE

Percutaneous nephrostomy drainage can also be done under ultrasound guidance. Advantages include rapid decompression of the obstructed kidney and percutaneous access to the urinary tract. This access provides a way to irrigate the tube to help maintain patency and can be used for antegrade radiology studies in the postpartum period, if necessary. Disadvantages include an external apparatus, which is cumbersome and will inevitably be colonized by bacteria. Obstruction of the tube by debris also makes frequent tube changes necessary. Because of these disadvantages, it is recommended that, before 22 weeks of gestation, a percutaneous nephrostomy tube be placed with conversion to an internal stent later in pregnancy but that a ureteral stent be placed after 22 weeks of gestation.[6,27] From an obstetric standpoint, the cutoff of 22 weeks appears somewhat arbitrary, and either approach could be considered, although generally favoring stent placement at later gestational ages.

URETEROSCOPY WITH LITHOTRIPSY

Ureteroscopy, a procedure involving direct visualization of the ureter for fragmentation and extraction of kidney stones, is becoming more common. Grenier and coworkers reported that the procedure should be performed at 20–34 weeks of gestation.[7] However, in the third trimester, the procedure tends to be more difficult.[11] Thinner endoscopes that obviate dilation of the urethral meatus and improved intracorporeal lithotripsy technology have made it easier to successfully access and fragment stones within the urinary tract.[6,7] Once ureteroscopic access has been achieved, laser lithotripsy can be performed safely.[11] If a stent is required, it can easily be placed at the time of the procedure.[7] Most stones can be retrieved with forceps, thus eliminating the need for indwelling stents. Stones larger than 1 cm are considered a contraindication to the use of ureteroscopy during pregnancy.[28] When fragmentation is needed, laser or pneumatic lithotripsy can be performed safely.[4] The difficulty in measuring the energy generated by the intracorporeal lithotripsy does have some researchers concerned about possible hazards to the fetus.[6] Use of the holmium laser, the pulsed-dye laser, and the pneumatic lithotriptor may be more appropriate for pregnancy. When used correctly, they deliver energy to a very localized area on the stone.[6] More data are needed before this approach can be recommended.

What's the Evidence?

Evans and Wollin summarized the recent data on the use of ureteroscopy in pregnant women.[6] Ultrasound guidance and flexible or rigid endoscopes were used in each study. In some cases, laser was needed to break up the stone before retrieval. Of the 44 patients reported, in various series 38 patients were stone free after the procedure, for a success rate of 86%. Although most studies reported no complications, two studies reported complications of fever (three patients), ureteral perforation (one patient), premature contractions (one patient), and urinary tract infection (two patients). Because of the high success rate of ureteroscopy, the procedure may become favored over the indwelling ureteral stent or percutaneous nephrostomy tube, but data at this time are limited.

Guiding Questions in Approaching the Patient

- Does the patient have a history of renal stones?
- Has the patient had a fever?
- Is hematuria present?
- Is her presentation typical for nephrolithiasis (colicky flank pain or CVA tenderness)?
- Are there peritoneal signs, making nephrolithiasis unlikely?
- Are obstetric causes for pain ruled out?

Conclusion

Nephrolithiasis occurs in fewer than 1% of pregnancies. Many physiologic changes of pregnancy may predispose to stone formation, although the incidence of nephrolithiasis during pregnancy is not significantly higher than in the nonpregnant population. Nephrolithiasis may be difficult to diagnose due to the wide differential diagnosis. The most commonly used imaging studies include abdominal radiographs, limited IVP, ultrasound of the kidney and ureter, and CT. These tests can lead to greater than 95% sensitivity for stones. Most cases can be successfully treated conservatively, with pain medication, hydration, and antiemetics. Fewer than 20% of cases require surgical intervention by percutaneous nephrostomy or ureteral stent placement. Intracorporeal lithotripsy has potential risks and is not recommended during pregnancy. Ureteroscopy has great potential for selected cases, but data on this procedure during pregnancy are limited.

Cases for Discussion

CASE 1: FLANK PAIN AND VOMITING IN PREGNANCY

A 23-year-old gravida 1, para 0 at 25 weeks of gestation presents to labor and delivery with complaints of back pain, nausea and vomiting. The pregnancy has been uncomplicated thus far. The patient reports pain that started yesterday and was intermittent and sharp in nature and started in the lower back and radiated to the groin. She also reports urinary frequency but no fever or chills. Physical examination is remarkable for a low grade fever of 99.0°F, normal fetal heart tones, rare contractions, no abdominal tenderness, and no CVA tenderness.

What testing, if any, would you recommend at this point?

Complete blood cell count, clean-catch urinalysis, blood urea nitrogen (BUN) and creatinine, and urine culture.

The complete blood cell count shows mild leukocytosis but no left shift. Urinalysis shows microscopic hematuria and a specific gravity of 1.020. BUN and creatinine levels are normal.

What is the initial management?

Admit for intravenous hydration, transabdominal and transvaginal ultrasound. Treat with antibiotics if there is positive urine culture or significant fever (≥100.4°F). Treat with antiemetics as needed.

Ultrasound examination shows mild hydronephrosis of the right kidney. A urinary stone is seen in the right ureter. The left urinary tract appears normal.

What is the next step in management?

Conservative measures are warranted in this patient. These include hydration, pain medication, and antiemetics, if necessary. Antibiotics are not indicated in this patient because there is a negative urine culture and the patient does not have a fever. The patient should be encouraged to strain all urine in an effort to collect the stone. If the stone is collected, analysis of the components can be considered. If the stone does not pass with conservative measures and the patient continues to be symptomatic with pain, a ureteral stent placement is recommended.

How should this patient be followed up?

Continue routine urine evaluation (dipstick) in the office and look specifically for hematuria. Reevaluate if there are any recurrent symptoms. If formation of a stone occurred previously, consider stent placement for the remainder of the pregnancy.

CASE 2: FLANK PAIN AND FEVER IN PREGNANCY

A 32-year-old gravida 3, para 1011 at 18 weeks of gestation presents with complaints of intermittent back pain, lower abdominal pain, and fever to 102.0°F. This pregnancy is complicated by two previous urinary tract infections for which she is using Nitrofurantoin for suppression. The pain is intermittent and sharp and has been increasing in intensity over the past 3 days. The fever has been present for the past 24 hours. Physical examination shows left costovertebral angle tenderness, maternal tachycardia, fetal tachycardia, but no discernible contractions.

What is the next step at this time?

This patient should be admitted for antibiotic therapy because she has a significant fever and likely pyelonephritis. The intermittent nature of the pain is also suspicious for a kidney stone.

What tests would you order at this point?

Complete blood cell count, clean-catch urinalysis, BUN and creatinine, urine culture, and transabdominal and transvaginal ultrasound.

The complete blood cell count shows a high white blood cell count with left shift. Urinalysis shows microscopic hematuria and is positive for nitrites leukocytes. BUN and creatinine levels are normal. Ultrasound examination shows significant hydronephrosis of the left kidney, minimal hydronephrosis of the right, and a kidney stone in the left ureter.

What would you recommend for initial management?

This patient needs conservative management and therapy for the coexistent pyelonephritis. However, because of the significant hydronephrosis, a percutaneous nephrostomy tube may be necessary if creatine levels increase.

How should this patient be followed?

The fever, costovertebral angle tenderness, and infected urine are characteristic of pyelonephritis and there is also a stone present. This patient should be treated with antibiotics (see Chap. 13, Pyelonephritis in Pregnancy) and be placed on prophylactic antibiotics to cover the organism identified in the urine. The urine should also be strained for stones. When discharged from the hospital, the patient should continue urine testing (dipstick) in the office and reevaluation for any sign or symptom of recurrence. If repeated stone formation occurs, consider percutaneous nephrostomy tube and/or ureteral stent placement for the remainder of the pregnancy.

REFERENCES

1 Biyani CS, Joyce AD. Urolithiasis in pregnancy. I: pathophysiology, fetal considerations and diagnosis. *BJU Int* 1999;89:811.

2 Marlow RA. Nephrolithiasis in pregnancy. *Am Fam Phys* 1989;40:185.

3 Butler EL, Cox SM, Eberts EG, et al. Symptomatic nephrolithiasis complicating pregnancy. *Obstet Gynecol* 2000;96:753.

4 Gorton E, Whitfield HN. Renal calculi in pregnancy. *Br J Urol* 1997;80(suppl 1):4.

5 Lewis DF, Robichaux AG, Jaekle, RK, et al. Urolithiasis in pregnancy: diagnosis, management and pregnancy outcome. *J Reprod Med* 2003;48:28.

6 Evans HJ, Wollin TA. The management of urinary calculi in pregnancy. *Curr Opin Urol* 2001;11:379.

7 Grenier N, Pariente JL, Trillaud H, et al. Dilatation of the collecting system during pregnancy: physiologic vs obstructive dilatation. *Eur Radiol* 2000;10:271.

8 Cunningham FG, Gant NF, Leveno KJ, et al. *Williams Obstetrics*, 21st ed. New York: McGraw-Hill, 2001.

9 Andreoli TE, Bennett JC, Carpenter CC, et al. *Cecil Essentials of Medicine*, 3rd ed. Philadelphia: W.B. Saunders/Harcourt Brace Jovanovich, 1993.

10 Walsh PC, Retik AB, Vaughan D, et al. *Campbells Urology*, 8th ed. Philadelphia: W.B. Saunders, 2002.

11 Loughlin KR, Kerr LA. The current management of urolithiasis during pregnancy. *Urol Clin North Am* 2002;29:701.

12 Rose BD. Nephrolithiasis during pregnancy. UpToDate version 11.1.

13 Boridy IC, Maklad N, Sandler CM. Suspected urolithiasis in pregnant women: imaging algorithm and literature review. *AJR* 1996;167:869.

14 Houshiar AM, Ercole CJ. Urinary calculi during pregnancy: when are they cause for concern? *Postgrad Med* 1996;100:131.

15 Swanson SK, Heilman RL, Eversman WG. Urinary tract stones in pregnancy. *Surg Clin North Am* 1995;75:123.

16 Dafnis E, Sabatini S. The effect of pregnancy on renal function: physiology and pathophysiology. *Am J Med Sci* 1992;303:184.

17 Stothers L, Lee LM. Renal colic in pregnancy. *J Urol* 1992;148: 1383–1387.

18 *ACOG Committee Opinion #158: Guidelines for Diagnostic Imaging During Pregnancy: 2003 Compendium of Selected Publication.* Washington, DC: American College of Obstetrics and Gynecology, 2003; p. 34.

19 Ellenbogen PH, Schelble FW, Talner LB, et al. Sensitivity of gray scale ultrasound in detecting urinary tract obstruction. *AJR* 1978;130:731.

20 Butler EL, Cox SM, Eberts EG. Symptomatic nephrolithiasis complicating pregnancy. *Obstet Gynecol* 2000;96:753.

21 Hertzberg BS, Carroll BA, Bowie JD, et al. Doppler assessment of maternal kidneys: analysis on intrarenal resistivity indexes in normal pregnancy and physiologic pelvocaliectasis. *Radiology* 1993;186:689.

22 Drago JR, Rohner TJ, Chez RA. Management of urinary calculi in pregnancy. *Urology* 1982;20:578.

23 Klein EA: Urologic problems of pregnancy. *Obstet Gynecol Surv* 1984;39:605.

24 Waltzer WC. The urinary tract in pregnancy. *J Urol* 1981;125:271.

25 Smith RC, Rosenfield AT, Choe KA, et al. Acute flank pain: comparison of non-contrast-enhanced CT and intravenous urography. *Radiology* 1995;194:789.

26 Murthy LN. Urinary tract obstruction during pregnancy: recent developments in imaging. *Br J Urol* 1997;80:1.

27 Denstedt JD, Razvi H. Management of urinary calculi during pregnancy. *J Urol* 1992;148:1072.

28 Biyani CS, Joyce AD. Urolithiasis in pregnancy. II: management. *BJU Int* 2002;89:819.

Management of Acute Pyelonephritis in Pregnancy

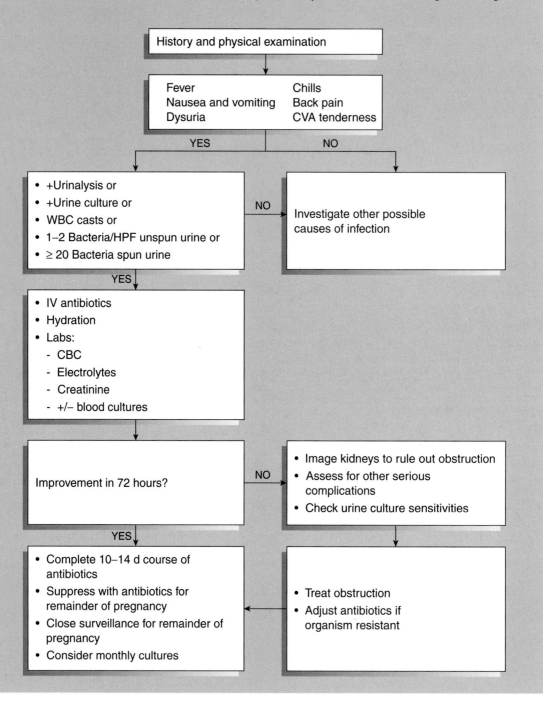

13 Pyelonephritis in Pregnancy

Barbara M. O'Brien

Introduction

Acute pyelonephritis is the one of the most common serious medical conditions that complicates pregnancy. Occurring in approximately 1–2% of all pregnancies, acute pyelonephritis can result in significant maternal and neonatal morbidity and mortality. Pyelonephritis is the leading cause of antepartum nonobstetric hospitalizations each year, affecting approximately 100,000 women per year in the United States alone. It is estimated that 80% of cases occur in the antepartum period and 20% occur in the postpartum period. The incidence of pyelonephritis depends on the prevalence of asymptomatic bacteriuria (ASB) and whether women with ASB are treated. The incidence of acute pyelonephritis has decreased since the introduction of screening for ASB in early pregnancy.

This chapter focuses on pyelonephritis, but because of the overlap in symptoms and the ascending nature of infections of the urinary tract, it is important to differentiate ASB, urinary tract infections (UTIs), cystitis, and pyelonephritis. UTIs are defined as the establishment and multiplication of microorganisms within the urinary tract. Cystitis is a symptomatic, significant bacteriuria associated with an infection of the uroepithelium of the bladder in the absence of systemic symptoms. ASB, by definition, is present when a urine culture shows 100,000 colony-forming units (CFU) of an organism in an asymptomatic patient. An acute episode of pyelonephritis is a symptomatic, significant bacteriuria with systemic illness and associated inflammation of the renal parenchyma, calices, and pelvis.

KEY POINT

Pyelonephritis occurs in 1–2% of all pregnancies, and can result in significant maternal and neonatal morbidity.

Physiologic Changes of the Urinary Tract During Pregnancy

It is essential to understand the normal changes that occur in the urinary tract during pregnancy to fully comprehend the development and course of bacteriuria. The urinary tract accommodates morphologically and physiologically to the increased demands of pregnancy. Mechanical and hormonal factors account for the changes seen. Pregnancy is associated with the presence and persistence of bacteriuria and the development of symptomatic infection. Nonpregnant women are not as inclined to develop symptomatic infections.

During pregnancy, the kidney grows approximately 1–1.5 cm and increases in weight.[1] Renal plasma flow increases by 50% by the time of delivery. There is also hyperplasia of the renal calyceal musculature, which confers an increased capacity. The renal collecting system shows the greatest physiologic change. Dilation of the renal pelvis and hydroureter can be seen as early as the seventh gestational week; these structures return to their normal state on average by 2 months postpartum. The ureter changes by becoming a hydroureter, i.e., it increases in diameter, becomes hypomobile, and exhibits hypotonicity of the muscular layers. Edema and hypertrophy of the musculature are seen frequently in the second trimester but can start in the first trimester. Up to 90% of pregnant women exhibit this edema, and hypertrophy of the ureter and hydroureter is most commonly seen on the right side of the pelvis. This may be secondary to simple mechanical uterine dextrorotation, the effect of the sigmoid along the left ureter, or compression from the ovarian and iliac vessels crossing the right ureter at right angles.[2] The maximum increase in the hydroureter is seen in the sixth month of pregnancy. The hydroureter retains 50–200 mL of urine.

Another factor in the etiology of hydroureter in pregnancy is hormonal changes. Progesterone is thought to affect the ureteral musculature and cause hypotony through its mediation on smooth muscle relaxation. Hormonal stimulation also has an effect on the urothelium. The urothelium is congested by hyperplasia and an increase in vascularization. Vesical tone decreases and this in turn causes an increase in vesical capacity. The decrease in vesical tone is also thought to be secondary to progesterone, causing muscle relaxation. There is also a relative change in bladder position, with the bladder becoming more of an abdominal rather than a pelvic organ.[1] Pregnancy-related increases in glomerular filtration rates result in glucosuria and aminoaciduria, which provide an excellent proliferation medium for bacteria and thus contribute to the bacteriuria seen in pregnancy.[3]

The large amount of urine output in pregnancy produces what has been referred to as a "washout effect," with an important role in the maintenance of bladder sterility. The urinary tract also secretes its own immunoglobulins (IgA and IgG) that serve as a mechanism of defense. Immunoglobulin A is secreted by the posterior urethra and the vesical wall. It acts to impede bacterial adherence and aid in the prevention of bacterial growth in the urinary tract. The urolethium is lined by glycosaminoglycans, which make the surface of the mucosa inappropriate for bacterial adherence. Other urinary products such as urea and mucoproteins also inhibit bacterial proliferation.

Risk Factors and Significance of Bacteriuria in Pregnancy

KEY POINT

Approximately 5–10% of pregnant women have asymptomatic bacteruria.

KEY POINT

A large percentage of cases of acute pyelonephritis occur in pregnant women with ASB.

ASB is defined as a urine culture with a single isolate of more than 100,000 CFU of a uropathogen without the patient presenting with symptoms. Approximately 5–10% of pregnant women have ASB. Approximately 33–66% of cases of acute pyelonephritis occur in pregnant women with preexisting ASB. Risk factors for ASB are important because 20–40% of cases of untreated ASB are associated with the development of acute pyelonephritis during pregnancy; risk factors for ASB are therefore risk factors for pyelonephritis. Risk factors for ASB include sexual activity, advancing age, parity, low socioeconomic status, sickle cell disease or trait (with associated renal parenchymal damage),[4] a history of UTI, diabetes mellitus, paralysis from spinal cord injury, and functional or anatomic abnormalities in the nonpregnant and pregnant state. The shortness of the female urethra, which is 3–4 cm long, and its proximity to the vagina contribute to the predisposition toward bacteriuria. The urethra is commonly colonized with microbes from the gastrointestinal tract, and bacteriuria is usually a result of this colonization as opposed to being acquired as a new organism during the pregnancy.[5] Pastore and coworkers reported that the presence of UTIs before 20 weeks of gestation or a history of UTI before pregnancy posed at least a twofold increased risk of symptomatic UTI during pregnancy.[6]

Swapp and associates reported that acute pyelonephritis developed in approximately 14% of pregnant patients with untreated bacteriuria and found that postpartum UTIs were also more common in patients with bacteriuria in pregnancy.[7]

In a meta-analysis of this topic, Romero and colleagues found a 50% decrease in the risk of preterm delivery and greater than 30% lower risk of low-birth-weight infants in nonbacteriuric patients compared with bacteriuric patients.[8] This difference in risk has led the American College of Obstetricians and Gynecologists to recommend routine screening for ASB in early pregnancy.[9] Since the initiation of routine screening and therapy for ASB, a decrease in the incidence of pyelonephritis from 4% to 0.8% has been demonstrated.[10–12] If ASB is identified and treated, the rate of persistent bacteriuria also decreases, from 86% to 11%.[11,12] Although ascending infection is the most common route of developing pyelonephritis, in rare cases, the etiology can be hematogenous spread in the presence of systemic infection or renal lesions.

An important part of the first prenatal visit consists of screening for ASB and pyuria by using a urine culture and an office dipstick. Other tests, such as a urinalysis, Gram stain of centrifuged urine, evaluation of leukocyte esterase, and the nitrite test, can also be used for screening if a patient complains of symptoms later in the pregnancy. However, ASB is defined by urine culture results, so a urine culture is recommended in early pregnancy. The diagnosis is based on a positive culture from urine collected midstream or by a catheter. Although urine cultures are expensive and time consuming, they remain the gold standard screening tool.[11]

The most common pathogens responsible for ASB, cystitis, and pyelonephritis are similar. *Escherichia coli* is found in 75–80% of infected pregnant patients. Wing and colleagues identified *E. coli* in 79% of urine cultures and 77% of blood cultures from women with pyelonephritis.[13] In addition, susceptibility testing demonstrated 46% resistance to ampicillin. The incidence of *E. coli* was lower (~50%) in patients with nosocomial infection who underwent instrumentation. Other pathogens, such as *Klebsiella*, *Proteus*, and *Enterococcus*, are more likely to be present in this group.[2]

The significance of low colony counts (i.e., $<10^5$ organisms/mL) of gram-positive organisms isolated from asymptomatic pregnant patients is uncertain. However, symptomatic UTIs have been reported with low colony counts of many gram-positive isolates.[5] Gram-positive bacteria have also been associated with urinary tract pathology other than infection, such as stone formation, especially coagulase-negative staphylococcus. Other pathogens that have been isolated in urinary tract infections, often in low concentrations, are *Gardnerella vaginalis*, lactobacilli, *Chlamydia trachomatis*, and *Ureaplasma urealyticum*.[11] More advanced culture techniques are required to isolate these organisms. Although clinically improved outcomes have been reported with treatment for *G. vaginalis* and *U. urealyticum*, their pathogenic potential remains unclear.[11]

Diagnosis

KEY POINT

Diagnosis of pyelonephritis depends on clinical findings, urinalysis, and urine culture.

Cystitis typically presents with symptoms of dysuria, urgency, frequency, hematuria, retropubic discomfort, and pressure. In contrast, clinical signs and symptoms of acute pyelonephritis include fever, shaking chills, flank pain, nausea and vomiting, costovertebral (CVA) tenderness, and symptoms of dysuria and frequency. Shaking chills, nausea, vomiting, migraine, myalgias, and signs and symptoms of UTIs are present in approximately 50% of cases. The release of endotoxins in a small minority of cases can lead to the development of sepsis. The diagnosis of pyelonephritis is confirmed by urine culture obtained by midstream collection or by catheterization. White blood cell casts also confirm the diagnosis. One to two bacteria per high-power field on an unspun catheterized specimen or greater than or equal to 20 bacteria per high-power field on a spun specimen are closely correlated with more than 100,000 CFU/mL bacteria on urine culture.[14]

In addition to urinalysis and urine culture, a complete blood cell count and a serum chemistry evaluation should be obtained. Evidence of hemolysis may lead to increased lactate dehydrogenase. Electrolyte abnormalities are also common. A decrease in creatinine clearance by at least 50% can also be seen,[14] but in the setting of acute pyelonephritis, renal insufficiency is usually transient.

Blood cultures may be positive in up to 15% of cases. Blood cultures are recommended if the patient appears septic or has a fever above 39°C. Data from three randomized trials on the clinical utility of urine and blood cultures in the clinical management of pregnant patients with acute pyelonephritis were reviewed by

Wing and coworkers.[13] Positive blood cultures directly influenced management by prolonging the duration of hospitalization. Decisions to change antibiotic therapy were affected more by clinical course than by culture results. Because of these findings, the investigators suggested eliminating the use of urine culture and blood cultures to simplify management and result in significant cost savings without compromising patient care.

Maternal and Fetal Complications

KEY POINT

Pyelonephritis is associated with preterm delivery, and can lead to serious maternal complications.

Pyelonephritis in pregnancy has been associated with hypertensive disorders of pregnancy, diabetes mellitus, preterm rupture of the membranes, clinical or subclinical chorioamnionitis, maternal postpartum fever, and neonatal infection.[15] Studies have shown a wide variation in the incidence of premature delivery associated with pyelonephritis, ranging from 6% to 50%.[14] In one study, 10% of pregnant patients with pyelonephritis who were at 26 weeks of gestation or greater and who had an average of eight or more uterine contractions per hour delivered prematurely.[16] The strength of the association between pyelonephritis and preterm delivery and low birth weight is less clear when many confounding factors are considered, especially socioeconomic status.[17] Nevertheless, a meta-analysis reported a significant decrease in the rate of low-birth-weight infants when patients who received therapy for ASB were compared with untreated controls (15% vs. 10%).[18] Proposed theories of how pyelonephritis leads to preterm labor include microorganisms that produce arachidonic acid, phospholipase A_2, and prostaglandins that may soften the cervix and increase myometrial free calcium content.[19]

Pyelonephritis in pregnancy may lead to many serious maternal complications such as septic shock, respiratory insufficiency, acute respiratory distress syndrome (ARDS), chronic renal insufficiency, disseminated intravascular coagulation, electrolyte and fluid balance disorders, and even death. ARDS is one of the most serious complications of pyelonephritis in pregnancy. In some series, ARDS was more common in women who were treated aggressively with intravenous hydration and β-sympathomimetic tocolytic therapy.[14] In patients with pyelonephritis and sepsis, bacterial endotoxin-mediated damage can lead to altered alveolar-capillary membrane permeability, which can progress to pulmonary edema and respiratory insufficiency in 2–8% of patients.[11,20] ARDS presents with symptoms of dyspnea, tachypnea, and hypoxia, and chest radiograph shows evidence of pulmonary edema. ARDS is managed with supportive measures such as supplemental oxygen, diuresis, and, if necessary, mechanical ventilation.[14]

Septic shock is another serious complication of pyelonephritis in pregnancy. Endotoxin-mediated damage to capillary endothelium results in decreased vascular resistance and subsequent changes in cardiac output. Therapy for septic shock requires hospitalization in an intensive care unit with central monitoring, often with pulmonary artery catheterization. Maintenance of blood pressure and fluid management are essential, as are immediate initiation of antibiotics and fluid resuscitation.[14]

KEY POINT

Alterations in renal function are relatively common with pyelonephritis, but are usually transient.

Abnormalities in renal function can also be seen as a complication of pyelonephritis, with a reported incidence of approximately 25–50% in pregnancy.[11] Fortunately, this is usually transient, with resolution occurring within a few days. Maternal anemia has been reported to occur in 25–66% of pregnant patients with pyelonephritis.[11,21] Anemia is thought to be due to an endotoxin-mediated, lipopolysaccharide-induced damage of red blood cell membranes. This also resolves with eradication of the infection. Pyelonephritis recurs in about 20% of women before delivery. Thus, careful observation after treatment and suppressive antimicrobial therapy is recommended until delivery.

Treatment Regimens

Pregnant patients with pyelonephritis have traditionally been treated in the hospital. More recently, a few studies have shown effective outpatient treatment of pyelonephritis in pregnant patients who were not bacteremic.[11,22] Similar rates of persistent or recurrent bacteriuria and recurrent pyelonephritis have been observed in selected pregnant patients treated as inpatients versus outpatients.[22] However, most pregnant patients are still being treated as inpatients with intravenous antibiotics, hydration, and evaluation of renal function. Antibiotics should be selected carefully to cover the most likely pathogens.

UTIs and pyelonephritis can be effectively treated with many antibiotics, with different spectrums of coverage and duration of therapy. Most of the data regarding effectiveness of drug regimens have been extrapolated from nonpregnant women with UTIs and pyelonephritis. In general, commonly used antibiotic regimens for pyelonephritis include a cephalosporin or penicillin with an aminoglycoside because the frequency of *E. coli* resistance to ampicillin.

KEY POINT

Intravenous antibiotic therapy is continued until the patient is afebrile and improving for 48 hours. Oral antibiotics are continued to complete a 10-14 day course of therapy.

Intravenous or intramuscular antimicrobial therapy should be given until the patient is afebrile for 48 hours and is clinically improved.[23] Oral antibiotics are then continued to complete a 10- to 14-day course. Antibiotic prophylaxis is then recommended until delivery to decrease the risk of recurrent infections.[24] After 48–72 hours of antibiotic therapy, some investigators recommend a urine culture to evaluate bacterial growth. If the culture is positive with any number of colony-forming units, the antibiotic therapy is inadequate and necessitates change. A follow-up urine culture should be obtained after 2 weeks of a clinical cure. If the culture is negative, monthly surveillance cultures are reasonable until delivery.[11] Some investigators recommend an imaging study of the kidneys and ureters in the postpartum period for patients who are diagnosed with pyelonephritis during pregnancy.

Most patients improve greatly within 72 hours of treatment. If there is no remission of the initial symptoms 72 hours after initial therapy of acute pyelonephritis, an imaging study such as a renal ultrasound should be considered to rule out obstructive nephrolithiasis. One should consider pyelonephritis with a stone in patients with recurrent UTIs, persistent microscopic hematuria, obstruction of the urinary tract, or a history of diseases involving the formation of stones.

What's the Evidence?

A meta-analysis published in 2003 in the Cochrane Database analyzed the best available evidence from randomized controlled trials on which therapies were most effective for symptomatic UTIs during pregnancy. The meta-analysis evaluated cure rates, rate of recurrence, incidence of preterm delivery and preterm rupture of the membranes, admission to the neonatal intensive care unit, need for change of antibiotics, and incidence of prolonged pyrexia. Five studies were included and the main treatment comparisons were as follows:

1. Intravenous plus oral antibiotics versus intravenous only
2. Outpatient versus inpatient antibiotics

3. Intramuscular cephazolin versus intravenous ampicillin plus gentamicin
4. Intramuscular ceftriaxone versus intravenous ampicillin plus gentamicin
5. Intramuscular ceftriaxone versus intravenous cephazolin
6. Cephalosporins once-a-day versus multiple doses
7. Oral ampicillin versus oral nitrofurantoin

There were no significant differences among the different antibiotic regimens regarding cure rates, recurrent infection rates, incidence of preterm delivery, admission to the neonatal intensive care unit, need for change of antibiotic, or incidence of prolonged pyrexia. All regimens were found to achieve high cure rates, and adverse events were reported in only a few cases.

Guiding Questions in Approaching the Patient

When first evaluating a patient with suspected pyelonephritis, the following questions aid in diagnosis and management:

- Does the patient appear ill?
- Is the patient febrile?
- Does the patient have flank pain? Dysuria? Nausea? Chills?
- On physical examination, does the patient have CVA tenderness?
- What do the urinalysis and urine culture show?
- What are the complete blood cell count, serum electrolyte, and creatinine results?
- Which antibiotics cover the most common pathogens in pyelonephritis and can be used safely in pregnancy?
- Is this a recurrent infection of the urinary tract? If so, are sensitivities available from previous urine cultures?

Conclusion

Acute pyelonephritis is one of the most common medical conditions that complicates pregnancy and has serious implications for mother and fetus. Patients should be screened for asymptomatic bacteriuria at the first prenatal visit because control of ASB can significantly decrease the incidence of acute pyelonephritis. If acute pyelonephritis develops in a pregnant patient, standard therapy includes hydration and appropriate antibiotic therapy.

If the patient does not improve within 72 hours, imaging of the urinary tract is warranted to rule out an obstructive uropathy. Prompt diagnosis and management of acute pyelonephritis in pregnancy can protect the mother from serious complications and potentially prevent preterm labor and delivery.

Discussion of Cases

CASE 1: ACUTE PYELONEPHRITIS IN PREGNANCY

A 28-year-old gravida 2, para 1 at 28 weeks of gestation presents with complaints of nausea, vomiting, chills, and right-side flank pain of 3 days' duration. On examination, her temperature is 39°C, and right-side costovertebral tenderness is noted. Urinalysis shows 50 white blood cells per high-power field and 20 red blood cells per high-power field. She also reports irregular contractions but no cervical change.

What is her diagnosis?

Acute pyelonephritis.

What therapy should be initiated?

Therapy consists of ampicillin and gentamicin and intravenous hydration.

What tests should be performed?

Complete blood cell count, blood urea nitrogen, (BUN), and creatine level.

A complete blood cell count, chem-7, and levels of BUN and creatinine were checked. The white blood cell count was 30.0 and all other laboratory values were normal. A urine culture was sent, but no blood culture was taken. The patient improved clinically and remained afebrile for 48 hours and was discharged home.

How should she be managed after discharge?

The patient should receive antibiotics, nitrofurantoin every night for the remainder of the pregnancy for suppression, and urine culture.

She completed a 14-day course of antibiotics and was then placed on nitrofurantoin every night for the remainder of her pregnancy for suppression. A urine culture was checked after 2 weeks of therapy and monthly until delivery.

CASE 2: PYELONEPHRITIS WITH PERSISTANT FEVER

A 19-year-old gravida 2, para 0 at 18 weeks of gestation presents with complaints of nausea, vomiting, and dysuria with bilateral back pain for 4 days. On examination, her temperature is 38.5°C, and she has bilateral CVA tenderness.

What tests should be requested?

Urinalysis and laboratory tests. Urinalysis showed more than 100 white blood cells on microscopic examination. Her white blood cell

count was 26,000 and her creatinine level was 1.0. Her potassium level was 3.0 mEq/L.

What is the diagnosis?

Acute pyelonephritis.

She was started on ampicillin and gentamicin but remained febrile for the next 3 days.

What is your next step?

Review of the initial culture and ultrasound examination.

The initial culture was reviewed and showed an organism sensitive to ampicillin and gentamicin. Renal ultrasound identified a 5-mm stone in the right ureter with severe right-side hydronephrosis. Urology was consulted and recommended stent placement to relieve the obstruction. She improved clinically and, after the stent was placed, remained afebrile for 48 hours. She completed a 2-week course of antibiotics and was given antibiotic suppression for the remainder of her pregnancy.

REFERENCES

1 Krieger JN. Complications and treatments of urinary tract infections during pregnancy. *Urol Clin North Am* 1986;13:685–693.

2 Santos JF. Urinary tract infections in women. *Int Urogynecol J* 2002; 13:204–209.

3 Lindheimer MD. The kidney in pregnancy. *N Engl J Med* 1970;283: 1095–1097.

4 Pritchard JA, Scott DE, Whalley PJ, et al. The effects of maternal sickle cell hemoglobinopathies and sickle cell trait on reproductive performance. *Am J Obstet Gynecol* 1973;117:662–670.

5 Patterson TF, Andriole VT. Bacteriuria in pregnancy. *Infect Dis Clin North Am* 1987;1:807–822.

6 Pastore LM, Savjitz DA, Thorp JM Jr. Predictors of symptomatic urinary tract infection at the first prenatal visit. *Epidemiology* 1999;10: 282–287.

7 Swapp GH. Asymptomatic bacteriuria, birthweight, and length of gestation in a defined population. In: Brumfitt W, Asscher AW, eds. *Urinary Tract Infection.* London: Oxford University Press, 1965; pp. 92–102.

8 Romero R, Oyarzun E, Mazor M, et al. Meta-analysis of the relationship between preterm delivery/low birth weight. *Obstet Gynecol* 1989;73:576–582.

9 *Gridelines for Perinatal Case 4th ed.* Hauth JC, Merenstein GB, Eds. American Academy of Pediatrics and the American College of Obstetricians and Gynecologists, 1997; p. 75.

10 Harris RE. The significance of eradication of bacteriuria. *Obstet Gynecol* 1979;53:71–73.

11 Connolly A, Thorp JM. Urinary tract infections in pregnancy. *Urol Clin North Am* 1999;26:779–787.

12 Elder HA, Santamarina BAG, Smith S, et al. The natural history of asymptomatic bacteriuria during pregnancy: the effect of tetracycline on the clinical course and the outcome of pregnancy. *Am J Obstet Gynecol* 1971;111:441–462.

13 Wing DA, Park AS, DeBuque L, et al. Limited utility of blood and urine cultures in the treatment of acute pyelonephritis during pregnancy. *Am J Obstet Gynecol* 2000;182:1437–1440.

14 Wing DA. Pyelonephritis. *Clin Obstet Gynecol* 1998;41:515–526.

15 Vazquez JC, Villar J. Treatments for symptomatic urinary tract infections during pregnancy. *Cochrane Database Syst Rev* 2003;1.

16 Graham JM, Oshiro BT, Blanco JD, et al. Uterine contractions after antibiotic therapy for pyelonephritis in pregnancy. *Am J Obstet Gynecol* 1993;168:577–580.

17 Millar LK, Cox SM. Urinary tract infections complicating pregnancy. *Infect Dis Clin North Am* 1997;11:13–26.

18 Smaill F. Antibiotic versus no treatment for asymptomatic bacteriuria. In: *Pre-Cochrane Reviews: The Cochrane Pregnancy and Database.* Oxford: BMJ Publishing Childbirth Group, 1995.

19 McGrady GA, Daling JR, Peterson DR. Maternal urinary tract infection and adverse fetal outcomes. *Am J Epidemiol* 1985;121:377–381.

20 Cunningham FG, Lucas MJ, Hankins GDV. Pulmonary injury complicating antepartum pyelonephritis. *Am J Obstet Gynecol* 1987;156: 797–807.

21 Gilstrap LC, Leveno KJ, Cunningham FG. Renal infection and pregnancy outcome. *Am J Obstet Gynecol* 1981;141:709.

22 Millar LK, Wing DA, Paul RH, et al. Outpatient treatment of pyelonephritis in pregnancy: a randomized controlled trial. *Obstet Gynecol* 1995; 86:560–564.

23 Angel JL, O'Brien WF, Finan MA, et al. Acute pyelonephritis in pregnancy: a prospective study of oral versus intravenous antibiotic therapy. *Obstet Gynecol* 1990;76:28–32.

24 Leveno KJ, Harris Gilstrap LC, et al. Bladder versus renal bacteriuria during pregnancy: recurrence after treatment. *Am J Obstet Gynecol* 1981;139:403–406.

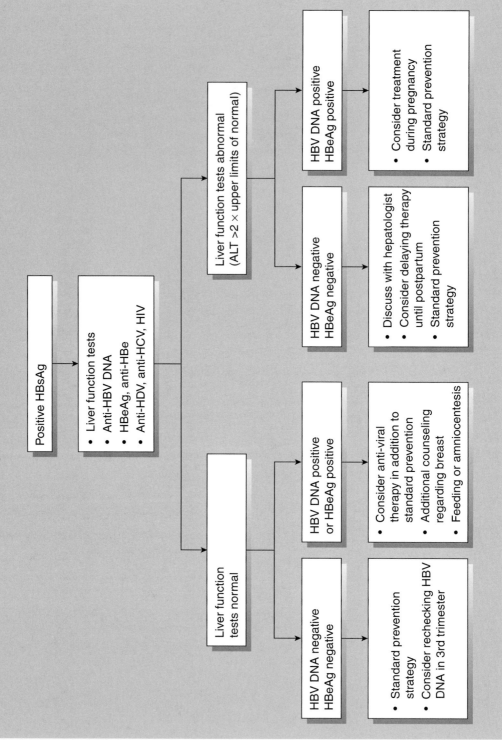

Management of Positive HBsAg

14 Hepatitis in Pregnancy

Laura Goetzl

Introduction

Hepatitis B (HBV) and hepatitis C (HCV) infections impose a significant health care burden in the United States, not only from acute hepatitis but from the sequelae of chronic infection: cirrhosis, liver failure, and hepatocellular carcinoma. Although most infections in the United States are acquired in adulthood, perinatally acquired hepatitis is more likely to result in chronic infection. Pregnancy represents a critical opportunity to identify individuals with chronic hepatitis. Women of childbearing age have reached their peak incidence for HBV and HCV, and pregnancy prompts health care utilization in young women who might not otherwise seek medical care. Therefore, it is imperative for obstetricians to understand the screening guidelines for hepatitis in pregnancy. Early identification of chronic carriers will allow for optimal treatment to prevent progression to cirrhosis and screening for hepatocellular carcinoma. In addition, identification of carriers during pregnancy allows for implementation of public health prevention strategies to prevent perinatal transmission. Studies to prevent perinatal transmission of human immunodeficiency virus (HIV) have led to substantial insights into the prevention of vertical transmission of viral infections. Further research is sorely needed to determine the optimal strategies to minimize perinatal transmission of HBV and HCV.

Hepatitis B

EPIDEMIOLOGY

Chronic hepatitis B is the most common global cause of cirrhosis and hepatocellular carcinoma.[1] Currently, it is estimated that 1.25 million individuals in the United States are infected with chronic

219

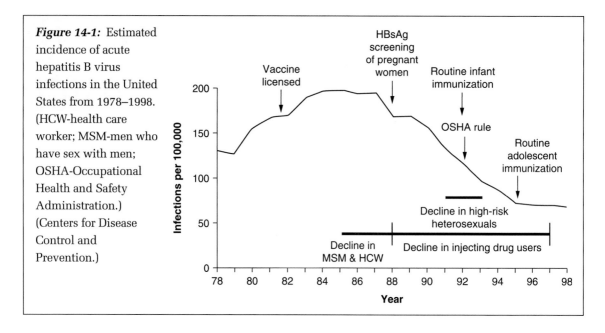

Figure 14-1: Estimated incidence of acute hepatitis B virus infections in the United States from 1978–1998. (HCW-health care worker; MSM-men who have sex with men; OSHA-Occupational Health and Safety Administration.) (Centers for Disease Control and Prevention.)

HBV.[2] The incidence of hepatitis B has decreased dramatically in the past decade due to several public health interventions, including routine infant immunizations and universal screening of pregnant women (Figure 14-1). Despite these interventions, 7,843 cases of acute HBV were reported in 2001 and the Centers for Disease Control and Prevention (CDC) has estimated that the actual number of new infections was 78,000.[3] Tragically, HBV remains the third leading cause of vaccine-preventable death after pneumococcal infections and influenza. The estimated prevalence of hepatitis B surface antigen (HBsAg) in pregnant women in the United States in unselected populations is 0.4–1.5%.[4] The CDC estimates that 20,000 infants (95% CI 15,000 to 32,000) are born to HBsAg-positive mothers each year.[2]

CLINICAL COURSE AND MANIFESTATIONS

The infectious agent for HBV is a small double-stranded DNA hepadnavirus. In adults, transmission occurs primarily after sexual or blood exposures (typically through sharing of infected needles or occupational exposure). The typical incubation period is 60–90 days. The clinical onset can be insidious, but a significant proportion of adults will develop symptoms such as nausea, vomiting, right upper quadrant pain, and jaundice; transaminases are typically high. The fatality rate for symptomatic acute hepatitis is 0.5–1%.

After an episode of acute hepatitis, approximately 2–10% of individuals will become chronically infected with HBV. Most patients will eventually undergo hepatitis B e antigen (HBeAg) seroconversion. This seroconversion is marked by loss of HBeAg, decreased HBV DNA to undetectable levels, normalization of alanine aminotransferase (ALT) levels, and substantially decreased risk of progression to cirrhosis. However, 10–40% of HBeAg-negative patients retain high levels of HBV DNA, and liver damage continues.[5] In addition, approximately 0.5% of HBsAg carriers will clear HBsAg each year. There is no evidence that pregnancy increases the mortality rate from acute HBV infection or the rate of progression to chronic disease.

DIAGNOSIS OF HBV

The most important screening test for HBV is HBsAg, which is positive in the setting of acute symptomatic HBV or chronic HBV infection. Anti-core IgM may also be helpful in confirming the diagnosis of acute infection. Chronic HBV infection is defined as HBsAg persisting longer than 6 months. Chronic HBV infection is further categorized by its attributes: (1) virologic (HBeAg negative or positive; with or without HBV DNA detectable in serum), (2) biochemical (with or without increased ALT levels), and (3) histologic status (activity and degree of liver fibrosis).[6]

PERINATAL TRANSMISSION AND PREVENTION

Perinatal transmission of HBV is extremely efficient, and, if untreated, the rate of perinatal transmission is approximately 90% in women with HBV DNA or HBeAg detectable in their serum.[7] Rates are considerably lower (10%) in women without HBeAg, and transmission is rare, but not unreported, in women without detectable HBV-DNA levels. The majority of transmission is thought to occur during labor and delivery. Perinatally acquired HBV tends to be mild and is almost always asymptomatic. Despite this indolent course, up to one third of children demonstrate significant liver fibrosis that can lead to long-term consequences.[8] Infants who become infected by perinatal transmission have a 90% risk of chronic infection, and up to 25% will die of chronic liver disease as adults.[9]

KEY POINT

Perinatal transmission of HBV is highly efficient if untreated.

KEY POINT

Universal screening with HBSAg is recommended during pregnancy.

To aid in the prevention of perinatal transmission of HBV, the American College of Obstetricians and Gynecologists and the CDC recommend universal screening of pregnant women with HBsAg in the first trimester of pregnancy.[10,11] For women who present in

KEY POINT

Ninety-five percent of perinatal HBV transmission can be prevented with neonatal administration of HBIG and HBV vaccination.

KEY POINT

In women with high viral loads, significant perinatal transmission persists despite prevention strategies.

labor with unknown HBsAg status, intrapartum screening may identify patients at risk.[12] Further, it is recommended that infants born to women who are positive for HBsAg be treated with hepatitis B immunoglobulin (HBIG) and receive the first in a series of three hepatitis B vaccines within 12 hours after birth.[11] If the entire vaccination series is completed, this regimen is 95% effective in preventing perinatal transmission.[13,14] However in the subset of infants born to highly viremic mothers, almost 30% have been reported to become persistently positive for HBsAg within 1 year.[15]

Treatment with antiviral therapy during pregnancy in patients with high viral load to potentially further decrease perinatal transmission has not been well studied. Two potential treatments have been used to successfully treat nonpregnant patients with chronic hepatitis B: interferon-α and lamivudine. Lamivudine is a pyrimidine nucleoside analog with antiviral activity against HBV and HIV that has been used extensively in pregnancy for the control of HIV. Interferon-α use in pregnancy has been reported, although not for this indication. Although it is category C, its large molecular weight prevents interferon-α from crossing the placenta into the fetus[16,17] or maternal breast milk.[18] Interferon use in pregnancy has been associated with a 22% rate of intrauterine growth restriction, but this finding may be due to the underlying disease process rather than to secondary to interferon therapy.[19] Lamivudine has been used to decrease viral load in pregnant women during pregnancy; however, although decreased viral loads were observed, vertical transmission was not universally prevented.[20,21] Although further research is needed to determine whether treatment of viremic mothers further decreases perinatal transmission, it would be reasonable to discuss the risks and benefits of lamivudine therapy (150 mg/day by mouth) at the end of the third trimester with patients with high levels of HBV DNA.

Small observational studies have not reported an increased risk of HBV transmission associated with breast feeding.[22,23] However, self-selection inevitably results in underlying differences between breast-feeding and formula-feeding cohorts, which may underestimate the risk in the breast-feeding group and overestimate the risks in the formula-feeding group. Currently it is not known whether breast feeding increases risk in women with a high viral load. The limitations of the data should be discussed with women in this category. Similarly, little is known regarding the role of amniocentesis in HBV transmission. Although rates of HBV perinatal transmission appear to be similar in women who have undergone amniocentesis, HBV DNA levels and HBeAg status may be helpful in counseling women with regard to the relative risks and benefits of prenatal diagnostic procedures.[24]

What's the Evidence?

Information regarding transmission rates and effectiveness of prevention measures is taken from prospective cohort studies and case control studies. Data on treatment of pregnant women with hepatitis are limited to case reports, small case control studies, and extrapolation from studies performed on nonpregnant patients.

PREVENTION OF HBV INFECTION AFTER KNOWN EXPOSURE

Pregnant health care workers may be exposed to needle sticks from HBsAg-positive patients during the course of their daily activities. The risks of developing clinical hepatitis after a parenteral blood exposure are 22–31% if the source is HBeAg positive and 1–6% if the source is HBeAg negative.[25] If the patient has undergone previous HBV vaccination and has anti-HBs levels of least 10 mIU/mL, no treatment for hepatitis B is necessary. In patients who have not been vaccinated or who have known low levels of anti-HBs despite vaccination, one dose of HBIG should be given (0.06 mL/kg intramuscularly) and HBV vaccination performed. HBIG and HBV vaccines are thought to be safe in pregnancy. Current HBV vaccines induce protective levels of antibody to HBsAg (anti-HBs) in 90% of adults.[26,27] The efficacy of combination of HBIG and HBV vaccination in preventing HBV after occupational exposure has not been evaluated but is thought to be higher than 75%.

KEY POINT

Vaccination and immunoglobulin for hepatitides A and B are safe in pregnancy and should be given when indicated.

MANAGEMENT OF HBV

In nonpregnant patients, the decision to treat patients without cirrhosis is generally made on the basis of (aminotransferase) ALT levels.[6] Treatment is considered in patients with increased levels of ALT. Response rates are low in patients with ALT levels less than two times the upper limit of normal; in these patients therapy is best deferred. Response rates to treatment, defined as sustained elimination of viremia, are higher that 50% in patients with ALT levels greater than five times the upper limit of normal;

in these patients therapy is recommended unless there is evidence of spontaneous loss of HBeAg after a 2- to 3-month observation period. Response rates are not as high (20–35%) in patients with ALT levels two to five times the upper limit of normal; in these patients, liver histology, age, and other health issues should be weighed in the decision to initiate treatment. In pregnant patients therapy with interferon should be deferred until after pregnancy unless high levels of HBV DNA are present. In the setting of high HBV DNA, it is reasonable to discuss the risks and benefits of interferon-α or lamivudine treatment.

Hepatitis C

EPIDEMIOLOGY

Hepatitis C is the most common blood-borne disease in the United States. Dubbed the "silent epidemic," HCV infects an estimated 1.8% of Americans (3.9 million), 74% of whom have chronic infection.[28] Although rates of transfusion-acquired HCV have decreased from 4% to 0.001% per unit due to improved testing protocols,[29] HCV infection continues to be a major public health problem. The incidence of new HCV infections cannot be determined accurately; no reliable serologic markers exist to distinguish between acute and chronic HCV infection. Similar to HBV infection, chronic HCV infection can result in serious long-term health sequelae: 7–16% of individuals progress to cirrhosis, approximately 1% develop hepatocellular carcinoma, and 1.3–3.7% die from liver-related disease.[30] The United Network for Organ Sharing reports that more than 33% of liver transplants are secondary to HCV-mediated liver failure. The prevalence of HCV in pregnant women in the United States has been reported as 2.3%, similar to the national infection rate.[31]

CLINICAL COURSE AND MANIFESTATIONS

Hepatitis C infection is caused by a single-stranded RNA virus primarily transmitted by parenteral exposures. Injection drug use currently accounts for at least 60% of HCV infections in the United States.[32] Because most patients with HCV are asymptomatic and unaware of their infection, detection depends on risk factor-based screening programs. After acute HCV infection, most individuals will progress to chronic infection (70%).[33] Younger age at infection and female sex are positive predictors of improved outcome with HCV infection. Two large studies have prospectively followed two cohorts of women infected with HCV after administration of contaminated RhoGAM.[34,35] Twenty years after infection, the rate of cirrhosis was only 1–2%, significantly lower than in an unselected population. Of note, since 1994 all RhoGAM and other immunoglobulins had to be negative for HCV RNA or include a viral inactivation procedure during production. Factors that increase the chances of progression to cirrhosis include further liver damage from ongoing alcohol consumption and other liver infections. Patients should be tested for hepatitides A and B and immunized as indicated.

Pregnancy may transiently worsen the clinical course of hepatitis C. Viral load increases over the course of pregnancy, peaking in the third trimester, whereas ALT levels generally decrease over pregnancy; both return to nonpregnant levels postpartum.[36] The rate of symptomatic cholestasis of pregnancy may be higher in women with chronic HCV.[37] There is no evidence that pregnancy worsens long-term prognosis of chronic HCV infection.[38]

DIAGNOSIS OF HCV

Antibody testing to diagnose acute HCV infection is difficult because approximately 30% of individuals with acute infection will be negative for anti-HCV; antibody may not be present for 6–16 weeks after infection.[39] Suspected acute HCV infection can be confirmed by the presence of HCV-RNA, which can detected by polymerase chain reaction (PCR) in all individuals within 1–2 weeks of infection. Chronic HCV infection is largely detected by risk factor-based screening tests. Indications for screening in adults are listed in Table 14-1. Initial screening should be performed using enzyme immunoassay, followed by recombinant immunoblot for confirmation. Viremia can be assessed with quantitative testing for HCV RNA. Diagnosis of perinatal transmission is determined by anti-HCV persisting longer than 18 months or detectable HCV-RNA after age 3–6 months.

PERINATAL TRANSMISSION AND PREVENTION

Prevention of perinatal transmission of HCV infection is limited; an effective vaccine has not been developed and anti-HCV in immunoglobulin preparations are not protective. In the absence of effective prevention measures, universal screening for HCV in pregnant women is not recommended.[32] Perinatal transmission in anti-HCV–positive women is almost universally confined to women with detectable serum HCV RNA. In this subset, rates of vertical transmission are further determined by viral load.

Table 14-1. TESTING OF ADULTS FOR HCV INFECTION

Adults who should be routinely tested for HCV infection
History of injection of illegal drugs (even once, many years previously)
Known HIV positivity
History of clotting factor concentrates before 1987
History of long-term hemodialysis
Persistently abnormal results on liver function tests
History of blood transfusion or organ transplant before July 1992
History of exposure to blood from an individual known to have HCV
History of incarceration

Adults who can be considered for HCV testing (need uncertain)
In vitro fertilization from anonymous donors
History of intranasal cocaine or other noninjectable illegal drug use
History of tattooing or body piercing
Known sexually transmitted disease or multiple partners
Steady sex partner of known HCV-positive individual
Steady sex partner of individual with history of injection drug use

HCV = hepatitis C virus; HIV = human immunodeficiency virus.

KEY POINT

Anti-HCV–positive pregnant women should be counseled on their risk of perinatal transmission based on the presence of HCV RNA in their serum.

Therefore, sensitive qualitative testing based on PCR may be useful to determine the presence of HCV RNA, followed by quantitative levels in RNA-positive women. Overall transmission rates in HCV RNA positive women are estimated at 4.3–6.2%.[40,41] Multiple studies have established that transmission rates are significantly higher in women with higher viral loads.[42–44] Although a safe cutoff for viral load has not been determined, studies have reported an increased risk of transmission at viral loads larger than 10^6 copies/mL.[45,46] Combining these two small studies, vertical transmission in the setting of a viral load larger than 10^6 was 22% (11 of 49 patients). Although higher rates of transmission have been reported in women coinfected with HIV or with concurrent injection drug use, higher viral loads in these relatively immunosuppressed subsets may explain this observation.[47,48]

The role of antiviral therapy or elective cesarean delivery in women with higher viral loads has not been adequately studied. Although most studies have not found an association between mode of delivery and risk of perinatal transmission, inadequate information regarding the proportion of cesarean delivery performed elective and level of maternal viremia limit the usefulness of these data. One small study has reported HCV transmission rates of 0% (0 of 31 patients) after elective cesarean delivery compared with a rate of 7.4% (26 of 393 patients) after vaginal delivery or emergency cesarean.[49] Although an HIV model suggests that maximum protection would result from a combination of antiviral medication and cesarean delivery for women with a persistently high viral load, further studies are needed to support this inference in HCV infections.

The role of breast feeding in perinatal transmission of HCV has not been adequately studied. As with HBV transmission, studies of breast feeding and HCV are plagued by small numbers, unknown confounders, and failure to control for maternal HCV RNA status or viral load. HCV can certainly be detected in breast milk and is more likely to be present in significant levels in the setting of high maternal viral load.[50] One small study has reported an increased risk of perinatal HCV transmission in women with HCV RNA-positive breast milk; however, because women with breast milk positive for HCV RNA are more likely to have higher serum viral loads, the independent contribution of breast feeding cannot be determined.[42] In women with high viral loads, the limitations of the data in excluding breast feeding as a possible source of infection should be discussed. Similarly, little is know regarding the risks of amniocentesis in the HCV-infected patient. Counseling should be based on the individual patient's indication for prenatal diagnosis in conjunction with data on that individual viral load. Because the sexual transmission of HCV is thought to be very low, it is not recommended that HCV-infected individuals change their sexual practices or use barrier methods with steady partners.

KEY POINT

There is insufficient evidence to determine whether breast feeding increases the risk of perinatal transmission of HBV or HCV.

PREVENTION OF HCV INFECTION AFTER KNOWN EXPOSURE

Prophylactic treatment is not available after occupational or other HCV exposures. The average conversion rate after a percutaneous needle injury from a known HCV-positive source is estimated at 1.8%.[25] Transmission in health care workers has not been reported after exposure of intact or nonintact skin to blood. Therapy with immunoglobulins or antiviral medications is not currently recommended.

TREATMENT OF HCV

Interferon-α and ribavirin have been used in the management of HCV infection. Ribavirin has been associated with teratogenicity in multiple animal experiments and is contraindicated in pregnancy. Interferon does not cross the placenta and is pregnancy category C. Traditionally, no therapy has been offered during pregnancy.

There are two potential treatment strategies that may be beneficial in pregnancy. First, in the setting of acute hepatitis C, therapy may decrease maternal progression to chronic hepatitis C. Second, in the setting of high maternal viral load, therapy may decrease the rate of perinatal transmission. Although interferon therapy to treat HCV infection in pregnancy has been described, the efficacy for these strategies has not been evaluated.[51–53] In nonpregnant patients, treatment with interferon monotherapy (3 mU three times a week for 12 weeks) is associated with an almost 30% decrease in the progression to chronic HCV infection. Therefore, because of the significant morbidity and mortality rates associated with chronic HCV infection, patients with known acute hepatitis C can be considered for a short course of interferon therapy. Similarly, in treatment-naive nonpregnant patients, Peginterferon monotherapy (1–1.5 ng/kg every other week) is associated with a 10–39% rate of sustained viral response (elimination of detectable HVC RNA from serum).[54] Therefore, in patients with high viral load, interferon therapy can be considered as an option that may decrease perinatal transmission. The success of antiviral therapy in pregnancy may be underestimated because female sex and younger age correlate with a higher likelihood of effective management.[55] However, interferon is associated with significant rate of side effects including fatigue, influenza-like symptoms, nausea, and depression. In addition, interferon therapy can be associated with infrequent neutropenia and/or thrombocytopenia, so the patient's hematologic parameters should be monitored.[56]

Hepatitis A

Although hepatitis A (HAV) is a significant contributor to acute hepatitis in pregnancy, mortality is rare and infection does not result in perinatal transmission or a chronic carrier state. The incidence of HAV in pregnancy is approximately 1 in 1000.[10] HAV is caused by an RNA virus; the primary route of transmission is oral-fecal. The average incubation period is 4 weeks, and the usual clinical manifestation is a gastroenteritis-like illness with jaundice in 70% of cases.[57] Diagnosis is confirmed by serum testing for anti-HAV IgM. Anti-HAV IgG without IgM indicates immunity. If acute infection is diagnosed, household and sexual contacts should receive HAV immunoglobulin; prophylaxis of infants born to women with acute HAV in the third trimester is reasonable. Treatment is largely supportive, and antiviral therapy is not indicated. An effective vaccine for HAV is available and is currently recommended in children. The childhood vaccination program has significantly decreased the incidence of HAV infection. In adults, vaccination is recommended for pregnant women who plan to travel to countries with endemic infection or who have chronic liver disease. The efficacy of the vaccine in adults is 94–100%.[58]

Other Causes of Hepatitis in Pregnancy

Other potential causes of infectious hepatitis in pregnancy include hepatitis E, cytomegalovirus (CMV), herpes simplex, and mononucleosis. Hepatitides D and G are mainly seen in individuals already infected with HBV and need not be considered separately. Hepatitis E is seen only rarely in the United States and is similar to HAV. Treatment is largely supportive, and no chronic carrier state results. CMV is the most common congenital infection. Although largely asymptomatic, it can cause elevations in liver function tests (Table 14-2). If suspected, the diagnosis should be confirmed with anti-CMV IgM and/or IgG seroconversion due to the potentially significant counseling implications. Herpes simplex

Table 14-2. **MOST COMMON CAUSES FOR ELEVATED LIVER FUNCTION TESTS IN PREGNANCY**

Preeclampsia/HELLP syndrome
Fatty liver of pregnancy
Vomiting (first trimester)
Gallbladder disease
Cholestasis of pregnancy
Hepatitis A
Hepatitis B ± hepatitis D
Hepatitis C
Hepatitis E
Hepatitis G
Cytomegalovirus
Mononucleosis
Herpes simplex
Autoimmune hepatitis
Drug-induced hepatitis

HELLP = hemolysis, elevated liver enzymes, and low platelets.

Table 14-3.   DRUGS ASSOCIATED WITH DRUG-INDUCED HEPATITIS COMMONLY USED IN PREGNANCY

Dihydralazine
Methyldopa
Nitrofurantoin
Phenytoin
Propylthiouracil
Amoxicillin-clavulanic acid
Erythromycin
Sulfonamides

(HSV) is a rare cause of hepatitis in pregnancy; however, only 50% of patients with HSV hepatitis manifest typical herpetic lesions.[59] Therefore, in cases of fulminant hepatitis, the diagnosis should be suspected, so that prompt antiviral therapy with acyclovir can be initiated. Although self-limited, mononucleosis in pregnancy can cause liver function test abnormalities and can be diagnosed by the presence of heterophile antibody.

Noninfectious hepatitis in pregnancy can be caused by specific drug exposures that induce autoimmune-mediated liver damage. Drug-induced hepatitis occurs predominantly in women and should be suspected as a diagnosis of exclusion.[60] Common clinical features include fever, rash, and/or eosinophilia. Drugs associated with liver disease are listed in Table 14-3. Immune- mediated liver injury typically appears within a few weeks of treatment initiation and should improve shortly after the offending agent is discontinued.

Guiding Questions in Approaching the Patient

- Does the patient have risk factors for hepatitis B or C?
- What are her liver function tests, specifically the ALT?
- What was the result of her screening HBSAg early in pregnancy?
- Has the patient started new medications associated with hepatitis?

Conclusion

Viral hepatitis remains a significant public health issue in the United States. Hepatitis B has a high perinatal transmission rate, so universal screening with HBsAg is recommended during pregnancy. Using neonatal administration of HBIG and HBV vaccinations can prevent 95% of perinatal HBV transmission. Screening for hepatitis C is based on risk factors. The risk of perinatal transmission of hepatitis C is related to the patient's viral load. There are no proven treatment strategies to decrease hepatitis C transmission. There is insufficient evidence to determine whether breast feeding significantly increases the risk of perinatal transmission of HBV or HCV. Further studies are needed to determine whether there is any role for antiviral therapy or cesarean delivery for prevention of perinatal transmission in the setting of a high viral load.

Cases for Discussion

CASE 1: POSITIVE HBSAG SCREEN

This patient's routine prenatal test returns with a positive HBsAg result.

How should this patient be evaluated?

This patient is likely to have chronic hepatitis B. The initial evaluation of this patient would include testing for markers of hepatitis B activity (HBeAg, anti-HBe, and HBV-DNA levels, and ALT) and for associated infections (HIV testing, anti-HCV, and anti-HDV) and abdominal ultrasound examination.

Tests show the patient is positive for HBeAg, negative for anti-HBe, and positive for HBV-DNA. Testing for associated infections is negative. Abdominal ultrasound in normal. ALT is mildly elevated (two times normal).

How should this patient be managed?

The patient should be informed that she has infectious hepatitis. Sexual and household contacts should be tested with HBsAg and anti-HBs and vaccinated if not immune. Sharing of needles should be avoided, as should unprotected intercourse. Alcohol intake should be limited. Vaccination should be given for HAV (2 doses 6–18 months apart). Because of the low level of ALT elevation, this patient would not be a candidate for antiviral treatment. ALT and HBV DNA levels should be rechecked in the early third trimester. A discussion of the risks and benefits of antiviral therapy should occur if HBV DNA levels remain high.

How is the patient's care during labor altered?

Care should be taken to minimize intrapartum exposure to infection. Early rupture of membranes, internal heart rate monitoring, and operative vaginal delivery should be avoided, if possible. The pediatrician caring for the newborn should be notified of the mother's HBsAg status so that the proper treatment with HBIG and HBV vaccination can be given.

CASE 2: ABNORMAL LIVER FUNCTION TESTS

A patient presents to obstetrics triage with right upper quadrant pain and elevated liver function tests.

What elements of the patient's history may be useful in determining the diagnosis?

Histories of household or sexual contacts with infectious hepatitis, injection drug use, pre-eclampsia symptoms, including headache and edema, generalized pruritus, flu-like symptoms, and recent travel.

What additional evaluation should you consider (see flow chart)?

Bilirubin, amylase, and lipase levels; right upper quadrant ultrasound; full evaluation for preeclampsia in the second or third trimester; and bile salts in the setting of pruritus.

How would you initially evaluate this patient for acute infectious hepatitis?

Measure values for anti-HAV IgM and IgG, HBsAg and anti HB-core IgM, anti-HCV and HCV RNA and consider measuring levels of anti-CMV IgM and IgG, heterophile antibody, and HSV IgM.

What is the primary therapy for viral hepatitis?

Intravenous hydration, nutritional support, appropriate consultation for acute hepatitis B or C infection, and identification, testing, and prophylaxis of contacts as appropriate.

REFERENCES

1 Lee WM. Hepatitis B virus infection. *N Engl J Med* 1997;337:1733–1745.

2 *Guidelines for Viral Hepatitis Surveillance and Case Management.* Atlanta: Centers for Disease Control and Prevention, 2002.

3 Centers for Disease Control and Prevention. Summary of notifiable diseases. *MMWR* 2001;50:1–108.

4 Dinsmoor MJ. Hepatitis in the obstetric patient. *Infect Dis Clin North Am* 1997;11:77–91.

5 Hadziyannis SJ. Hepatitis B e antigen negative chronic hepatitis B: from clinical recognition to pathogenesis and treatment. *Viral Hepat Rev* 1995;1:7–36.

6 Lok AS, McMahon BJ. Practice Guidelines Committee, American Association for the Study of Liver Diseases: chronic hepatitis B. *Hepatology* 2001;34:1125–1141.

7 Stevens CE, Neurath RA, Beasley RP, et al. HBeAg and anti-HBe detection by radioimmunoassay: correlation with vertical transmission of hepatitis B virus in Taiwan. *J Med Virol* 1979;3:237–241.

8 Bortolotti F, Jara P, Crivellaro C, et al. Outcome of chronic hepatitis B in Caucasian children during a 20-year observation period. *J Hepatol* 1998;29:184–190.

9 Beasley RP, Hwang L-Y. Epidemiology of hepatocellular carcinoma. In: Vyas GN, Dienstag JL, Hoofnagle JH, eds. *Viral Hepatitis and Liver Disease.* New York: Grune & Stratton, 1984; p. 209–224.

10 American College of Obstetricians and Gynecologists. *Viral Hepatitis in Pregnancy. Educational Bulletin No. 248.* Washington, DC, 1998.

11 Centers for Disease Control and Prevention. Hepatitis B virus: a comprehensive strategy for eliminating transmission in the United States through universal childhood vaccination: recommendations of the immunization practices advisory committee (ACIP). *MMWR* 1991;40:1–19.

12 Petermann S, Ernest JM. Intrapartum hepatitis B screening. *Am J Obstet Gynecol* 1995;173:369–374.

13 Stevens CE, Toy PT, Tong MJ, et al. Perinatal hepatitis B virus transmission in the United States: prevention by passive-active immunization. *JAMA* 1985;253:1740–1745.

14 Stevens CE, Taylor PE, Tong MJ, et al. Yeast-recombinant hepatitis B vaccine: efficacy with hepatitis B immune globulin in prevention of perinatal hepatitis B virus transmission. *JAMA* 1987;257:2612–2616.

15 Canho R del, Grosheide PM, Mazel JA, et al. Ten-year neonatal hepatitis B vaccination program, The Netherlands, 1982–1992: protective efficacy and long-term immunogenicity. *Vaccine* 1997;15:1624–1630.

16 Waysbort A, Giroux M, Mansat V, et al. Experimental study of transplacental passage of alpha interferon by two assay techniques. *Antimicrob Agents Chemother* 1993;37:1232–1237.

17 Pons JC, Lebon P, Frydman R, et al. Pharmocokinetics of interferon-alpha in pregnant women and fetoplacental passage. *Fetal Diagn Ther* 1995;10:7–10.

18 Kumar AR, Hale TW, Mock RE. Transfer of interferon alfa into human breast milk. *J Hum Lact* 2000;16:226–228.

19 Hiratsuka M, Minakami H, Koshizuka S, et al. Administration of interferon-alpha during pregnancy; effects on fetus. *J Perinat Med* 2000;28:372–376.

20 Van Nunen AB, deMan RA, Heijtink RA, et al. Lamivudine in the last 4 weeks of pregnancy to prevent perinatal transmission in highly viremic chronic hepatitis B patients. *J Hepatol* 2000;32:1040–1041.

21 Kazim SN, Wakil SM, Khan LA, et al. Vertical transmission of hepatitis B virus despite maternal lamivudine therapy. *Lancet* 2002;359:1488–1489.

22 Wang JS, Zhu QR, Wang XH. Breastfeeding does not pose any additional risk of immunoprophylaxis failure on infants of HBV carrier mothers. *Int J Clin Pract* 2003;57:100–102.

23 Hill JB, Sheffield JS, Kim MJ, et al. Risk of hepatitis B transmission in breast-fed infants of chronic hepatitis B carriers. *Obstet Gynecol* 2002;99:1049–1052.

24 Davies G, Wilson RD. Amniocentesis and women with hepatitis B, hepatitis C or human immunodeficiency virus. Society of Obstetricians and Gynaecologists of Canada Practice Guidelines. *J Obstet Gynaecol Can* 2003;25:145–148.

25 Centers for Disease Control and Prevention. Updated U.S. public health service guidelines for the management of occupational exposures to HBV, HCV, and HIV and recommendations for postexposure prophylaxis. *MMWR* 2001;50:1–42.

26 Mast EE, Mahoney FJ, Alter MJ, et al. Progress toward elimination of hepatitis B virus transmission in the United States. *Vaccine* 1998;16: S48–S51.

27 Lemon SM, Thomas DL. Vaccines to prevent viral hepatitis. *N Engl J Med* 1997;336:196–204.

28 Alter MJ, Kruszon-Moran D, Nainan OV, et al. The prevalence of hepatitis C virus infection in the United States, 1988 through 1994. *N Engl J Med* 1999;341:556–562.

29 Burns D, Minkoff H. Hepatitis C: screening in pregnancy. *Obstet Gynecol* 1999;94:1044–1048.

30 Seeff L. Natural history of chronic hepatitis C. *Hepatology* 2002;36: S35–S46.

31 Bohman VR, Stettler RW, Little B, et al. Seroprevalence and risk factors for hepatitis C virus antibody in pregnant women. *Obstet Gynecol* 1992;80:609–613.

32 Centers for Disease Control and Prevention. Recommendations for prevention and control of hepatitis C virus (HCV) Infection and HCV-related chronic disease. *MMWR* 1998;47:1–39.

33 Di Bisceglie AM, Goodman ZD, Ishak KG, et al. Long-term clinical and histopathological follow-up of chronic post-transfusion hepatitis. *Hepatology* 1991;14:969–974.

34 Kenny-Walsh E, for the Irish Hepatology Research Group. Clinical outcomes after hepatitis C infection from contaminated anti-D immune globulin. *N Eng J Med* 1999;340:1228–1233.

35 Wiese M, Berr F, Lafrenz M, et al. Low frequency of cirrhosis in a hepatitis C (genotype 1b) single-source outbreak in Germany: a 20-year multicenter study. *Hepatology* 2000;32:91–96.

36 Gervais A, Bacq Y, Bernuau J, et al. Decrease in serum ALT and increase in serum HCV RNA during pregnancy in women with chronic hepatitis C. *J Hepatol* 2000;32:293–299.

37 Paternoster DM, Fabris F, Palu G, et al. Intra-hepatic cholestasis of pregnancy in hepatitis C virus infection. *Acta Obstet Gynecol Scand* 2002;81:99–103.

38 Fontaine H, Nalpas B, Carnot F, et al. Effect of pregnancy on chronic hepatitis C: a case-control study. *Lancet* 2000;356:1328–1329.

39. Farci P, Alter HJ, Wong D, et al. A long-term study of hepatitis C virus replication in non-A, non-B hepatitis. *N Engl J Med* 1991;325:98–104.

40 Roberts E, Yeung L. Maternal–infant transmission of hepatitis C virus infection. *Hepatology* 2002;36:S106–S113.

41 Dore G, Kaldor J, McCaughan G. Systematic review of role of polymerase chain reaction in defining infectiousness among people infected with hepatitis C virus. *BMJ* 1997;315:333–337.

42 Ruiz-Extremera A, Salmeron J, Torres C, et al. Follow-up of transmission of hepatitis C to babies of human immunodeficiency virus-negative women: the role of breast-feeding in transmission. *Pediatr Infect Dis J* 2000;19:511–516.

43 Ceci O, Margiotta M, Marello F, et al. Vertical transmission of hepatitis C in a cohort of 2,447 HIV-seronegative pregnant women: a 24-month prospective study. *J Pediatr Gastroenterol Nutr* 2001;33: 570–575.

44 Thomas D, Riester K, Mofenson L, et al. Perinatal transmission of hepatitis C virus from human immunodeficiency virus type 1–infected mothers. *J Infect Dis* 1998;177:1480–1488.

45 Ohto H, Terazawa S, Sasaki N, et al. Transmission of hepatitis C virus from mothers to infants. *N Engl J Med* 1994;330:744–750.

46 Moriya T, Sasaki F, Mizui M, et al. Transmission of hepatitis C virus from mothers to infants: its frequency and risk factors revisited. *Biomed Pharmacother* 1995;49:59–64.

47 Tovo PA, Palomba E, Ferraris G, et al. Increased risk of maternal-infant hepatitis C virus transmission for women coinfected with human immunodeficiency virus type 1. Italian Study Group for HCV Infection in Children. *Clin Infect Dis* 1997;25:1121–1124.

48 Resti M, Azzari C, Galli L, et al. Maternal drug use is a preeminent risk factor for mother-to-child hepatitis c virus transmission: results from a multicenter study of 1372 mother–infant pairs. *J Infect Dis* 2002;185:567–572.

49 Gibb D, Goodall R, Dunn D, et al. Mother-to-child transmission of hepatitis C virus: evidence for preventable peripartum transmission. *Lancet* 2000;356:904–907.

50 Lin HH, Kao JH, Hsu HY, et al. Absence of infection in breast-fed infants born to hepatitis C virus–infected mothers. *J Pediatr* 1995;126: 589–591.

51 Özaslan E, Yilmaz R, Simsek H, et al. Interferon therapy for acute hepatitis C during pregnancy. *Ann Pharmacother* 2002;36:15–18.

52 Hiratsuka M, Minakami H, Koshizuka S, et al. Administration of interferon-alpha during pregnancy; effects on fetus. *J Perinat Med* 2000;28:372–376.

53 Trotter J, Zygmunt A. Conception and pregnancy during interferon-alpha therapy for chronic hepatitis C. *J Clin Gastroenterol* 2001;32: 76–78.

54 Chander G, Sulkowski MS, Jenckes MW, et al. Treatment of chronic hepatitis C: a systematic review. *Hepatology* 2002;36:S135–S144.

55 Alberti A Boccato S, Vario A, et al. Therapy of acute hepatitis C. *Hepatology* 2002;36:S195–S200.

56 Fried MW. Side effects of therapy of hepatitis C and their management. *Hepatology* 2002:36:S237–S244.

57 Lednar WM, Lemon SM, Kirkpatrick JW, et al. Frequency of illness associated with epidemic hepatitis A virus infection in adults. *Am J Epidemiol* 1985;122:226–233.

58 Centers for Disease Control and Prevention. Prevention of hepatitis A through active or passive immunization recommendations of the Advisory Committee on Immunization Practice (ACIP). *MMWR* 1999;48:1–12.

59 Kang AH, Graves CR. Herpes simplex hepatitis in pregnancy: a case report and review of the literature. *Obstet Gynecol Surv* 1999;54: 463–468.

60 Liu ZX, Kaplowitz N. Immune-mediated drug-induced liver disease. *Clin Liver Dis* 2002;6:155–174.

Assessment of Gastroenteritis

History of illness
- Symptoms: frequency of stools or vomiting, duration, fever, pain, neurologic symptoms, headache, lethargy, arthralgia
- Exposure to foodborne pathogens?
- Travel history?
- Other contacts ill?
- Animal exposure?
- Recent antibiotics or chemotherapy?
- Length of illness

Physical assessment
- Vital signs
- Hydration status: orthostatic vital signs, skin turgor, mucous membrane examination
- Abdominal tenderness or distention
- Jaundice, hepatomegaly

Initial assessment
- Severe illness?
- Dehydration, fever, >48 hrs, severe abdominal pain
- Bloody diarrhea

YES

NO

Stool evaluation
- Inflammatory cells

Therapy
- Oral fluids & electrolytes
- Intravenous fluids prn
- Diet modification
- Avoid antimotility agents

Illness continues

Illness resolves

Inflammatory cells present
Differential Dx: *Salmonella*, *Campylobacter*, *Shigella*, EHEC, *C. difficile*

No inflammatory cells
Differential Dx: *S. aureus*, *B. cereus*, ETEC, *C. perfringens*, norovirus, other causes

Further evaluation
- Routine stool cultures
- Directed stool cultures
- Stool toxin screens
- Consider empiric antibiotic therapy unless EHEC suspected

Therapy
- Continue supportive therapy and fluid replacement
- Further evaluation if illness continues

Directed therapies
- Consider specific antibiotic therapy for specific pathogen identified if illness not resolving
- Consider other diagnostic possibilities if no clear diagnosis

15 *Gastroenteritis*

Stanley J. Stys

Introduction

Acute gastroenteritis is one of the most common illnesses experienced around the world, probably second only to the common cold. Pregnant women are as vulnerable to gastroenteritis as is the general population, and, in some cases, they are particularly vulnerable to complications from an illness that is most often self-limiting and inconvenient rather than a serious health risk. Gastroenteritis usually presents with several of the following characteristics: nausea, vomiting, diarrhea, abdominal cramps, fever, chills, myalgia, and headache. The illness typically persists 24–72 hours. The economic effect worldwide is enormous, and morbidity and mortality are considerable.

The specific etiologic agent that causes gastroenteritis is often not identified because the disease is usually self-limiting without a need for therapeutic intervention. In the United States, viral gastroenteritis is more common than bacterial or protozoan etiologies. In underdeveloped countries, bacterial and protozoan causes are common, leading to significant morbidity and mortality, and are linked to poor hygiene and contaminated water. Viral gastroenteritis is commonly spread by fecal-to-oral vectors such as surface contamination, hand-to-hand transmission, and during food preparation and consumption. Some of the more serious bacterial causes of gastroenteritis are specifically food-borne and develop in clusters. Although rare, *Listeria* infection is a food-borne illness that is uniquely dangerous to pregnant women and can lead to pregnancy loss.

239

Etiology

Acute gastroenteritis in often referred to as "intestinal flu" by the public but should not be confused with influenza. Influenza is a seasonal, epidemic acute respiratory illness. The significant majority of cases of viral gastroenteritis are caused by rotavirus, norovirus, enteric adenovirus, and astrovirus.[1-4] The noroviruses predominate as the infectious agent in adults and older children; the others infect infants and young children most often. Bacteria that cause acute gastroenteritis include *Salmonella, Shigella, Campylobacter, Escherichia coli, Listeria monocytogenes, Staphylococcus aureus, Bacillus cereus,* and *Clostridium perfringens.*[1] Parasitic agents can also cause gastroenteritis, including *Cryptosporidium parvum, Cyclospora cayetanensis, Entamoeba histolytica,* and *Giardia lambia.*[1]

VIRAL GASTROENTERITIS

Viral gastroenteritis is present at all times of the year and infects all age groups. Hundreds of thousands of deaths per year are attributed worldwide to viral gastroenteritis, in particular rotavirus. In contrast, only a few hundred deaths occur annually in the United States.[2] Morbidity, even in the United States, is considerable, with thousands of hospital admissions attributed annually to rotavirus and norovirus infections. Viral gastroenteritis presents in two epidemiologic patterns: endemic disease in children, usually caused by rotavirus, and epidemic patterns in adults and older children usually associated with norovirus. Norovirus is often a food-borne infection.

ROTAVIRUS

By age 3 years, nearly all children have experienced rotavirus gastroenteritis. Reinfections are common but usually less severe. Malnourished children are particularly vulnerable. More than 100 million children are infected annually worldwide, with mortality greater than 500,000. Infection occurs less commonly in adults. Pregnant women can be exposed to the virus as a result of inadequate hygiene while changing diapers or through other fecal-to-oral pathways. Rotavirus is most prevalent in winter in temperate climates. The incubation period for rotavirus is 1–3 days; the illness persists 4–8 days. Symptoms include vomiting, watery diarrhea, and low-grade fever.[1] Treatment is supportive and is directed toward fluid and electrolyte replacement.

In general, there is no unusual risk for a pregnant woman from rotavirus.

NOROVIRUS

Noroviruses, previously known as Norwalk-like viruses, are the primary causes of epidemic viral gastroenteritis but can be the cause of endemic diarrhea.[1,3,4] Twenty million people are infected annually in the United States; unfortunately, immunity is short-lived. The incubation period is 18–72 hours. Initial symptoms can present gradually or abruptly as abdominal cramps and nausea and progress to vomiting and/or diarrhea. Diarrhea is usually moderate, with four to eight loose to watery stools daily. Generalized myalgia, malaise, and headache are prominent symptoms, with a fever of 101–102°F among 50% of patients. Despite these symptoms, most patients are not seriously ill and recover fully in 48–72 hours. Norovirus accounts for 90% of the outbreaks of gastroenteritis reported to the Centers for Disease Control and Prevention (CDC). The venues most often reported are restaurants or catered meals; long-term care facilities and hospitals; schools, day-care centers, and camps; and vacation destinations including cruise ships.

ADENOVIRUS

Enteric adenovirus infection is uncommon in adults but accounts for 3–10% of endemic gastroenteritis cases in children. The incubation period is 8–10 days; the disease persists 5–12 days and primarily infects children younger than 2 years. Transmission is usually person to person. There is no significant seasonal variation in rates of infectivity. Adenovirus has less medical and financial effects on the population than do infections caused by rotavirus or norovirus.

ASTROVIRUS

Astrovirus is the cause of endemic childhood gastroenteritis in 5–10% of cases, affects elderly and immunocompromised patients, but rarely causes epidemic gastroenteritis. The incubation period is 36–48 hours. Vomiting is less common than are diarrhea, headache, malaise, nausea, and low-grade fever. Symptoms generally persist for 3 days but can continue longer. Healthy adults experience fewer significant symptoms than do children or the elderly.

FOOD-BORNE ILLNESSES

The CDC estimates that 350 million episodes of diarrhea occur annually in the United States, with more than 20% of these from food-borne contamination. Food-borne illness leads to 5000 deaths annually and more than 300,000 hospitalizations.[5] On average each person has diarrhea one to two times per year, with a food-borne illness occurring once every 3 or 4 years.

A substantial portion of cases of food-borne diseases is caused by norovirus.[5] A wide variety of bacteria can also be transmitted as food-borne pathogens.[1] Clinicians need to distinguish the milder forms of food-borne gastroenteritis from the more pathogenic forms, for which therapies are available and appropriate.

The pathogenic mechanisms and resulting symptom complexes[1] often assist in the differential diagnosis of food-borne disease. Some pathogenic organisms make a toxin in the food. When contaminated food is consumed, symptoms occur rapidly, are often localized to the upper intestinal tract, and present as nausea and vomiting within 6–12 hours. Diarrhea can also be present in these illnesses. Gastroenteritis caused by ingestion of toxin-contaminated food is often due to *S. aureus* or *B. cereus*. *Clostridium botulinum* causes botulism also by producing toxin in food but presents with non-gastrointestinal symptoms. There are several other food-borne pathogens that produce toxins with neurologic manifestations.

Another group of pathogens produce toxin after the contaminated food has been ingested. The onset of illness occurs at least 24 hours after food ingestion. These organisms may cause watery or bloody diarrhea. A third group of bacteria cause illness by damaging the epithelial layer of the gastrointestinal tract, thus initiating watery or inflammatory diarrhea. With *L. monocytogenes*, the intestinal cell barrier is breached, leading to systemic illness, including possible fetal loss.

The CDC has suggested a scheme for differential diagnosis of food-borne disease based on timing and type of symptoms. Important historical elements in establishing a differential diagnosis are the nature of the presenting symptoms, exposure to a food that is associated with food-borne disease, and the interval between exposure and onset of symptoms.[1] The CDC presents an exhaustive list of organisms, incubation periods, food vectors, types and duration of symptoms, potential laboratory tests, and therapies for food-borne disease.[1]

EARLY ONSET GASTROENTERITIS

Ingestion of food contaminated by a preformed toxin usually leads to a quick onset (6–12 hours) of nausea, vomiting, and, sometimes, diarrhea and fever. Common organisms associated with vomiting as the presenting symptom are *S. aureus*, *B. cereus*, and noroviruses.[1]

The enterotoxin from *S. aureus* develops in foods left at room temperature after the organism has been introduced during food preparation by a carrier of the organism. The toxin develops in unrefrigerated or improperly refrigerated meats, potato and egg salads, and cream pastries.[1] Stool, vomitus, and the food can be tested for the toxin or cultured for the organism. Most diagnoses are made clinically. Treatment is supportive care; antibiotics are not indicated.

Bacillus cereus produces an enterotoxin in improperly refrigerated and cooked and fried rice and meats.[1] The illness is usually limited to 24 hours. This organism can produce a diarrheal toxin, during an incubation period of 10–16 hours, and causes abdominal cramps, watery diarrhea, and nausea. Meats, stews, gravies, and vanilla sauce are the associated foods. Laboratories can test for both toxins, although the illness is usually self-limiting, and testing is not often initiated.

Noroviruses are a common cause of food-borne illnesses. They have been associated with large outbreaks on cruise ships. Norovirus is readily transmitted by vomitus and can be transmitted in aerosol form. Food handlers transmit the virus during food preparation. Poorly cooked shellfish, contaminated ready-to-eat foods, salads, sandwiches, ice, cookies, and fruit are potential vectors.[1] There are no routine laboratory tests available for noroviruses. Therapeutic care is supportive, with a focus on fluid and electrolyte replacement to counter vomiting and large-volume watery diarrhea.

NONINFLAMMATORY DIARRHEA

Noninflammatory, watery diarrhea is a result of mucosal hypersecretion or decreased absorption of the small intestine and is not usually associated with mucosal destruction. Watery diarrhea is to be contrasted with inflammatory diarrhea, which often presents as a more severe form of diarrhea with blood or mucus, severe abdominal pain, and fever. Watery diarrhea is also a common presentation of many food-borne pathogens. Most patients with watery diarrhea develop only mild dehydration and illness.

Clostridium perfringens causes illness after ingestion of spores with subsequent production of toxin in the host. The spores germinate in meats, poultry, gravy, and dried or precooked foods.[1] The incubation period in the host is 8–16 hours, followed by watery diarrhea, nausea, and abdominal cramps; fever is rare. Reference laboratories can test for the toxin in the stool or food source. The illness is usually limited to 24–48 hours.

Enterotoxigenic *E. coli* (ETEC) is a common cause of traveler's diarrhea and also occurs in outbreaks within the United States. The incubation period is 1–3 days after ingestion of water or food contaminated with human feces.[1] Symptoms are usually watery diarrhea, abdominal cramping, and some vomiting. The illness often persists for 3–7 days. ETEC is not distinguishable from other *E. coli* on standard laboratory media.

Cryptosporidium parvum is a parasitic organism that causes persistent chronic diarrhea in immunocompromised patients and can cause large outbreaks in the general population. Symptoms appear after an incubation period of 7–28 days. The source is contaminated water, fresh produce, unpasteurized milk, or person-to-person spread. The illness persists from days to weeks. Diarrhea is the primary symptom, but fever and vomiting may be present and may be relapsing.[1]

Although most causes of watery diarrhea are associated with mild illness, cholera, caused by *Vibrio cholerae*, is an important exception that usually causes voluminous watery diarrhea. Cholera is uncommon in the United States but continues to be endemic in Asia, Latin America, and Africa. Rehydration, correction of fluid and electrolyte imbalance, and antibiotic therapy are critical for managing victims of this potentially fatal illness.

INFLAMMATORY DIARRHEA

Inflammatory diarrhea is a result of mucosal invasion, usually of the colon, by invasive cytotoxigenic bacteria with subsequent inflammation, fever, abdominal pain, myalgia, malaise, vomiting, and mucoid or bloody diarrhea. Stool specimens usually demonstrate many fecal leukocytes or markers, such as lactoferrin. Neither test is able to exclude invasive pathogens if negative. Common pathogens for inflammatory diarrhea include *Salmonella*, *Campylobacter*, *Shigella*, and enterohemorrhagic *E. coli*.[6]

There are numerous types of *Salmonella* that cause a variety of illnesses. In the United States, *Salmonella* infections usually cause diarrhea, fever, abdominal cramps, and vomiting.[1] The incubation period is 1–3 days, with the illness usually abating in 4–7 days.

KEY POINT

Inflammatory diarrhea is a result of mucosal invasion and can lead to serious sequelae.

Salmonella are found in the intestines of many animals and in eggs. Potential sources of infection include contaminated eggs, poultry, unpasteurized milk or juice, cheese, or cross-contaminated raw fruits and vegetables.[1] Infection occurs as a result of under-cooking meat and poultry products or cross-contamination of other foods during food preparation. Other infections occur as a result of contact with carriers such as pet reptiles or ducklings. *Salmonella* infects up to 4 million individuals per year in the United States. The dose of organisms needed to cause infection is smaller in patients who use antacids or H_2 blockers, medications often used by pregnant women. The diagnosis is confirmed by stool cultures; antibiotics are not usually indicated for treatment, which is supportive.

Campylobacter jejuni is another potential cause of inflammatory diarrhea.[1] This organism is also borne by food and infects more than 2 million individuals annually in the United States. The incubation period is 2–5 days after ingestion of contaminated food, under-cooked poultry, or unpasteurized milk. *Campylobacter* contaminates 70–80% of retail poultry. Stool cultures are a reliable diagnostic tool. *Campylobacter* gastroenteritis typically begins as abdominal pain and diarrhea, which is often bloody; however, the illness may begin instead as fever and malaise. The diarrheal stage of the illness is accompanied by periumbilical abdominal pain, which can be confused with appendicitis because a mild leukocytosis is common. Once diarrhea begins, it usually persists for 4–5 days. Most patients who are cultured are improveing when the culture results are reported, so antibiotics are not often needed. Erythromycin is the preferred antibiotic during pregnancy. Rare complications of *Campylobacter* infection are cholecystitis, pancreatitis, hepatitis, peritonitis, and hemolytic-uremic syndrome (HUS).

Shigella is the classic cause of dysentery in underdeveloped countries; nevertheless, there are nearly 500,000 cases in the United States annually. *Shigella* colonizes only in humans and other primates. Transmission occurs from fecal contamination of food or water. *Shigella* is acid resistant, thus allowing passage of a small inoculum through the stomach into the small intestine, where the organisms multiply. Subsequently, the much larger number of *Shigella* pass into the colon and attack the colonic cells. Symptoms include abdominal pain, mucoid, watery, or bloody diarrhea, fever, vomiting, and tenesmus. Stool frequency is typically 8–10 per day but may be as high as 100 per day. Stools are of small volume, and significant fluid loss is not usually an issue. Symptoms resolve in 4–7 days.[1] Antibiotic therapy is not usually necessary, but antibiotics do shorten shedding of *Shigella*, which may persist for 6 weeks. *Shigella* is highly contagious because ingestion of 10–100 organisms can produce disease. The diagnosis is confirmed by stool culture.[6]

Enterohemorrhagic *E. coli* (EHEC) is a pathogenic strain also known as *Shigatoxin*-producing *E. coli*. The *Shiga* toxin contributes substantially to disease complications. The most prevalent serotype in the United States is *E. coli* 0157:H7. Approximately 20,000 cases are identified annually. The clinical illness begins after an incubation period of 1–8 days after ingestion of undercooked beef, unpasteurized milk and juice, and cross-contaminated raw fruits and vegetables. The most common symptom is severe diarrhea, often bloody, in addition to abdominal pain and vomiting.[1,6] Fever is not a common symptom. Hospitalization is required in 25–50% of patients, and the mortality rate is 1–2%. HUS is the most serious complication of EHEC and is manifested by acute renal failure, microangiopathic hemolytic anemia, and thrombocytopenia. HUS most often affects children younger than 10 years[7] and is the most common cause of acute renal failure in children.

KEY POINT

HUS is a serious potential complication of EHEC infection.

Stool cultures should be screened for *E. coli* 0157:H7; often the diagnosis is confirmed initially by direct detection of *Shiga* toxin in stool. Control of EHEC gastroenteritis does not include antibiotic therapy, which potentially increases production or release of toxin. Antiperistaltic agents also increase the risk of systemic infections. Therapy for EHEC infection is supportive while monitoring for HUS. Prevention of EHEC infection is aimed at decreasing fecal soilage of meat during slaughter and processing. Meats should be cooked so that internal temperatures exceed 155°F to neutralize contamination.

Clostridium difficile is not a food-borne pathogen because it is part of normal human fecal flora, but it can cause inflammatory diarrhea.[1,6] Diarrhea from this organism is usually triggered by an overgrowth after use of antibiotics or chemotherapeutic agents. Healthy individuals are rarely affected; hospitalized patients, including pregnant patients, immunocompromised individuals, and the elderly, are susceptible to this infection. Discontinuation of the inciting antibiotic is usually sufficient to quell the diarrhea, but oral metronidazole and oral vancomycin are indicated in severe cases. Antimotility agents are dangerous in *C. difficile* diarrhea and are contraindicated.

FOOD-BORNE ILLNESSES WITH NEUROLOGIC MANIFESTATIONS

Some food-borne illnesses present with neurologic symptoms[1] rather than with gastroenteritis. These illnesses follow ingestion of improperly canned or stored foods, contaminated seafood, poisonous mushroom varieties, or chemical poisons. Patients with paresthesias, respiratory depression, and bronchospasm require immediate attention to the differential diagnosis and therapeutic interventions including hospital admission, respiratory support, and appropriate antitoxin therapy.

Botulism develops 12–72 hours after ingestion of food in which *C. botulinum* spores have germinated and produced toxin.[1,8] Symptoms include vomiting, diarrhea, cranial neuropathies including blurred vision, diplopia, dysphagia, and descending muscle weakness. The primary cause of death in patients is respiratory failure. Careful monitoring of respiratory status is critical, with prompt intubation and mechanical ventilation with early signs of respiratory failure. Botulinum antitoxin is available from state health departments and the CDC. Potential sources of botulinum toxin are home-canned foods with low acid content, improperly canned commercial foods, fermented fish, herb-infused oils, and foods held warm for extended periods.

Illness from *Ciguatera* fish toxin is associated with consumption of a variety of large reef fish such as grouper, red snapper, amberjack, and, most commonly, barracuda.[1] Abdominal pain, nausea, vomiting, and diarrhea often present within 2–6 hours, but these symptoms are followed within a few hours by paresthesias and reversal of hot and cold, pain, and weakness. Cardiovascular symptoms of bradycardia and hypotension can develop several days later.

Shellfish can contain toxins that cause diarrheal, neurotoxic or amnesic symptoms that occur within 30 minutes of ingestion. Mushroom toxins can produce gastrointestinal symptoms and neurologic symptoms, including hallucinations and confusion. Other agents cause different symptoms, most often gastrointestinal. Included are antimony, arsenic, cadmium, copper, thallium, tin, and zinc. Nitrite poisoning can cause vomiting, headache, dizziness, and loss of consciousness.

FOOD-BORNE GASTROINTESTINAL ILLNESSES WITH SYSTEMIC MANIFESTATIONS

Some food-borne illnesses present with systemic symptoms and can have significant consequences, particularly to a pregnant woman and her fetus. Hepatitis A infection has an incubation period of 15–50 days after ingestion of foods contaminated naturally, such as shellfish harvested from contaminated waters, or raw or cooked foods contaminated by infected food handlers. Symptoms include diarrhea, dark urine, jaundice and flu-like symptoms.[1] The illness persists from 2 weeks to 3 months. Most cases in pregnant patients do not result in adverse outcomes for mother or fetus. Vertical transmission is usually confined to the neonatal period in women who are still shedding virus after their children are born. Fatalities from hepatitis A infection increase with age, with rates exceeding 1% in patients older than 40 years.

Infection from *L. monocytogenes* is uncommon; approximately 1000–2000 cases are reported annually in the United States.[1,9] One third of reported cases occur in pregnant women. Although serious complications of listeriosis, including meningoencephalitis, cerebritis, and rhombencephalitis, can occur in adults and children, the unique adverse outcomes during pregnancy may contribute to identification of listeriosis in this population.

Symptoms associated with listeriosis during pregnancy are nonspecific, flu-like symptoms such as fever, myalgia, nausea, and vomiting. Symptoms begin within 48 hours after consumption of contaminated foods. Flu-like symptoms coincide with the bacteremic phase of listeria infection. Antibiotic therapy at this time can prevent fetal infection. Unfortunately, the symptom complex is nonspecific, and the opportunity to perform blood cultures and to initiate therapy is often missed. Invasive disease usually takes 2–6 weeks to develop and frequently presents as premature labor or premature rupture of membranes with signs of chorioamnionitis. Intrauterine fetal demise often occurs before the development of obstetric symptoms. Fetuses who survive birth often succumb to infection in the neonatal period. The diagnosis of listeriosis is often made only when neonatal cultures or postmortem examinations are performed.

KEY POINT

Listeriosis is often caused by eating unpasteurized milk or cheese or deli meats.

Listeriosis is linked to ingestion of fresh soft cheeses, unpasteurized milk, and ready-to-eat deli meats, or hot dogs. The organism can grow at temperatures as low as 3°C. Pregnant women should be counseled to avoid soft cheeses and unpasteurized milk. Ready-to-eat meats and hot dogs should be heated significantly before consumption. Likewise, pregnant women should be questioned about possible consumption of these foods whenever they report a flu-like illness. History of fever and other systemic symptoms should be a trigger to obtain blood cultures and to initiate antibiotic therapy if *Listeria* is cultured. Amniocentesis can provide evidence of chorioamnionitis before a positive blood culture.

What's the Evidence?

Gastroenteritis is caused by multiple organisms and is most often managed symptomatically and empirically without identification of the causative organism.[1,6] Few evidence-based therapeutic guidelines exist for the various causes of gastroenteritis. A meta-analysis has reported on 12 trials that studied the effects of antibiotic management of *Salmonella*.[10] There was no clinical benefit from antibiotic therapy in nonsevere *Salmonella* infections; moreover, adverse drug reactions and relapses were more common in groups treated with antibiotics.

Other studies have documented the effectiveness of antibiotics and *Lactobacillus* management in endemic infantile diarrhea; both treatments proved beneficial.[11,12] The effectiveness of antibiotic therapy in traveler's diarrhea, often caused by enterotoxigenic *E. coli* and *Shigella* strains, has also been demonstrated in several randomized trials.[13] A meta-analysis has been initiated to evaluate the effectiveness of preventative and therapeutic interventions for HUS, often caused by *E. coli* 0157:H7. There is no current consensus regarding prevention or treatment modalities for this serious illness.[14,15]

Clinical Recommendations

The most significant risk of gastroenteritis is dehydration caused by large-volume vomiting or diarrhea. Initial therapy should focus on fluid, electrolyte, and glucose replacement. Oral hydration is sufficient management of diarrhea of short duration.[6] In more severe dehydration, intravenous fluid, electrolyte, and glucose replacement are indicated. Oral hydration can be accomplished in mild cases simply by ingesting extra clear liquids. Patients who have more severe diarrhea with light-headedness and oliguria will benefit from oral rehydration solutions, such as Pedialyte or generic versions. The popular sweat-replacement fluids are inadequate for oral hydration in moderate to severe diarrhea. A more beneficial oral hydration fluid can be prepared by adding $1/2$ teaspoon of salt, $1/2$ teaspoon of baking soda, and 4 tablespoons of sugar to 1 L water.

Most cases of diarrhea will be mild to moderate and persist for only 1–2 days. A more thorough assessment must be made whenever diarrhea is profuse, dehydrating, bloody, or accompanied by fever.[6] A thorough history of the illness and potential vectors of infectious exposure is crucial for determining the etiology of the illness. A directed physical examination will provide data regarding the patient's status and possible causative agents.

KEY POINT

Fecal testing is warranted when inflammatory diarrhea is suspected.

Fecal testing is warranted in cases suggestive of inflammatory diarrhea. Fecal leukocytes and lactoferrin are suggestive, but not diagnostic, of inflammatory diarrhea. Stool cultures identify specific bacterial pathogens, but routine cultures will miss some pathogens. Consultation with the clinical laboratory regarding specific testing will enhance the potential for identification of the pathogen. Stool analysis for toxins is an important diagnostic pathway, particularly when the patient has been taking antibiotics or is exhibiting neurologic symptoms.

The risks and benefits of antibiotic usage for the control of infectious gastroenteritis must be carefully considered.[6] Although antibiotic treatment will be useful in shortening symptoms in some cases, many diarrheal illnesses are not benefited by antibiotic therapy. Use of antibiotics is suspected of inducing or worsening HUS in *E. coli* 0157:H7 infection. Antimotility agents may also cause adverse effects in the most serious types of inflammatory diarrhea. Antibiotic and antimotility therapies should be reserved for diarrheal illnesses in which the causative agent is documented and clear therapeutic benefits have been established.

Guiding Questions in Approaching the Patient

- What symptoms are being reported by the patient and what is the course of the illness?
- Have there been fever, myalgia, and/or neurologic symptoms?
- Are there other contacts who have developed a similar illness?

- Has the patient had contact with large groups such as day-care facilities, schools, or communal living facilities?
- Has the patient traveled to areas where untreated water is consumed?
- Does the patient have contact with animals that might be a source for infection?
- Has the patient consumed food that might be a source of infection?
- Should the illness be reported to the local or state health department or to the CDC?

Conclusion

Infectious gastroenteritis and food borne illness are as common in pregnant women as in the general population. Supportive care is usually all that is indicated. A primary goal is to prevent dehydration. Whenever diarrhea is profuse, dehydrating, bloody, or accompanied by fever, the patient should be evaluated carefully. If an inflammatory diarrhea is suspected, fecal cultures should be done. Antibiotics and antimotility agents should only be given if a specific illness is diagnosed, and benefit is likely to be gained based on prior research.

Discussion of Cases

CASE 1: NEONATAL LISTERIA SEPSIS

A 26-year-old gravida 2, para 1001, currently at 30 weeks of gestation, reports that she developed fever, chills, headache, myalgia, and sore throat 2 weeks previously. She was on vacation from her job as a sandwich maker in a small deli and sought care at an urgent care clinic. She had a group A *Streptococcus* test, a test for mononucleosis, and a urinalysis; all were reported as negative. She was asked to report any worsening of symptoms, but her illness resolved over a few days. At the current visit, she has no unusual findings. Her fundal height is an appropriate size for gestational age, and fetal heart tones are present.

What additional history or evaluation would you seek?

The patient is asked if her family or other contacts have been ill, if she has traveled recently, if she has animal exposures, and if she has eaten uncooked deli meats or soft cheeses. Her son attends day care, but the children have been well as have other contacts. She often has a meal at her place of work, usually making herself a sandwich with cold cuts.

Two weeks later the patient calls to report rupture of her membranes. Labor progresses and she delivers 8 hours after admission. The patient has a normal postpartum course, but her premature newborn begins to show signs of sepsis. Despite full efforts in the intensive care nursery, the newborn continues to deteriorate and dies on the third day of life.

What are the potential causes of the newborn's sepsis and death?

Group B *Streptococcus* and *E. coli* account for a large percentage of early onset neonatal sepsis, although a number of other organisms can cause a similar illness. The laboratory reports that the neonatal blood cultures grew *L. monocytogenes*.

What elements of the patient's history and clinical presentation are consistent with listeriosis?

The symptoms of listeriosis are often nonspecific and may be similar to those of influenza. Blood cultures are diagnostic and should be performed when a pregnant patient has fever without a clear etiology. This patient had ample exposure to suspect foods and no clear etiology of her fever and illness. Fetal and neonatal infections result from transplacental transmission and can be prevented with maternal antibiotic therapy. Pregnant women should be advised to avoid foods that increase the risk of listeriosis.

CASE 2: *E. COLI* GASTROENTERITIS

A 28-year-old woman, gravida 3, para 1011, currently at 16 weeks of gestation, calls to report that her family has been ill the past 2 days with diarrhea. What is particularly alarming to the patient is that her 4-year-old daughter has had blood in her diarrheal stools. The patient, her husband, and daughter have had severe abdominal cramps with this illness.

What additional history would you seek?

The patient is asked where she has traveled in the past few days, what foods she and her family have consumed, and if she knows of others who are ill. The patient reports that her family attended a family reunion picnic 3 days previously, where hot dogs and hamburgers were grilled by a relative. The pot luck meal also included fried chicken, salads, and snack foods. The family also has had meat loaf, eggs sunny side up, cereal, sandwiches, and pizza in recent days.

What diagnostic tests are indicated?

Bloody diarrhea suggests possible infection with a *Shiga* toxin-producing *E. coli* such as *E. coli* 0157:H7 (EHEC), *Campylobacter*, *Salmonella*, or *Shigella*. Routine stool cultures will detect common enteric pathogens such as *Campylobacter*, *Salmonella*, and *Shigella*. Most clinical laboratories require a special request to test for *E. coli* 0157:H7. Cultures should be obtained whenever *E. coli* 0157:H7 is part of the differential diagnosis.

Stool cultures obtained from family members grew *E. coli* 0157:H7.

What treatment is needed?

Management of *E. coli* 0157:H7 is supportive. Oral or intravenous hydration is important, particularly to decrease the effects of volume depletion on the kidneys. Hospitalization should

be considered for patients who appear ill. Antibiotic therapy is controversial and may even be harmful. Antibiotics may lead to the release of toxin as *E. coli* organisms are killed. The toxin is absorbed systemically and may increase the risk of HUS. Antimotility agents should also be avoided. Delayed clearance of pathogens allows for increased time for absorption of toxins and increases the risk and severity of HUS. Careful monitoring of patients infected by *E. coli* 0157:H7, especially children, is crucial to identify early signs and symptoms of HUS or other complications such as thrombotic thrombocytopenic purpura.

REFERENCES

1 Diagnosis and management of foodborne illnesses: a primer for physicians. *MMWR* 2001;50(RR-2):1–69.

2 Blacklow NR, Greenberg HB. Viral gastroenteritis. *N Engl J Med* 1991; 325:252–264.

3 Hedberg CW, Osterholm MT. Outbreaks of foodborne and waterborne viral gastroenteritis. *Clin Microbiol Rev* 1993;6:199–210.

4 Norwalk-like viral gastroenteritis in U.S. Army trainees—Texas, 1998. *MMWR* 1999;48(11):225–227.

5 Mead PS, Slutsker L, Dietz V, et al. Food-related illness and death in the United States. *Emerg Infect Dis* 1999;5:607–625.

6 Guerrant RL, Van Gilder T, Steiner TS, et al. Practice guidelines for the management of infectious diarrhea. *Clin Infect Dis* 2001;32: 331–350.

7 Wong CS, Jelacic S, Habeeb RL, et al. The risk of the hemolytic-uremic syndrome after antibiotic treatment of *Escherichia coli* 0157:H7 infections. *N Engl J Med* 2000;342:1930–1936.

8 Shapiro RL, Hatheway C, Swerdlow DL. Botulism in the United States: a clinical and epidemiologic review. *Ann Intern Med* 1998;129: 221–228.

9 Silver HM. Listeriosis during pregnancy. *Obstet Gynecol Surv* 1998; 53:737–740.

10 Sirinavin S, Garner P. Antibiotics for treating salmonella gut infections. *Cochrane Database Syst Rev* 2003;3.

11 Thoren A, Wolde-Mariam T, Stintzing G, et al. Antibiotics in the treatment of gastroenteritis caused by enteropathotic *Escherichia coli*. *J Infect Dis* 1980;141:27–31.

12 Lactobacillus is safe and effective for treating children with acute infectious diarrhea. *ACP J Club* 2002;137(3):96.

13 DuPont HL, Ericsson CD, Reves RR, et al. Antimicrobial therapy for travelers' diarrhea. *Rev Infect Dis* 1986;8(suppl 2):S217–S222.

14 Elliott E, Ridley G, Craig J, et al. Interventions for preventing haemolytic uraemic syndrome/thrombotic thrombocytopenic purpura. *Cochrane Database Syst Rev* 2003;3.

15 Elliott E, Ridley G, Hodson E, et al. Interventions for established haemolytic uraemic syndrome/thrombotic thrombocytopenic purpura. *Cochrane Database Syst Rev* 2003;3.

Management of IBD Flare

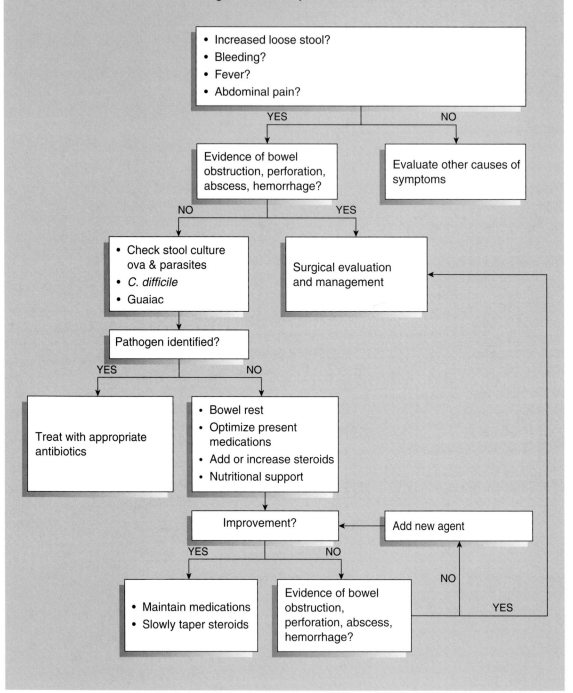

- Increased loose stool?
- Bleeding?
- Fever?
- Abdominal pain?

YES → Evidence of bowel obstruction, perforation, abscess, hemorrhage?

NO → Evaluate other causes of symptoms

NO →
- Check stool culture ova & parasites
- *C. difficile*
- Guaiac

YES → Surgical evaluation and management

Pathogen identified?

YES → Treat with appropriate antibiotics

NO →
- Bowel rest
- Optimize present medications
- Add or increase steroids
- Nutritional support

Improvement?

Add new agent

YES →
- Maintain medications
- Slowly taper steroids

NO → Evidence of bowel obstruction, perforation, abscess, hemorrhage?

NO / YES

16 Inflammatory Bowel Disease

Dorothy Beazley

Introduction

Inflammatory bowel disease (IBD) is a chronic, idiopathic disorder of the gastrointestinal tract. The two main types of IBD are Crohn's disease and ulcerative colitis. These two entities share clinical and epidemiologic characteristics and are managed similarly. IBD is associated with patterns of relapse and remission. The peak age of onset occurs in adolescence and early adulthood, so most women with IBD are of childbearing age. The activity of disease at conception is important for determining pregnancy outcome. Most women will have a normal pregnancy outcome, although recent studies have suggested that there are increased risks of preterm birth and low birth weight independent of disease activity. Most medications used to control IBD are safe during pregnancy. This chapter focuses on the etiology and pathophysiology of IBD, the effect of the disease on pregnancy, the effect of pregnancy on the disease, delivery issues, and methods of treatment.

The combined prevalence of ulcerative colitis and Crohn's disease in the United States is approximately 200–300 cases per 100,000 population. IBD is more common in Caucasian populations, with a north-to-south gradient. The cause is not known, but there is strong evidence from twin studies, familial risk data, and segregation analysis that IBD, especially Crohn's disease, has a genetic component. There is an increased risk of IBD among Ashkenazi Jews and monozygotic twin pairs and it is seen in family clusters. IBD has been linked to chromosomes 16, 12, 7, 3, and 1, and various human leukocyte antigen alleles may also play a role.[1] Approximately 10% of patients with ulcerative colitis or Crohn's disease have a first-degree relative with IBD. First-degree relatives of patients with Crohn's disease have a 5.2% risk of developing the disease, whereas the risk is 1.6% with ulcerative colitis. This risk is higher in Jewish families (7.8% vs. 4.5%, respectively). If both parents have IBD, the risk of recurrence in offspring is estimated at 37%.[2] However, inheritance of IBD does not follow simple Mendelian genetics. It is considered a complex genetic trait; immunologic, infectious, and environmental factors cause dysregulated intestinal mucosal function in genetically predisposed individuals.[3]

Diagnosis

IBD should be suspected when patients present with prolonged diarrhea or bloody diarrhea, persistent perianal sepsis, or abdominal pain. Atypical presentations also occur, such as fever of unknown origin, liver abnormalities, malabsorption syndromes, intermittent intestinal obstruction, and fistula formation. The early symptoms of disease may be mild and nonspecific. Crohn's disease and ulcerative colitis share several extraintestinal manifestations of the skin, eyes, and joints that are related to inflammatory disease activity. The diagnosis is made by radiologic, endoscopic, and pathologic findings. Several autoantibodies have been detected in patients with IBD, such as atypical perinuclear antineutrophil cytoplasmic antibodies, anti–*Saccharomyces cerevisiae* antibodies, anti-goblet cell autoantibodies, anti-colon autoantibodies, and anti-pancreatic autoantibodies. Some of these may be prove useful in the differential diagnosis and management of patients with IBD.

ULCERATIVE COLITIS   The major symptoms of ulcerative colitis are diarrhea, rectal bleeding, tenesmus, passage of mucous, and abdominal pain. Diarrhea may be nocturnal and/or postprandial. Severe cramping and abdominal pain occur with severe attacks of the disease. Other symptoms include anorexia, nausea, vomiting, fever, and weight loss. Ulcerative colitis is characterized by nonspecific, superficial inflammation of the mucosa of the rectum and colon. The rectum is involved in 95% of cases. Ulcerative colitis usually extends proximally from the rectum in a continuous, uniform distribution without intervening areas of normal mucosa. The layers beneath the mucosa are not typically involved. Recurrent inflammation may lead to fibrosis, longitudinal retraction, and loss of the normal haustral pattern that leads to the "lead pipe" appearance of the colon on barium study. Regenerating mucosa surrounded by areas of ulceration may appear as inflammatory "pseudopolyps." Patients with ulcerative colitis are also at increased risk of colon cancer related to duration and extent of disease.

Ulcerative colitis can be described as mild, moderate, or severe. Patients with disease confined to the rectum or rectosigmoid may have intermittent rectal bleeding, passage of mucus, and diarrhea with fewer than four small loose stools per day. Crampy pain, tenesmus, and constipation are common, but severe abdominal pain, profuse bleeding, fever, and weight loss are not part of mild disease. Moderate disease is characterized by inflammation that extends to the splenic flexure. Clinically, patients have frequent loose, bloody stools (four to six per day), mild anemia, abdominal pain, and low-grade fever. Nutrition is usually adequate. Severe disease is defined by extensive colonic, involvement often to the cecum, more than six loose stools per day, severe cramping, weight loss, volume depletion, fever, and bleeding that may require blood transfusion. Patients with acute, severe toxic symptoms, such as fever, anorexia, and abdominal pain, in addition to bloody diarrhea are at risk for toxic megacolon and bowel perforation and should be admitted to the hospital.

Active disease can be associated with increased C-reactive protein, platelet count, erythrocyte sedimentation rate, and decreased hemoglobin levels. Albumin levels may also decrease rapidly in severely ill patients. Increased white blood counts can also occur. The diagnosis is based on patient history, clinical symptoms, negative stool culture for bacteria, ova and parasites, *Clostridium difficile* toxin, sigmoidoscopic findings, and biopsy specimens. In patients with severe disease, a supine film of the abdomen will show edematous and irregular colonic thickening. Toxic dilation may also be seen on plain radiograph. Barium enema, computed tomography, and magnetic resonance imaging may also be useful.

CROHN'S DISEASE

The cardinal symptom of Crohn's disease is prolonged diarrhea, with or without gross bleeding. It is more likely to cause abdominal pain and systemic symptoms such as fever and weight loss than is ulcerative colitis. Crohn's disease is characterized by chronic, transmural inflammation that extends through all layers of the intestinal wall and into the mesentery and regional lymph nodes.

As a result of serosal inflammation, the bowel wall thickens and narrows the intestinal lumen. Peritoneal fibrosis occurs, which can lead to local sepsis and abscess formation. Fistulous tracts may also form between different segments of intestine and between the intestine and various other structures such as the bladder, vagina, or skin. The site of disease influences the clinical manifestations. Unlike ulcerative colitis, Crohn's disease may affect any part of the alimentary tract but frequently affects the terminal ileum and colon. The rectum is spared in approximately 50% of cases. Crohn's disease is characterized by areas of normal bowel or "skip areas" that are interspersed between diseased segments. Mural thickening of the small bowel, mesenteric fat stranding, perianal disease, adenopathy, and granuloma formation are also characteristic. An inflammatory mass may be palpated in the right lower quadrant of the abdomen. There is also an increased risk of colon cancer and small bowel cancer with Crohn's disease.

The inflammatory process of Crohn's disease typically leads to a fibrostenotic obstructive pattern or a fistulous pattern. The site of the disease influences the clinical picture. As with ulcerative colitis, laboratory abnormalities may include a high sedimentation rate, C-reactive protein, anemia, hypoalbuminemia, and leukocytosis.

KEY POINT

As gestational age advances, the terminal ileum and appendix migrate toward the right upper quadrant. Abdominal pain in this area may be associated with flare.

What's the Evidence?

Most evidence related to IBD in pregnancy has been reported in observational and epidemiologic reports, cohort studies, and case series. There are no controlled trials of treatment in pregnancy. In addition, much of the literature does not distinguish between characteristics of disease such as the regions of bowel affected, the type of therapy administered, or complications of the disease. IBD first diagnosed in pregnancy is rare, so this entity is poorly studied.

Fertility

Early studies on IBD in pregnancy have suggested decreased rates of fertility. However, many of the studies did not take into account patient choice about pregnancy.[4] Recent studies have suggested that the fertility rate among women with ulcerative colitis is probably normal because infertility rates are the same as those among the general population, i.e., approximately 8–10%.[5,6] Among women who have had surgery, the infertility rate is somewhat decreased, presumably due to adhesion formation.[7,8] Impaired fertility is also more likely with active Crohn's disease.[9] Control of Crohn's disease restores normal fertility.

Factors that influence fertility include ileal inflammation, which may cause adhesions of the tubes and ovaries, perianal disease, which may result in dyspareunia and decreased libido, and the systemic effects of inflammation such as fever, abdominal pain, and malnutrition. Relationship difficulties, body image problems, fear of pregnancy, and inappropriate medical advice may also contribute to a decision to not have children.[10] Infertility in men can be caused by sulfasalazine but reverses when treatment is stopped.

Effect of Pregnancy on IBD

ULCERATIVE COLITIS

The course of ulcerative colitis in pregnancy is related to the activity of the disease at conception. Between 25% and 100% of patients will worsen unless drug therapy is initiated or more vigorously used.[11–14] Mogadam and coworkers found that 50% of gravidas with active disease at conception worsen or remain unchanged.[15] Conversely, 62–75% of gravidas with quiescent disease at conception remain without relapse during pregnancy.[13,15,16] Pregnancy does not seem to affect the relapse rate for patients with ulcerative colitis. In any given year, the risk of exacerbation in a fertile woman is approximately 32% compared with 34% in pregnancy.[17]

KEY POINT

The course of IBD in pregnancy is related to disease activity at the time of conception.

The early literature suggested that disease tends to flare during the first trimester, but this effect was observed before the recommendation to continue pharmacologic therapy during pregnancy. Pregnancy has also been reported to decrease disease activity or induce clinical remission.[17] Termination of pregnancy has not been shown to reverse the course of disease. Postpartum relapse is not common.[6,12]

Ulcerative colitis first diagnosed during pregnancy is rare. Several case series have described it as extremely severe and potentially lethal.[11,13,18] Colitis that requires emergency colectomy has been reported in pregnancy.[19–21] Postpartum colitis also has been reported but is rare, and in one series was described as mild in all cases.[6]

CROHN'S DISEASE

As with ulcerative colitis, the course of Crohn's disease in pregnancy depends on the level of disease activity at conception.[15] Of patients who have active disease and conceive, approximately one third will worsen, one third will improve, and one third will remain unchanged.[12] Relapse rates vary from 9% to 39%.[16,22,23] The activity of disease after pregnancy tends to be similar to that at delivery. Crohn's disease first diagnosed during pregnancy is rare.[24] Modern medical management has improved outcomes for mother and fetus.[25]

A history of childbearing may affect the natural history of Crohn's disease. In a study by Nwokolo and associates,[26] parous women had fewer resections or longer intervals between resections than did women who had no children but otherwise similar disease. The investigators suggested that this effect might be mediated through decreased immune responsiveness, through the production of relaxin, a hormone produced in pregnancy, which resulted in less fibrosis and stricture formation, or inhibition of macrophages.[26]

Effect of IBD on Pregnancy

Data on the effects of IBD on pregnancy are mixed. Early studies suggested that IBD in pregnancy carried a poor prognosis.[27,28] Other studies concluded that neither ulcerative colitis nor Crohn's disease had any unfavorable effect on the outcome of pregnancy.[6,16,18,29] In contrast, active disease at the time of conception appeared to increase the risk of complications in pregnancy. In those with active disease, complications were reported to occur in about 66% of patients.[30] Active IBD doubled the risk of spontaneous abortion[31] and increased the risk of preterm birth (<37 weeks).[4,32] Stillbirth was found to be more frequent in one study[30] but not in another.[17]

The most recent data have suggested that IBD does place the pregnancy at increased risk for adverse outcome.[6,32] These studies have demonstrated an increased risk of prematurity (<37 weeks) and low birth weight (<2500 g) among women with IBD that is independent of disease activity.[4,9,32–37] Another study has reported an increased risk of small-for-gestational-age infants and congenital malformations in babies of mothers with ulcerative colitis (7.9%) compared with gravidas with Crohn's disease (3.4%) or controls (1.7%).[38] There was no clear explanation for the increase in congenital malformations in the offspring of mothers with ulcerative colitis. In general, major birth defects are reported to occur in 2–3% of pregnancies.

First-trimester exacerbation of IBD has been associated with prematurity and multiple exacerbations with low birth weight.[32] There is no increased risk of hypertension or proteinuria with IBD.[39] If first hospitalized during pregnancy, there also appears to be an increased risk of preterm birth and intrauterine growth restriction.[17,33]

Management During Pregnancy

Women of childbearing age should be made aware of the most recent information about IBD in pregnancy. If possible, a preconception consultation with an obstetrician gynecologist or perinatologist familiar with IBD should be arranged. Otherwise, the patient should seek prenatal care as early as possible in the first trimester of pregnancy. An obstetrician or perinatologist and gastroenterologist can then follow the patient.

In general, it is recommended that women be in remission for 3 months before pregnancy. The patient's medications should be reviewed before conception, if possible, with changes made before pregnancy. Patients should be discouraged from discontinuing medications abruptly when pregnant due to possible exacerbation of disease. Depending on the medications used, they may pose less risk than a severe flare. In addition, a patient's previous IBD complications and surgeries should be reviewed and a delivery plan outlined. Patients should also be aware of the recommendation that all women of childbearing age take a multivitamin that contains folic acid 400 μg to decrease the risk of birth defects such as spina bifida and that additional folic acid (2 mg/day) is recommended if on sulfasalazine.

Pregnant women with IBD should be screened for anemia and nutritional deficiencies. There is an increased risk of vitamin D deficiency, calcium malabsorption, and malnutrition. Deficiencies of vitamin B_{12} and fat-soluble vitamins may occur after ileal resection or with ileal disease. Supplemental iron to prevent or treat iron deficiency and additional folate are recommended. A detailed ultrasound in the second trimester to assess for birth defects is prudent, as is monitoring fetal growth because of the possible increased risk of growth restriction. Antenatal fetal testing to confirm fetal well-being should also be considered for gravidas with significant or active disease and for those with growth restriction.

Weight gain and abdominal symptoms in pregnancy should be monitored. Weight loss may signal disease activity. If this occurs, the patient should be questioned about symptoms of disease including diarrhea, fever, abdominal pain, and bleeding. Moreover, vomiting, particularly after the first trimester, may signal obstruction and should be investigated thoroughly.

It should also be remembered that many normal pregnant women experience abdominal discomfort, changes in bowel habits, and reflux. The differential diagnosis of abdominal symptoms should include IBD, the pregnancy, and other organ systems. Cholelithiasis, pancreatitis, appendicitis, nephrolithiasis, abruptio placenta, chorioamnionitis, and preterm labor should be considered. Due to absorptive changes in the intestinal mucous membrane, patients with IBD have a greater incidence of cholelithiasis and nephrolithiasis. Moreover, pregnancy causes physiologic changes such as increased sedimentation rates, alkaline phosphatase levels, and lower hemoglobin and albumin levels, which can cloud the clinical picture.

Evaluation of a potential flare should include a careful history, selected laboratory tests, and assessment of clinical symptoms. A workup should include stool cultures for bacteria, ova and parasites, *C. difficile* toxin, and tests for occult blood. Empiric treatment is recommended. Pregnant women with IBD rarely need radiologic or endoscopic evaluation to confirm active disease. Radiologic and endoscopic procedures can be performed to establish the diagnosis or to define the extent or severity of disease, especially if there is an emergency or if surgery is being considered. Sigmoidoscopy with biopsy and upper endoscopy are safe, and there is no evidence that sigmoidoscopy causes preterm labor.[40–42] Colonoscopy has been performed successfully during pregnancy, but the experience is limited and fetal monitoring is recommended.

In gravidas who are sick, abdominal films can be obtained. The risks of fetal exposure to ionizing radiation should be balanced against the risks of not performing the study. In general, low doses (<5 rad) are preferred and have not been associated with adverse outcome.[43] Ultrasound is considered safe in pregnancy, and magnetic resonance imaging for diagnosis of Crohn's disease has been reported.[44] If intestinal dilation is diagnosed, nasogastric decompression and insertion of a rectal tube are recommended. Colectomy should be considered for patients with toxic megacolon (colon >6 cm in patients who appear toxic) or who do not respond to therapy in 72 hours.

KEY POINT

Pregnant women with IBD rarely need radiologic or endoscopic evaluation to confirm active disease. Evaluation of potential flare should include a careful history, stool cultures, and tests for occult blood. Empiric therapy is recommended.

KEY POINT

Indications for surgery for IBD in pregnancy are the same as those for nonpregnant patients: obstruction, perforation, abscess, and hemorrhage.

The indications for surgery for IBD in pregnancy are the same as those for nonpregnant patients and include obstruction, perforation, abscess, and hemorrhage.[46] Under these circumstances, continued medical management may further increase the risk to the mother and fetus.[46,47] Various surgical procedures have been performed in pregnancy and include proctocolectomy, subtotal colectomy with ileostomy, hemicolectomy, segmental resection, and subtotal colectomy. Primary anastomosis carries a greater risk of postoperative complications, so a temporary ileostomy is generally preferred. If surgery is required, cesarean section should be considered if the neonatal outcome after delivery is expected to be good. For example, the risk of fetal mortality in patients with fulminant ulcerative colitis that requires emergent colectomy is estimated at 50–60%.[19,46] Surgery performed in the second trimester does not appear to increase the risk of perinatal mortality.[48]

Guiding Questions in Approaching the Patient

- What was the status of the patient's disease at conception?
- Is the patient's IBD currently active, controlled, or inactive?
- Which medications have been effective in the past?
- What specific symptoms have signaled flare for the patient in the past?
- Is there any indication for surgical intervention (e.g., evidence of obstruction, perforation, abscess, or hemorrhage)?
- Does the patient have significant anemia, weight loss, or nutritional deficiency?
- Are the patient's current medications considered safe in pregnancy?

Delivery

There is no consensus about the best mode of delivery in women with IBD. However, there is a perception that vaginal delivery and episiotomy in patients with active perianal disease could be complicated by disease extension, rectovaginal fistulas, and nonhealing perineal wounds. A retrospective study reported no increased risk of active perineal disease after vaginal delivery, and cesarean section (C/S) did not prevent women with Crohn's disease from having recurrent perianal or perineal disease.[49] Further, in women with no existing perianal disease, 18%

developed active perianal disease after vaginal delivery and episiotomy.[50] Hence, the rate is higher in women with IBD. Vaginal delivery and C/S seem to be safe for patients with an ileal pouch/anal anastomosis.

Previous surgery for ulcerative colitis, including panproctocolectomy with ileostomy, need not interfere with a normal pregnancy.[51] Women with panproctocolectomy and ileal pouch/anal anastomosis also appear to do well in pregnancy.[52] Patients have a higher rate of C/S, but pregnancy does not affect anastomotic function. Patients had a lower rate of pouch-related complications during pregnancy than did those with a knock pouch or ileostomy. In addition, women with an ostomy tend to do well, although they may experience prolapse of the site.

With current management, most patients with either form of IBD who are pregnant will have a normal, uncomplicated pregnancy. It is generally believed that the chance of complications is greater in those with active disease at conception, those who relapse, or those with an initial diagnosis in pregnancy. Abscess or intestinal obstruction carries the greatest risk to the fetus.[53,54]

Treatment

KEY POINT

Active IBD is associated with poor pregnancy outcome. Appropriate medications should be continued during pregnancy and flares should be aggressively managed.

Active IBD is associated with poor outcomes during pregnancy. It is recommended that medical therapy continue throughout the pregnancy and that flares be aggressively managed. The use of the various drugs should be based on their relative safety and the extent and severity of disease. Women with severe disease should have bowel rest, nutritional support, and parental steroids.

Antidiarrheal agents may be effective for symptomatic relief but should not be used in the acutely ill patient because of the risk of precipitating toxic megacolon. They are useful in patients with diarrhea without systemic symptoms despite therapy directed at colitis. Their use should be monitored closely because increased stool frequency may indicate disease activity. Loperamide is the preferred drug because of its safety and efficacy.

5-Amniosalicylic acid (5-ASA) is a first-line medication for management of IBD. It is effective for acute treatment and long-term maintenance therapy. 5-ASA comes in oral and topical preparations (suppositories and enemas). The oral form of 5-ASA is an alternative to sulfasalazine, which has been used for more than

KEY POINT

Medication selection should be based on the drug's relative safety, previous effectiveness, and severity of disease.

50 years for the management of IBD. The metabolite of 5-ASA, *N*-acetyl-5-ASA, crosses the placenta. Most studies on the use of 5-ASA in pregnancy have been small with no control groups but have demonstrated relative safety and no increased risk of birth defects.[55–57] One prospective cohort study did find a statistically significant increased risk of preterm birth (13% vs. 5%) and decreased birth weight (3.4 vs. 3.2 kg) but no increased risk of birth defects, stillbirth, or fetal distress with a mean daily dose of 2.0 g/day.[58] Another study assessed the risks of adverse outcome in a cohort of 88 Danish pregnant women taking 5-ASA ascertained by a prescription registry over a 10-year period. The data were controlled for age, parity, and smoking status but not disease activity. The investigators found an increased risk of stillbirth and preterm birth in women with ulcerative colitis but not in those with Crohn's disease. There was no substantial increased risk of fetal malformation or growth restriction in either group. Whether the increased risk of stillbirth and preterm birth in women with ulcerative colitis is caused by disease activity, patient compliance, or other factors is not known.[59] The topical preparation of 5-ASA is presumed to be safe in pregnancy.[56]

KEY POINT

Sulfasalazine, corticosteroids, and 5-ASA are commonly used for medical management of IBD and can be used in pregnancy with relative safety.

Sulfasalazine and its metabolite, sulfapyridine, are absorbed in small amounts and cross the placenta. Sulfapyridine can displace bilirubin from plasma protein; however, it is not associated with jaundice or kernicterus. Based on several large studies, it is considered safe during pregnancy and nursing.[5,6,33,39,59,60] Sulfasalazine interferes with folate absorption, and pregnant women or those attempting to get pregnant are advised to take supplemental folic acid 2 mg/day, which is twice the recommended dose.

Corticosteroids are used for the control of moderate to severe IBD in pregnancy. Steroid foams, enemas, and parenteral forms are available. They are used when patients do not respond to other medications. The usual starting dose of prednisone is 40–60 mg/day, which is typically effective within 10–14 days. Because there is no evidence that chronic steroid therapy maintains remission, a slow taper is usually instituted (5 mg/week). Maintenance therapy with topical steroid foam does not appear to prevent relapse in those with distal disease. It should be remembered that parenteral and topical steroids may produce systemic steroid side effects. Patients taking steroids during pregnancy should receive stress dose steroids in labor or perioperatively if delivered by C/S.

Steroids cross the placenta, but the rate depends on the formulation. The placenta more effectively metabolizes prednisone and prednisolone than dexamethasone and betamethasone. Fetal levels of theses drugs approximate 10% of maternal levels.[61] High doses of corticosteroids have been associated with fetal growth restriction and cleft lip and palate in animals but rarely in humans.[63] Most of the data suggest that corticosteroids are safe in pregnancy and not harmful to the fetus. Mogadam and colleagues specifically examined the use of corticosteroids to control IBD in pregnancy and found no increase in stillbirth, prematurity, spontaneous abortion, or birth defects.[15] Conversely, Norgard and associates found that women on 5-ASA and steroids had a greater risk of stillbirth than did women on 5-ASA and no steroids, but the study was limited by a small sample size. The researchers suggested that their results indicate the importance and disadvantage of disease activity.[59] Prednisone can be used while breast feeding.

Antibiotics may be helpful for specific indications in IBD. They are presumably effective because they treat an undetectable pathogen, bacterial overgrowth, or an unsuspected perforation. Metronidazole and ciprofloxacin are the most frequently used antibiotics. Although they have no role in the management of active or quiescent ulcerative colitis, they are useful in controlling pouchitis (colectomy and ileal pouch/anal anastomosis). They are also useful in controlling inflammatory, perianal, and fistulous Crohn's disease. Antibiotics should also be given to patients with fulminant disease with high fever, leukocytosis with bandemia, and peritoneal signs or megacolon. Metronidazole and ciprofloxacin are the most common antibiotics used in IBD. They are probably safe in pregnancy but should be used only if clearly indicated and in short courses. There is controversy over their safety while breast feeding.

Azathioprine and its metabolite, 6-mercaptopurine, are purine analogs that inhibit the immune response. These drugs are effective and typically used in corticosteroid-dependent IBD, but there are no formal guidelines for use in pregnancy. Both drugs cross the placenta. Animal studies have suggested an increased risk of fetal wastage and multiple abnormalities such as cleft palate, hydrocephalus, skeletal defects, and ocular abnormalities in offspring. The data in human pregnancy are sparse with no prospective controlled trials. Data from the transplant literature have suggested that the risk of anomalies is approximately 4%.[63] Two studies on IBD in pregnancy found no increased risk of prematurity, spontaneous abortion, or congenital anomalies.[64,65] In contrast, another study found that, in exposed pregnancies, there is an increased risk of congenital abnormalities, perinatal mortality, preterm birth, and low birth weight compared with controls.[66] Ultimately, the risks and benefits of active disease versus drug use must be discussed with each patient. Azathioprine is not recommended while breast feeding.

Methotrexate is a folic acid antagonist that is effective in inducing remission in refractory Crohn's disease. It is pregnancy category X because it is toxic to embryonic and trophoblastic tissue as demonstrated by the use of this drug as an abortifacient and for management of ectopic pregnancies. Methotrexate is also associated with congenital anomalies such as spina bifida and craniofacial defects. Methotrexate is contraindicated while breast feeding.

Cyclosporine alters the immune response by inhibiting interluekin-2, and it affects cell proliferation and turnover. It is effective for the treatment of severe ulcerative colitis. Much of the data on cyclosporine in pregnancy are from the transplant literature. There have been reports of increased rates of low birth weight and prematurity; however, rates of neonatal complications were low and there were no birth defects.[67–69] Cyclosporin may be considered for use in severe colitis, to avoid surgery, and to reach a gestational age when the fetus may be safely delivered. It is considered contraindicated during breast feeding.

Newer medical therapies for controlling IBD are emerging, although they have not been studied in pregnancy. Anti–tumor necrosis factor antibody is effective in decreasing intestinal inflammation in Crohn's disease. Tacrolimus, an immunomodulator similar to cyclosporine, is effective in patients with refractory IBD. Mycophenolate mofetil, an inhibitor of intracellular guanosine monophosphate, is effective in decreasing glucocorticoid requirements in patients with IBD. Anti-inflammatory cytokines, interluekin-10, interleukin-12, and interleukin-11 are effective in decreasing inflammation in animal models of colitis. Thalidomide, a potent teratogenic compound that causes severe malformations of the limbs and other systems, also appears efficacious in glucocorticoid refractory and fistulous Crohn's disease. Thalidomide is contraindicated in pregnancy and it should not be prescribed to women of childbearing age except to those who undergo extensive counseling, use two types of reliable contraception, and have negative monthly pregnancy tests. It is also contraindicated during breast feeding.

Conclusion

Ulcerative colitis and Crohn's disease are common, chronic disorders that affect women in their childbearing years. The course of these inflammatory bowel diseases during pregnancy largely depends on disease activity at conception, and they can be associated with pregnancy complications. Management requires continuation of appropriate medications and close surveillance, with aggressive treatment of any flare. Several commonly used medications for IBD have been shown to be safe in pregnancy. With current management, most women with IBD will have normal pregnancy outcomes.

Discussion of Cases

CASE 1: NEW ONSET OF BLOODY DIARRHEA

A 28-year-old gravida 2, para 1 you are following at 20 weeks of gestation complains of a 2-week history of diarrhea. She reports six to eight loose stools per day. She denies abdominal pain, fever, or vomiting but has noted blood in her stool.

What other information would you like from her history?

It would be important to know whether she has any previous similar episodes, a family history of IBD, and whether or not she has lost weight.

What would you look for on physical examination?

She may have abdominal pain, an abdominal mass, rectal mass, or no remarkable physical findings.

What laboratory evaluation would you order?

A complete blood cell count should be drawn, stool should be checked for occult blood, and stool should be sent for culture and evaluation of ova and parasites.

Her hematocrit is 34%, occult blood was confirmed, and stool cultures were negative. She continues to have symptoms, which have been present now for 3 weeks.

What would be the next step in your evaluation?

If she continues to have diarrhea but has no evidence of a surgical emergency, referral to a gastroenterologist for further evaluation would be appropriate.

The gastroenterologist agrees that this is likely IBD and asks for your opinion regarding the safety of endoscopy.

Sigmoidoscopy, biopsy, and colonoscopy have been performed safely in pregnancy. These procedures can be performed to establish the diagnosis of Crohn's disease or ulcerative colitis, which will be important in the patient's ongoing care. New onset of IBD in pregnancy is relatively rare and may be associated with a quite severe course in some cases. Recognition of the condition, evaluation, and appropriate medical management seem to afford the best available care. At 21 weeks of gestation, the patient may be at the best point to perform a diagnostic procedure. Some investigators have recommended fetal monitoring if colonoscopy is performed after viability.

CASE 2: PRECONCEPTION COUNSELING WITH ULCERATIVE COLITIS

A 30-year-old nulliparous woman with ulcerative colitis presents for preconception counseling. She was diagnosed 10 years previously, and the colitis is currently fairly well controlled with sulfasalazine, but she has required corticosteroids during several flares. She has approximately four loose stools per day and occasional bleeding, and she has not required surgery.

How would you counsel her regarding pregnancy?

The course of her IBD during pregnancy is somewhat related to disease activity at the time of conception; disease will worsen or remain active in around 50% of women with active disease at conception, and 25–40% of those with quiescent disease at conception will relapse. In general, relapse rates are similar among fertile women and pregnant women in any given year. Active disease at conception may also have an affect on the risk of pregnancy complications, including spontaneous abortion, preterm delivery, and fetal growth restriction.

Pregnancy management involves continuing most medications or changing to medications considered safe in pregnancy, treating flares aggressively, assessing fetal growth, and screening for anemia and nutritional deficiencies. Mode of delivery is usually not affected by a history of IBD. Most patients with IBD will have normal, uncomplicated pregnancies.

She asks whether or not her ulcerative colitis will affect her fertility.

The infertility rate among women with ulcerative colitis appears to be around 8–10%, the same as the rate seen in the general population.

If she opts to pursue pregnancy, how would you counsel her to plan for pregnancy?

It is important to inquire about her method of contraception because she needs a reliable and effective method to be able to avoid pregnancy until her disease is well controlled. She should be advised to take supplemental folic acid 2 mg/day because of the potential interference by sulfasalazine on folate absorption.

REFERENCES

1 Online Mendelian Inheritance in Man (OMIM) (TM). McKusick-Nathans Institute for Genetic Medicine, Johns Hopkins University (Baltimore, MD) and National Center for Biotechnology Information, National Library of Medicine (Bethesda, MD), 2000. Available at: http//www.ncbi.nlm.nih.gov/omim/

2 Yang H, Taylor KD, Rotter JI. Inflammatory bowel disease 1. Genetic epidemiology. *Mol Genet Metab* 2001;74:1–21.

3 Karlinger K, Gyorke T, Mako E, et al. The epidemiology and the pathogenesis of inflammatory bowel disease. *Eur J Radiol* 2000;35: 154–167.

4 Baird DD, Narendranathan M, Sandler RS. Increased risk of preterm births for women with inflammatory bowel disease. *Gastroenterology* 1990;99:987–994.

5 Woolfson K, Cohen Z, McLeod RS. Crohn's disease and pregnancy. *Dis Colon Rectum* 1990;33:869–873.

6 Willoughby CP, Truelove SC. Ulcerative colitis and pregnancy. *Gut* 1980;21:469–474.

7 Hudson M, Flett G, Sinclair TS, et al. Fertility and pregnancy in inflammatory bowel disease. *Int J Gynaecol Obstet* 1997;58:229–237.

8 Olsen KO, Juul S, Berndtsson, et al. Ulcerative colitis: female fecundity before diagnosis, during disease and after surgery compared to a population sample. *Gastroenterology* 2002;122:15–19.

9 Fonager K, Sorensen HT, Olsen J, et al. Pregnancy outcomes for women with Crohn's disease: a follow up study based on linkage between national registries. *Am J Gastroenterol* 1998;93:2426–2430.

10 Moody G, Mayberry JF. Perceived sexual dysfunction amongst patients with inflammatory bowel disease. *Digestion* 1993;54:256–260.

11 Abramson D, Jankelson IR, Milner LR. Pregnancy and colitis. *Am J Obstet Gynecol* 1951;61:121–129.

12 Crohn BB, Yarmis H, Grohn EB, et al. Ulcerative colitis and pregnancy. *Gastroenterology* 1956;30:391–403.

13 McDougall I. Ulcerative colitis and pregnancy. *Lancet* 1956;ii: 641–643.

14 DeDombal FT, Watts JM, Watkinson G, Golisher JC. Ulcerative colitis and pregnancy. *Lancet* 1965;2:599–602.

15 Mogadam DM, Korelitz BI, Ahmed SW, et al. The course of inflammatory bowel disease during pregnancy and post partum. *Am J Gastroenterol* 1981;75:265–269.

16 Miller JP. Inflammatory bowel disease in pregnancy: a review. *J R Soc Med* 1986;79:221–225.

17 Nielsen OH, Andreasson B, Bondesen S, Jarnum S. Pregnancy in ulcerative colitis. *Scand J Gastroenterol* 1983;18:735–742.

18 Banks BM, Korelitz BI, Zetzel L. The cause of nonspecfic ulcerative colitis; a review of 20 years experience and late results. *Gastroenterology* 1957;32:983–1012.

19 Bohe MG, Ekelund GR, Genell SN, et al. Surgery for fulminating colitis during pregnancy. *Dis Colon Rectum* 1983;26:119–122.

20 Cooksey G, Gunn A, Wotherspoon WC. Surgery for acute ulcerative colitis and toxic megacolon during pregnancy. *Br J Surg* 1985;72:547.

21 Anderson JB, Turner GM, Willliamson RCN. Fulminating ulcerative colitis in late pregnancy and post partum. *J R Soc Med* 1987;80:492–494.

22 Nelson H, Dozois RR, Kelly KA, et al. The effect of pregnancy and delivery on the ilial pouch anal anastomosis function. *Dis Colon Rectum* 1989;32:384–388.

23 Homan WP, Morbjarnason B. Crohn's disease and pregnancy. *Arch Surg* 1976;3:545–547.

24 Marinbeau PW, Welch JS, Weiland LH. Crohn's disease and pregnancy. *Am J Obstet Gynecol* 1975;122:746–749.

25 Morton MR. Inflammatory bowel disease presenting in pregnancy. *Aust N Z J Obstet Gynecol* 1992;32:40–42.

26 Nwokolo C, Tan WC, Andrews HA, et al. Surgical resections in parous patients with distal ileal and colonic Crohn's disease. *Gut* 1994;35:220–223.

27 Imrie AH. Pregnancy & Crohn's disease. *BMJ* 1970;2:299.

28 Schofield PF, Turnbull RB, Hawk WA. Crohn's disease and pregnancy. *BMJ* 1970;2:364.

29 Lindhagen T, Bohe M, Ekelund G, Valentis L. Fertility and outcome in pregnancy in patients operated on for Crohn's disease. *Int J Colorect Dis* 1986;1:25–27.

30 Baiocco PJ, Korelitz BI. The influence of inflammatory bowel disease and it's treatment on pregnancy and fetal outcome. *J Clin Gastroenterol* 1984;6:211–216.

31 Donaldson RM. Management of medical problems in pregnancy. Inflammatory bowel disease. *N Engl J Med* 1985;312:1616–1619.

32 Fedorkow DM, Persaud D, Nimrod CA. Inflammatory bowel disease: a controlled study of late pregnancy outcome. *Am J Obstet Gynecol* 1989;160:98–1001.

33 Kornfeld D, Cnattignuis S, Ekbom A. Pregnancy outcomes in women with inflammatory bowel disease. A population based cohort study. *Am J Obstet Gynecol* 1997;177:942–946.

34 Larzillier I, Beau P. Chronic inflammatory bowel disease a case control study. *Gastroenterol Clin Biol* 1998;22:1056–1060.

35 Tennebaum K, Marteau P, Elefant et al. Pregnancy outcome in inflammatory bowel disease. *Gastroenterol Clin Biol* 1999;23:464–469.

36 Norgard B, Fonager K, Sorensen HT, et al. Birth outcomes of women with ulcerative colitis: a nationwide Danish cohort study. *Am J Gastroenterol* 2000;95:3165–3170.

37 Moser MA, Okun NB, Mayes DC. Crohn's disease, pregnancy and birth weight. *Am J Gastroenterol* 2000;95:1021–1026.

38 Dominitz JA, Young JC, Buyko EJ. Outcome of infants born to mothers with inflammatory bowel disease: a population based cohort study. *Am J Gastroenterol* 2002;97:641–648.

39 Porter RJ, Stirrat GM. The effects of inflammatory bowel disease on pregnancy: a case controlled retrospective analysis. *Br J Obstet Gynecol* 1986;93:1124–1131.

40 Cappel MS. The fetal safety and clinical efficacy of gastrointestinal endoscopy during pregnancy. *Gastroenterol Clin North Am* 2003;32: 123–179.

41 Cappell MS, Sidhom OA. Multicenter multiyear study of safety and efficiency of flexible sigmoidoscopy during pregnancy in 24 females with follow up of fetal outcome. *Dig Dis Sci* 1995;40:472–479.

42 Cappell MS, Colon VJ, Sidhom O. A study at 10 medical centers of the safety of 8 flexible sigmoidoscopies and 8 colonoscopies during pregnancy with follow up of fetal outcome and with comparison to control groups. *Dig Dis Sci* 1996;41:2353–2361.

43 Brent RL. The effect of embryonic and fetal exposure to x-ray, microwaves and ultrasound: counseling the pregnant and nonpregnant patient about these risks. *Semin Oncol* 1989;16:347–368.

44 Shoenut JP, Senelka RC, Silverman K, et al. MRI in the diagnosis of Crohn's disease in two pregnant women. *J Clin Gastroenterol* 1993;17: 244–247.

45 Firstenberg MS, Malansoni MA. Gastrointestinal surgery during pregnancy and gastrointestinal disorders. *Gastroenterol Clin North Am* 1998;27:73–88.

46 Anderson JB, Turner FM, Williamson RC. Fulminant ulcerative colitis in late pregnancy and the puerperium. *J R Soc Med* 1987;80:492–494.

47 Subhani JM, Hamilton MI. Review article: the management of inflammatory bowel disease during pregnancy. *Aliment Pharmacol Ther* 1998;12:1039–1053.

48 Kelly M, Hunt TM, Wicks ACB, et al. Fulminant ulcerative colitis and parturition: a need to alter current management? *Br J Obstet Gynecol* 1994;100:166–167.

49 Rogers RG, Katz VL. Cause of Crohn's disease during pregnancy and its effect on pregnancy outcome: a retrospective review. *Am J Perinatol* 1995;12:262–264.

50 Brandt LJ, Estabrook SG, Reinus JF. Results of a survey to evaluate when vaginal delivery and episiotomy lead to perinatal involvement in women with Crohn's disease. *Am J Gastroenterol* 1995;90:1918–1923.

51 Priest FO, Gilchrist RK, Long JS. Pregnancy in the patient with ileostomy and colectomy. *JAMA* 1959;169:213.

52 Juhasz ES, Fozard B, Dozors RR, et al. Ileal pouch and anal anastomosis function following childbirth. An extended evaluation. *Dis Colon Rectum* 1995;38:159.

53 Korelitz BI. Epidemiology and psychosocial aspects of inflammatory bowel disease with observations in children, families and pregnancy. *Am J Gastroenterol* 1982;77:929.

54 Singer AJ, Branat LJ. Pathophysiology of the gastrointestinal tract during pregnancy. *Am J Gastroenterol* 1991;86:1695.

55 Martineau P, Tennenbaum R, Elefant E, et al. Foetal outcome in women with inflammatory bowel disease treated during pregnancy with oral mesalazine microgranules. *Aliment Pharmacol Ther* 1998; 12:1101–1108.

56 Bell CM, Habal FM. Safety of topical 5-aminosalicylic acid in pregnancy. *Am J Gastroenterol* 1997:92;2201–2202.

57 Habal FM, Hui G, Greenberg GR. Oral 5-aminosalicylic acid in pregnancy: safety and clinical course. *Gastroenterology* 1993:105;1057–1060.

58 Diav-Citrin O, Park YH, Veerasuntharm G, et al. The safety of mesalamine in human pregnancy: a prospective controlled cohort study. *Gastroenterology* 1998;114:23–28.

59 Norgard B, Fonager K, Pedersen L, et al. Birth outcome in women exposed to 5-aminosalicylic acid during pregnancy: a Danish cohort study. *Gut* 2003;52:243–247.

60 Norgard B, Cxeizel AE, Rockenbauer M, et al. Population based case control study of the safety of sulphasalazine use during pregnancy. *Aliment Pharmacol Ther* 2001;15:403–406.

61 Bietens I, Bayard F, Anses IG, et al. The transplacental passage of prednisone in pregnancy near term. *J Pediatr* 1972;81:936–945.

62 Carmichael SL, Shaw GM, Maternal corticosteroids use and the risk of selected congenital abnormalities. *Am J Med Genet* 1999;86:242–244.

63 Carach V, Carmona F, Monleon FJ, et al. Pregnancy after renal transplantation: 25 years experience in Spain. *Br J Obstet Gynaecol* 1993; 100;122–125.

64 Almstead EM, Ritchie JK, Lennard-Jones JE, et al. Safety of azathioprine in pregnancy in inflammatory bowel disease. *Gastroenterology* 1990;99:443–446.

65 Francella A, Dayan A, Rubin P, et al. 7-Mercaptopurine (6-MP) is safe therapy for childbearing patients with inflammatory bowel disease: a case controlled study. *Gastroenterology* 1996;110(suppl):A909.

66 Norgard B, Pedersen L, Fonager S, et al. Azathioprine, metcaptopurine and birth outcome: a population-based cohort study. *Aliment Pharmacol Ther* 2003;17:827–834.

67 Armenti VT, Ahlswede KM, Ahlswede BA, et al. National Transplant Pregnancy Registry: outcomes of 154 pregnancies in cyclosporine-treated female kidney transplant recipients. *Transplantation* 1994;57: 502–506.

68 Sgro MD, Barozzino T, Mirghani HM, et al. Pregnancy post renal transplantation. *Teratology* 2002;65:5–9.

69 Haugen G, Farchald P, Sodal G, et al. Pregnancy outcome in renal allograft recipients in Norway: the importance of immunosuppressive drug regimens and health status before pregnancy. *Acta Obstet Gynecol Scand* 1994;73:541–546.

ICP: Diagnosis & Management

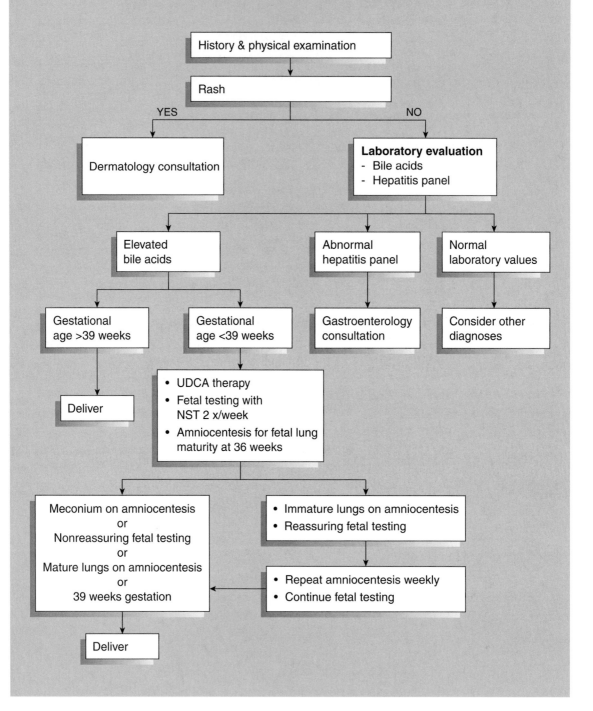

17 Intrahepatic Cholestasis of Pregnancy

Karen M. Davidson

Introduction

Intrahepatic cholestasis of pregnancy (ICP) is the most common liver disease of pregnancy. The primary features of ICP include pruritus and laboratory evidence of cholestasis in the setting of no other underlying liver disease. Once thought to be benign for mother and fetus, recent evidence supports an association between ICP and an increased risk of fetal morbidity and mortality. Alterations in the usual obstetric and medical management of pregnancy are necessary to decrease the risks to the fetus.

Clinical Course and Diagnosis

ICP is characterized by skin pruritus without evidence of skin lesions in the second half of pregnancy. The pruritus typically begins on the palms and soles and then spreads to the trunk and extremities. It is common for the itching to be most intense at night, leading to sleep deprivation and fatigue. Some patients also report vague symptoms of anorexia, nausea, and vomiting. Physical examination shows skin excoriations from intense scratching and, in 20% of patients, mild jaundice. Abdominal examination is remarkable for lack of abnormalities, with a nontender liver of normal size.

In patients with ICP, approximately 80% develop symptoms after 30 weeks of gestation. Patients with the diagnosis of ICP before the third trimester should be screened for hepatitis because an early and/or severe presentation of ICP is more common in patients with

279

chronic hepatitis C.[1] Symptoms resolve in all patients within days of delivery. Laboratory abnormalities may take 4–6 weeks to normalize. If symptoms and laboratory abnormalities do not resolve after delivery, other forms of cholestasis and other liver disorders must be considered.

Serum and urine bile acids are uniformly abnormal in ICP, with most values increased to 100 times above the normal range. If a pregnant patient is being evaluated for pruritus, the finding of normal bile acids virtually excludes the diagnosis of ICP. Increases in serum bile acids have been shown to precede the onset of clinical symptoms of ICP by several weeks in a cohort of patients followed prospectively.[2] Mild to moderate increases in serum aminotransferases are seen in 20–60% of patients.[2,3] In contrast to other types of cholestasis, γ-glutamyl transpeptidase and 5′-nucleotidase are not increased in ICP.[3] In patients with clinical jaundice, direct bilirubin levels are mildly to moderately increased and only rarely exceed 10 mg/dL.[3]

KEY POINT

The diagnosis of ICP requires the exclusion of other causes of pruritus and liver function abnormalities (Table 17-1).

A right upper quadrant ultrasound can be useful in identifying patients with gallstone disease, especially those with biliary colic and jaundice. Patients with ICP do not develop high fevers, a tender upper abdomen, or markedly increased bilirubin levels, all of which are more consistent with acute hepatitis. Profuse vomiting, mental status changes, severe coagulopathies, or hypertension should raise the suspicion of acute fatty liver of pregnancy (AFLP) or preeclampsia. AFLP has been reported to coexist in one series of

Table 17-1. **DIFFERENTIAL DIAGNOSIS OF PRURITUS AND ELEVATED LIVER FUNCTION TESTS**

ICP	All symptoms resolve completely after delivery
Cholelithiasis/CBD obstruction	Jaundice, colicky abdominal pain, abnormal RUQ US
Acute hepatitis	Fever, tender upper abdomen, abnormal hepatitis panel
AFLP	Coagulopathy, encephalopathy, liver failure
Preeclampsia/HELLP	HTN, proteinuria
Primary biliary cirrhosis	Cholestasis without resolution after delivery

AFLP = acute fatty liver of pregnancy; CBD = commonbile duct; HELLP = hemolysis, elevated liver enzymes, and low platelets; HTN = hypertension; ICP = intrahepatic cholestasis of pregnancy; RUQ = right upper quadrant; US = ultrasound.

seven patients, where the presence of ICP was credited in the early diagnosis of AFLP because the patients' symptoms of ICP brought them to medical attention.[4] ICP has not been implicated as causative of AFLP, but it is important to be aware that the two diagnoses may occur simultaneously.

ICP occurs with a strikingly uneven prevalence throughout the world. In most countries, including the United States, ICP is relatively rare, occurring with an incidence of 1 in 1000 to 1 in 10000 deliveries. There is a markedly increased incidence in Sweden and Chile, where the disease occurs in 2% and 14% of deliveries, respectively.[5] ICP also shows seasonal variations, with an increased incidence in the winter months.[5] ICP occurs equally among all maternal ages and parities. It appears more commonly in women with multiple gestations and in those who developed cholestasis in a previous pregnancy or while taking oral contraceptives.

Pathogenesis

KEY POINT

The development of ICP likely involves the interaction of pregnancy with a number of other factors, including a genetic predisposition.

The etiology of ICP is unclear, but there is much indirect evidence, especially from epidemiological data, to suggest that estrogen may play a pivotal role in the development of cholestasis. ICP occurs only in pregnancy and resolves promptly after delivery. Patients with increased estrogen levels, such as those carrying twins, have an increased incidence of the disease. In experimental models, estrogen is capable of altering bile excretion to a variable degree in normal volunteers.[6] Patients with a history of ICP show a more dramatic alteration in bile excretion in response to estrogen ingestion. However, ICP does not recur in subsequent pregnancies in all patients.

Because of the high incidence of ICP in certain countries, such as Chile and Sweden, and the finding of some family pedigrees with many generations of women affected by ICP, a genetic predisposition to ICP has been proposed. Jacquemin and associates studied families with rare, inborn cholestatic syndromes related to dysfunction of biliary transporters.[7] ICP was noted to be more common in women heterozygous for gene mutations coding for transporter proteins. The researchers speculated that heterozygous women have a baseline mild dysfunction of canalicular transporters, which causes no problems outside of pregnancy. During pregnancy, the transporters' capacity to secrete substrates such as estrogen is exceeded, leading to the onset of clinical symptoms. It is also hypothesized that fetal inheritance of a mutation that affects bile acid transport across the placenta may predispose the fetus to increased risk of intrauterine death. Clearly, further studies are necessary to establish the etiology of ICP.

Maternal Outcome

Although long-term outcome is good for mothers affected with ICP, morbidity can be considerable. Nocturnal itching can lead to severe fatigue, whereas anorexia and nausea can lead to poor weight gain. Cholestasis can lead to malabsorption of fat-soluble vitamins, worsening maternal nutritional status. ICP has been associated with up to a 20% incidence of postpartum hemorrhage[8–10] and an increased risk of epidural hematoma.[11] This tendency toward bleeding is thought to be due to the inadequate absorption of vitamin K, which prevents normal synthesis of coagulation factors by the liver. No maternal deaths have been reported as a result of ICP.

Fetal Morbidity and Mortality

Early reports of ICP considered the disease to be benign for mother and fetus. Subsequent reports have shown a consistent pattern of increased rates of fetal morbidity and mortality. ICP is associated with increased rates of preterm delivery, perinatal mortality, intrapartum non-reassuring fetal heart rate patterns, and meconium staining of the amniotic fluid (Table 17-2).

Although no association has been found between severity of maternal disease and rate of meconium passage by the fetus, the presence of meconium most sensitively correlates with poor fetal outcome. Meconium passage has been reported in 86% of cholestasis-associated fetal deaths.[12] This is a significantly higher rate of meconium passage than seen in fetal deaths of other etiologies, which has been reported at approximately 23%.[12] Passage

KEY POINT

Severity of maternal signs and symptoms does not correlate with the likelihood of fetal morbidity or mortality.

Table 17-2.   FETAL MORBIDITY AND MORTALITY RATES WITH INTRAHEPATIC CHOLESTASIS OF PREGNANCY

Perinatal mortality	10–11%
Thick meconium	27–58%
Preterm delivery	36–44%
Fetal distress	22–33%

of meconium in ICP is not associated with a decrease in amniotic fluid volume or a higher rate of fetal growth restriction, suggesting that it is not likely to be related to chronic fetal hypoxia or placental dysfunction. This is further substantiated by the finding of reassuring fetal monitoring up until a few hours before intrauterine fetal demise. Nonstress tests (NSTs) have been reported as normal up to 1 day before fetal demise, and maternal monitoring of fetal movement has been normal up to a few hours before fetal demise.[13]

The mechanism by which ICP leads to poor fetal outcome is not clear but is likely related to toxic effects of maternal bile acids. Fetomaternal bile acid homeostasis requires normal placental transfer of bile acids from the fetus back to the mother, where a normally functioning maternal hepatobiliary system can detoxify and excrete these toxic metabolites. Marked increases in maternal serum bile acid concentrations are thought to impair placental clearance of fetal bile acids. This leads to an accumulation of bile acids within the fetal liver and alterations in fetal liver metabolism. In sheep models, infusion of bile acids increased colonic motility and meconium passage.[14] In other animal experiments, bile acids were found to stimulate prostaglandin release in the rat, increase myometrial contractility, and increase myometrial responsiveness to oxytocin. It is hypothesized that these events may combine to initiate premature labor.

The etiology of intrauterine fetal death in ICP is not clear. Chronic placental insufficiency is unlikely to be a key component of the etiology because most fetuses of women with ICP are not growth restricted and have normal Doppler studies of the umbilical artery. Meconium has been shown in experimental models to cause acute umbilical vein constriction, leading to an acute decrease in umbilical blood flow and subsequent fetal death.[15] Autopsy studies in cases of fetal death related to ICP have shown pericardial, pleural, and pulmonary petechiae consistent with acute anoxia.[16] Further studies are needed to elucidate a more conclusive mechanism of fetal death in patients with ICP.

What's the Evidence?

OBSTETRIC MANAGEMENT	Because of the significant risks of fetal morbidity and mortality, many obstetric management protocols have been proposed to improve fetal outcome. Fisk and Storey reviewed perinatal outcome

with ICP at their institution from 1965 to 1974 and noted a perinatal mortality rate of 107 per 1000.[16] During this period, a policy of expectant management was used, with no antepartum fetal surveillance. In contrast, the perinatal mortality rate in the subsequent 10-year period at the same institution was 35 per 1000 after a protocol including intensive fetal monitoring and delivery once fetal lung maturity was achieved. However, fetal deaths occurred in several cases soon after reassuring fetal testing, indicating that traditional fetal testing may not be adequate in predicting all fetal deaths associated with ICP.

Rioseco and colleagues retrospectively reviewed fetal outcome after the institution of a standard obstetric management protocol of patients with ICP.[13] Patients were monitored with weekly NSTs starting at 34 weeks of gestation. Induction of labor was performed at 38 weeks with documented lung maturity or at 36 weeks with mature indices in patients with more severe clinical disease. Their perinatal mortality rates were not different from those of the general obstetric population in their institution. However, they noted that each of the fetal deaths in patients with ICP occurred within 1 week of a reactive NST, again suggesting that the precipitant behind fetal death associated with ICP may be an acute and unpredictable event. Similarly, Alsulyman and colleagues noted an increase in perinatal mortality rate when patients with ICP were followed only with weekly NSTs and delivered at term or after term for the usual obstetric indications.[17] They also concluded that traditional fetal surveillance is not adequate for predicting fetal death associated with ICP.

The most recently studied management protocol[12] recognizes that traditional monitoring of fetal well-being does not predict most cases of fetal death in ICP, likely due to ICP-related stillbirths showing no evidence of chronic hypoxia. Meconium passage is very commonly associated with these stillbirths but occurs in more than 80% of cases.[12] Their protocol was therefore based on the search for meconium and elective delivery as soon as fetal lung maturity was documented because most fetal deaths occur after 37 weeks of gestation. Patients with ICP were followed with weekly amniocentesis and amnioscopy starting no later than 36 weeks and induced for mature lung indices, meconium, 37 completed weeks, or evidence of intrauterine growth restriction. These patients were also followed with twice weekly NSTs and assessment of amniotic fluid volumes and delivered for any evidence of non-reassuring fetal testing using

KEY POINT

Traditional fetal surveillance is not adequate for predicting fetal death associated with ICP.

these traditional tests. There were no fetal deaths in their study population of 206 patients with ICP. Induction of labor occurred in 71%, with no difference noted in the cesarean section rate as compared with the general population. Meconium was noted in 18% of patients before 37 weeks of gestation. None of these patients had oligohydramnios, fetal growth restriction, or other evidence of placental insufficiency. Of note, three patients underwent immediate cesarean section due to the presence of a non-reassuring NST. This finding of an abnormal result on fetal testing in a small proportion of patients underscores the continued need for traditional fetal testing with NSTs in obstetric management protocols for ICP. Until the mechanism of fetal death associated with ICP becomes clearer, it appears that an aggressive protocol including traditional fetal testing, the search for meconium, and early induction of labor for mature fetal lung indices, meconium, or non-reassuring fetal testing is warranted (see algorithm).

MATERNAL MEDICAL MANAGEMENT

The goal of medical treatment of patients with ICP is to decrease maternal symptoms and to normalize high bile acid concentrations that may be involved in poor fetal outcome. Ideally, treatment should work quickly, involve no adverse side effects to mother or fetus, and decrease poor perinatal outcomes. At this time, no medication clearly fills all of these criteria.

Some cases of mild pruritus improve simply with physical and psychological rest and a low-fat diet. Likewise, antihistamines, benzodiazepines, and minor tranquilizers can decrease the discomfort of pruritus mainly through their sedating qualities. However, none of these therapies improve the laboratory abnormalities associated with ICP or affect fetal outcome.

Early studies of medications to relieve ICP symptoms included phenobarbital and dexamethasone. Phenobarbital acts to induce microsomal enzymes, leading to a decrease in bile acid synthesis and an increase in bile acid secretion. Some studies have shown improvements in pruritus, whereas others have shown no clinical improvements and no study has shown any improvement in the laboratory evidence of cholestasis.[18] Dexamethasone theoretically improves ICP by suppression of fetoplacental estrogen production. In clinical use, dexamethasone has provided mixed results. One small study has shown clinical and laboratory improvement, whereas another study has shown marked worsening of symptoms after initiation of dexamethasone therapy.[19,20]

Cholestyramine is a widely used therapy for ICP-related symptoms. It functions as an exchange resin by binding to bile acids in the intestinal lumen and increasing bile acid fecal excretion. Although capable of providing symptomatic relief to patients with pruritus, cholestyramine has not been shown to improve laboratory abnormalities or fetal outcome. Importantly, cholestyramine has been shown to worsen the malabsorption of fat-soluble vitamins, especially vitamin K.[18,21,22] Because ICP and cholestyramine independently worsen vitamin K absorption, the risk of coagulopathy is significant. Patients treated with cholestyramine for ICP should therefore receive parenteral vitamin K prenatally and have coagulation studies monitored periodically.

A more widely studied medication used in patients with ICP is S-adenyl-L-methionine (SAMe). In experimental models, SAMe renders bile acids water soluble by methylation and sulfuration, increases the flow of bile acids and biliary lipid metabolism, and prevents the negative effects of ethinyl estradiol on bile flow.[23–26] SAMe is therefore theoretically capable of not only preventing but also reversing the impaired bile secretion of ICP. One small observational study and two small randomized controlled studies have showed a symptomatic improvement and an improvement in laboratory parameters in patients who were treated with parenteral SAMe.[27–29] No maternal side effects were noted. The studies were too small to note any change in fetal outcome. In contrast, Ribalta and coworkers performed a larger, randomized, controlled trial that compared parental SAMe with placebo and found no significant improvement in symptoms or bile acid levels between groups.[30] There were no side effects and no differences in fetal outcome. Of note, this study enrolled only patients with early onset, relatively severe disease that was refractory to other therapies. The investigators hypothesized that SAMe may not be effective if cholestasis is well established at the onset of treatment. The parenteral dosing of SAMe also makes is difficult to use in the outpatient setting.

The most promising medication currently in use for patients with ICP is ursodeoxycholic acid (UDCA; Actigall). UDCA is a naturally occurring dihydroxy bile acid that had been used for more than 40 years in the treatment of nonpregnant patients with acute and chronic hepatic disorders, such as primary biliary cirrhosis, cholelithiasis, chronic hepatitis, and autoimmune hepatitis. UDCA acts to displace toxic bile acids and stimulate bile acid secretion by hepatocytes and bile duct cells. UDCA also confers cytoprotective and immunomodulatory effects on the hepatocytes and bile duct cells.

The earliest study of UDCA in ICP involved a nonrandomized pilot trial with eight patients who showed improvement in maternal pruritus scores and decreases in bile acid concentrations and liver function abnormalities.[31] Three subsequent, small, randomized, controlled trials also found improvements in maternal symptoms and bile acid levels in those patients treated with UDCA compared with placebo.[32–34] No side effects were noted in any of these patients. Fetal outcome could not be well evaluated due to the small size of these studies.

In two larger, randomized, controlled studies that compared UDCA with placebo, patients who received UDCA reported significant improvements in pruritus symptoms and had significant decreases in bile acid concentrations in serum and amniotic fluid.[35,36] The UDCA group delivered at a significantly later gestational age due to a decrease in preterm labor and in indicated deliveries for poor fetal testing or meconium. No maternal side effects of the medication were noted in either study.

Two randomized, controlled studies have compared the efficacy of UDCA with that of SAMe. Floreani and associates randomized 20 patients with ICP to oral UDCA versus parenteral SAMe.[37] UDCA was found to be superior to SAMe in decreasing pruritus symptoms and bile acid concentrations. No differences were noted in neonatal outcome and there were no maternal side effects in either group. Nicastri and colleagues randomized 32 patients with ICP to one of four treatment arms: oral UDCA, parenteral SAMe, both medications, or placebo.[38] All four groups, including the placebo group, reported decreased pruritus during the study. The patients who received a combination of UDCA and SAMe or UDCA alone were found to have a significant decrease in bile acid concentration during the study period compared with the placebo group or the group receiving SAMe alone. There were no significant differences in neonatal outcome and there were no maternal side effects noted in any group.

Recently, two retrospective reviews compared outcomes of ICP patients managed with UDCA with those managed with "traditional therapies."[39,40] Significant improvements were noted in maternal pruritus symptoms and laboratory abnormalities in the patients treated with UDCA. Neither study was large enough to

Table 17-3.   DOSING RECOMMENDATIONS FOR URSODEOXYCHOLIC ACID IN PREGNANCY

Start with initial dose of 300 mg orally twice daily
If symptoms persist after 1 week, increase evening dose to 600 mg
If symptoms persist after 2 weeks, increase to a maximum dose of 600 mg twice daily

KEY POINT

UDCA appears to decrease the intense maternal symptoms of pruritus and decrease maternal serum bile acid concentrations better than all other available treatment options.

detect any significant differences in neonatal outcome, although there was a trend toward longer gestations in those patients treated with UDCA.

Although none of the available studies on UDCA in ICP have shown a clear improvement in neonatal outcome, several studies have suggested that UDCA is theoretically capable of decreasing fetal morbidity and mortality. Serrano and coworkers studied bile acid transport in placental membranes of patients with ICP and found that UDCA has a beneficial effect on the impaired placental bile acid transport seen in ICP.[41] Rodrigues and colleagues studied bile acid composition in amniotic fluid, cord blood, and meconium in patients with ICP and found that UDCA decreases bile acid concentrations in amniotic fluid and cord blood.[42] UDCA therapy did not alter bile acid concentrations in meconium. The investigators theorized that UDCA may not be able to alter bile acid concentrations in meconium because these concentrations have already accumulated in the fetus. They suggested that providers should consider starting UDCA soon after the diagnosis of ICP to theoretically prevent the build-up of bile acids in the fetus.

Dosing recommendations for UDCA in pregnancy are listed in Table 17-3. It works quickly in all but the most severe and well-established cases, is well tolerated by most women, and does not appear to result in any severe maternal or fetal side effects. In theory, UDCA has the potential to decrease the perinatal morbidity and mortality rates associated with ICP, but larger studies are necessary to further assess this possibility.

Guiding Questions in Approaching the Patient

Diagnosing ICP

- Does the patient have prolonged pruritus without evidence of visible skin pathology?

- Are bile salts increased?
- Is there evidence of any other underlying liver disease?

Assessing the need for delivery

- Does the patient have a diagnosis of ICP?
- Are the symptoms of pruritus persistent?
- What is the gestational age?
- Is the fetal testing reassuring?
- Are the lungs mature on amniocentesis?
- Is there meconium on amniocentesis?

Conclusion

ICP is a disease characterized by the onset of pruritus and increases in bile acids primarily late in pregnancy, with prompt resolution soon after delivery. The pathogenesis is unknown but may involve a genetic hypersensitivity to estrogen or a predisposition to poor bile acid metabolism. Maternal morbidity is minimal, but fetal morbidity and mortality can be substantial. Meconium is associated with poor fetal outcome and is unlikely associated with chronic fetal hypoxia or placental dysfunction. Traditional fetal surveillance does not adequately predict fetuses at risk for intrauterine fetal demise. Optimal obstetric management includes delivery after establishment of fetal lung maturity. UDCA decreases maternal symptoms and reverses laboratory abnormalities. Further research is necessary to establish the efficacy of UDCA in decreasing perinatal morbidity and mortality rates.

Discussion of Cases

CASE 1: PRURITUS IN THE THIRD TRIMESTER

A 25-year-old gravida 1, para 0 presents to your office at 32 weeks of gestation with itching that has increased in intensity for the past 1–2 weeks. She reports that the itching is most intense at night and primarily affects her abdomen, the palms of her hands, and the soles of her feet. She denies any other symptoms. Her physical examination shows excoriations from scratching but no other skin lesions or rash.

What evaluation, if any, would you perform at this point?

Right upper quadrant ultrasound to rule out gallstone disease, and laboratory evaluation of

bile acids, hepatitis panel, and liver function tests.

Results from her ultrasound, hepatitis panel, and liver function tests are normal. You are informed by the laboratory that her bile acids will take 1–2 weeks to return.

Would you do anything in the next 2 weeks while you wait for the bile acid results?

Because the clinical symptoms are representative of ICP and no other cause of the patient's itching has been found, a preliminary diagnosis of ICP can be made, pending the bile acid results. Because the gestational age is less than 39 weeks, consider starting therapy with UDCA 300 mg twice daily orally. Start fetal testing with NSTs twice weekly.

One week later, bile acid levels are found to be markedly high. The patient is still itching and unable to sleep. The fetal testing is reassuring.

What would you do now?

Increase the UDCA oral dose to 300 mg every morning and 600 mg every evening. Continue twice-weekly fetal testing.

Over the course of the next week, the patient's itching decreases.

Do you need to do any further fetal testing now that the itching has decreased?

The itching likely decreased due to the larger dose of UDCA. Because of the limited information in the literature on the ability of UDCA to improve fetal outcome, it is still necessary to continue fetal testing.

The patient is now at 36 weeks of gestation. Her fetal testing has thus far been reassuring.

Would you change anything about her current management?

Fetal death in ICP is not predictable using traditional fetal testing in most cases. Therefore, amniocentesis is recommended at 36 weeks, with delivery for mature lungs or the finding of meconium.

You perform an amniocentesis that shows clear fluid and evidence of immature lungs.

What would you do now?

Continue UDCA and twice weekly fetal testing with NSTs. Repeat the amniocentesis within 1 week if the fetal testing is reassuring.

One week later, a repeat amniocentesis shows clear fluid and evidence of mature lungs.

What would you do now?

Deliver the patient by induction of labor. Reserve cesarean section for the usual obstetric indications.

The patient undergoes an uncomplicated induction of labor and delivers a healthy infant. Her itching subsides entirely by 48 hours after delivery. She returns for a 6-week postpartum visit and wants to know about the risk of recurrence of ICP in a future pregnancy.

What would you tell her?

Although there is no exact figure quoted in the literature concerning risk of recurrence, it appears that there is a high risk of recurrence in a subsequent pregnancy. In addition, many patients with ICP find that their symptoms recur while on birth control pills.

CASE 2: PRIMIGRAVIDA WITH JAUNDICE AND PRURITUS

An 18-year-old gravida 1, para 0 presents at 37 weeks complaining of itching and abdominal pain. Physical examination shows icteric sclera, no evidence of skin rash, and a gravid abdomen with tenderness in the right upper quadrant. Her temperature is 101.3°F and blood pressure is 100/70 mm Hg.

What is your differential diagnosis for this patient?

Intrahepatic cholestasis of pregnancy, acute hepatitis, cholelithiasis or common bile duct obstruction, and AFLP.

What further evaluation will you perform at this point?

Laboratory evaluation for hepatitis panel, liver function tests, bile acids, complete blood cell count, ammonia, and glucose and right upper quadrant ultrasound.

Her liver function tests show marked increases in the transaminases (10 times normal) and a bilirubin level that is three times the normal level. Her complete blood cell count and glucose and ammonia levels are normal. Her hepatitis panel and bile acid concentrations are pending. Her right upper quadrant ultrasound is normal.

How do these results narrow your differential diagnosis?

A normal right upper quadrant ultrasound makes gallbladder disease unlikely. Normal levels of glucose and ammonia make AFLP unlikely. Fever and markedly increased transaminases and bilirubin make ICP unlikely. ICP is less likely because of tenderness in the right upper quadrant. The most likely diagnosis is acute viral hepatitis.

One day later, the patient's hepatitis panel shows evidence of acute hepatitis B. One week later, bile acid concentrations are found to be normal, thus virtually ruling out ICP.

Does this patient need to be delivered?

No. Acute viral hepatitis is not considered an indication for delivery and is not expected to improve with delivery.

REFERENCES

1 Locatelli A, Roncaglia N, Arreghini A, et al. Hepatitis C virus infection is associated with a higher incidence of cholestasis of pregnancy. *Br J Obstet Gynaecol* 1999;106:498.

2 Heikkinen J. Serum bile acids in the early diagnosis of intrahepatic cholestasis of pregnancy. *Obstet Gynecol* 1983;61:581.

3 Lunzer M, Barnes P, Byth K, et al. Serum bile acid concentrations during pregnancy and their relationship to obstetric cholestasis. *Gastroenterology* 1986;91:825.

4 Reyes H, Sandoval L, Wainstein A, et al. Acute fatty liver of pregnancy: a clinical study of 12 episodes in 11 patients. *Gut* 1994;35:101.

5 Reyes H. Intrahepatic cholestasis of pregnancy: an estrogen related disease. *Semin Liver Dis* 1993;13:289.

6 Reyes H, Ribalta J, Gonzalez MC, et al. Sulfobromophthalein clearance tests before and after ethinyl estradiol administration in men and women with familial histories of intrahepatic cholestasis of pregnancy. *Gastroenterology* 1981;81:226.

7 Jacquemin E, Cresteil D, Manouvrier S, et al. Heterozygous non-sense mutation of the MDR3 gene in familial intrahepatic cholestasis of pregnancy. *Lancet* 1999;353:210.

8 Reid R, Ivey KJ, Rencoret RH, et al. Fetal complications of obstetric cholestasis. *Br Med J* 1976;1:870.

9 Shaw D, Frohlich J, Wittman BA, et al. A prospective study of 18 patients with cholestasis of pregnancy. *Am J Obstet Gynecol* 1982; 142:621.

10 Fisk N, Bye KB, Storey GNB. Maternal features of obstetric cholestasis: 20 years experience at King George V Hospital. *Austr N Z J Obstet Gynecol* 1988;28:172.

11 Yarnell RW, D'Alton ME. Epidural hematoma complicating cholestasis of pregnancy. *Curr Opin Obstet Gynecol* 1996;8:239.

12 Roncaglia N, Arreghini A, Locatelli A, et al. Obstetric cholestasis: outcome with active management. *Eur J Obstet Gynecol Reprod Biol* 2002;100:167.

13 Rioseco A, Ivankovic M, Manzur A, et al.: Intrahepatic cholestasis of pregnancy: a retrospective case-control study of perinatal outcome. *Am J Obstet Gynecol* 1994;170:890.

14 Marin JJE, Villaneuva GR, Esteller A. Diabetes-induced cholestasis in the sheep: possible role of hyperglycemia and hypoinsulinemia. *Hepatology* 1988;8:332.

15 Altshuler G, Hyde S. Meconium induced vasoconstriction: a potential cause of cerebral and other fetal hypoperfusion and of poor pregnancy outcome. *J Child Neurol* 1989;4:137.

16 Fisk NM, Storey GNB. Fetal outcome in obstetric cholestasis. *Br J Obstet Gynaecol* 1988;95:1137.

17 Alsulyman OM, Ouzounian JG, Ames-Castro M, et al. Intrahepatic cholestasis of pregnancy: perinatal outcome associated with expectant management. *Am J Obstet Gynecol* 1996;175:957.

18 Heikkinen J, Maentausta O, Ylostal OP, et al. Serum bile acid levels in intrahepatic cholestasis of pregnancy during treatment with phenobarbital or cholestyramine. *Eur J Obstet Gynecol Reprod Biol* 1982; 14:153.

19 Hirvioja M-L, Tuimala R. The treatment of intrahepatic cholestasis of pregnancy by dexamethasone. *Br J Obstet Gynecol* 1992;99: 109.

20 Kretowicz E, McIntyre HD. Intrahepatic cholestasis of pregnancy, worsening after dexamethasone. *Austr N Z J Obstet Gynecol* 1994; 34:211.

21 Laatikainen T. Effect of cholestyramine and phenobarbital on pruritus and serum bile acid levels in cholestasis of pregnancy. *Am J Obstet Gynecol* 1978;132:501.

22 Acuna R, Gonzalez MC. Hypoprothrombinemia and bleeding associated to treatment with cholestyramine. *Rev Med Chile* 1977; 105:27.

23 Stramentinoli G, DiPadova C, Gualano M, et al. Ethynyl estradiol-induced impairment of bile secretion in the rat: protective effects of S-adenosyl-L-methionine and its implications in estrogen metabolism. *Gastroenterology* 1981;80:154.

24 Boelsterli UA, Rakhit G, Balazs T. Modulation by S-adenosyl-L-methionine of hepatic NaKATPase, membrane fluidity, and bile flow in rats with ethynyl estradiol-induced cholestasis. *Hepatology* 1983; 3:12.

25 Marchesini G, Bianchi GP, Lolli R, et al. Effect of S-adenosyl-L-methionine (SAMe) on plasma levels of sulfur-containing amino acids (SCAA) in patients with liver cirrhosis. *J Hepatol* 1988;7:5148.

26 Vendemiale G, Altomare E, Altavilla R, et al. S-adenosyl-L-methionine (SAMe) improves acetaminophen metabolism in cirrhotic patients. *J Hepatol* 1989;9:S240.

27 Bonfiarro G, Chieffi O, Quinti R, et al.: S-adenosyl-L-methionine (SAMe)-induced amelioration of intrahepatic cholestasis of pregnancy. Results of an open study. *Drug Invest* 1990;2:125.

28 Frezza M, Centini G, Cammareri G, et al. S-adenosyl-L-methionine for the treatment of intrahepatic cholestasis of pregnancy. Results of a controlled clinical trial. *Hepatogastroenterology* 1990;37:122.

29 Frezza M, Pozzato G, Chiesa L, et al. Reversal of intrahepatic cholestasis of pregnancy in women after high dose S-adenosyl-L-methionine administration. *Hepatology* 1984;4:274.

30 Ribalta J, Reyes H, Gonzalez MC, et al. S-adenosyl-L-methionine in the treatment of patients with intrahepatic cholestasis of pregnancy: a randomized, double-blind, placebo-controlled study with negative results. *Hepatology* 1991;13:1084.

31 Palma J, Reyes H, Ribalta J, et al. Effects of ursodeoxycholic acid in patients with intrahepatic cholestasis of pregnancy. *Hepatology* 1992; 15:1043.

32 Meng LJ, Reyes H, Palma J, et al. Effects of ursodeoxycholic acid on conjugated bile acids and progesterone metabolites in serum and urine of patients with intrahepatic cholestasis of pregnancy. *J Hepatol* 1997;27:1029.

33 Brites D, Rodrigues CMP, Oliveira N, et al. Correction of maternal serum bile acid profile during ursodeoxycholic acid therapy in cholestasis of pregnancy. *J Hepatol* 1998;28:91.

34 Javitt NB. Cholestasis of pregnancy: ursodeoxycholic acid therapy. *J Hepatol* 1998;29:827.

35 Diaferia A, Nicastri PL, Tartagni M, et al. Ursodeoxycholic acid therapy in pregnant women with cholestasis. *Int J Obstet Gynecol* 1996;52:133.

36 Palma J, Reyes H, Ribalta J, et al. Ursodeoxycholic acid in the treatment of cholestasis of pregnancy: a randomized, double-blind study controlled with placebo. *J Hepatol* 1997;27:1022.

37 Floreani A, Paternoster D, Grella V, et al. Ursodeoxycholic acid in intrahepatic cholestasis of pregnancy. *Br J Obstet Gynaecol* 1994; 101:64.

38 Nicastri PL, Diaferia A, Tartagni M, et al. A randomised placebo-controlled trial of ursodeoxycholic acid and S-adenosyl-L-methionine in the treatment of intrahepatic cholestasis of pregnancy. *Br J Obstet Gynaecol* 1998;105:1205.

39 Berkane N, Cocheton JJ, Brehier D, et al. Ursodeoxycholic acid in intrahepatic cholestasis of pregnancy. A retrospective study of 19 cases. *Acta Obstet Gynecol Scand* 2000;79:941.

40 Laifer SA, Stiller RJ, Siddiqui DS, et al. Ursodeoxycholic acid in the treatment of intrahepatic cholestasis of pregnancy. *J Matern Fetal Med* 2001;10:131.

41 Serrano MA, Brites D, Larena MG, et al. Beneficial effect of ursodeoxycholic acid on alterations induced by cholestasis of pregnancy in bile acid transport across the human placenta. *J Hepatol* 1998;28:829.

42 Rodrigues CMP, Marin JJG, Brites D. Bile acid patterns in meconium are influenced by cholestasis of pregnancy and not altered by ursodeoxycholic acid treatment. *Gut* 1999;45:446.

Management of Biliary Tract Disease in Pregnancy

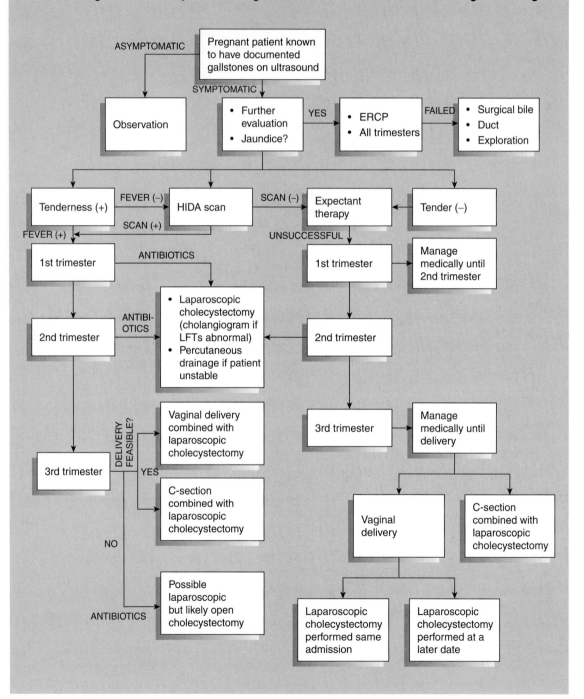

18 Biliary Complications in Pregnancy

Sahar A. Kinney
Steven D. Schwaitzberg

Epidemiology

KEY POINT

Biliary tract disease follows appendicitis as the second most common general surgical condition women are faced with during pregnancy.

Biliary tract disease follows appendicitis as the second most common general surgical condition women are faced with during pregnancy. Gallstones are found to be present in 4.5–12% of all pregnancies by ultrasound.[1] However, symptomatic cholelithiasis and cholecystitis occur in only 5–10 of every 10,000 births, and of these, 40% of patients will fail medical management and require cholecystectomy during their pregnancy.[2] As such, obstetricians and surgeons are often faced with the unique dilemmas that this entity poses during pregnancy.

What's the Evidence?

Much of the evidence regarding surgical procedures in pregnancy is taken from case reports and case series, many of which are described in this chapter. Some case control studies have been performed to evaluate gall bladder function during pregnancy. There are no randomized trials regarding the treatment of biliary disease in pregnant patients, and as with many conditions, treatment is based on extrapolation of information obtained from nonpregnant patient populations. Evidence of the physiologic effects of laparoscopy during pregnancy is largely derived from animal experiments, and is outlined in the text.

Pathophysiology

PREGNANCY AND GALLBLADDER DISEASE

Clinicians have long believed that the earliest symptoms of gallbladder disease in women often occur during pregnancy or in the puerperium.[3] As early as 1880, it was reported that 90% of women having gallstone disease had been gravid at least once.[4] A later report demonstrated a slightly lesser (80%) incidence, which was roughly the proportion of women who had been pregnant in the general population.[5] Contrary to frequent teaching, the patient need not be "fair, fat and forty" to have gallstones. Thin young women in their twenties, particularly those who have borne children, may present with symptoms of cholelithiasis. In 1968, Glenn reported that of 300 females aged 12–25 undergoing surgery for cholelithiasis 219 had been pregnant at least once, 12 had never been pregnant, and 69 were inconclusive. Furthermore, 81% had developed biliary symptoms within one year of onset of pregnancy.[6]

GALLBLADDER MOTILITY

KEY POINT

Gallbladder motility is impaired during pregnancy.

Many studies have revealed that there is impaired gallbladder motility during pregnancy. A healthy gallbladder will usually excrete in excess of 75% of its contents in response to a stimulus to contract. Following the introduction of cholecystography in 1924, Gerdes demonstrated significantly reduced gallbladder emptying of only 38% during the second and third trimesters, with recovery to 71% at 6 to 8 weeks post partum. His hypothesis was that delayed gallbladder emptying was due to a spastic sphincter of Oddi from increased intra-abdominal pressure, increased vagal stimulation, and increased levels of progesterone in pregnancy.[4] Braverman and Stauffer used real-time ultrasonography to assess gallbladder kinetics in pregnant women and nonpregnant controls. After the first trimester, the gallbladder volume during fasting and residual volume after contraction was twice as large in the pregnant group. The rate and percentage of emptying were also decreased, perhaps leading to bile stasis in the gallbladder.[7,8]

HORMONES OF PREGNANCY

Most of the aforementioned findings can be attributed to the hormones associated with pregnancy. By administering 1 mg daily of synthetic estrogen, Kreek was able to induce jaundice in a woman with recurrent cholestatic jaundice of pregnancy who was asymptomatic upon delivery.[9] Estrogen has been shown to decrease the activity of the sodium pump in the gallbladder mucosa, and this can lead to decreased water absorption from the gallbladder mucosa and, hence, increased fasting gallbladder volume.[10] This is consistent with the fact that oral contraceptive use is associated with increased risk of gallbladder disease.[10] Furthermore, specific progesterone receptors have been identified in the human gallbladder[11] and their presence may be related to the "biliary stasis" that occurs during pregnancy. Progesterone may impair gallbladder contraction by inhibiting cholecystokinin-mediated smooth muscle contraction or by reducing the responsiveness of the gallbladder to cholecystokinin.[10] This is consistent with the increased gallbladder volume that occurs during the second and third trimesters of pregnancy, when levels of progesterone are high. As one author perfectly summarized, "the muscle-relaxing action of progesterone, bile duct hypotonia, biliary stasis, cholesterol saturation and increased endoabdominal pressure are physiological conditions of pregnancy that can favor the formation of gallstones."[12] This apparent impact of estrogen and progesterone may explain why women are four times more likely to have gallbladder disease than men.

KEY POINT

The physiologic changes of the gallbladder during pregnancy favor the formation of gallstones and are largely due to hormonal effects.

Complications of Biliary Calculi

Whether during pregnancy or not, far and away the most common complications of biliary calculi are limited to diseases of the gallbladder. This is fortunate since the treatment of stones that migrate into the common bile duct is complicated and poses greater hazards for the mother and fetus. There are three basic diseases of the gallbladder that are the result of cholelithiasis. They are biliary colic, acute cholecystitis, and noninfected obstruction of the cystic duct, also known as hydrops of the gallbladder. Biliary colic not only is the most common form of gallbladder disease, it is also the most elusive to diagnose since many of the symptoms of pregnancy, particularly as noted below, resemble those of biliary colic. This may ultimately lead to a delay in the diagnosis of symptomatic cholelithiasis. Furthermore, just because the patient has the appropriate symptoms and gallstones, it does not always follow that the stones are causing any one of the patient's symptoms. It is generally held that the symptoms of biliary colic are due to the intermittent obstruction of the cystic duct by mobile gallstones. When the gallbladder contracts against this temporarily obstructed cystic duct, the increased intraluminal pressure in the gallbladder is the source of pain and subsequent symptomatology. This may be relatively straightforward in situations where a patient reports having right upper quadrant pain within a few hours of having a fatty meal, but there is a wide variety of presentations for symptomatic cholelithiasis even in nonpregnant patients.[13] Patients who are having biliary colic in the absence of acute cholecystitis or hydrops would generally not be tender, would not have fever, and would manifest normal laboratory values.

Evaluation of these laboratory values can be particularly problematic in the pregnant patient. Patients who develop acute cholecystitis, whether they are pregnant or not, will have a symptom complex of fever, elevated white count, and right upper quadrant (RUQ) tenderness. Since elevated white counts can be a normal part of pregnancy, it is the fever and RUQ tenderness that should lead the clinician towards a diagnosis of acute cholecystitis during pregnancy.

Cholecystitis may be difficult to distinguish from hydrops of the gallbladder due to cystic duct obstruction but not infection. Gallbladders that have been subject to this latter condition will have bile inside of them that is clear instead of green, representing a reabsorption of the bile pigment by the biliary mucosa with only mucus remaining in the gallbladder. Since patients generally do not exhibit fever or elevated white count with this condition, it is sometimes mistaken erroneously for biliary colic despite the RUQ tenderness elicited upon physical examination. Other less common complications of gallbladder calculi include partial obstructions of the common bile duct caused by a stone in the cystic duct that actually impinges onto the common bile duct (Mirrizzi syndrome).

KEY POINT

Patients who develop acute cholecystitis will have a symptom complex of fever, elevated white count, and right upper quadrant tenderness.

Complications of Common Bile Duct Stones

Choledocholithiasis is almost always symptomatic. Even nonobstructing stones form a nidus for bacterial infection and lead to the possibility of cholangitis. In addition, those stones that are small enough to pass through the ampulla of Vater and into the intestines may cause severe pain during their passage and may cause pancreatitis.

Stones which obstruct the common bile duct represent a surgical emergency. Charcot's triad of fever, jaundice, and RUQ tenderness must not be ignored. Elevations of white blood cell count, total bilirubin, and alkaline phosphatase are significant. An ultrasound will generally demonstrate extra hepatic biliary dilatation. The identification of a stone in the common bile duct is significant but the ultrasonographic absence of the stone may simply represent a falsely negative test. Immediate intervention to relieve the common bile duct obstruction is mandatory, regardless of the trimester of the pregnancy, with the subsequent thoughtful consideration of how to remove the source of the gallstones once the bile duct is decompressed.

A more problematic but fortunately less common form of this disease is seen in the Asian population with an entity known as Oriental cholangiohepatitis. While the etiology of this condition is unclear, the primary formation of stones in the intra- and extra-hepatic ducts is the hallmark of this disease. It is not uncommon to require a partial hepatectomy to eradicate the calculus disease, although stenting of the common bile duct may sufficiently temporize the obstruction during a pregnancy.

Gallstone Pancreatitis

Cholelithiasis is present in almost every patient when pancreatitis complicates pregnancy.[14] Common bile duct obstruction is not a prerequisite to the development of pancreatitis. Transient choledocholithiasis may be sufficient to incite the inflammatory cascade. If not treated by cholecystectomy and clearance of the common bile duct, gallstone pancreatitis has a high relapse rate during pregnancy, approaching 72%.[15] In addition it has been associated with maternal and fetal mortality rates of 15% and 60%, respectively. Hence, the consequences of delay in intervention can be severe, and surgical intervention is indicated, even during pregnancy, if cholelithiasis is an etiologic factor. In most cases the diagnosis is made by a rise in serum amylase in the setting of cholelithiasis. The majority of patients have a short-lived course of pancreatitis with serum amylase returning to normal within a few days. These patients could undergo surgery (laparoscopic cholecystectomy) immediately from a biliary standpoint, pregnancy issues notwithstanding. A minority of patients will have persistent pancreatitis requiring critical care. In these patients an endoscopic retrograde cholangiopancreatography (ERCP) to evaluate and remove a stone in the distal common bile duct may be required.

Diagnosis

Abdominal pain is a common complaint during pregnancy. Fortunately, general surgical emergencies are less common.[16] The diagnosis of gallstone disease in pregnancy is quite difficult. Symptoms of excessive flatulence, heartburn, and fatty food intolerance, once thought to be indicitive of gallbladder disease, are no longer thought to be reliable critieria for the diagnosis.[17] Some of the signs and symptoms of acute abdomen, such as nausea, vomiting, and anorexia, may simply be pregnancy induced. Conversely, pregnant patients who present with recurrent episodes of nausea and vomiting may be diagnosed with hyperemesis gravidarum, when really suffering from cholelithiasis. The change in the signs and symptoms of common acute abdominal disease due to pregnancy related alteration in the anatomy and physiology adds to further the confusion and causes a delay in diagnosis. The enlarging uterus may displace the organs away from the anterior abdominal wall, distorting the clinical picture.[16] In the final 3 months of pregnancy, changes in location mean that pain reported in a typical site may be incorrectly interpreted as contractions of the uterus.[12] This may lead to error and delay in diagnosing a pancreatic pathology, which is a serious matter even outside of pregnancy, and during gestation may jeopardize fetal outcome and seriously increase maternal morbidity. In addition, acute peptic ulcer, pancreatitis, hepatitis, pneumonia, pyelonephritis, early herpes zoster, and appendicitis can mimic this disease and should be considered in the differential diagnosis.

Unfortunately, objective information may be difficult to obtain. Laboratory values are nonspecific in pregnancy because white blood cell count and alkaline phosphatase are already increased during pregnancy. The physical examination may add further difficulty; few pregnant patients will have a positive Murphy's sign. Therefore, cholecystitis is diagnosed clinically and verified by the presence of calculi on ultrasound. Ultrasound has been demonstrated to be accurate in the diagnosis of gallstones in excess of 90% of cases.[17] This procedure has replaced oral cholecystography and intravenous cholangiography in the radiologic

KEY POINT

Cholecystitis is diagnosed clinically and verified by the presence of calculi on ultrasound.

diagnosis of gallbladder disease, thus eliminating hazards of radiation exposure. Although hepatobiliary iminodiacetic acid cholescintigraphy (HIDA scan) has been used at half the normal dose,[18] some recommend avoiding this procedure if possible. Animal and human data support the assertion that exposures below 5 rads do not increase the incidence of anatomic malformations, growth retardation, mental retardation, or abortion.[19] The estimated dose to the uterus-embryo with HIDA scan diagnostic procedure is 0.15 rads,[20] well below this range. The purpose of the HIDA scan in this setting is to determine if the cystic duct is obstructed, and it would be used in a setting where a positive study would lead to an intervention. Indicated radiologic studies or other diagnostic modalities should not be delayed because of possible adverse effects on the fetus, because delay may only complicate matters further. Early diagnosis and treatment is essential for successful pregnancy outcome.

Treatment Options

The management of symptomatic gallstones during pregnancy continues to be controversial. Medical treatment may be prolonged and result in repeated hospitalizations, whereas surgical management exposes the mother and fetus to the intrinsic risks of surgery and general anesthesia.[10] This dilemma poses great challenges for the general surgeon and obstetrician.

Guiding Questions

KEY POINT

Most pregnant patients with biliary colic can be managed with a nonfat diet and pain medications until delivery.

- What is the nature of the patient's symptoms and are they recurrent?
- Are her physical findings consistent with gallbladder disease?
- What are her WBC, total bilirubin, and amylase results?
- What does the right upper quadrant ultrasound examination reveal?
- Is there any evidence of a condition requiring immediate surgical treatment (obstruction of the common bile duct, gallstone pancreatitis, acute cholecystitis failing medical treatment, or peritonitis)?
- Is a trial of conservative management appropriate and has it been tried in the past?
- If elective surgery is an option, what is the gestational age at this point?

NONOPERATIVE MANAGEMENT

Most pregnant patients with biliary colic, particularly those late in the course of their pregnancy, can be managed with a nonfat diet and pain medications until delivery. Those early in the course of pregnancy may not respond to such therapy for a prolonged period. The management of acute cholecystitis during pregnancy is also initially conservative, and has been shown to be successful in up to 84% of pregnant patients with acute cholecystitis.[21] This comprises the combination of restriction of oral intake, intravenous antibiotics and hydration, bed rest, and adequate pain relief. However, care should be taken in choosing the appropriate antibiotic for the pregnant patient. Therapy should be directed against *E. coli, Klebsiella*, and enterococci, since these are the predominant pathogens. Anaerobic infections are rare. Chenodeoxycholic acid has been linked to liver injury and possible teratogenicity in lower animals. Because bile acids cross the placenta, pregnant women have generally been excluded from study of this medication, and it is therefore not an option in pregnancy.[17]

> **KEY POINT**
>
> *The management of acute cholecystitis during pregnancy is initially conservative, and has been shown to be successful in up to 84% of pregnant patients.*

PROBLEMS ASSOCIATED WITH NONOPERATIVE MANAGEMENT

Although most women respond well to nonoperative management, there can be serious consequences for women who are not treated definitively during the initial presentation. Problems include the recurrent nature of biliary disease, the increased cost of medical management due to repeated hospitalizations, inevitable surgery under more serious circumstances, and increased maternal and fetal morbidity.

Cholecystectomy for failed medical management occurs frequently. Davis demonstrated that almost half of patients managed conservatively needed more than one admission.[22] Similarly, Dixon reported a 58% recurrence rate among 44 women treated medically.[23] Finally, Swisher showed that nonoperative management of symptomatic gallstones in pregnancy is frequently initially successful, but that as many as 69% of patients will develop recurrent symptoms. These recurrent attacks require repeated hospitalizations and chronically expose the patient to possible complications of the disease process. Complications included the need for emergency surgery, the development of preterm contractions due to underlying biliary disease, and the need to induce labor to relieve severe symptoms. In contrast, there were no relapses in patients who were initially treated with surgery.[24] Failed medical management has led to significant pregnancy loss, predominantly during the first trimester. Spontaneous abortion is more frequent in patients with symptomatic gallstones who were initially treated conservatively compared with those who were initially treated surgically.[23]

SURGERY AND OTHER INTERVENTIONS

As noted above, the complications of choledocholithiasis can significantly increase morbidity and mortality. This fact and the associated high recurrence rate have caused many authors to advocate surgery as the initial treatment of choice of symptomatic gallstones in pregnancy.[23] Proponents of earlier surgical intervention report successful outcomes, shorter hospital stays, and lower cost. Further, it may be argued that the greatest danger to a fetus is not surgery, but a mother who is doing poorly because of associated illness. Regardless, the need to perform a cholecystectomy during pregnancy is rare, but it can be performed with minimal risk to the fetus irrespective of gestational age. There is no apparent increase in maternal mortality from surgery for uncomplicated cholecystitis.[17] Fetal morbidity is less than 5% following cholecystectomy, especially in the 2nd and 3rd trimesters, but approaches 60%[24a] when pancreatitis secondary to biliary tract disease is left untreated.

KEY POINT

The need to perform a cholecystectomy during pregnancy is rare, but it can be performed with minimal risk to the fetus irrespective of gestational age.

KEY POINT

The optimal time for surgery is during the second trimester, when organogenesis is complete and the uterus is not large enough to obstruct safe access to the abdomen and gallbladder.

The optimal time for surgery is during the second trimester, when organogenesis is complete and the uterus is not large enough to obstruct safe access to the abdomen and gallbladder. The most common indications for surgery, in decreasing order, are acute cholecystitis, gallstone pancreatitis, common bile duct stones, and persistent biliary colic. Other motives to surgically intervene are persistent or recurrent symptoms despite antibiotics and analgesics, or failure to gain weight resulting in a potential risk to the fetus. Most authors agree that surgery is indicated in any trimester for obstructive jaundice, acute cholecystitis failing medical treatment, gallstone pancreatitis, suspected peritonitis, or when diagnosis is in question in an ill patient.[18]

PRETERM LABOR AND SPONTANEOUS ABORTION

It is clear that concern about fetal death in utero is one of the major reasons for the conservative management of symptomatic gallstones during pregnancy. In 1963, a risk of fetal loss of up to 15% was reported when open cholecystectomy was performed during pregnancy.[25] Some thought that the risk was different for each trimester. Thirty years later, a spontaneous abortion rate for open cholecystectomy of 12% during the first trimester, declining to 5.6% and 0%, respectively, in the second and third trimesters was reported. The incidence of preterm labor was found to be 0 in the second trimester, increasing to 40% in the third.[26]

On the other hand, emergent procedures for cholecystitis or obstructive jaundice are associated with an increased risk of fetal loss.[25] Preterm delivery rates increase after an emergency procedure as compared with an elective procedure (21.3 vs 6.5% respectively, $p < 0.07$).[27] Because the sickest patients undergo surgery, occasionally after suffering complications of disease progression, surgery is associated with more adverse outcomes. While modern ultrasound techniques have alleviated much of this problem, the historically high loss rate in the literature may also have been related to the significant number of women undergoing elective pregnancy termination from fear of first trimester radiation exposure. With the traditional emphasis on waiting as long as possible, increased losses in older series may have been related to the severity of the underlying disease once surgery was finally undertaken.[22] The incidence of prematurity and fetal loss does not seem to be increased when elective non-obstetric operation is performed during pregnancy.

LAPAROSCOPIC CHOLECYSTECTOMY

Many authors argue that laparoscopy will diminish the risk of preterm labor or spontaneous abortion associated with open cholecystectomy during pregnancy. Most of the general surgeons who began performing laparoscopic cholecystectomies in 1989 and 1990 felt that pregnancy was a relative contraindication to the procedure. Pregnancy was felt not only to cause potential difficulties in exposure to the operative field but also carried the added concerns of possible adverse effects on the developing fetus from increased carbon dioxide in the environment and pressure accompanying the pneumoperitoneum. However, gynecologists have performed laparoscopic procedures during pregnancy for decades. In recent years, numerous authors have reported favorable outcomes with laparoscopic procedures performed during pregnancy.[18]

Laparoscopic cholecystectomy is the most common laparoscopic procedure performed in pregnant women. Up until 1991, cholecystectomy was traditionally performed via a laparotomy incision either in the upper midline or in the right upper quadrant. Laparoscopic cholecystectomy has many advantages over

KEY POINT

Laparoscopic cholecystectomy is the most common laparoscopic procedure performed in pregnant women.

traditional cholecystectomy, including shorter hospital stay, early return to normal activity and a reduction in medical expenses. These advantages may be more critical in the pregnant patient because rapid return to full activity could reduce the frequency of maternal thrombosis and embolic events, which are the leading cause of maternal mortality in this country. Furthermore, laparoscopic surgery decreases post-operative pain leading to decreased fetal exposure to narcotics. Also, there is a decreased incidence incisional hernia or dehiscence following labor, and return to full diet sooner with no nutritional stress. With upper abdominal disease visualization and accessibility are not compromised by the expanding uterus.[15] Since minimal or no uterine manipulation is required during laparoscopic cholecystectomy, the risk of preterm labor should be minimized. Insufflation pressures seem less of a risk to the fetus than manual retraction of the uterus, which may be necessary in conventional cholecystectomy.

That pregnancy might be a relative contraindication to laparoscopic cholecystectomy is mainly based on three major concerns. First is the danger in the initial entry into the abdomen. Most surgeons gain initial access to the abdomen during pregnancy by the open Hasson technique. Although Veress needle entry has been used successfully, laceration of the uterus has been reported.[28] This can be avoided by using the open Hasson technique or by using modified (cephalad) sites of insertion, and by being aware of the location of the fundus of the uterus. This is important particularly after 18 weeks' gestation, when the uterus may rise above the umbilicus.

The potential fetal effects of the carbon dioxide pneumoperitoneum and the pressure by which it is delivered are also of concern. Pneumoperitoneum affects the fetus in two ways—by directly increasing pressure on the uterus and by altering maternal hemodynamics and acid-base balance.[29] In theory increased intra-abdominal pressure could cause fetal acidosis, hypotension, and hypoxia due to decreased uterine blood flow. In addition, reversed Trendelenburg, the position employed in cholecystectomy, will cause decreased maternal venous return and cardiac output. Increased intra-abdominal pressure in addition to Trendelenburg will cause added reductions in materal total lung capacity and functional residual capacity. These effects can be minimized by employing positive pressure ventilation and lower insufflation pressures.

Although it is not proven in humans, carbon dioxide pneumoperitoneum may cause fetal acidosis secondary to maternal hypercarbia. In a study of 8 pregnant women who underwent insufflation, arterial blood gases were measured at baseline, during 15 mm Hg insufflation, and after insufflation. There were no significant changes in the maternal arterial to end-tidal carbon dioxide pressure difference ($PaCO_2$—$PetCO_2$) during CO_2 pneumoperitoneum as compared with pre-insufflation values during laparoscopic surgery.[30] It can be argued that the absence of maternal effects may negate any fetal effects.

Accurate interpretation of fetal physiology requires invasive monitoring, and has not been researched for this purpose in the human fetus. However, recent animal studies have assessed the fetal response to carbon dioxide pneumoperitoneum. In 1995, Barnard studied the fetal response to carbon dioxide pneumoperitoneum in the pregnant ewe. Five ewes underwent a 1-hour laparoscopy with insufflation pressures of 20 mm Hg and manual ventilation to maintain a constant maternal carbon dioxide pressure range of 37.1 ± 3.3 mm Hg. Fetal blood flows and blood gases were obtained at 30 and 60 minutes of insufflation, as well as at 40 minutes of desufflation. Although it was found that maternal placental blood flow fell significantly (by 22%), there were no changes in fetal placental perfusion pressure and blood flow, pH, or blood gas values. Therefore, it was asserted that fetal acid-base disturbances were caused by high insufflation pressures rather than carbon dioxide absorption.[31] In a similar study the same year, Hunter found that carbon dioxide pneumoperitoneum did indeed induce fetal acidosis as well as fetal tachycardia and hypertension in the pregnant ewe.[29] These effects were found to be increased in a "stepwise" manner; that is, as the insufflation pressures were increased, fetal effects were increased. This is an additional indication to minimize insufflation pressures. Furthermore, because these effects were not seen with nitrous oxide pneumoperitoneum, Hunter argued to the contrary of Barnard that fetal tachycardia and hypertension were caused by hypercarbia and not by increased intra-abdominal pressure. Regardless, 7/8 ewes survived, with one fetal demise secondary to preoperative illness. Another study of helium pneumoperiteum did not cause maternal or fetal acidosis, also indicating that the metabolic effects seen with CO_2 are the result of the specific gas used.[32] In another controlled study of the short- and long-term effects of CO_2 pneumoperitoneum in pregnant ewes, Curet reported statistically significant increases in maternal heart rate, amniotic pressure, $EtCO_2$, PCO_2, fetal blood pressure, and fetal PCO_2, with decreases in uterine blood flow and maternal and fetal pH.[33] There were no long-term adverse outcomes, and all ewes delivered healthy lambs at full-term gestation. Hence, it may be argued that short-term fetal acidosis, even if severe, may not lead to long-term deleterious effects.[34]

There are a small number of studies in which human fetal heart rate is assessed during laparoscopy. Contrary to those effects found in animals, Glasgow found that there was no maternal hypercarbia, nor was there any significant change in the fetal heart rate in response to positioning the patient on the operating table, induction of anesthesia, insufflation of and maintenance of pneumoperitoneum, or during recovery.[2] There are some alternatives to standard pneumoperitoneum such as a combination low-pressure pneumoperitoneum with an "abdominal wall lift"[35] or a gasless laparoscopic cholecystectomy "Laprolift" (Origin Medsystems, Menlo Park, Ca.) abdominal wall suspension device.[18] Despite these successful reports, abdominal wall suspension devices may be limited by providing less exposure to the operative field and causing increased postoperative pain due to extensive retraction. Moreover, with the increasing number of successful cases of laparoscopic cholecystectomy reported in the pregnant patient using standard techniques, these alternatives have become less appealing.

Despite these concerns, hundreds of laparoscopic cholecystectomies in pregnant patients have been reported in the medical literature and it has become the procedure of choice in pregnant patients with biliary disease. The key technical points are outlined in Table 18-1. The only adverse outcome was reported in a study by Amos in 1996, where 3 out of 4 cases resulted in fetal demise.[36] This study contains key flaws. Although Amos claims that fetal demise was due to carbon dioxide pneumoperitoneum, there is no information supplied showing that there was hypercarbia or acidosis. Moreover, the patients in this study had severe disease including gallstone pancreatitis and perforated appendicitis, both of which could have contributed to fetal loss.

The timing of cholecystectomy remains controversial. We recommend that surgery be performed during the second trimester of

Table 18-1. **GUIDELINES FOR PERFORMING LAPAROSCOPIC CHOLECYSTECTOMY DURING PREGNANCY**

- Whenever possible, the procedure should be deferred to the second trimester.
- It is imperative to include the possibility of preterm labor and fetal loss in the informed consent.
- A very experienced surgeon should obtain pneumoperitoneum access with the open Hasson technique.
- Intra-abdominal pressures should not exceed what is needed to visualize the operative field. Many procedures can be well visualized with insufflation pressures in the 9–10 mm Hg range (Figures 18-1 and 18-2).
- Maternal end-tidal CO_2 should be monitored and maintained by relative hyperventilation.
- Consider rotating the operating table to displace the uterus from the inferior vena cava. Pre- and postoperative fetal and uterine monitoring is recommended when appropriate for gestational age.
- Intra-operative monitoring via transvaginal ultrasound may be considered once the pregnancy reaches viability.
- Pneumatic compression devices must be implemented to prevent venous stasis leading to deep venous thrombosis.
- Use of a lead shield is advocated when performing intraoperative cholangiogram.
- The routine use of prophylactic tocolytics is controversial.
- Preoperative glucocorticoids are recommended 48 hours before surgery to enhance lung maturity in cases performed between 24 and 34 weeks' gestation.

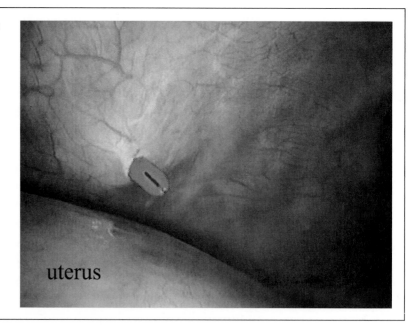

Figure 18-1: Laparoscopic cholecystectomy in a 24-week twin pregnancy. Adequate exposure and access to the gallbladder is illustrated.

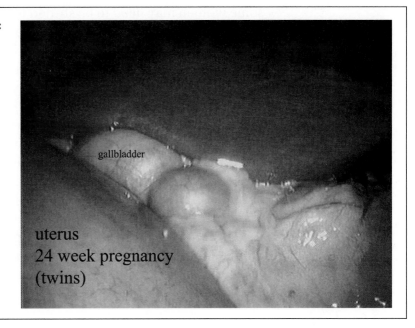

Figure 18-2: Laparoscopic cholecystectomy in a 24-week twin pregnancy. Primary access is gained using the open Hasson trocar technique.

gallbladder

uterus
24 week pregnancy
(twins)

pregnancy (ideally around 17–18 weeks, but can be accomplished later), when organogenesis is complete, the uterine size is not large enough to obstruct the operative field, and the risk of spontaneous abortion and preterm labor is low. Patients presenting in the first trimester should ideally be managed conservatively until the second trimester, when elective laparoscopic cholecystectomy should be performed. Furthermore, patients in their third trimester should, whenever possible, be treated conservatively and have surgery delayed until the post-partum period. Unfortunately, some conditions, such as unrelenting and debilitating biliary colic, choledocholithiasis, severe or recurrent gallstone pancreatitis, or severe cholecystitis (gangrene, pneumatosis, empyema), demand urgent action despite the stage of pregnancy and must be dealt with in a timely and expeditious manner.

Fortunately, laparoscopic cholecystectomy has been successfully performed in all trimesters.[18] The reports that include third trimester procedures repeatedly suggest that gallbladder exposure is essentially effortless, although no pregnancy has been beyond 33 weeks' gestation at the time of surgery. Cannula placement in some women may need to be shifted many centimeters cephalad, depending on the degree of uterine enlargement. As this space occupancy dilemma worsens, the obvious considerations must include delay of the surgical procedure until spontaneous term delivery, induction of labor, or delivery by caesarean section with simultaneous performance of the intra-abdominal operation. Laparoscopic cholecystectomy can be performed at the time of cesarean section. We have also performed laparoscopic cholecystectomy prior to hospital discharge following uncomplicated vaginal delivery. Mythic fears of increased bleeding due to hyperemia are unfounded. Many women would rather have definitive therapy at the time of delivery or immediately thereafter since surgery later in the postpartum period separates them from the newborn infant and may interfere with breastfeeding.[22] In addition, the child care logistics are simplified when delivery is followed by immediate cholecystectomy.

ERCP

In addition to medical and surgical treatment, endoscopy represents a third option to treat certain biliary complications in pregnancy.[37] ERCP and sphincterotomy can be performed safely during all stages of pregnancy by taking specific measures to minimize fetal exposure to radiation. Despite success with ERCP during pregnancy, this procedure can be quite cumbersome. Prone positioning can be difficult during the later stages of pregnancy, when a more lateral or even supine position is required.[37] Furthermore, it is difficult to ascertain a safe period of intrauterine exposure to radiation, as no upper limit has been set and its late effects are unknown. Finally, ERCP does not necessarily ensure a definitive solution to the biliary problem, since the source of calculi remains intact.

Nonetheless, ERCP is an attractive option in patients with escalating pancreaticobiliary disease such as acute cholangitis and gallstone pancreatitis. As with operative management, the second trimester is the most favorable period for endoscopic treatment of symptomatic ductal stones. Retrograde stone extraction is the procedure of choice. If possible, women in their first trimester should be managed conservatively to avoid possible teratogenic effects of radiation. However, if conservative management fails, endoscopic sphincterotomy can generally be safely accomplished. With adequate lead shielding, the amount of radiation exposure to the fetus in minimal.[38] If possible, patients in the mid- to late-third trimester should be managed conservatively until delivery, because of the inability to appropriately shield the fetus from radiation as well as difficulty in positioning the patient in the prone position. Theses patients could alternatively undergo endoscopic sphincterotomy with stenting with minimal or no fluoroscopy.[38] When ERCP fails, surgical bile duct exploration is indicated.

Conclusion

Regardless of etiology, cholelithiasis is relatively common in women of child bearing age. Fortunately, these calculi invoke significant symptoms in only a small percentage of pregnancies. Operative intervention should be performed (laparoscopically whenever possible) in cases of acute cholecystitis or hydrops of the gallbladder. Clinically significant common bile duct stones can be retrieved by experienced endoscopists with a minimum of fluoroscopic radiation. The challenge for the surgeon and obstetrician is to determine the significance of symptoms in those cases of biliary colic where operative intervention is contemplated. Elective surgery can be performed with a minimum risk of fetal loss when symptoms rise to the level of operative intervention. Surgery for the treatment of acute inflammatory processes should not be delayed at any stage of pregnancy as disease progression or failed conservative therapy is a greater risk for inciting pre-term labor than the surgical procedure itself.

CASE 1: RIGHT UPPER QUADRANT PAIN IN SECOND TRIMESTER

A 24-year-old G2P2 woman at 16 weeks' gestation presents to the emergency department complaining of right upper quadrant pain of three hours duration. She had complained of significant amounts of nausea with occasional vomiting since early in her pregnancy. Careful questioning reveals some fatty food intolerance. The pain is location just below the ribcage and radiates to the right flank. In addition, she complains of mild nausea and hiccups. Her vitals are: heart rate 100, respiratory rate 24, and temperature 37.5°C. On physical examination she is in obvious discomfort. The uterus is palpable 3 cm below the umbilicus. The abdomen is mildly tender in the right upper quadrant. Her laboratory examination is remarkable for an elevated white blood cell count of 15.3 thousand without left shift. The liver function studies are normal. The serum amylase is very mildly elevated. The urinalysis demonstrates 5–10 white blood cells per high powered field, a few squamous cells, and a few bacteria per high powered field.

What is the key differential diagnosis of a pregnant woman with significant right upper quadrant pain?

This is a fairly typical presentation for a pregnant woman with symptomatic cholelithiasis. It is clear that some of the symptoms are very similar to those observed in early pregnancy, but on careful questioning a history suggestive of biliary colic can be elucidated, especially if the woman has been pregnant before. While she is clearly in pain there is no particular feature suggestive of acute infection. Mild amylase elevation should not be misconstrued as signs of pancreatitis.

What additional diagnostic testing, if any, is indicated in this scenario?

The diagnostic test of choice here is an ultrasound of the right upper quadrant, especially to visualize the gallbladder and biliary tree, the kidney, and the pancreas. This test is both sensitive and specific for the detection of gallstones and hydronephrosis. Ultrasound is less acute for diagnosing acute cholecystitis. If this is suspected, a HIDA scan is the test of choice.

If symptomatic cholelithiasis is the leading diagnosis, what is (are) the appropriate therapeutic intervention(s) at this point?

The initial management of biliary colic would be geared toward symptomatic relief. The patient should be counseled to adopt a low fat diet. If her symptoms are successfully managed in this fashion, then cholecystectomy should be performed post partum. This could be performed in conjunction with cesarean section, the day after delivery, or at a convenient point of election. On the other hand there are occasional patients whose biliary colic is so severe that consideration must be given to operative intervention.

If these symptoms persist, what are the indications for cholecystectomy? How is an operative plan impacted by the progression of the pregnancy?

Classically the second trimester is the preferred time for non-emergent operations. However, successful cholecystectomy is reported in all trimesters with uncomplicated pregnancy outcomes. The limitation for performing the cholecystectomy laparoscopically is a function of the growing uterus obstructing access to the gallbladder. Originally the prevailing wisdom was to offer laparoscopic procedures until approximately 18 weeks' gestation when the uterus reaches the umbilicus. In experienced hands, safe entry cephalad to the umbilicus can be performed using careful open techniques as late as 26 weeks or so, depending on body habitus.

CASE 2: JAUNDICE IN THE FIRST TRIMESTER

A twenty-year-old G1P0 woman has become jaundiced during the eighth week of her otherwise uncomplicated pregnancy. She is febrile and tender in the right upper quadrant completing Charcot's triad. A presumptive diagnosis of ascending cholangitis is made. This is supported by an ultrasound that demonstrates cholelithiasis and intrahepatic biliary dilatation.

What are the key modalities that can be employed to treat this urgent medical problem, and what are the pros and cons of each of these choices?

There are three methods for decompressing the extrahepatic bile, which needs to be done in addition to the immediate initiation of intravenous antibiotics aimed at covering gram negative rods and enterococci. Surgical common bile duct exploration and therapeutic ERCP in conjunction with biliary sphincterotomy can be employed to remove obstructing choledocholithiasis. Poor surgical candidates could be decompressed via percutaneous transhepatic cholangiography with catheter placement. The latter two modalities involve radiation, usually in the form of fluoroscopy. Hard limits on the amount of fluoroscopy need to be determined pre-procedure and if reached would mitigate surgical decompression. If ERCP is successful then a decision is made as to whether or not a cholecystectomy is needed during the pregnancy. Since the patient's symptoms were caused by bile duct not gallbladder obstruction, the definitive procedure to remove the source of calculi can be postponed until after delivery. If right upper quadrant pain persists then cholecystectomy should be performed. If an operative procedure is performed to remove the common bile duct stone, choledoscopy or a single shot radiograph can be used verify stone clearance in order to minimize radiation exposure.

REFERENCES

1 Sungler P, Heinerman PM, Steiner H, et al. Laparoscopic cholecystectomy and interventional endoscopy for gallstone complications during pregnancy. *Surg Endosc* 2000;14:267–271.

2 Glasgow RE, Visser BC, Harris HW, Patti MG, Kilpatrick SJ, Mulvihill SJ. Changing management of gallstone disease during pregnancy. *Surg Endosc* 1998;12:241–246.

3 Tegenfeldt EG, Kirtland HB, Brown RG. Gallstones, pancreatitis and pregnancy. *Am Surg* 1967;33:88–90.

4 Gerdes M, M, MD, Boyden E, A, PhD. The rate of emptying of the human gall bladder in pregnancy. *Surg Gynecol Obstet* 1932:145–155.

5 Friley MD, Douglas G. Acute cholecystitis in pregnancy and the puerperium. *Am Surg* 1972;38:314–317.

6 Glenn F, McSherry CK. Gallstones and pregnancy among 300 young women treated by cholecystectomy. *Surg Gynecol Obstet* 1968; 127:1067–1072.

7 Braverman DZ, Johnson ML, Kern F, Jr. Effects of pregnancy and contraceptive steroids on gallbladder function. *N Engl J Med* 1980; 302:362–364.

8 Stauffer RA, Adams A, Wygal J, Lavery JP. Gallbladder disease in pregnancy. *Am J Obstet Gynecol* 1982;144:661–664.

9 Kreek MJ, MD, Sleisenger M, H, MD, Jeffries G, H, MRCP. Recurrent cholestatic jsundice of pregnancy with demonstrated estrogen sensitivity. *Am J Med* 1967;43:795–803.

10 Ghumman E, Barry M, Grace PA. Management of gallstones in pregnancy. *Br J Surg* 1997;84:1646–1650.

11 Basso L, McCollum PT, Darling MR, Tocchi A, Tanner WA. A study of cholelithiasis during pregnancy and its relationship with age, parity, menarche, breast-feeding, dysmenorrhea, oral contraception and a maternal history of cholelithiasis. *Surg Gynecol Obstet* 1992; 175:41–46.

12 Paternoster DM, Floreani A, Sacco NS, Ancona E. Chronic recurrent pancreatitis in pregnancy. *Minerva Ginecol* 1995;47:561–564.

13 Berger MY, van der Velden JJIM, Lijmer JG, de Kort H, Prins A, Bohnen AM. Abdominal symptoms: Do they predict gallstones? *Scand J Gastroenterol* 2000;35:70–76.

14 Block P, Kelly TR. Management of gallstone pancreatitis during pregnancy and the postpartum period. *Surg Gynecol Obstet* 1989;168: 426–428.

15 Andreoli M, Sayegh SK, Hoefer R, Matthews G, Mann WJ. Laparoscopic cholecystectomy for recurrent gallstone pancreatitis during pregnancy. *South Med J* 1996;89:1114–1115.

16 Gurbuz AT, Peetz ME. The acute abdomen in the pregnant patient. Is there a role for laparoscopy? *Surg Endosc* 1997;11:98–102.

17 Simon J, A, MD. Biliary tract disease and related surgical disorders during pregnancy. *Clin Obstet Gynecol* 1983;26: 810–821.

18 Iafrati MD, Yarnell R, Schwaitzberg SD. Gasless laparoscopic cholecystectomy in pregnancy. *J Laparoendosc Surg* 1995;5:127–130.

19 Brent R, L. Utilization of developmental basic science principles in the evaluation of reproductive risks from pre- and postconception environmental radiation exposures. *Teratology* 1999;59:182–204.

20 Leveno K, L, Cunningham F, G, Gant N, F, et al. In: Seils A, Noujaim S, R, Davis K, eds. *Williams Manual of Obstetrics*. New York: McGraw-Hill, 2003:826.

21 Landers D, Carmona R, Crombleholme W, Lim R. Acute cholecystitis in pregnancy. *Obstet Gynecol* 1987;69:131–133.

22 Davis A, Katz VL, Cox R. Gallbladder disease in pregnancy. *J Reprod Med* 1995;40:759–762.

23 Dixon NP, Faddis DM, Silberman H. Aggressive management of cholecystitis during pregnancy. *Am J Surg* 1987;154:292–294.

24 Swisher SG, Hunt KK, Schmit PJ, Hiyama DT, Bennion RS, Thompson JE. Management of pancreatitis complicating pregnancy. *Am Surg* 1994;60:759–762.

24a Jouppila P, Mokka R, Larmi TK. Acute pancreatitis in pregnancy. *Surg Gynecol Obstet* 1974;139:879–882.

25 Greene J, Rogers A, Rubin L. Fetal loss after cholecystectomy during pregnancy. *Can Med Assoc J* 1963;88:576–577.

26 McKellar DP, Anderson CT, Boynton CJ, Peoples JB. Cholecystectomy during pregnancy without fetal loss. *Surg Gynecol Obstet* 1992; 174:465–468.

27 Kort B, MD, Katz V, L, MD, Watson W, J, MD. The effects of nonobstetric operation during pregnancy. *Surg Gynecol Obstet* 1993;177: 371–376.

28 Barnett MB. Complication of laparoscopy during early pregnancy. *BMJ* 1974;23:328.

29 Hunter JG, Swanstrom L, Thornburg K. Carbon dioxide pneumoperitoneum induces fetal acidosis in a pregnant ewe model. *Surg Endosc* 1995;9:272–277; discussion 277–279.

30 Bhavani-Shanker K, Steinbrook RA, Brooks DC, Datta S. Arterial to end-tidal carbon dioxide pressure difference during laparoscopic surgery during pregnancy. *Anesthesiology* 2000;92:370–370.

31 Barnard JM, Chaffin D, Droste S, Tierney A, Phernetton T. Fetal response to carbon dioxide pneumoperitoneum in the pregnant ewe. *Obstet Gynecol* 1995;85:669–674.

32 Curet MJ, Weber DM, Sae A, Lopez J. Effects of helium pneumoperitoneum in pregnant ewes. *Surg Endosc* 2001;15:710–714.

33 Curet MJ, Vogt DA, Schob O, Qualls C, Izquierdo LA, Zucker KA. Effects of CO_2 pneumoperitoneum in pregnant ewes. *J Surg Res* 1996; 63:339–344.

34 Curet M, J, MD. Special problems in laparoscopic surgery. Previous abdominal surgery, obesity, and pregnancy. *Surg Clin North Am* 2000; 80:1093–1108.

35 Edelman DS. Alternative laparoscopic technique for cholecystectomy during pregnancy. *Surg Endosc* 1994;8:794–796.

36 Amos JD, Schorr SJ, Norman PF, et al. Laparoscopic surgery during pregnancy. *Am J Surg* 1996;171:435–437.

37 Liberman MA, Phillips EH, Carroll B, Fallas M, Rosenthal R. Management of choledocholithiasis during pregnancy: a new protocol in the laparoscopic era. *J Laparoendosc Surg* 1995;5:399–403.

38 Jamidar PA, Beck GJ, Hoffman BJ, et al. Endoscopic retrograde cholangiopancreatography in pregnancy. *Am J Gastroenterol* 1995;90: 1263–1267.

Pathway for the Management of HSV

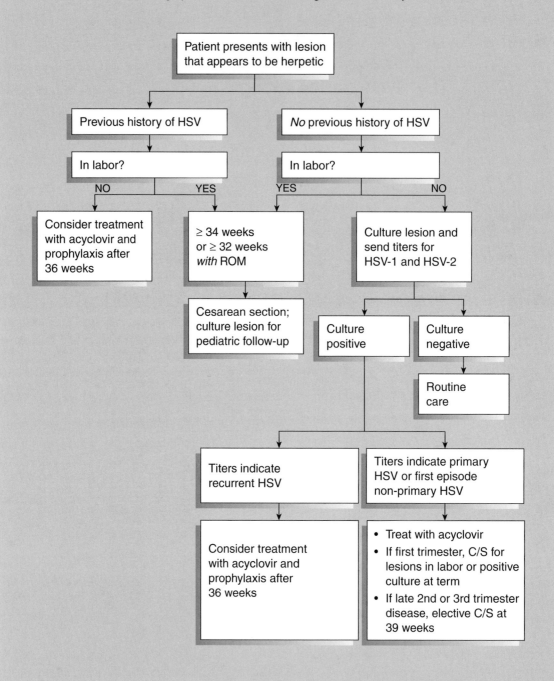

19 Herpes Simplex Virus

Steven J. Ralston

Introduction

Herpes simplex (HSV) is one of the most prevalent viral infections in pregnancy. Aside from the social stigma of being a sexually transmitted infection, the physical effects on maternal well-being are rarely important: the symptoms of HSV may be annoying and emotionally distressing but are usually self-limited and infrequent. However, the neonatal consequences of vertical transmission during pregnancy and childbirth can be devastating, with mortality rates as high as 50% and poor neurologic outcome in many survivors. Prevention of neonatal infection is the paramount goal of the management of HSV in pregnancy.

Virology

KEY POINT

HSV-1 and HSV-2 can cause genital herpes and neonatal infections.

Herpes simplex is a member of the Herpes family of viruses that includes varicella (chicken pox), Epstein-Barr virus (mononucleosis), and cytomegalovirus. These are double-stranded DNA viruses that produce of variety of medical illnesses in humans. There are two major subtypes, HSV-1 and HSV-2. HSV-1 primarily affects the oral mucosa, whereas HSV-2 is mainly a genital disease, and both subtypes can be sexually transmitted and can infect the vaginal mucosa, cervix, or vulva. In addition, both subtypes have been associated with neonatal herpetic infections of similar severity. Nevertheless, 90% of genital herpes infections in women are caused by HSV-2; thus HSV-2 is the more common pathogen of the two subtypes in the neonatal period.

321

Epidemiology

Studies of pregnant women in the United States have shown that 20–25% have serologic evidence of previous HSV-2 infection. The incidence of new maternal infections in pregnancy is 1–2%.[1] Neonatal herpes infection occurs in 1 in 7,500–15,000 births in the United States.

The terminology used to describe herpes infections can be confusing. *Primary disease* is an infection that occurs in someone with *no previous history* of HSV infection of either subtype. *First episode, nonprimary disease* is an infection in someone with previous HSV infection but of the heterologous subtype (i.e., a new infection of subtype 2 in someone who previously had subtype 1 or vice versa). *Recurrent infection* is a reactivation of disease in someone previously infected with HSV.

Neonatal Disease

Most newborns who acquire HSV do so during delivery; however, 5–10% become infected by a transplacental route. The virus can attack the neonate through the mucosal membranes or where there has been a loss of skin integrity. Vaginal delivery when the mother is shedding virus or has active lesions is the greatest risk factor; however, cesarean section is not entirely protective: in some series, up to 30% of newborns with HSV were delivered by cesarean section.[2]

Newborns who become infected with HSV can manifest the disease in a variety of ways. Mild disease accounts for 45% of cases of neonatal herpes; it is localized to the skin or eyes and typically these babies have good outcomes.[3] One third of babies present with central nervous system involvement, which is more of a concern because it is associated with a 15% mortality risk and a 40–60% risk of poor neurologic outcome in survivors. Moreover, 25% of babies present with disseminated disease; this portends a mortality rate higher than 50%, with poor neurologic outcomes in most survivors. Advances in antiviral medications have improved outcomes for babies with neonatally acquired HSV infections, but it remains a disease of significant morbidity and mortality.

There has been a good deal of published epidemiologic data demonstrating that transmission of HSV to the neonate is much more common with primary maternal infections than with recurrent infections.[4] This is likely due to the higher degree and longer duration of viral shedding in primary disease and the lack of protective maternal immunoglobulin (Ig) G given to the neonate transplacentally in primary disease. Published attack rates for neonates born vaginally to women with a primary infection (or nonprimary first episode) during labor are as high as 50%.[5] Recurrent disease in the mother confers a transmission rate of 1–3%. Previous maternal infection with HSV-1 does not appear to adequately protect the neonate against infection with HSV-2 (although previous infection with HSV-1 *may* protect the mother from acquiring HSV-2).[6]

Maternal Clinical Manifestations

KEY POINT

HSV should be suspected in any woman with a vulvar lesion that presents as a vesicle or ulcer. It is difficult to distinguish primary from recurrent disease on clinical grounds.

Genital herpes should be suspected in any woman complaining of a vulvar lesion. The differential diagnosis of such lesions is quite long (Table 19-1), however, the appearance and clinical course of herpetic lesions help to distinguish HSV from most other vulvar diseases. Classically, the herpetic lesion begins as a small papule that soon progresses to a vesicle or pustule and may occur anywhere on

Table 19-1. **DIFFERENTIAL DIAGNOSIS OF VULVAR LESIONS**

Infections
Herpes
Syphilis
Chancroid
Lymphogranuloma venereum
Granuloma inguinale
Candidiasis
Zoster
Folliculitis
Vaccinia
Molluscum contagiosum

Inflammatory conditions
Contact dermatitis
Inflammatory bowel disease
Stevens-Johnson syndrome

Autoimmune diseases
Behçet's disease

Neoplasms
Vulvar cancer

the vulva, thighs, vaginal mucosa, or cervix. As in chicken pox, the classic lesion appears as a small vesicle on a red base ("dewdrop on a rose petal"). After about 6 days, the vesicle or pustule will ulcerate and in about a week will begin crusting over. Concurrently with vesicle formation and ulceration, patients often will have local symptoms of itching, pain, or dysuria. Many patients also experience a prodrome of itching or discomfort in the area where the vesicles are destined to erupt. Systemic manifestations can occur (especially in primary infections) including fever, malaise, and lymphadenopathy. Urinary retention, hepatitis, and meningitis are rarer manifestations. Shedding of the virus begins before lesion formation and continues until the lesions have crusted over.

Distinguishing between primary and recurrent infections can be difficult when solely using clinical criteria. Many patients will have lesions that are asymptomatic, and even primary infections can occur without the patient knowing; similarly, recurrent infection can present with systemic manifestations and in patients with no history of HSV infection. In a study by Hensleigh and associates,[7] more than 80% of women who presented with signs and symptoms of herpetic infections in pregnancy and who were thought to have a primary infection by their practitioner actually had serologic evidence of *old* infection and thus were having recurrent outbreaks.

Whether primary or secondary, the diagnosis of a herpetic lesion can usually be made on clinical grounds (especially in a patient with a history of recurrent attacks). However, in someone with no history of HSV infection, it is worth confirming the diagnosis by laboratory investigation (see below). There are many reasons to perform these confirmatory tests: a woman with a primary HSV infection should be counseled about and screened for other sexually transmitted infections; an incorrect diagnosis of herpes can have significant adverse consequences for the woman and her partner if suspicions of infidelity are raised needlessly; and the perinatal effect of a primary HSV infection in pregnancy can be devastating to the newborn and appropriate preventative measures need to be taken.

Diagnosis

The gold standard for the diagnosis of HSV infection is culture. The yield depends on the amount of virus being shed; best results occur when the lesion is still a vesicle. The virus lives in the

KEY POINT

Culture of the base of the herpes ulcer remains the gold standard for diagnosis. Serology and polymerase chain reaction testing may be useful adjuncts in select patients.

epithelium at the base of the vesicle, so proper culturing technique involves unroofing the vesicle and obtaining the culture sample from the base of the ulcer. Most herpetic lesions will yield a positive culture in 3 days, with 90% being positive by 1 week. Recurrent lesions are less likely to produce a positive culture result because the window of viral shedding is shorter, as is the total viral load.

Microscopy of a smear obtained from the lesions (Tzanck's prep or Papanicolaou's smear) will show cytologic evidence of herpes infection in 60–70% of lesions that are culture positive. The classic findings are multinucleated giant cells and vacuolization. These are not often used as a primary means of diagnosis, although Papanicolaou's smear results with findings suggestive of herpes infection should be investigated.

Serologic tests are only rarely useful in the diagnosis and management of herpes infections in pregnancy. Nevertheless, these tests have improved markedly over the past decade, currently adequately distinguish between HSV subtypes, and may be useful in distinguishing primary from recurrent infections with increasing IgG titers in paired acute and convalescent samples. For women whose partners are known to carry HSV, serologic testing can accurately identify those women at risk for acquiring the infection during pregnancy, and these women can be offered appropriate counseling to prevent transmission. Serologic testing may also prove useful in women whose Papanicolaou's smears are suggestive of herpes infection.

Detection of viral DNA is possible using polymerase chain reaction (PCR) techniques, which are now commercially available. These tests are usually not necessary for vulvar disease because culture is extremely sensitive. However, in patients whose lesions are old and viral shedding may be especially low, the added sensitivity of PCR may be clinically useful. PCR for herpes infections has proved to be especially useful in the diagnosis of neonatal encephalitis because very low levels of viral DNA can be detecting in the newborn's cerebrospinal fluid.

Effects of Herpes Infection on Pregnancy Outcome

In addition to the neonatal risks of HSV infection, primary (and nonprimary first episode) disease has been associated with an increased risk of spontaneous abortion, intrauterine growth restriction, and preterm delivery.[8]

Antiviral Treatment of Herpes Infections in Pregnancy

PRIMARY DISEASE

KEY POINT

Acyclovir appears to be safe in pregnancy and should be used when clinically indicated without fear of fetal effects.

KEY POINT

Primary disease in pregnancy should be treated with acyclovir to decrease the severity of the outbreak and to decrease the amount of viral shedding.

When a pregnant woman presents with a clinical presentation suspicious for a primary herpes infection, confirmation of the diagnosis should be made by culture and serology. Antiviral therapy with acyclovir (400 mg three times daily for 7–14 days) or one of its relatives should not be withheld for fetal indications because these medications are likely safe in pregnancy. Further, there are clear maternal benefits to antiviral treatment in cases of disseminated disease, hepatitis, pneumonia, or encephalitis.[9] Therapy for primary disease in pregnancy also decreases the length of the outbreak and the amount of viral shedding.

Because recurrences and asymptomatic shedding are much more common after a primary infection, some investigators have supported the use of suppressive antiviral therapy in women who present with primary herpes in pregnancy. Suppressive therapy (400 mg two or three times daily) can decrease viral shedding and the need for cesarean section,[10] but there have not been studies large enough to demonstrate a decrease in neonatal disease.

If the primary infection occurs late in the pregnancy, then cesarean section is recommended when the patient labors at term because cervical viral shedding can be quite high for weeks after the primary infection. If the primary infection occurs in the first or second trimester, then some researchers have supported the use of acyclovir prophylaxis. Serial cultures to document absence of viral shedding *may* be useful in this small subgroup.

RECURRENT DISEASE

KEY POINT

Patients with frequent recurrences may benefit from acyclovir prophylaxis to prevent lesions in labor and thus cesarean section.

The management of recurrent disease in pregnancy is more controversial because the risk of neonatal disease is so much lower, so studies are difficult to conduct that will show a decrease in transmission. However, recent published data have demonstrated a decrease in the number of days of viral shedding, the number of recurrences, and the need for cesarean section in women with a history of genital herpes who were placed on prophylactic suppressive acyclovir therapy at 36 weeks of gestation.[11] One decision analysis in the literature[12] has suggested that it is cheaper to administer acyclovir prophylaxis to these women to prevent shedding. My personal bias is to give prophylaxis to those women with a history of genital herpes who have frequent recurrences (six or more times per year) or for whom a cesarean section would pose significant morbidity. Prophylaxis may be started at 36 weeks of gestation or sooner if the patient has a history of preterm delivery. Patients who are coinfected with the human immunodeficiency virus have higher rates of recurrence and also may benefit from acyclovir prophylaxis.

Prevention of Vertical Transmission

KEY POINT

Cesarean section is indicated in any woman who presents in labor with a vulvar, vaginal, or cervical lesion that is thought to be herpetic.

Regardless of whether she has received antiviral prophylaxis, cesarean section should be performed for any woman who presents in labor with active herpetic lesions on the cervix, vagina, or vulva. The reason for this recommendation is twofold: cesarean section may protect against infection,[13] and neonatal disease acquired from recurrent lesions, although rare, is just as damaging to the neonate as that acquired from primary disease.

In patients who have herpes outbreaks that are nongenital (e.g., thigh or buttocks), cesarean section probably can be safely avoided if these are areas can be covered to avoid contamination of the newborn during delivery. Although cervical shedding is certainly possible with these distal lesions, this shedding probably poses more of a theoretical risk than a real danger to the fetus or neonate.

The use of fetal scalp electrodes, vacuum extraction, and forceps in these patients is controversial. Each of these devices is associated with trauma to the fetal scalp or skin, but there is no clear evidence that they increase the risk of neonatal transmission of the herpes virus. It may be best to avoid these interventions if possible, but they are not contraindicated.

As HSV screening has become more accurate in distinguishing between HSV subtypes 1 and 2, the role of HSV titers in preventing neonatal HSV has become more controversial. Some experts have suggested universal screening and counseling of couples at risk for transmission during pregnancy, but it is not clear that this large-scale endeavor would be cost effective. Certainly, if a woman's partner is known to have a history of HSV-2 and she is shown to be HSV-2 antibody negative, it would be wise to counsel her about the prevention of transmission by abstention or condom use, especially during the third trimester.

What's the Evidence?

There is ample evidence that neonatal herpes is more common in women who have active lesions or who are asymptomatically shedding virus at the time of their labor.[1,8] There is also excellent data supporting the efficacy of acyclovir therapy in decreasing the amount of viral shedding at the time of delivery in women with a history of herpes.[10,11] However, there are no clear data showing the cost effectiveness of universal prophylaxis with acyclovir. Research is ongoing regarding the use of acyclovir in pregnancy and/or the possibility of vaccine development to prevent primary disease. It should also be noted that, although there are data showing that cesarean section is not fully protective in preventing neonatal herpes, a recent study supports the notion that cesarean section may be useful in the management of this disease.[13]

Guiding Questions in Approaching the Patient

- Does a woman who presents with a vulvar lesion have a herpes infection?
- Is this a primary or recurrent infection?
- Is she a candidate for antiviral therapy?
- Is the neonate at risk and is a cesarean section indicated?

Conclusion

HSV is a common infection in pregnant women and the results of neonatal transmission can be devastating. Patients who have primary infections in pregnancy are at highest risk of transmitting the disease to their babies; these women should be offered primary cesarean sections if their infection occurs late in pregnancy, if they have active lesions in labor, or if they have evidence of shedding during labor. Patients with recurrent HSV can be reassured that their risk of transmission is low, but they also should be offered cesarean section if they have active lesions in labor. Acyclovir prophylaxis is probably safe in pregnancy and may be cost effective in preventing cesarean sections in women with frequent outbreaks.

Discussion of Cases

CASE 1: VESICULAR LESION IN LABOR

A 35-year-old gravida 5, para 4 presents in labor at term with membranes that ruptured 6 hours previously; dilation is 8 cm and the patient has a history of four spontaneous vaginal deliveries. Physical examination shows a vesicular lesion with an erythematous base on the vulva. She has no history of herpes infections and is otherwise feeling well with no systemic manifestations or regional lymphadenopathy.

Should this patient be offered a cesarean section?

Because there is no diagnostic test that can rapidly rule out herpes in this patient, a cesarean section is indicated. Even though the risk of neonatal transmission is low with recurrent herpes, the consequences may be devastating, so every effort should be made to prevent transmission; the risk of a cesarean section to the vast majority of women is low.

Does the period of membrane rupture affect your decision-making process in these patients?

No. Neonates can become infected with membrane rupture of any interval; conversely, cesarean section may be protective even after prolonged membrane rupture.

CASE 2: PRIMARY HSV IN PREGNANCY

A 24-year-old gravida 2, para 1 presents at 34 weeks with what appears to be a herpetic lesion on her vulva. She has no history of herpes.

What tests would you order?

Culturing the base of the lesion is the most important step in the management of this patient. If the lesion is herpetic, then therapy with acyclovir is indicated. She should also be screened for other sexually transmitted diseases including HSV. In addition, serologic testing for HSV-1 and HSV-2 IgG and IgM should be considered. If this is serologically a *primary* infection, then the patient should continue with acyclovir and primary cesarean section at term should be recommended because the risk of the viral shedding at term is so high in patients with primary disease late in pregnancy.

CASE 3: PARTNER WITH HSV

A 28-year-old gravida 1, para 0 presents for her first prenatal visit. She has no history of herpes, but her husband does and he has outbreaks every 3–4 months.

What tests would you order?

Serologic testing should be done to determine whether the patient has ever been exposed to HSV.

How would you counsel her?

If her serologic findings show previous HSV infection, then you can reassure her that she is unlikely to transmit the disease to her infant unless she has lesions in labor. She does not need to modify her behavior during pregnancy. If her serologic findings show that she has *not* been exposed to herpes, then she is at risk of acquiring primary infection during her pregnancy. She should be told to refrain from sexual relations from her husband whenever he begins to have a herpetic prodrome until the time his lesions crust over; they should also consider using condoms during the pregnancy. If he has frequent outbreaks, it is probably safest for them to abstain from sex entirely during the pregnancy.

REFERENCES

1 Brown ZA, Selke S, Zeh J, Kopelman J, et al. The acquisition of herpes simplex virus during pregnancy. *N Engl J Med* 1997;337:509–515.

2 Sánchez PJ, Siegle JD. Herpes simplex virus. In: McMillan J, et al, eds. *Oski's Pediatrics*, 3rd ed. Philadelphia: Lippincott Williams & Wilkins, 1999; p. 433–436.

3 Hensleigh PA, Nguyen LK. Genital herpes simplex virus. In: Gonik B, ed. *Viral Diseases in Pregnancy.* New York: Springer-Verlag, 1994; p. 52–68.

4 Prober CG, Sullender WM, Yasukawa LL, et al. Low risk of herpes simplex virus infections in neonates exposed to virus at the time of vaginal delivery with recurrent herpes simplex virus infections. *N Engl J Med* 1987;316:240–244.

5 Brown ZA, Benedetti J, Ashley R et al. Neonatal herpes simplex virus infection in relation to asymptomatic maternal infection at the time of labor. *N Engl J Med* 1991;324:1247–1252.

6 Mertz GL, Benedetti J, Ashley R, et al. Risk factor for the sexual transmission of genital herpes. *Ann Intern Med* 1992;116:197–202.

7 Hensleigh PA, Andrews WW, Brown ZA, et al. Genital herpes during pregnancy; inability to distinguish primary and recurrent infections clinically. *Obstet Gynecol* 1997;89:891–895.

8 Brown ZA, Vontver LA, Bendetti J, et al. Effects on infants of a first episode of genital herpes during pregnancy. *N Engl J Med* 1987; 312:1246.

9 Lagrew DC Jr, Furlow TG, Hager WD, et al. Disseminated herpes simplex virus infection in pregnancy. Successful treatment with acyclovir. *JAMA* 1984;252:2058–2059.

10 Scott LL, Sanchez PJ, Jackson GL, et al. Acyclovir to prevent cesarean delivery after first-episode genital herpes. *Obstet Gynecol* 1996;87: 69–73.

11 Watts DH, Brown ZA, Money D, et al. A double-blind, randomized, placebo-controlled trial of acyclovir in late pregnancy for the reduction of herpes simplex virus shedding and cesarean delivery. *Am J Obestet Gynecol* 2003;188:836–843.

12 Randolph AG, Hartshorn RM, Washington AE. Acyclovir prophylaxis in late pregnancy to prevent neonatal herpes: a cost-effectiveness analysis. *Obstet Gyncol* 1996;88:603–610.

13 Brown ZA, Wald A, Morrow RA, et al. Effect of serologic status and cesarean delivery on transmission rates of herpes simplex virus from mother to infant. *JAMA* 2003;289:203–209.

Approach to Pregnant Women with HIV

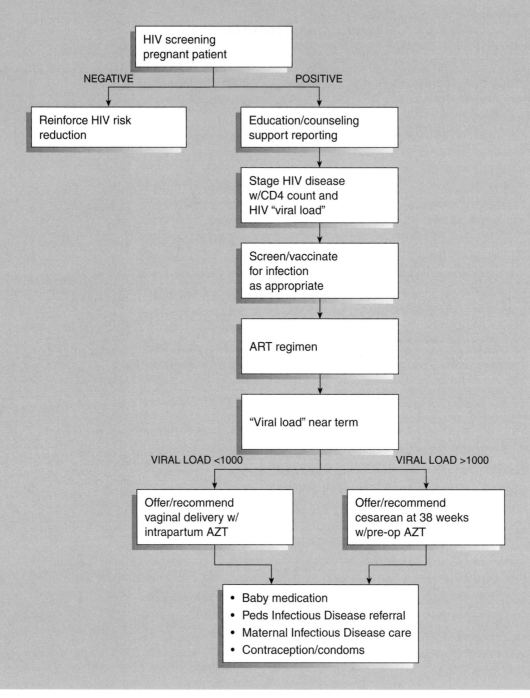

20 Care of the HIV-Infected Pregnant Woman

Elizabeth G. Livingston

Introduction

Infection with human immunodeficiency virus (HIV) has been recognized for just over two decades. Currently, nearly 1 million Americans live with HIV infection. Worldwide, 42 million people are believed to live with HIV infection, with 70% of those individuals living in sub-Saharan Africa. In the United States, HIV has become the leading cause of death for women 25–44 years old in some urban areas and the third leading cause for death in this age group nationwide. Of the estimated 40,000 new infections occurring in the United States each year, 25% are in women.[1] Of those women, fewer than 50% are younger than 25 years old and more than 50% are infected heterosexually. Deaths in the United States due to HIV and acquired immunodeficiency syndrome (AIDS) and the incidence of HIV vertical transmission have plummeted over the past 10 years due to better therapies. Currently, 280–370 infected infants are born in the United States each year.[2] Despite accurate information regarding the cause of HIV/AIDS and its method of spread, the incidence of new infections remains constant in this country and continues to increase in the developing world.

Pathophysiology

HIV is a single-stranded RNA virus in the family of retroviruses. HIV infection is usually contracted through sexual contact (vaginal, anal, or oral), contact with blood (intravenous drug use, health care occupational exposure, and blood products), and vertical transmission from mother to child (during intrauterine life, delivery, and breast feeding).

COURSE OF ILLNESS

After gaining entry to the body, HIV infects predominately T lymphocytes and macrophages by fusing with surface CD4 receptors and coreceptors. The RNA virus uses the enzyme reverse transcriptase to make a DNA copy of its genome, which is inserted into the host cell DNA. New viruses are released, destroying the CD4 lymphocyte. HIV infections cause gradual immunologic decline of the host through destruction of CD4 (T helper) cells.

After initial HIV infection, most individuals develop a flu-like primary illness characterized by high levels of virus for a few weeks. There is no HIV antibody during this period, and diagnosis of the infection may be difficult unless the index of suspicion is high and the clinician orders tests looking for virus rather than for antibody.

Next, the individual develops a lengthy, asymptomatic latent infection. Antibody is present, and conventional tests may be used to diagnose infection. The infected individual can transmit the virus during this latent period that may last for longer than a decade. For a few lucky individuals, known as long-term nonprogressors, immune decline does not occur. However, in most people, there is eventual immune decline as CD4 cells decrease. As the CD4 count decreases below 200/mL, the individual develops AIDS and is prone to life-threatening infections such as *Pneumocystis* pneumonia. Average time from diagnosis of AIDS to death, if untreated, is about 2 years.

STAGING ILLNESS WITH VIRAL LOAD AND CD4 COUNT

Clinically, a physician may measure the number of CD4 cells and the level of free circulating virus ("viral load") measured by polymerase chain reaction (PCR). The clinician uses these measurements to understand the degree to which infected individuals' immune systems have been affected, their need for medical intervention, and their risk of opportunistic infection. An absolute CD4 count of 200 or less is considered immunocompromised and meets the case definition for AIDS, whereas a CD4 count of 500 or more indicates relatively preserved immune function. A viral load lower than 500 indicates a low risk of disease progression, whereas a load higher than 30,000 is associated with a more rapid decline in CD4 cells.

Identification of the HIV-Infected Pregnant Patient

SCREENING
STRATEGIES

KEY POINT

HIV testing should be recommended to all pregnant women in the United States.

With the possibility of treatment for the mother and the ability to prevent vertical transmission, most professional groups advocate for the availability of HIV testing to all pregnant women in the United States. Screening based on patient-reported risk factors has been repeatedly shown to exclude many seropositive women. The United States Public Health Service (USPHS), Institute of Medicine, American College of Obstetrics and Gynecology (ACOG), and American Academy of Pediatrics support universal testing as a routine component of prenatal care. These groups suggest that an extensive pretest counseling process may hinder efforts to test most patients. The ACOG and American Academy of Pediatrics recommend patient notification of the testing and the right of refusal of the test.

DIFFERENT
APPROACHES

Laws vary from state to state regarding HIV testing. Most approaches fall under three types of testing strategies. *Opt-in* testing is where women are offered pretest counseling, and the woman must specifically consent to the HIV test. This approach results in pregnancy testing rates of 25–69%.[3] *Opt-out* refers to notifying women that HIV will be included in a battery of tests, and they may refuse HIV testing. The opt-out approach is associated with higher testing rates of 71–85% of pregnant women. *Mandatory* testing is the routine testing of newborns if the mother has declined previous testing. Testing rates in those states range from 81–93%. Because not all women will obtain prenatal care, no testing strategy will achieve 100% testing rates. An additional testing strategy includes offering a second test late in pregnancy to women in high HIV prevalence communities, where seroconversion during pregnancy occurs more frequently.

RAPID TESTING

Rapid HIV testing of women who present in labor without prenatal care offers an opportunity to administer intrapartum and neonatal medication for the prevention of vertical transmission. Positive findings need confirmation with standard testing. In 2002, the United States Food and Drug Administration approved the OraQuick

(Abbott Diagnostics, Abbott Park, IL) rapid HIV-1 antibody test, which allows for testing with a median turnaround time of 45 minutes. Rapid testing with medication intervention in labor is a strategy that appears promising for resource-poor settings.

DIAGNOSTIC TESTS   The most common screening test for HIV detection looks for the presence of antibodies with an enzyme-linked immunosorbent assay (ELISA). If positive, the test is repeated to eliminate laboratory errors. If repeatedly positive, a confirmatory test, usually a western blot, is performed. For the western blot test, specific viral proteins are separated by electrophoresis. Reaction of antibody to three proteins must occur to be considered positive.

False-negative results can occur early in the course of infection, but overall an ELISA has about 98% sensitivity. For the patient with recent or ongoing exposure to HIV, repeat testing every 6 months may be worthwhile. False-positive results are uncommon, although the incidence increases when testing is performed in groups with a low incidence of HIV infection. False-positive results have been noted after some vaccinations. Western blot has about a false-positive rate of 1 in 20,000. An indeterminate result occurs when one or two bands are positive on the western blot rather than the three required for a positive result. In low-risk populations, indeterminant results generally revert to negative over several months.

COUNSELING AFTER TESTING   All patients with negative results should receive the results of their HIV testing. For those engaging in risky behaviors, HIV testing may be an opportunity to promote behavioral change. All HIV-positive patients need to be told clearly about their diagnosis. All HIV-infected patients, pregnant or not, need to understand their duties to others including informing their sexual partners, using latex condoms for intercourse, avoiding blood and organ donation, and not sharing razors or toothbrushes. The pregnant patient needs to have the risk of vertical transmission and the benefits of intervention with antiretroviral therapy explained.

Effect of Pregnancy on HIV Infection

Despite the evidence that pregnancy is associated with an overall decreased immune response, pregnancy is not usually associated with hastening of the immunocompromise associated with HIV infection. A meta-analysis of previous studies indicated that inter-current pregnancies do not appear to increase the rate of progression to AIDS.[4] Follow-up of 400 women with second pregnancies in the Women Infants Transmission Study showed similar CD4 status when compared with women with single pregnancies.[5] A transient depression of the CD4 count has been noted in late pregnancy but usually recovers after delivery.[6]

Effect of HIV Infection on Pregnancy

Aside from the risk of vertical transmission, a pregnant HIV-infected woman in the United States can anticipate a pregnancy outcome similar to that of her uninfected peers. Although higher rates of prematurity and low birth weight have been noted in HIV-infected women when compared with the United States population at large, this result does not persist when compared with adequately selected control groups. Poor pregnancy outcome in HIV-infected women in the United States appears to be related to other risk factors such as socioeconomic status, ongoing illicit drug use, and coexistent sexually transmitted diseases.[7] HIV is not known to be teratogenic. In general, HIV-infected women do not have higher recorded rates of anomalies due to cytomega-lovirus or toxoplasmosis.[7]

General Principles Guiding Medication Use

INITIATION IN NONPREGNANT INDIVIDUALS

In the late 1990s, the combined use of three or more antiretroviral drugs was found to be highly successful at suppressing viral replication. These drug combinations, known as highly active anti-retroviral therapy (HAART), can halt replication of virus and allow recovery of the immune system. Unfortunately, HIV cannot be completely eliminated from the body even with long-term suppression of viral replication due to long-lived infected lymphocytes within nodes. Although not curative, medications allow HIV infection to be managed as a chronic illness. Until viral resistance to medications occurs or complications due to the medications occur, immune compromise can be indefinitely deferred, and life span can be extended. Current USPHS guidelines suggest initiation when the CD4 count decreases to lower than 350/mm^3 or the HIV RNA PCR "viral load" levels exceed 55,000 copies/mL.

CATEGORIES OF MEDICATIONS

The most commonly used medications fall into three categories: nucleoside/nucleotide reverse transcriptase inhibitors, non-nucleoside reverse transcriptase inhibitors, and protease inhibitors. Updated information about safety and teratogenicity of these medications can be found in the document "Safety and Toxicity of Individual Antiretroviral Agents in Pregnancy" that is available on the Internet (http://aidsinfo.nih.gov/drugs/).[8]

USE OF HAART

COMBINATION STRATEGIES Because of the many available antiretroviral medications, there are many potential combinations for HAART. Clinicians' choice of medications depends on the patient's degree of immunocompromise, previous drug exposures, viral resistance testing, toxicity profiles, other medications, and drug expense. A common HAART combination would consist of two nucleoside agents and a protease inhibitor. There is no single best regimen that optimizes viral suppression and ease of use and minimizes side effects. With an increasing array of drugs, recommendations are not static. An Infectious Disease consultation should be considered before initiating therapy. The USPHS recommendations for treatment are maintained and regularly updated on an Internet Web site (http://www.aidsinfo.nih.org/).[9]

MONITORING HAART The CD4 count and viral load are measured every 3–4 months on HAART to determine effectiveness of the regimen. The best clinical responses occur when the viral load decreases below detectable levels (<50 with ultrasensitive HIV RNA PCR assays), which should occur in 6 months. Usually, an effective drug regimen will result in a 0.6 log decrease in virus in the first 1–2 months.[9] In general, the first set of drugs taken by the patient will be the most effective regimen.

BARRIERS TO HAART EFFECTIVENESS

ADHERENCE For patients who do not achieve optimal viral suppression, there are several potential causes. Adherence is the ability of the patient to take regimens as recommended by the care provider. Side effects of the medications, complexity of the regimen, denial of the seriousness of the illness, lack of education on the importance of consistent use of the drugs, depression, and drug use can make adherence to a complicated antiretroviral drug regimen difficult. Enrollees in HIV clinical trials generally achieve adherence in the range of 90%. In HIV-infected pregnant patients, reported adherence rates have been as high as 80% to as low as 34.2%. A 95% adherence rate may be necessary for optimal HAART results.

RESISTANCE Another cause of regimen failure is viral resistance to the medications in the regimen. Antiretroviral resistance can occur when there is ongoing viral replication in the presence of the selection pressure of subtherapeutic medication levels. Use of antiretroviral monotherapy or taking a medication at improper intervals may increase the likelihood that resistance occurs by incompletely suppressing viral replication and allowing selection for resistant virus. Some individuals or neonates may be primarily infected with resistant HIV. Most experts agree that eventually all HIV medication regimens will fail over time. Hence, it is necessary to emphasize proper adherence to the HAART regimen and careful choice of the sequence of treatment regimens to avoid resistance and prolong their effectiveness.

Commercial assays are available to evaluate for drug resistance. Utility of resistance assays is limited by a requirement that the viral load be over 1000. Recommendations for the optimal use of these assays usually suggest evaluating resistance after regimen failure or if treatment occurs during the primary infection episode. An International AIDS Society–USA Panel has recommended resistance testing for pregnant women with viremia when the woman has a history of antiretroviral exposure, or there are high rates of drug resistant virus in the community.[10] Most groups in the United States recommend using resistance testing in pregnancy for the same indications as outside pregnancy: a high likelihood there is infection with resistant virus by history of medication failure or infection in an area with high prevalence of resistant virus.[9] Patients should be taught that if they are unable to tolerate or adhere to a regimen, they are benefited more by abruptly discontinuing medications than by skipping doses, which might promote viral resistance.

SIDE EFFECTS OF HAART

Side effects of antiretroviral medications can range from merely annoying to deadly. Nucleoside agents can cause headaches and malaise. In 70% of patients, zidovudine (ZDV; formerly AZT; Retrovir, GlaxoSmithKline, Research Triangle Park, NC) administration will result in a mild megaloblastic anemia. With regimens that contain protease inhibitors, gastrointestinal disturbances are common. Nevirapine (Viramune, Roxane Laboratories, Columbus, OH) can cause a Stevens-Johnson syndrome type of rash in a small percentage of patients. It has also been associated with hepatitis. Metabolic complications are observed on HAART regimens including the development of insulin resistance, hyperlipidemia, lactic acidosis, hepatic steatosis, osteopenia, centripetal obesity, buffalo hump, and breast enlargement. Nucleoside reverse transcriptase inhibitors can bind to mitochondrial DNA polymerase gamma and cause inhibition of mitochondrial replication and function, leading to lactic acidosis and liver failure.

Whether these side effects of antiretroviral medications are more common in pregnancy is unclear. Higher baseline pregnancy rates in HIV-negative women of nausea, vomiting, glucose intolerance, lipidemia, cholestasis, and acute fatty liver suggest a need for vigilance. A small number of cases of death due to liver failure in pregnancy in women taking stavudine (d4T, Zerit, Bristol Myers Squibb, New York, NY) and didanosine (ddI, Videx, Bristol Myers Squibb) in combination have been reported. Other deaths due to liver failure have been noted in pregnant women on ZDV/lamivudine (Combivir, GlaxoSmithKline), nelfinavir (Viracept, Agouron Pharmaceuticals, LaJolla, CA), and nevirapine (Virammune, Roxane Laboratories, Columbus, OH; manufacturer's drug safety information).

Additional Maternal Care

In addition to antiretroviral therapy, the HIV-infected pregnant woman may require other health interventions. As in all pregnancies, screening for other sexually transmitted diseases such as syphilis, gonorrhea, and Chlamydia is indicated. Herpes prophylaxis can be given as in uninfected pregnancies. Routine evaluation for hepatitis C should be performed in HIV-positive women. Higher rates of vertical transmission of hepatitis C may be seen in the setting of HIV infection. Patients should be screened for hepatitis B carrier status and vaccinated, if indicated. Influenza and pneumococcal vaccinations are also indicated. Tuberculosis skin testing should be conducted. Most clinicians have abandoned anergy testing and use a 5-mm purified protein derivative (PPD) result as positive. If there is a strong concern for tuberculosis, the diagnosis should be pursued even with a negative skin test. A Papanicolaou's smear should be done because the HIV-infected population has a high incidence of dysplasia.

Most clinicians obtain baseline liver and renal function tests before initiating medications. Screening and intervention for substance use should be performed. Although baseline serologies for toxoplasmosis and cytomegalovirus may prove useful in patients who have severe immunocompromise and develop complications, delaying these tests until after delivery is reasonable to avoid maternal anxiety regarding perinatal infection. For patients with low CD4 counts, prophylaxis for opportunistic infections such as *Pneumocystis* pneumonia (same as in nonpregnant patients) or *Mycobacterium avium* (azithromycin is used in place of clarithromycin, which has teratogenicity issues) may be required.[7,9]

Vertical Transmission

RISK FACTORS

Despite the tremendous advances during the past decade in the understanding and prevention of vertical HIV infection from mother to child, our knowledge of the pathophysiology of transmission is far from complete. Reported rates of transmission without intervention in the industrialized world are 14–25%. The maternal clinical factor portending the greatest risk of vertical transmission is advanced maternal disease state.[11] Reflective of this risk, high maternal HIV RNA viral load has been correlated with a higher risk of vertical transmission, whereas lower levels are associated with decreased risk.[12]

Other research on vertical transmission suggests that most (~70%) infections to the fetus occur intrapartum, with fewer cases (~30%) occurring before labor. Higher rates of vertical transmission have been noted when membranes are ruptured for longer than 4 hours before birth, presumably due to prolonged exposure of the fetus to virus in maternal vaginal secretions. Prematurity, chorioamnionitis, use of scalp electrodes, or scalp sampling are also associated with higher risks of vertical transmission. The exact mechanisms of viral transfer, either antepartum or intrapartum, is unknown.

VERTICAL
TRANSMISSION
PREVENTION WITH
MEDICATIONS

KEY POINT

*Optimal therapy
with medications
can decrease
HIV vertical
transmission rates
to 1–2%.*

Antiretroviral drugs, alone or in combination, decrease mother-to-child HIV transmission rates. The 1994 AIDS Clinical Trial Group 076 reported that ZDV could interrupt HIV infection from mother to the infant.[13] Subsequently, some modified shortened courses of ZDV have been demonstrated to be nearly as effective.[7] The exact mechanisms of protection by ZDV is not clear because follow-up reports suggest protection independent of modest decreases in viral load.[14] The assumption is that drug levels in the fetus confer postexposure protection analogous to occupationally exposed health care workers on medication by preventing initial viral replication.

Another single-agent antiretroviral therapy, nevirapine, dramatically decreased vertical transmission rates in an African study, HIVNET 012.[15] A simple cost-saving regimen of a single intrapartum dose of nevirapine to the mother and a postnatal dose to the baby was more effective than a shortened ZDV regimen. Of concern, even after a single dose of nevirapine, high rates of viral resistance to nevirapine have been observed, making this drug less useful if required for future maternal treatment. Similarly, investigation of Combivir (combination ZDV/lamivudine tablets, GlaxoSmithKline) for dual therapy for prevention of vertical transmission demonstrated lamivudine viral resistance to these medications in 40% of mothers.[16]

All pregnant women should be recommended to take antiretroviral therapy to decrease the risk of vertical transmission. Combination therapy improves the chance that viral levels will be decreased to undetectable levels and minimize vertical transmission.[7,9] Women on three or more agents, HAART, and undetectable HIV RNA viral loads have vertical transmission rates of 1–2%.[7] No regimen has resulted in absence of vertical transmission of virus.

Looking beyond the limited scope of vertical transmission, the use of HAART has potential long-term health benefits for the HIV-infected mother because it may slow progression of HIV infection and prolong life. A USPHS publication has stated that pregnancy should not preclude the use of antiretroviral agents as prescribed for nonpregnant individuals.[9]

Nonpregnant patients with a CD4 count higher than 500×10^6/L and HIV RNA levels below 5000 copies/mL are at low risk of clinical progression over the next 3 years and may not need immediate HAART for their well-being.[9] Review of older data suggest that

ZDV monotherapy may be a reasonable alternative to HAART in these patients. Vertical transmission rates have been reported in the 1% range with low viral loads and ZDV monotherapy.[17] Due to the low level of viral replication, development of resistance is unlikely. Individual considerations regarding the best regimen for prevention of vertical transmission and the role of medication in lifelong treatment need to be balanced.

OBSTETRIC COMPLICATIONS OF MEDICATIONS Early data that assessed pregnancy outcome of women treated with combination therapy suggested a higher rate of side effects. Follow-up studies suggested that, if outcome were controlled for stage of disease, previous poor pregnancy outcome outside therapy, and drug use, the risk of preterm delivery, low birth weight, low Apgar scores, and stillbirth would be unaltered.[18]

Teratogenicity data have been limited. Several pharmaceutical companies have established an Antiviral Pregnancy Registry (www.APRegistry.com) that has more than 2000 reported exposures to date. Birth defect rates have paralleled the general population rates.[19] One agent that has raised teratogenic concern is efavirenz. The FDA has recently changed the pregnancy to category D given retrospective reports of neural tube defects in women exposed to efavirenz in the first trimester.[20] In utero exposure to tenofovir has resulted in bone lesions in monkey offspring, although no human lesions have been reported. The USPHS recommends that pregnant women already on antiretroviral medications at the time of conception continue the medications, except for those with specific fetal concerns, whereas those patients diagnosed during early pregnancy should delay treatment until after the first trimester.

NEONATAL MITOCHONDRIAL TOXICITY Recently, concern has been raised over a risk of mitochondrial toxicity to the offspring of a mother on retroviral therapies. Large retrospective reviews of exposed infants failed to confirm the risk. Concerns regarding toxicity must be balanced against the risk of vertical transmission. Nucleoside agents may be inserted into nonviral DNA chains, raising concerns for carcinogenicity in exposed children. This has not been observed in practice to date, and a National Institutes of Health expert consensus statement suggested that the real benefit of medication exposure greatly outweighed the theoretical risks. Only 10 years of follow-up are available for children exposed to ZDV and fewer for combination therapies; hence, long-term consequences are unknown.

KEY POINT

Cesarean section may play a role in decreasing vertical transmission risk in some HIV-infected women.

POTENTIAL BENEFITS Preventing the fetus from being exposed to vaginal secretions of the HIV-infected mother seems logical, but early studies on the effectiveness of cesarean section in the prevention of vertical transmission had inconsistent results. Recent studies have controlled for the use of antiretroviral drugs, labor, and ruptured membranes and have suggested a benefit from cesarean section. A meta-analysis of 15 prospective cohort studies in Europe and North America involving 8000 women found that cesarean section before onset of labor decreased the risk of vertical transmission by 50% with ZDV alone.[21] Among patients who received ZDV, vertical transmission occured in 2.0% of those who delivered by elective cesarean section and 7.3% of those with other modes of delivery. A European, prospective, randomized, controlled trial suggested that there is a 1.8% risk of infection associated with cesarean sections compared with a 10.5% risk of infection for vaginal deliveries.[22] With these studies in hand, the ACOG drafted a committee opinion that HIV-infected pregnant women with viral loads higher than 1000 should be counseled regarding the potential benefit of cesarean section for prevention of vertical infection.[23] This publication acknowledges that the cesarean benefit is not clear in women with viral loads below 1000 or for pregnancies after onset of labor or rupture of membranes. If cesarean section is selected as the mode of delivery, the ACOG recommends the procedure be done at 38 weeks to avoid onset of labor. Preoperative ZDV intravenous infusion should be administered. Current data suggest the logical stance of avoiding fetal contact with HIV through the use of HAART or by a combination of antiretroviral medications plus cesarean section.

COMPLICATIONS OF CESAREAN SECTION Although HAART is not always entirely safe or well tolerated, cesarean section also has its risks. The European Collaborative Study on cesarean section addressed this issue and found no serious morbidities but did find significantly higher rates of febrile morbidity (6.7% vs. 1.1%) and anemia (hemoglobin <8 mg/dL in 4 of 225 women vs. 2 of 183 women) in cesarean section deliveries compared with vaginal deliveries. When compared with HIV-negative cesarean patients, no differences in major morbidities were found, with a slightly higher risk of febrile morbidity.[22] A retrospective comparison among HIV seropositive mothers showed the highest rates of morbidity among emergent cesarean deliveries when compared with vaginal deliveries and elective cesareans. When analyses were performed including emergent cesareans for unsuccessful labor in the vaginal delivery group, vaginal deliveries, and elective cesarean sections showed similar rates of morbidity.[24]

There is risk to the operative team while performing a cesarean section on an HIV-infected patient. Although the use of sharp instruments cannot be avoided, the liberal use of cautery, blunt-tipped needles, and double gloving and assembling experienced operating room teams for an elective daytime procedure may decrease occupational risk.[25] A "dryer" operative field may also have the advantage of decreasing the risk of vertical transmission.

POSTNATAL CARE OF THE INFANT

After birth, the infant should be cleaned of maternal secretions. HIV cultures and HIV PCR should be obtained from neonatal blood draw rather than from the cord, where false-positive findings are prone to occur. Prophylaxis with ZDV syrup should begin shortly after birth. Controversy exists over whether more potent neonatal drugs should be given for prophylaxis if the mother had advanced disease at birth or if the mother is known to have ZDV-resistant virus. Breast feeding is discouraged. Identification of the vertically infected child can generally be confirmed by age 4 months. Rather than awaiting the disappearance of maternal antibody, PCR or culture techniques allow the identification of virus from the infant's blood.

BREAST FEEDING

Controversy also surrounds the risk of breast feeding. The estimated risk of HIV transmission with breast feeding is about 14% higher than the antepartum or intrapartum risk.[9] Whether the risk of infectious diarrhea with formula feeding outweighs the risk of HIV transmission is unclear. The infant appears to be at risk throughout the duration of lactation and not just in critical periods that might be amenable to short-term drug interventions.

What's the Evidence?

Randomized clinical trials have demonstrated the usefulness of medication for prevention of vertical transmission. ZDV administered by the ACTG 076 study antepartum, intrapartum, and to the neonate decreased HIV transmission from 25% to 6%.[13] Nevirapine administered by the HIVNET 012 study intrapartum and to the neonate demonstrated that a simpler method could be used to prevent vertical transmission in the developing world.[15] Some clinical trials have supported the use of cesarean section to prevent vertical transmission. The European Mode of Delivery Collaboration, a randomized trial, demonstrated the benefit of cesarean section in the prevention of vertical transmission.[24] More information is needed on the risk of hepatic failure in pregnant women on antiretrovirals. Better information on practices that promote adherence to medications in pregnancy are required. More long-term follow-up studies of infants exposed to drugs in pregnancy are warranted. The role of cesarean section in women with low HIV viral loads should be investigated. Cheap, effective, and acceptable therapies that can be implemented should be devised.

Guiding Questions in Approaching the Patient

The newly diagnosed patient

- Does she have other medical illnesses?
- Is she at risk for viral resistance?
- What is the stage of her illness?
- Does she have barriers such as depression or substance abuse that might affect her ability to adhere to a medication regimen?

Choosing a medication regimen

- Does she have a contraindication to ZDV use?
- Has she been exposed previously to antiretroviral medications?
- Does her virus have known resistance to certain medications?
- Does she have other medical illnesses that might affect her ability to tolerate certain medications?
- Would it be advantageous to the patient to save a category of antiretroviral medications?

Choosing a delivery route

- What is the patient's HIV viral load?
- Does she have obstetric indications for a cesarean section?
- Does she have a medical illness that might make a cesarean more hazardous?

Conclusion

Hope for a cure for HIV infection has diminished, but medications have emerged to make it a manageable albeit expensive chronic illness. The development of a vaccine truly preventive of new infection lies in the future. As a consequence, providing universal access to HIV screening and providing patients with the knowledge to avoid contracting or spreading HIV infection should be a goal of every practicing health care provider.

Discussion of Cases

CASE 1:

You are seeing a 24-year-old primigravida for her second obstetric visit at 16 weeks of gestation. She consented to and received HIV testing as part of her obstetric laboratory tests that were performed the previous week. The laboratory reports a positivity to HIV by ELISA and western blot. You share the results of the test with her. After she recovers from the news, she begins to talk about her concerns that a former partner experimented with street drugs, and she worries that he may have been HIV positive. She is anxious and has many questions about her diagnosis.

How do you counsel her regarding avoiding transmission to others?

She should not donate blood, semen, or organs. She should not share toothbrushes or razors where small quantities of blood may be present. She should avoid vaginal, oral, and anal sex or practice "safer" sex with latex condoms and dental dams. She should inform past and current sexual partners directly or by a public health contact tracing, so that they may be tested. She should be told that hugging, "dry" kissing, eating utensils, coughing, and used diapers cannot transmit the infection.

She is worried about the risk of transmission to the baby.

What risk do you quote?

With no treatment, the risk of vertical transmission is 25–30% in the United States. With optimal antiretroviral treatment and a suppressed HIV viral load below 1000, the risk is 1–2%.

Which laboratory tests might be helpful?

Stage HIV disease with CD4 count and HIV viral load; screening for sexually transmitted disease (syphilis, gonorrhea, and Chlamydia) if it was not done as part of prenatal care; Papanicolaou's smear; screen for hepatitides C and B (vaccinate for hepatitis B); baseline complete blood cell count (anemia is common on medications) and renal and liver function tests (since medications are cleared by those organs); tuberculosis screening with PPD (no anergy panel), with a finding of 5 mm considered positive (if negative and the index of suspicion high, obtain chest radiograph and sputum cultures); consider serologies for cytomegalovirus and toxoplasmosis if there is

specific concern for maternal health (i.e., very immunocompromised and new onset neurologic or ophthalmologic symptoms); and consider HIV resistance testing (if the viral load is >1000 and she is at risk for having contracted resistance virus because, e.g., her boyfriend was on an antiretroviral regimen that did not suppress viral replication).

Her CD4 count is 275/mL and her HIV viral load is 68,000.

What are her medication options?

The regimen should consist of at least three medications chosen to optimize viral suppression, enhance patient adherence to the regimen, and minimize side effects. ZDV should be included in the regimen unless there is a specific contraindication because it is the retroviral best studied to prevent vertical transmission. Let her know that there is no perfect regimen. All have side effects and toxicities.

CASE 2: PRECONCEPTUAL CONSULTATION FOR AN HIV-INFECTED WOMAN

A 28-year-old para 2 HIV-infected woman comes to your office with her second husband who is HIV negative. She has done well on her regimen of ZDV, lamivudine, and lopinavir-ritonavir and has increased her CD4 count steadily to 580 over the 2 years on her regimen and has maintained her HIV viral load at less than 50 on an ultrasensitive assay. They want to have a baby.

Should she stop taking her medicines to avoid exposing the baby?

Because of the risk of developing resistance with stopping and starting medications, current USPHS recommendations are that she should continue with her drugs. Although there are few data, the current cases in the Antiretroviral Pregnancy Registry suggest that rates of malformation are no higher than background rates with current medications. Efavirenz was associated with central nervous system birth defects in apes so changing that drug before conception or in early pregnancy could be considered. A National Institutes of Health expert panel has suggested that the risk of vertical transmission without medications outweighs the potential risk of fetal medication exposure.

When should the husband stop using condoms?

Never! Even with her suppressed HIV viral load, there is no way to ensure that he will not be infected during unprotected intercourse.

Will the patient's health be compromised by the pregnancy?

Current data in the United States suggest that pregnancies do not hasten immunocompromise or worsen the course of HIV infection.

REFERENCES

1 Centers for Disease Control. HIV and AIDS—US 1981–2001. *MMWR* 2001;50:430–434.

2 Centers for Disease Control. Revised recommendations for HIV screening of pregnant women. *MMWR* 2001;50(RR-19).

3 HIV testing among pregnant women—US and Canada. *MMWR* 2002; 51:1013–1016.

4 French R, Brocklehurst P. The effect of pregnancy on survival in women infected with HIV: a systemic review of the literature and meta-analysis. *BJOG* 1998;105:827–835.

5 Minkhoff H, Hershow R, Watts DH, et al. The relationship of pregnancy to HIV disease progression. *Am J Obstet Gynecol* 2003;189: 552–559.

6 Dinsmoor MJ, Christmas JT. Changes in T-lymphocyte subpopulations during pregnancy complicated by HIV infection. *Am J Obstet Gynecol* 1992;167:1575–1579.

7 Watts DH. Management of HIV infection in pregnancy. *N Engl J Med* 2002;346:1879–1890.

8 Safety and toxicity of individual antiretroviral agents in pregnancy. Available at: http://aidsinfo.nih.gov/drugs/. Accessed March 23, 2004.

9 Panel on clinical practices for treatment of HIV infection, guidelines for the use of antiretroviral agents in HIV-infected adults and adolescents. Recommendations for use of antiretroviral drugs in pregnant HIV-1 infected women for maternal health interventions to reduce perinatal HIV-1 transmission in the US. Available at: http://aidsinfo.nih.gov/. Accessed September 22, 2003.

10 Hirsch MS, Brun-Vezinet F, Clotet B, et al. Antiretroviral drug resistance testing in adults infected with HIV type 1: 2003 recommendations of an International AIDS Society–USA Panel. *Clin Infect Dis* 2003;37:113–128.

11 Kliks S, Wara DW, Landers DV, Levy JA. Features of HIV-1 that could influence maternal–child transmission. *JAMA* 1994;272:468–474.

12 Garcia PM, Kalish LA, Pitt J, et al. Maternal levels of plasma HIV type 1 RNA and the risk of perinatal transmission. Women and Infants Study Group. *N Engl J Med* 1999;341:385–393.

13 Connor EM, Sperling RS, Gelber R, et al: Reduction of maternal–infant transmission of HIV-1 with zidovudine treatment. Pediatric AIDS Clinical Trials Group 076. *N Engl J Med* 1994;331:1173–1180.

14 Sperling RS, Shapiro DE, Coombs RW, et al. Maternal viral load, zidovudine treatment, and the risk of transmission of HIV-1 from mother to infant. Pediatric AIDS Clinical Trials 076 Study Group. *N Engl J Med* 1996;335:1621–1629.

15 Guay LA, Musoke P, Fleming T, et al. Intrapartum and neonatal single dose nevirapine compared with zidovudine for prevention of mother-to-child transmission of HIV-1 in Kampala, Uganda: HIVNET012 randomised trial. *Lancet* 1999;354:795–802.

16 Mandelbrot LM, Landreau-Mascaro A, Rekacewicz C, et al. Lamuvidine–zidovudine combination for prevention of maternal–infant transmission of HIV-1. *JAMA* 2001;285:2083–2093.

17 Ionnidis JPA Abrams EJ Ammann A, et al. Perinatal transmission of HIV1 by pregnant women with viral loads <1000. *J Infect Dis* 2001;183:539–545.

18 Tuomala RE, Shapiro DE, Mofenson LM, et al. Antiretroviral therapy during pregnancy and the risk of an adverse outcome. *N Engl J Med* 2002;346:1863–1870.

19 Covington DL, Tilson H, Elder J, Doi PA. Assessing teratogenicity of antiretroviral drugs: monitoring and analysis plan of the Antiretroviral Pregnancy Registry. *Pharmacoepidemiol Drug Saf* 2002;11:S137.

20 Fundaro C, Genovese O, Redeli C, et al: Myelomeningocoele in a child with intrauterine exposure to efavirenz. *AIDS* 2002;16:299–300.

21 International Perinatal HIV Group. The mode of delivery and the risk of vertical transmission of HIV type 1. *N Engl J Med* 1999;340: 977–987.

22 Elective caesarean-section versus vaginal delivery in prevention of vertical HIV-1 transmission: a randomised clinical trial. The European Mode of Delivery Collaboration. *Lancet* 1999;353:1035–1039.

23 ACOG Committee Opinion. Scheduled cesarean delivery and the prevention of vertical transmission of HIV infection. 2000;234.

24 Marcollet A, Goffinet F, Firtion G, et al. Differences in postpartum morbidity in women who are infected with the human immunodeficiency virus after elective cesarean delivery, emergency cesarean delivery, or vaginal delivery. *Am J Obstet Gynecol* 2002;186:784–789.

25 Livingston E. Management of HIV in pregnancy. *Curr Women Health Rep* 2002;2:247–252.

Management of Toxoplasma gondii in Pregnancy

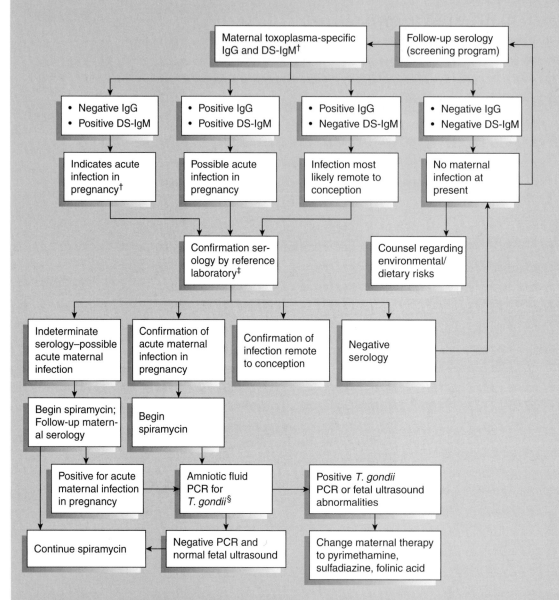

† IgG by ELISA or Dye Titer; IgM by Double-Sandwich ELISA; testing performed for clinical findings (maternal mononucleosis-like illness or lymphadenopathy), fetal anomalies (intracranial clacifications; hydrocephalus), or as part of an antenatal screening program (possible screening times 8–12 weeks, 16–20 weeks, 24–30 weeks).

‡ In the United States confirmation serologies can be obtained at the Toxoplasma Serology Laboratory, Palo Alto Medical Foundation (http://www.pamf.org/serology; telephone 650–853–4828), and if positive spiramycin may be obtained on a treatment IND protocol.

§ Polymerase chain reaction (PCR) to be performed by reference laboratory

Continued on Page 354

21 Management of Cytomegalovirus and Toxoplasma gondii in Pregnancy

Nicholas Guerina

Introduction

It is well recognized that infectious complications in pregnancy can adversely affect the mother, fetus, or newborn. As recently as the 1940s, many infections now known to affect the fetus were thought to be blocked against in utero transmission by the placenta.

This section reviews the epidemiology and management of two infectious diseases, cytomegalovirus (CMV) and *Toxoplasma gondii*.[1] These agents differ greatly not only in CMV being a herpes virus and *T. gondii* being a protozoan parasite but also in their epidemiology and pathogenesis. CMV may be transmitted in utero or postnatally through breast milk, and transmission may occur when mothers have primary infection, reinfection, or reactivation of remote infection. Congenital toxoplasma infection occurs almost exclusively with primary maternal infection during pregnancy, and postnatal vertical transmission does not occur. CMV is species specific with no nonhuman reservoirs, whereas toxoplasma can infect many mammals and avian species. Nevertheless, these agents share

Management of Cytomegalovirus (CMV) in Pregnancy

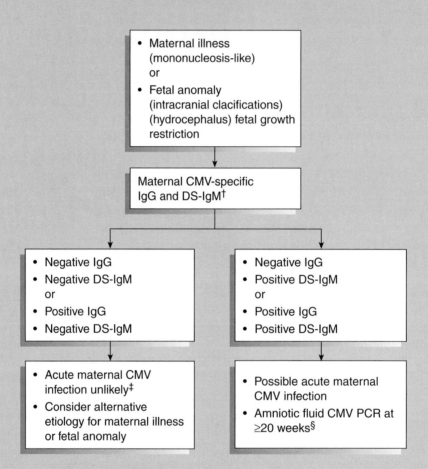

- Maternal illness
  (mononucleosis-like)
  or
- Fetal anomaly
  (intracranial clacifications)
  (hydrocephalus) fetal growth
  restriction

Maternal CMV-specific
IgG and DS-IgM†

- Negative IgG
- Negative DS-IgM
  or
- Positive IgG
- Negative DS-IgM

- Negative IgG
- Positive DS-IgM
  or
- Positive IgG
- Positive DS-IgM

- Acute maternal CMV
  infection unlikely‡
- Consider alternative
  etiology for maternal illness
  or fetal anomaly

- Possible acute maternal
  CMV infection
- Amniotic fluid CMV PCR at
  ≥20 weeks§

† Double-sandwich IgM enzyme-linked immunosorbent assay (ELISA)

‡ CMV reactivation with fetal transmission possible for mothers with positive
IgG; if fetal anomaly is present, amniotic fluid polymerase chain reaction
(PCR) may be useful since symptomatic congenital CMV can rarely occur with
remote maternal primary infection.

§ The combination of acute maternal CMV infection, fetal anomaly, and positive
PCR would suggest symptomatic congenital CMV infection and an increased
risk for severe fetal disease; in the absence of a fetal anomaly, most fetuses
will have subclinical infection, even in the setting of primary maternal infection.

some common features: both cause chronic infection in all hosts they infect and may cause multiorgan injury to the infected fetus.

Cytomegalovirus

Even if primary maternal infection can be determined, it is difficult to predict fetal outcome.

CMVs are herpes viruses that derive their name from the cytopathology they produce. Infected cells become enlarged and contain characteristic intranuclear and cytoplasmic inclusions. Infection results from exposure to infected breast milk or blood products or from intimate personal contact with a partner or other individual who is shedding virus. Most individuals will become infected at some time in their lives, but the highest risk for seroconversion occurs in four groups beyond the neonatal period: young children in day care, mothers of young children in day care, day-care providers, and sexually active adolescents.[2] In some regions of the world, the seropositivity rate by the end of the second decade is higher than 90% (e.g., Chile, Japan, and Ivory Coast), whereas the rate in Europe and the United States varies from 50% to 85%, with the higher rate being found in populations of lower socioeconomic status. Prospective studies in the United States have shown that childbearing women of middle and upper socioeconomic background acquire CMV at a rate of approximately 2% per year, whereas those of lower socioeconomic background acquire CMV at a rate of approximately 6% per year. CMV has been recognized for decades as a prevalent cause of congenital infection, but it continues to pose diagnostic and therapeutic dilemmas.[3]

GUIDING QUESTIONS IN APPROACHING THE PATIENT

- Is the woman in a high-risk group for CMV or toxoplasma infection?
- Does she have an immunodeficiency?
- Are there abnormal ultrasound findings including fetal growth restriction, echogenic bowel, microcephaly, intracranial calcifications, and ventriculomegaly?
- If toxoplasma infection is considered, have serologic studies been sent to a reference laboratory?

WHAT'S THE EVIDENCE?

Vertical (mother-to-infant) transmission of CMV can occur in utero, presumably by transplacental transfer, from exposure to infected genital secretions at delivery and postnatally through infected breast milk. Approximately 1% of all newborns are infected with CMV, but only 0.1% develops symptomatic disease.[4] This translates to about 8,000 infants born with symptomatic CMV infection in the United States. Congenital and perinatal CMV infections are common in infants born to women with remote (preconception) infection despite the presence of CMV-specific maternal immunity, presumably from reactivated shedding of endogenous virus, but symptomatic fetal and newborn disease is rare in this setting.[5] Severe congenital CMV disease typically occurs from in utero fetal transmission after primary maternal infection during pregnancy. However, it is very difficult to determine primary versus reactivated disease in pregnancy, unless the serologic status of the mother is known immediately before conception. The difficulties arise from many factors:

1. Most CMV infections acquired after the newborn period are asymptomatic, so primary infection during pregnancy is usually not clinically apparent.
2. Although site-specific viral shedding may occur for longer duration after primary infection, variable shedding rates can occur throughout pregnancy with primary and reactivated CMV infections. Thus maternal cultures alone are poor predictors of primary versus reactivated maternal infection.
3. It is difficult to predict congenital transmission based on maternal antibody levels. Vertical transmission commonly occurs despite preexisting and substantial humoral immunity, presumably due to CMV reactivation during pregnancy. In addition, vertical transmission after primary maternal infection occurs at a higher rate in mothers with high antibody titers against CMV-specific proteins; the higher antibody response may reflect higher viral replication resulting in a greater chance of transmission.

When symptomatic adult infection occurs, symptoms are typically those of a mononucleosis syndrome with fever, sore throat, and lymphadenopathy. Myalgias, headache, and splenomegaly may be present, in addition to malaise, anorexia, and, in rare cases, hepatitis presenting as abdominal pain and jaundice. Acute (primary) CMV infection should be considered in any pregnant women presenting with such symptoms, especially if heterophile antibody is negative. Symptomatic infection may also be very mild and limited to fever and sore throat or adenopathy.

Even if primary maternal infection can be determined, it is difficult to predict fetal outcome because symptomatic fetal disease is unlikely. The rate of intrauterine transmission is estimated to be 30–40% with primary maternal infection, but fewer than 15% of infected newborns develop significant disease. Several studies that followed subsequent pregnancies in women who gave birth to infants with symptomatic CMV infection have demonstrated that fetal infection may again occur, but the infected infants are asymptomatic.[6] The overall rate of CMV shedding in pregnant women (~9% cervix and 4% urine) does not appear to be significantly different from that in nonpregnant women, but the rate of shedding does appear to increase with gestational age. CMV shedding also appears to decrease with advancing maternal age.

Fetal infection can occur with essentially equal frequency throughout pregnancy, but there is some evidence that symptomatic disease may be more severe when fetal infection occurs in the first half of pregnancy. Common clinical findings in the newborn with symptomatic CMV infection include petechiae (76%), jaundice (67%), hepatosplenomegaly (60%), microcephaly (53%), small for gestational age (50%), prematurity (<38 weeks gestation; 34%), and chorioretinitis (14%). Bone marrow suppression may result in extramedullary hematopoiesis, including cutaneous involvement resulting in red-purple focal lesions referred to as "blueberry muffin spots" (Figure 21-1). There is an unusually high incidence of inguinal hernia in males with symptomatic congenital CMV infection (~25%). Abnormalities in laboratory findings include increased hepatic transaminases, increased bilirubin levels, anemia, and thrombocytopenia. Abnormal ultrasound findings include intracranial calcifications, microcephaly, ventriculomegaly, and fetal growth restriction. There is a particular predilection for the intracranial calcifications to be in periventricular regions, although calcifications may occur anywhere in the brain. Approximately one-third of infants with symptomatic CMV infection die, but these infants generally have severe multiple organ system disease or severe central nervous system (CNS) involvement. Infants who survive symptomatic CMV infection are at high risk for developmental and neurologic dysfunctions, including mental retardation, sensorineural hearing loss (60%), language and learning disabilities, motor abnormalities, and visual disturbances. Infants with asymptomatic infection have virtually no mortality, but 5–15% may develop hearing

Figure 21-1: Photograph of newborn infant with congenital cytomegalovirus infection. Pictured are numerous raised (~3–8 mm in diameter), red-blue lesions of extramedulary hematopoiesis. Petichiae are visible. The infant also had jaundice at birth.

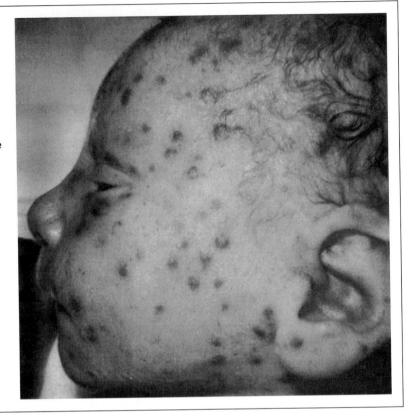

loss; rarely, mental retardation, motor spasticity, and microcephaly have been observed.[7,8]

MANAGEMENT STRATEGIES

KEY POINT

> *Screening for CMV infection in high-risk groups is not indicated.*

MATERNAL INFECTION Although there are identifiable groups of women who may have an increased risk for acquiring CMV in pregnancy (adolescents, day-care providers, and mothers with a toddler in day care), no specific recommendations can be made for universal CMV screening for any of these groups in the absence of maternal symptoms or observed fetal abnormalities. Testing is currently used in cases in which there are acute maternal symptoms of mononucleosis or hepatitis, or when fetal abnormalities are seen (microcephaly, intracranial calcifications, or ventriculomegaly). Not all cases of fetal growth restriction require CMV testing, but when this fetal finding is otherwise unexplained and the mother is in a high-risk group or has recent onset of fever, sore throat, or lymphadenopathy, CMV testing should be considered.

The principal tests used in the diagnosis of CMV infection are serology, viral isolation, and demonstration of viral antigens or nucleic acid in tissues or body fluids.[9] Serologic tests for the determination of CMV-specific immunoglobulin G (IgG) and immunoglobulin M (IgM) are readily available, but interpretation of results is not always straight forward. The only reliable method to identify serologically acute maternal CMV infection is by documenting seroconversion with serial IgG determinations during pregnancy. Thus it is not surprising that serology has been most useful in diagnosing previous CMV exposure and not acute infection.

KEY POINT

Serologic studies are more helpful in determining previous infection than in detecting acute infection.

The demonstration of a significant (fourfold or greater) increase in IgG titer may be useful in diagnosing acute maternal infection, but this is also unreliable and would require multiple determinations in hopes of identifying the acute increase. The presence of a positive CMV IgG titer early in the first trimester does not guarantee that the fetus will escape severe infection, but symptomatic fetal disease is unlikely to occur if seropositivity is documented at least several months before conception. The avidity of CMV-specific IgG can help to further investigate the timing of maternal infection.[10] High avidity IgG indicates that infection is most likely to have occurred at least 3 months previously, so the presence of high avidity IgG in the first trimester supports infection before conception.

Factors interfering with the specificity and sensitivity of CMV-IgM assays include the presence of high titer CMV IgG and nonspecific serum factors (e.g., rheumatoid factor). More recently, the IgM capture or double sandwich enzyme-linked immunosorbent assay (DS-IgM-ELISA) technique has been adopted for the measurement of CMV-specific IgM. Demonstration of CMV IgM in maternal serum may be indicative of a recent infection, but IgM antibody may persist for months, making it difficult to determine precisely when infection occurred.

After an acute maternal infection, it is likely that shedding of CMV occurs from multiple sites, including the kidneys. Thus it may be possible to isolate virus from maternal urine, but shedding can be erratic and recurrent even in the setting of remote maternal infection. The detection of CMV-specific early antigens by immunofluorescence ("shell vial" and similar assays) also has very good sensitivity and can detect virus within 24 hours from urine. It is important to refrigerate specimens for CMV testing at 4°C and transport them to the laboratory on ice because viral titers may decrease rapidly with freezing or when transported at ambient temperatures.

The buffy coat recovered from centrifuged peripheral blood can be spread on a microscope slide, the leukocytes lysed, and

CMV-specific (pp65) antigen detected by immunostaining. Although this procedure can be used to demonstrate viremia, a negative test does not rule out systemic spread of the virus. The buffy coat technique may be most useful for monitoring treatment efficacy in immunocompromised patients. Polymerase chain reaction (PCR) is increasingly replacing tissue culture and antigen detection methods as a sensitive and specific assay for the rapid detection of CMV-specific nucleic acid. PCR may be used on a variety of tissues and body fluids including biopsy tissue, blood, oral and respiratory secretions, and cerebrospinal fluid (CSF).

In general, the demonstration of CMV shedding from the cervix or in urine of pregnant women has been found to have a poor predictive value for fetal infection. Of greater significance is that, even with documented acute maternal CMV infection, most fetuses will not be infected or have asymptomatic infection. Rarely, symptomatic CMV disease has been reported in mothers despite clear documentation of remote (preconception) CMV infection.

FETAL INFECTION   The determination of fetal CMV infection is difficult and generally of uncertain utility. Even if acute (primary) maternal infection can be demonstrated and transmission to the fetus is documented, therapeutic options are limited. There is no effective therapy that can be administered to pregnant women to treat the fetus in utero. It is also difficult to counsel women with respect to pregnancy termination because most infected fetuses will not be severely affected by CMV, even in the setting of primary maternal infection.

The expected rate of symptomatic congenital CMV infection is ≤0.5/1000 births for lower socioeconomic groups and ≤1/1000 births for higher socioeconomic groups. For nonimmune women the risk of having an infant with symptomatic CMV infection is ≤2/1000, whereas the risk for immune women is ≤1/1000.

Recent studies have suggested that amniotic fluid culture and PCR may be useful in diagnosing fetal CMV infection. This may be particularly true for the symptomatic fetus in which CMV excretion is likely to occur. However, it may not be possible to detect virus reliably in amniotic fluid culture PCR before 20 to 22 weeks of gestation. Fetal abnormalities possibly associated with CMV infection include intracranial or hepatic calcification, enlarged lateral ventricles consistent with hydrocephalus, or other abnormalities of the brain parenchyma. A common consequence of symptomatic congenital CMV disease is growth restriction, but it is important to realize that the converse is not true.

Different reports have demonstrated an association between the antenatal ultrasound finding of echogenic bowel foci and congenital infection.[11] CMV is the principal agent in this association, but a firm link has not been established. The incidence of congenital CMV in fetuses with echogenic bowel has been reported to be approximately 2.5%. Because CMV occurs in 1% of newborns on average (with some epidemiologic groups having a higher rate), controlled studies with adequate power need to be performed before the significance of CMV in echogenic bowel can be determined. Nonetheless, the potential association with CMV has prompted some obstetricians to consider fetal infection in the differential of echogenic bowel. Consideration of maternal and fetal testing must be made on an individual basis taking into consideration proper parental counseling and ultrasound findings.

If it is determined that diagnosing maternal infection and fetal transmission is indicated, Table 21-1 presents a guide to the interpretation of maternal serology and the use of amniocentesis for CMV PCR testing. It must be emphasized that this is only a guide, and the results for any given patient should be reviewed with an infectious disease specialist. This is especially true for indeterminate serologic results where additional testing may be required.

Newborn infants with symptomatic and asymptomatic congenital CMV infections excrete large quantities of virus in oropharyngeal secretions and urine for many months. Although viral titers may steadily decrease over the first year of life, virus can be isolated from most infants for 2 to 4 years. Thus the diagnosis of neonatal CMV infection can usually be made by the combination of characteristic clinical symptoms and a positive urine culture or PCR. The absence of viral excretion during the first 2 postnatal weeks differentiates natal and postnatal infections from congenital infection. Because most cases of congenital CMV infection are asymptomatic, confirmation of congenital CMV in a symptomatic infant does not prove causation because other infectious agents may produce similar symptoms (e.g., *T. gondii*). Specific laboratory tests to rule out a second (concomitant) congenital infection should always be considered.

Table 21-1.   **GUIDE TO MATERNAL CMV SEROLOGICAL SCREENING AND AMNIOTIC FLUID CMV PCR TESTING**

TEST RESULT	INTERPRETATION	AMNIOTIC FLUID PCR AT 20–22 WK
IgM negative and IgG negative	No infection	No
IgM negative, IgG positive, and high IgG avidity	Likely to be remote infection to pregnancy at any gestation, but highest specificity is in first trimester.	Consider only if fetal abnormality strongly suggests fetal infection
IgM positive, IgG positive, and high IgG avidity	First trimester: infection before conception Second trimester: possible infection during pregnancy	No for first-trimester result Consider at 20–22 wk for second-trimester result
IgM positive, IgG positive, and low IgG avidity	Infection during pregnancy possible with first-trimester result and likely with second-trimester result	Consider at 20–22 wk

CMV = cytomegalovirus; IgG = immunoglobulin G; IgM = immunoglobulin M; PCR = polymerase chain reaction.

THERAPEUTIC OPTIONS

Although there are antiviral agents that are active against CMV, none have proved to be safe or effective in preventing or improving the outcome of fetal infection. Therefore, preventive measures hold the best promise for eliminating symptomatic congenital CMV infection. Recognition of risk factors associated with maternal infection may provide a means of counseling some women, but preventing acquired maternal infection in most cases will be difficult. Approximately 2% of women acquire acute primary CMV infection in pregnancy, but maternal infection is usually asymptomatic and goes undiagnosed.

The antiviral drug ganciclovir (9-1,3-dihydroxypropoxymethyl guanine) is very active against CMV in vitro and has proved beneficial in the management of certain clinical conditions resulting from CMV infection including treatment of newborns with CMV CNS disease such as hearing impairment.

Current data suggest relatively short-term benefit from neonatal ganciclovir therapy. Longer follow-up is needed because sensineural hearing loss may develop several years or more after birth. There are no studies that have attempted to alter fetal outcome by maternal treatment with ganciclovir or valganciclovir in pregnancy, and use of these drugs during pregnancy is not recommended in light of animal and in vitro evidence for carcinogenesis and for testicular atrophy.

Promising prophylactic therapies include passive immunization with hyperimmune anti-CMV immunoglobulin or active immunization with a live attenuated CMV vaccine. Hyperimmune globulin could be used for prophylaxis of high-risk women against primary infection in pregnancy or to attempt to alleviate or protect the newborn against symptomatic CMV disease. Attenuated live CMV vaccines have been developed, but their efficacy has not been established. Special consideration must be given to the possibilities of chronic infection with vaccine strains and viral reactivation with fetal transmission in pregnancy.

PREVENTION

Breast milk is a common source for perinatal CMV infection of the newborn infant, but symptomatic infection is rare, especially in term infants in which protection against disseminated disease may be provided by transplacentally derived maternal IgG. However, preterm infants may not be protected because of insufficient transplacental transfer of maternal IgG. There is no effective procedure to eliminate CMV from infected breast milk; freezing milk at −20°C may decrease, but not eliminate, the titer of active virus. It may be reasonable to screen mothers of preterm infants for CMV seropositivity and, if positive, minimize the viral load by pasteurization or freezing. However, it is generally recommended that the benefits of breast milk outweigh the exposure risk from infected breast milk.

Environments with the potential to be high risk for CMV exposure include day-care centers and hospitals. Studies have documented a high rate of horizontal transmission in day-care centers caring for infants and toddlers. However, studies on the rate of seroconversion among hospital personnel have not shown an increased risk for infection compared with the general population.[12] The practice of good handwashing and routine hospital infection control measures appear to be sufficient to control the spread of CMV to workers. Although such practices may be difficult to enforce in day-care settings, they should be encouraged, and pregnant women with toddlers in day care should be instructed to practice good handwashing when changing diapers or coming in contact with oral secretions.

Discussion of Case

CASE 1: ACUTE MATERAL CMV INFECTION AND FETAL GROWTH RESTRICTION

A 27-year-old gravida 2, para 1 woman had an antenatal fetal ultrasound in the first trimester that confirmed pregnancy, with dates consistent with the last menstrual period. She was well except for a recent sore throat that lasted about 1 week with no other symptoms. Her examination at the time was normal. There were no recent illnesses in the family, including her 3-year-old daughter who is attending day care. Follow-up ultrasound was performed at 18 weeks because of small size for dates, and the fetus was found to have a symmetrical growth restriction in the 10th percentile. No other fetal abnormalities were observed.

Is there any infectious disease etiology you would consider in your differential diagnosis of the fetal growth restriction?

Congenital CMV is the most likely infectious cause of fetal growth restriction. Obtain maternal serology for CMV-specific IgG, DS-IgM-ELISA, and IgG avidity.

Serology is positive for acute maternal CMV infection.

What would you do now?

Counsel the parents regarding the possibility that the fetal growth restriction is due to CMV infection. Most infants do not have symptoms from CMV infection, even when the mother becomes infected for the first time in pregnancy.

If the growth restriction is due to CMV infection, there is likely to be a greater risk for other complications, but it is still difficult to predict the outcome for this fetus. Offer amniotic fluid testing after 20 weeks of gestation.

The amniotic fluid PCR for CMV is positive. The fetal ultrasound survey shows continued growth at the 10th percentile and no other fetal abnormalities.

What do you do next?

Reiterate to the parents that, although there is likely to be an increased risk for serious complications from CMV, you cannot predict the outcome for their fetus. The absence of other fetal abnormalities, aside from growth restriction, does not rule out severe CNS disease.

The parents chose to continue the pregnancy. Expectant obstetric management shows the fetus to continue to grow at the 10th percentile with no ultrasound abnormalities. At 33 weeks, the mother presented with rapidly progressive preterm labor and preterm delivery with premature rupture of membranes. The male infant had a normal examination, except for being small for gestational age with weight, head circumference, and length at the 10th percentile. Urine culture on the infant was positive for CMV. A complete blood cell count showed thrombocytopenia with platelet counts of 50,000/mm^3. Hearing testing by brainstem-evoked responses was normal, computed tomography of the head was normal, and ophthalmologic evaluation was normal. Thrombocytopenia spontaneously resolved by 2 weeks. Repeated hearing screens are being performed to monitor for late onset hearing loss.

Case 1 underscores the difficulties in counseling parents regarding newborn outcomes from congenital CMV infection. Some studies have tried to correlate a positive amniotic fluid PCR or culture for CMV with newborn outcomes, but there are insufficient data to allow for an accurate assessment of risk. If additional abnormalities had been observed, such as microcephaly, intracranial calcifications, or ventriculomegaly, the risk of moderate to severe CNS disease could have been considered significant.

Toxoplasma gondii

Toxoplasma gondii is an obligate, intracellular protozoan parasite capable of infecting many mammals, including humans. The name is derived from its morphology (toxoplasma = "arclike form") and the North African desert rodent from which it was first isolated (*Ctenodactylus gondii*). The disease is usually self-limiting in healthy children and adults, but severe disease may occur in the immunologically "immature" fetus and young infant or in individuals with acquired immunodeficiency syndrome (AIDS).[13,14]

TOXOPLASMA GONDII LIFE CYCLE AND HUMAN TRANSMISSION

Toxoplasma gondii has sexual and asexual life cycles. The sexual cycle takes place only in the intestinal tract of cats (many species). Millions of *Toxoplasma* oocysts may be shed daily in cat feces over the initial weeks after infection. Oocysts typically have an octet of sporozoites and may remain viable for months to years (depending on climatic conditions). Over 24 hours, oocysts undergo meiosis to form highly infectious sporozoites.

After ingestion by a susceptible animal, the oocysts rupture, thereby releasing the sporozoites that multiply in intestinal cells and gastrointestinal lymph nodes. Acute parasitemia occurs when the sporozoites differentiate into a "rapidly" growing form of *T. gondii* (tachyzoites) that spread throughout the bloodstream. Tachyzoites can invade any organ including the eye, brain, heart, lung, and skeletal muscle. In hosts with adequate immunity, humoral and cell-mediated responses control further spread, but the tachyzoites already invading tissues combine with host cells to form tissue cysts. Within tissue cysts, the tachyzoites change into the "slowly" growing bradyzoites, which may remain viable in the tissue cysts throughout the life of the host. Any susceptible animal ingesting tissue cysts may also develop parasitemia and chronic infection, thus perpetuating the asexual cycle of *T. gondii*.

KEY POINT

*Approximately 90%
of adult infections
with* T. gondii *are
asymptomatic.*

KEY POINT

*Women who are
infected before
conception are very
unlikely to have an
infant with
congenital
toxoplasma
infection.*

EPIDEMIOLOGY   Infection of humans occur from direct ingestion or inhalation of oocysts from cat litter, unwashed produce, or contaminated water and soil, from ingestion of tissue cysts present in undercooked meat, or, rarely, from tachyzoites present in unpasteurized goat milk. Horizontal transmission between individuals does not occur, except in the rare situations of contaminated blood transfusion or organ transplantation. The resulting tissue cysts are microscopic and of no consequence to normal hosts, except that local inflammation may occur if cysts rupture.

Vertical transmission occurs through transplacental transfer of tachyzoites from mother to fetus. Although different strains of *T. gondii* have been isolated, immunologically normal individuals, including pregnant women, appear to be protected against reinfection. Thus women who are infected remote to conception are very unlikely to have an infant with congenital toxoplasma infection; only when acute maternal infection occurs during pregnancy is the fetus at a significant risk for congenital infection. In some cases, vertical transmission occurs after reactivated disease in pregnant women who have a severe immunodeficiency. Very rarely has fetal transmission occurred when an immunocompetent mother was infected remote to conception.

MATERNAL SEROPREVALENCE   Toxoplasma infection occurs throughout the world, but age-specific and overall seroprevalence varies by region and is influenced by environmental exposure, food sources, and customs. In regions where there is a relatively large number of cats that live outdoors and warm, humid temperatures, children are often exposed to oocysts in contaminated soil and water at a young age, and by adolescence the seropositivity rate may be as high as 50–75% (e.g., Central America). In some regions, the principal route of human transmission is eating undercooked meat, and exposure seroprevalence may begin outside of early childhood and continue through adulthood. Most regions of the world likely have a mixed pattern of exposure. The National Health and Nutritional Examination Survey has reported stable toxoplasma seroprevalence rates in the United States for the past 10 years; the overall seroprevalence rate has been estimated to be 15.8% for the 1999–2000 survey.

DIAGNOSIS　　The mainstay for the diagnosis of toxoplasma infection is the demonstration of specific serum antibodies against toxoplasma antigens.[15] Direct demonstration of *T. gondii* nucleic acid by PCR has also become an important tool for detecting toxoplasma in body fluids and tissues, including amniotic fluid. Other adjunctive tests that may be useful but are not widely available include the detection of toxoplasma antigens in tissues and body fluids, placental pathology and culture, and cultures of blood and CSF. In *many* cases, the combination of maternal serologic testing and, when indicated, amniotic fluid PCR allow for the determination of possible acute maternal toxoplasma infection in pregnancy and assessment of the risk of fetal disease and provide outcome guidance and treatment options. This is not to say that all cases can be easily resolved with certainty, and the interpretation of serologic studies and PCR results should be made with consultation of an infectious disease specialist. Further, it is strongly recommended that most serologic studies and PCR assay be performed by a toxoplasma reference laboratory. The principal laboratory in the United States is the Toxoplasma Serology Laboratory at the Palo Alto Medical Foundation Research Institute (Ames Building, 795 El Camino Real, Palo Alto, CA 94301-2302; telephone 650-853-4828; fax 650-614-3292; e-mail toxolab@pamf.org; URL http://www.pamf.org/ serology).

SEROLOGY　　There are highly specific and sensitive serologic assays for the measurement of IgG against toxoplasma. These include the Sabin-Feldman dye test, indirect fluorescent antibody assay, and ELISA. Most IgG assays have limited utility in determining acute infection, unless serial testing has been performed. Toxoplasma-specific IgG may be detected within 1 week of infection and often peaks at 3–8 weeks. For immunologically normal children and adults, IgG remains positive throughout life. Serial antibody testing showing a fourfold increase in IgG titers indicates recent infection, but the titers should ideally be run in tandem (simultaneous measurements). A high dye test titer at 2 months of gestation generally indicates maternal infection remote to conception. Because IgG is transferred efficiently across the placenta after 28 weeks of gestation and especially during the last 10 weeks of pregnancy, IgG testing in the early months of life can be difficult to interpret for newborn infants.

The diagnosis of acute toxoplasmosis is aided by the use of sensitive and specific IgM assays. Two such assays are the DS-IgM-ELISA and the IgM-immunosorbent agglutination assay (IgM-ISAGA). Both tests have high sensitivity and specificity. The DS-IgM-ELISA is becoming increasingly available commercially but is best performed by a toxoplasma reference laboratory. Determination of specific IgM is important not only for the assessment of acute maternal infection but also for the determination of congenital infection in newborn infants because their IgG titers may simply reflect transplacentally transferred antibody from infected mothers. Toxoplasma-specific IgM can be detected within 1 week of infection and typically peak at 3–4 weeks. IgM titers determined by DS-IgM-ELISA or IgM-ISAGA may be detected for months to over 1 year, so serial titer measurements may be needed. With regard to IgG titers, serial samples should be measured simultaneously. Additional serologic assays useful for the determination of acute toxoplasmosis are the toxoplasma-specific IgA-ELISA and IgE-ELISA, the differential agglutination (AC/HS) test, and the measurement of IgG avidity. All of these assays are routinely performed at the Palo Alto Medical Foundation Toxoplasma Serology Laboratory.

Amniotic fluid PCR   PCR has been used to detect *T. gondii* in amniotic fluid, CSF, blood, urine, ocular fluid, and bronchoalveolar lavage specimens. Amniotic fluid PCR appears to be more sensitive and specific in the diagnosis of congenital toxoplasma infection than invasive procedures such as cordocentesis.[16] The latter has been used to test fetal blood for specific (*T. gondii* culture, toxoplasma-specific antibody) and nonspecific indicators of infection (complete blood cell counts, liver function tests, total IgM). PCR can be used as soon as amniocentesis can be safely performed (after 15 weeks of gestation), although it may be more sensitive if performed closer to 20 weeks of gestation. With regard to serologic studies, interpretation of PCR results should be done in conjunction with the consultation of an infectious disease expert. Amniotic fluid specimens must be handled appropriately, and specific instructions regarding volume and handling should be reviewed with the receiving reference laboratory.

MANAGEMENT STRATEGIES

Clinical Symptoms and Treatment in Adults   It is uncommon for specific symptoms to develop in pregnant women that signal the occurrence of acute toxoplasmosis. Most cases are subclinical, and lymphadenopathy is the most frequently recognized finding in symptomatic adults. Some women develop a mononucleosis-like syndrome with fever, malaise, headache, and myalgia. An atypical lymphocytosis may be present, but a sore throat and hepatosplenomegaly are usually absent. Other symptoms may include fatigue, maculopapular rash, hepatitis, pneumonitis, myositis, myocarditis, pericarditis, and meningitis.[17]

Lymphadenopathy is typically localized to one area in adults, with the most common sites being cervical followed by axillary and inguinal. Affected nodes are firm and mobile and may be tender. They range from 2 cm or smaller to as large as 6 cm. The duration of lymphadenopathy is usually 2 months or less but sometimes may be present for 6 months or longer. The differential diagnosis for toxoplasma lymphadenopathy is broad. Biopsy differentiates from among the possibilities, but toxoplasma serology should always be obtained.

New onset chorioretinitis may be the presenting symptom of toxoplasmosis in adults. Symptoms include blurred vision, photophobia, epiphora, and conjunctival erythema. With macular involvement, vision loss may occur. Most cases of chorioretinitis are unilateral.

Adults with immunodeficiency may develop localized or disseminated disease from acute or reactivated toxoplasma infection. Fever with multiple organ involvement may be observed, but these findings are nonspecific for toxoplasma. However, disease progression may be fulminant so toxoplasmosis should always be considered in these patients. In patients with AIDS, toxoplasma encephalitis and interstitial pneumonitis may occur. Pregnant women with human immunodeficiency virus (HIV), and especially with AIDS, may reactivate toxoplasma and develop parasitemia, resulting in fetal infection.

In most immunocompetent adults with mild symptomatic toxoplasmosis, the disease is self-limiting and does not require therapy. More severe disease can be controlled with a brief course (2–4 weeks) of pyrimethamine and sulfadiazine plus *folinic acid* (given to protect against the antimetabolite effects of pyrimethamine). Pyrimethamine and sulfadiazine are synergistic in action against tachyzoites. They do not have significant activity against bradyzoites in tissue cysts, so treatment does not cure the host of chronic toxoplasma infection. Pyrimethamine is a folic acid antagonist, but the administration of exogenous folinic acid (leucovorin; *not* folic acid) can block and reverse the effects on the host. *Toxoplasma gondii* does not benefit from this therapy because it can not efficiently use exogenous folinic acid. Therapy is usually continued for approximately 2 weeks after resolution of clinical symptoms. Because of the antimetabolite effects of pyrimethamine, complete blood cell counts should be monitored with longer treatment courses, and the dose of folinic acid can be increased as needed if abnormal results are observed (typically neutropenia or anemia). The most common side effects of treatment are gastrointestinal symptoms that are often tolerable and may decrease over time. For patients with allergy to sulfa drugs, clindamycin can be used. Special consideration must be given to the intensity and duration of treatment and the use of long-term suppression in immunocompromised patients with toxoplasmosis.

Ocular toxoplasmosis is usually treated with pyrimethamine or sulfadiazine plus folinic acid, although regimens with clindamycin are preferred by some experts, and the macrolide atovaquone has also been used. Atovaquone has activity against bradyzoites in tissue cysts, so there is much interest in potential long-term benefits from treatment with this drug, especially in the decrease of recurrent ocular disease. If sight is threatened, most experts administer prednisone until approximately 2 weeks after inflammation has resolved.

Fetal Transmission   Rates of congenital toxoplasma infection in the United States have varied from as few as 0.1 in 1000 to 1–2 in 1000. It is estimated that the overall risk of fetal infection after acute maternal infection is 30–40%. The rate of transmission is proportional to gestational age. The average transmission during the first trimester is approximately 15%, but fetal morbidity and mortality rates are high. The average transmission rate doubles to 30% in the second trimester and doubles again to 60% in the third trimester.[18] Transmission is very low in the periconceptional period (~1%), begins to increase more sharply toward the end of the first trimester, and may approach 80% or higher at term. Mild or subclinical infection is seen for most fetal infections in the second trimester, and nearly all fetuses have subclinical disease when infection occurs in the third trimester.

KEY POINT

Most fetuses and neonates with congenital toxoplasma infection appear normal.

CLINICAL FINDINGS IN THE INFECTED FETUS AND NEWBORN Antenatal findings for fetuses with symptomatic disease may include ventriculomegaly or intracranial calcifications. However, calcifications may be difficult to determine on ultrasound. Toxoplasma infection should be considered for any fetus with hydrocephalus or any parenchymal brain lesions, but most infected fetuses will have no findings on antenatal ultrasound surveys. Further, most infants with congenital toxoplasmosis have no overt signs of infection at birth. These infants may have retinal and CNS disease that can be identified only by postnatal head CT, lumbar puncture, and indirect ophthalmoscopy. This has been clearly shown by an ongoing study of infants with congenital toxoplasmosis identified through a newborn screening program. The Massachusetts Department of Public Health uses the toxoplasma DS-IgM-ELISA to screen all newborn infants for congenital toxoplasma infection in Massachusetts and New Hampshire.[1] The incidence of detected newborn infection is close to 1 in 10,000 live births. Ninety percent of infected infants have normal routine newborn examinations, and they are discharged home for routine pediatric follow-up. Only through newborn screening are they identified as having congenital toxoplasma infection. Specific testing after serologic diagnosis identified CNS or retinal disease in as many as 40% of these infants. Approximately 20% had unilateral retinal scars, typically in the region of the fovea affecting vision, and active chorioretinitis was rarely noted. CNS disease was generally very mild with several focal calcified lesions or mildly increased CSF protein. Despite the overall subclinical presentation for most infants with congenital toxoplasma infection, several important studies have shown that, in the absence of extended combination antitoxoplasma therapy, these infants remain at high risk for developing long-term ophthalmologic and neurologic sequelae.

Overt neonatal disease is observed in 10% or fewer of newborn infants with congenital toxoplasma infection. Ophthalmologic and CNS complications are very common and include seizures, abnormal CSF profiles, intracranial calcifications, and chorioretinitis. Some infants also demonstrate signs and symptoms of generalized disease with hepatosplenomegaly, lymphadenopathy, jaundice, and anemia.

Sequelae of Untreated Congenital Toxoplasma Infection   The most common sequel of congenital toxoplasma infection is chorioretinitis. Retinal lesions are seen in approximately 20% of infected infants diagnosed by postnatal serology, and the risk of developing new retinal lesions persists into adulthood.[19] Prospective studies in infants not receiving extended antitoxoplasma therapy found that up to 90% develop new onset retinal disease, with the occurrence most often being in adolescence. Severe visual impairment and unilateral blindness developed in some patients. Similar results have been reported for newborn infants diagnosed with congenital infection by serologic screening and not treated with extended combination antitoxoplasma drugs, even when there was no evidence of CNS or ophthalmologic disease at birth. Deafness and severe neurologic outcomes have also been reported.

Antenatal Screening for Acute Maternal Infection   Reports from countries with antenatal screening programs have shown that the severity of fetal disease can be ameliorated by maternal treatment with antitoxoplasma therapy.[13] In these programs, mothers undergo serial testing for seroconversion beginning in the first trimester. When seroconversion is found, maternal treatment with the macrolide antibiotic spiramycin is initiated to decrease fetal transmission. Spiramycin does not effectively treat the fetus once infection has occurred, so techniques to assess the infection status of the fetus are used; if infection is confirmed or suspected, a change in therapy to pyrimethamine, sulfadiazine, and folinic acid is used. This approach appears to decrease significantly the incidence of severe fetal disease, even when infection occurs in the first trimester.

In the absence of an antenatal screening program for acute maternal toxoplasmosis in pregnancy, maternal infection is identified sporadically. In the United States there are no guidelines established for toxoplasma screening in pregnancy, and inconsistent approaches to the problem have been used. Many obstetricians only screen if fetal abnormalities suggesting infection are seen or the mother has symptomatology of toxoplasmosis in pregnancy. Other obstetricians obtain a single toxoplasma serologic test if a patient has a household cat. Because testing may be performed outside of a toxoplasma reference laboratory, the IgM results may be falsely negative or positive, and the infectious status of the mother may be misdiagnosed.

Some experts have called for universal maternal screening for toxoplasma in the United States, whereas others have argued that, for multiple reasons, universal screening may be too difficult and inappropriate. The arguments can be applied to most countries where resources permit maternal testing, but the incidences of maternal seroconversion and fetal disease are relatively low. Although government health agencies and national health organizations in many countries, including Centers for Disease Control and the American College of Obstetrics and Gynecology in the United States, have not recommended universal screening at this time, some form of limited maternal screening can be considered provided the necessary resources are available. Selected screening based on the presence of a household cat should probably be discouraged because maternal exposure to *T. gondii* can come from multiple environmental and dietary sources.

A possible approach to universal screening in countries such as the United States would be to use a combination of several time points for serologic testing in pregnancy coupled with prevention counseling. Mothers could be screened for toxoplasma IgG and IgM during the first obstetric visit and counseled regarding preventive measures to decrease potential exposure during the remainder of the pregnancy. Ideally tests should be performed by a toxoplasma reference laboratory, and retesting could be repeated in the second and third trimesters if a mother is found to be susceptible. Although this approach may not be as effective as the monthly testing performed in some universal screening programs, it has the potential to detect maternal seroconversion and allow for further assessment of fetal infection and therapeutic options. Testing as early as possible in the first trimester with counseling and repeated testing twice in the second trimester may be best to determine seroconversion during the period of greatest risk for severe fetal disease. It must be emphasized that such a screening program has not been evaluated.

THERAPEUTIC OPTIONS AND LONG-TERM OUTCOMES

Once acute maternal toxoplasmosis has been diagnosed, treatment with spiramycin should be initiated. This drug has been used in the first trimester without adverse effects on the fetus, but in the United States the drug is available only as an investigational new drug (IND) protocol. Maternal infection must be confirmed with the Palo Alto Medical Research Institute Toxoplasma Serology Laboratory, and the IND number can then be obtained from the Food and Drug Administration. A supply of drug can be shipped overnight for immediate use. Studies should also be undertaken to assess fetal infection, and, if infection is suspected or confirmed, drug therapy should be changed to pyrimethamine and sulfadiazine plus folinic acid. Complete blood cell counts should be monitored and the dose of folinic acid increased if abnormalities (e.g., neutropenia or anemia) are found.

Amniocentesis and percutaneous umbilical blood sampling have been used successfully to detect fetal infection in the setting of acute maternal toxoplasmosis in pregnancy. Before the development of the amniotic fluid PCR assay, fetal blood samples were cultured for toxoplasma and tested for toxoplasma-specific IgM, total IgM, complete blood cell counts, and liver function tests. Amniotic fluid obtained at the time of cordocentesis was also cultured for *T. gondii*. These studies coupled with fetal ultrasound surveys had a high sensitivity and specificity for congenital infection, at least when performed by experienced investigators in a research setting. Cordocentesis and amniotic fluid cultures have been replaced by amniotic fluid PCR for *T. gondii*. In a clinical study with experienced investigators using the assay in a reference laboratory, the test was found to perform better than cordocentesis and to have very high sensitivity (97%) with 100% specificity. A more recent study found the sensitivity to be only 64% (87.8% negative predictive value), with 100% specificity. Amniocentesis can be performed by 15 weeks of gestation, but the sensitivity of the toxoplasma PCR may suboptimal until 20 weeks of gestation. Because of potential limitations of toxoplasma PCR, some experts elect to treat with pyrimethamine and sulfadiazine plus folinic acid, beginning near the middle or end of the second trimester, even if fetal infection has not been confirmed and no fetal abnormalities have been detected. The fetus appears to tolerate this treatment very well, with normal growth and development. Amniocentesis should be avoided in HIV-positive mothers because of the risk of fetal HIV transmission; however, if these women are diagnosed with acute toxoplasmosis in pregnancy, treatment with pyrimethamine and sulfadiazine (plus folinic acid) may be indicated for their own benefit and that of their fetus.

Newborn infants diagnosed with congenital toxoplasma infection should also be treated with pyrimethamine and sulfadiazine plus folinic acid, even if no stigmata of infection can be found. The principal goals underlying current treatment programs are to initiate therapy as soon as possible after infection has been diagnosed and to extend therapy for at least 1 year. Recent reports from France and the United States confirm the substantial benefits of this approach.

PREVENTION OF MATERNAL INFECTION   Toxoplasma oocysts are very hardy and can resist drying and treatment with disinfectants, alcohols (95% ethanol and 100% methanol), and 10% formalin. Inactivation can be achieved by heating at 66°C (>150°F). Oocysts are also destroyed by freezing temperatures but survive for extended periods in tropical regions. Bradyzoites in tissue cysts can also be destroyed by heating to 66°C, by gamma irradiation, and by freezing at −20°C (−4°F). Tachyzoites are easily destroyed with drying or freeze-thawing and by digestive enzymes.

The prevention of congenital toxoplasmosis requires maternal counseling on environmental and dietary risk factors Box 21-1. Simple procedures may be helpful in minimizing maternal exposure to *T. gondii* during pregnancy. Ideally, women should be counseled on these preventive measures at the first obstetric visit.

Box 21-1.   GUIDE TO PREVENTIVE MEASURES TO HELP PREVENT OF INFECTION WITH TOXOPLASMA GONDII

Cats
- Keep indoors
- Empty litter daily (avoid if pregnant or wear gloves)
- Feed only dry, canned, or cooked food

Meat
- Avoid eating undercooked
  - Cook until no pink color remains in the center
- Freezing meat before preparing may decrease risk of infection

- Wear gloves when handling, or wash hands thoroughly after handling
- Keep cutting boards and utensils thoroughly clean

Vegetables
- Wear gloves when gardening
  - Avoid touching the face with a gloved hand
  - Change clothing and wash hands after completing yard/garden work
- Wash thoroughly before eating
- Wear gloves when handling or wash hands thoroughly after handling

Conclusion

While toxoplasmosis and cytomegalovirus rarely cause serious maternal illness, they can cause congenital infection and serious permanent sequelae. Cytomegalovirus can cause perinatal infection in-utero or by breast milk exposure and can occur with primary infection, reinfection, and reactivation of remote infection. Congenital toxoplasmosis results from in-utero exposure of a primary maternal infection.

For both illnesses maternal serology studies are helpful in making a diagnosis of infection. Amniocentesis studies can help determine whether fetal infection has occurred, but cannot establish prognosis. Medical treatment is available during pregnancy for toxoplasmosis, but not for cytomegalovirus. Abnormal ultrasound findings are useful for prediction of outcome, but in most cases prognosis is difficult to predict with accuracy.

Discussion of Cases

Case 2: Prenatal Diagnosis of Hydrocephalus

A 19-year-old gravida 1 woman had a fetal ultrasound performed at 26 weeks of gestation, which showed severe fetal ventriculomegaly (Figure 21-2). No other fetal anomalies were identified. There were no recent illnesses in the family. The patient denied eating undercooked meat, and all vegetables and fruits were store bought and washed before consumption. She lived in a city apartment with no garden and she had no pets. She only occasionally ate meat and stated that it was always store bought and frozen before preparation. There was no family history of congenital abnormalities.

Is there any infectious disease etiology you would consider in the differential of the fetal hydrocephalus?

Although congenital hydrocephalus most often results from noninfectious causes, congenital infection should always be considered. ***Toxoplasma gondii*** **and CMV should be considered. Obtain maternal serology for** ***T. gondii*** **and CMV. It may be best to have** ***T. gondii*** **serology performed at a reference laboratory, where an extended panel of tests can be performed to help determine recent from remote infection. CMV-specific IgG, DS-IgM-ELISA, and IgG avidity (if IgG positive) should be obtained.**

Serology was positive for acute *T. gondii* infection. Specific IgG, DS-IgM-ELISA, and IgA titers were highly positive, and the differential agglutination pattern was consistent with recent infection. CMV serology was negative.

What do you do next?

The severity of the hydrocephalus was concerning for severe brain damage; parenchymal

Figure 21-2: A:
Ultrasound image of
severe
ventriculomegaly in a
fetus with congenital
toxoplasma infection.
B: CT image of
ventriculomegaly
intracranial
calcifications.
C: Large retinal scar by
opthalmoscopy.

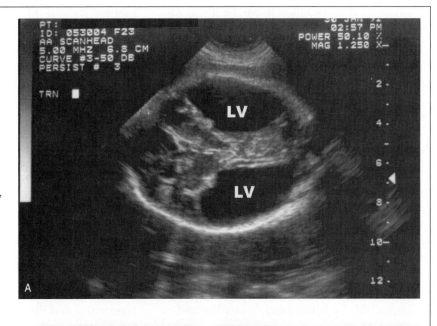

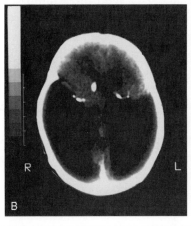

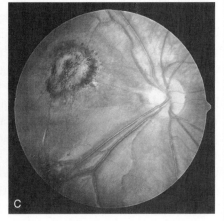

destruction cannot be ruled out. Start treatment with pyrimethamine and sulfadiazine plus folinic acid until delivery. Monitor maternal complete blood cell counts and adjust folinic acid if neutropenia or worsening anemia develops.

At birth the infant had unilateral microphthalmia but no other abnormalities on examination. Head CT showed severe hydrocephalus ex vacuo, and there were unilateral microphthalmia with vitreitis and a large retinal scar in the opposite eye by indirect ophthalmoscopy.

What is the source of the maternal infection and how do you counsel the mother regarding future pregnancies?

Not uncommonly, a specific source for infection cannot be identified. On more careful questioning of this mother, however, it was discovered that she had participated in the slaughter of a lamb at a farm. Although she did not consume any of the meat, she did assist with its cutting and processing. This took place at approximately 7 weeks of gestation. This may have been the source of the infection. The mother should be informed that unless she develops a severe immunodeficiency disease, it is extremely unlikely that she will have another child with congenital toxoplasma infection, especially if she waits an additional 6–9 months before her next conception.

CASE 3: ACUTE MATERNAL TOXOPLASMA INFECTION

A 36-year-old gravida 2, para 1 woman has no significant medical history and has had a normal pregnancy, now at 20 weeks of gestation. An amniocentesis had been performed for advanced maternal age and showed a 46,XY fetus. No fetal abnormalities by ultrasound were observed at that time. During the visit she mentions that her husband has just been diagnosed with a toxoplasma eye infection. He developed unilateral blurred vision 1 month previously, but only recently had he seen an ophthalmologist who diagnosed chorioretinitis. The ocular lesion was thought to be active, and he was started on "antibiotics." The family lives in the Caribbean most of the year, and they frequently eat a variety of meats. They usually cook their meat so that it is still "pink" in the middle, and they obtain fresh vegetables from a nearby farm. They have a 3-year-old daughter, no pets, and they frequently work, play, and lounge in their yard. There are "many" cats in the neighborhood. The mother's examination is completely normal, and she reports no illness in her daughter or herself.

Is this women at risk for acute toxoplasma in pregnancy? Would you do any testing?

Although most cases of ocular toxoplasma in adults have been thought to represent reactivation of congenital infection, it is now recognized that a significant number of these cases may result from acute acquired infection. Further, simultaneous infection of multiple family members has been well documented, presumably from a common source exposure. In this case there are multiple potential environmental and dietary risk factors. Perform a fetal ultrasound survey. Obtain toxoplasma-specific IgG and DS-IgM-ELISA serologies. Consider using a reference laboratory so additional testing can be performed to help confirm recent infection in pregnancy.

Toxoplasma-specific IgG and DS-IgM-ELISA serologies are positive, and additional testing shows low IgG avidity, positive IgA ELISA, and a differential agglutination pattern consistent with recent maternal infection.

The fetus is now at 22 weeks of gestation. What do you do next?

Repeat fetal ultrasound shows no abnormalities. Inform the parents that, although the fetal ultrasound remains normal, you cannot rule out fetal infection. Discuss with the parents the option to begin spiramycin and to perfom a repeat amniocentesis, this time to test for *T. gondii* by PCR. An ultrasound examination could also be performed at the same time to search further for fetal abnormalities. Explain that spiramycin may decrease the transmission of *T. gondii* to the fetus, but it would not likely effectively treat the fetus if infection has occurred. Explain that the amniotic fluid PCR performed at 22 weeks is likely to be highly sensitive for infection, but it is not 100% sensitive so there is a small chance that infection could be missed. Discuss the need to change to treatment with pyrimethamine and sulfadiazine plus folinic acid if fetal infection is determined, and that this treatment appears to improve the outcome of infected fetuses.

Based on the father's presentation, a common exposure may have happened in the early second trimester. The maternal serologies are consistent with this.

What additional information should you tell the parents? Are there alternative options to amniocentesis and spiramycin?

The risk of fetal transmission may be 15–30% based on the likely timing of maternal infection. Although there is typically a delay in transmission of *T. gondii* to the fetus, 6–8 weeks may have already passed since the onset of maternal infection. Discuss the fact that most fetal infections in the second trimester result in mild or subclinical infections. Retinal lesions affecting vision may be the major risk. Most infants at birth do not have retinal lesions. When lesions do occur, they are often unilateral. Discuss the use of empiric treatment with pyrimethamine and sulfadiazine plus folinic acid, although initiating spiramycin therapy and performing amniocentesis would be the more standard approach. The factors to consider in this decision include the possibility of false-negative PCR, maternal and fetal risks of the medication, and risks from amniocentesis.

The family chooses not to undergo an amniocentesis. Their rationale is that they would prefer to have empiric treatment for their fetus, even if laboratory monitoring (complete blood cell counts) are required. They prefer to have the potential benefit of full treatment even if the chance of a false-negative PCR may be very small, and complications from the amniocentesis would be a very low risk.

A 3.4-kg male infant is delivered at 39 weeks. The examination was normal, head CT was negative, and a pediatric ophthalmologic evaluation was negative. Toxo-plasma-specific IgG was positive but the DS-IgM ELISA and the IgM-ISAGA were negative (as determined by a toxo-plasma reference laboratory). Repeat serologies were obtained at 1 month, 3 months, 5 months, 7 months, and 1 year. The IgG titer steadily decreased and was negative at 7 months and 1 year.

This fetus escaped infection so treatment with pyrimethamine and sulfadiazine plus folinic acid was not necessary. Nonetheless, using empiric treatment was acceptable.

REFERENCES

1 Guerina NG, Hsu HW, Meissner HC, et al, for New England Regional Toxoplasma Working Group. Neonatal serologic screening and early treatment for congenital *Toxoplasma gondii* infection. *N Engl J Med* 1994;330:1858–1863.

2 Pass RF, Stagno S, Myers GJ, Alford CA. Outcome of symptomatic congenital cytomegalovirus infection: results of long-term longitudinal follow-up. *Pediatrics* 1980;66:758–762.

3   Stagno S. Cytomegalovirus. In: Remington JS, Klein JO, eds. *Infectious Diseases of the Fetus and Newborn Infant*, 4th ed. Philadelphia: Saunders, 2001; p. 389–424.

4   Stagno S, Pass RF, Cloud G, et al. Primary cytomegalovirus infection in pregnancy. Incidence, transmission to fetus, and clinical outcome. *JAMA* 1986;256:1904–1908.

5   Morris DJ, Sims D, Chiswick M, et al. Symptomatic congenital cytomegalovirus infection after maternal recurrent infection. *Pediatr Infect Dis J* 1994;13:61–64.

6   Krech U, Konjajev Z, Jung M. Congenital cytomegalovirus infection in siblings from consecutive pregnancies. *Helv Paediatr Acta* 1971; 26:355–362.

7   Pass RF, Hutto C, Ricks R, Cloud GA. Increased rate of cytomegalovirus infection among parents of children attending day-care centers. *N Engl J Med* 1986;314:1414–1418.

8   Pearl KN, Preece PM, Ades A, Peckham CS. Neurodevelopmental assessment after congenital cytomegalovirus infection. *Arch Dis Child* 1986;61:323–326.

9   Boppana SB, Britt WJ. Antiviral antibody responses and intrauterine transmission after primary maternal cytomegalovirus infection. *J Infect Dis* 1995;171:1115–1121.

10 Bodeus M, Van Ranst M, Bernard P, et al. Anticytomegalovirus IgG avidity in pregnancy: a 2-year prospective study. *Fetal Diagn Ther* 2002;17:362–366.

11 Kesrouani AK, Guibourdenche J, Muller F, et al. Etiology and outcome of fetal echogenic bowel. Ten years of experience. *Fetal Diagn Ther* 2003;18:240–246.

12 Balfour CL, Balfour H Jr. Cytomegalovirus is not an occupational risk for nurses in renal transplant and neonatal units. Results of a prospective surveillance study. *JAMA* 1986;256:1909–1914.

13 Lynfield R, Hsu HW, Guerina NG. Screening methods for congenital toxoplasma and risk of disease. *Lancet* 1999;353:1899–1900.

14 Remington JS, McLeod R, Thulliez P, Desmonts GI. Toxoplasmosis. In: Remington JS, Klein JO, eds. *Infectious Diseases of the Fetus and Newborn Infant,* 4th ed. Philadelphia: Saunders. 2001; p. 205–215.

15 Montoya JG. Laboratory diagnosis of *Toxoplasma gondii* infection and toxoplasmosis. *J Infect Dis* 2002;185(suppl 1):S73–S82.

16 Romand S, Wallon M, Franck J, et al. Prenatal diagnosis using polymerase chain reaction on amniotic fluid for congenital toxoplasmosis. *Obstet Gynecol* 2001;97:296–300.

17 Sever JL, Ellenberg JH, Ley AC, et al. Toxoplasmosis: maternal and pediatric findings in 23,000 pregnancies. *Pediatrics* 1998;82:181–192.

18 Gilbert R, Gras L. European Multicentre Study on Congenital Toxoplasmosis. Effect of timing and type of treatment on the risk of mother to child transmission of *Toxoplasma gondii. BJOG* 2003;110: 112–120.

19 McAuley J, Boyer K, Patel D, et al. Early and longitudinal evaluations of treated infants and children and untreated historical patients with congenital toxoplasmosis: the Chicago Collaborative Treatment Trial. *Clin Infect Dis* 1994;18:38–72.

VZV Infection Management in Pregnancy

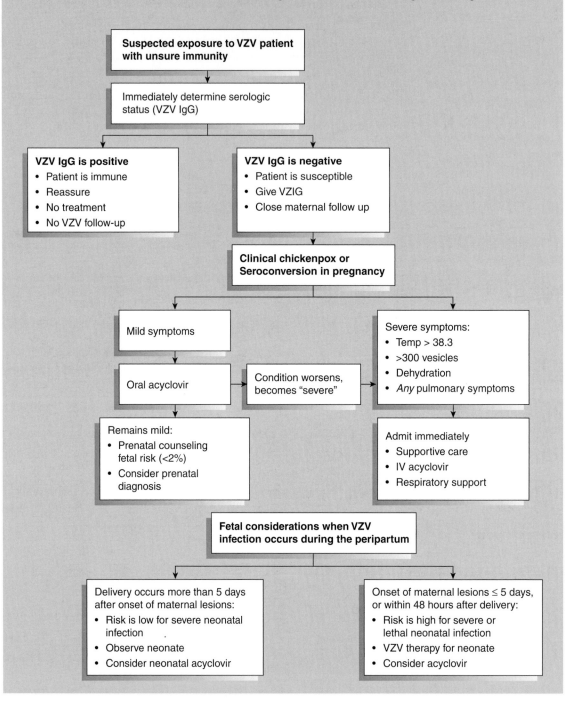

22

Varicella Zoster Virus in Pregnancy

Peter G. Pryde

Introduction

Varicella zoster virus (VZV), a member of the herpesvirus family of double-stranded DNA viruses, is the causative agent in two well-known clinical syndromes: *varicella*, or "chickenpox," and *herpes zoster*, commonly known as "shingles." Because of its highly contagious biology, VZV accounts for frequent epidemics that affect nearly all exposed, susceptible children. Fortunately, these nearly universal childhood infections, with rare exception, confer life-long immunity (demonstrable in the serology laboratory by presence of anti-VZV antibodies). As a consequence, North American prenatal serologic surveys have indicated that fewer than 5% of reproductive-age woman remain seronegative (indicating susceptibility to acute infection), and only about 2% of varicella cases occur among women ages 15 to 49 years.[1] Likewise, the population risk for *antenatal VZV infection* is quite low (estimated at 1–5 in 10,000 pregnancies). An important exception to this is among women who have emigrated from subtropical and tropical areas, where childhood VZV epidemics are considerably less common, leaving susceptibility (seronegativity) as high as 16%. Thus obstetricians should think of this subpopulation separately because they face a considerably higher individual risk for pregnancy-associated varicella.[2]

Biology and Clinical Manifestations of VZV Infection

Varicella, or chickenpox, is spread mainly by respiratory droplets (nasopharyngeal secretions) that are transmitted by coughing or fomites from viremic individuals to susceptible (seronegative) individuals by contact with the upper respiratory or conjunctival mucosa. Less commonly, the virus can be transmitted by direct contact with the virion-rich fluid that can be expressed, or may leak, from acute chickenpox vesicles. Due to the highly contagious nature of the virus, the attack rate after household or workplace exposure in susceptible (seronegative) adults approaches 90%. After exposure and establishment of infection, the virus rapidly replicates for several days within Waldeyer's ring and regional lymph nodes. Subsequently, over an "incubation period" of around 14 days (range 10 to 20 days), there occurs (1) a primary viremia, leading to (2) infectious involvement of internal organs, where (3) further viral replication ensues, after which (4) a secondary viremia occurs.

KEY POINT

The duration of infectivity is from 48 hours before clinical signs until all of the vesicles have crusted over.

It is during this secondary viremia that the host becomes symptomatic, first with fever and generalized malaise (lasting about 48 hours) and then with viral invasion of cutaneous tissues, eventuating in the well-known and easily recognized maculopapular, intensely pruritic, and ultimately vesicular exanthem. It is clinically important to recognize that infectivity begins with the onset of secondary viremia such that there are nearly 2 days of pre-rash contagiousness during which unsuspecting contacts may be exposed to a mildly ill child who is only later found to be evolving the disease. Contagiousness then lasts throughout the period of variably severe exanthem until all vesicles have crusted over.

Most cases, particularly in children, are self-limiting aside from the nuisance of the skin manifestations, which, in rare cases, can be severe with or without bacterial superinfection. However, further complications (Table 22-1) carrying significant risk for severe morbidity and even mortality can result and do so far more frequently in affected adults than in children. The most common of these complications, varicella pneumonitis, may affect as many as 20% of infected adults. This feared pulmonary manifestation of the disease, which is dangerous for all affected adults but apparently considerably more so among pregnant women, carries pre–acyclovir era mortality rates reportedly as high as 17% in adults generally and 40% in pregnant women.[3]

Table 22-1. **LIFE-THREATENING AND LONG-TERM COMPLICATIONS FROM VARICELLA**

Common
Pneumonia
Superinfection of skin vesicles

Uncommon
Encephalitis
Meningitis
Arthritis
Myocarditis
Glomerulonephritis

Rare
Reye's syndrome
Guillain-Barré syndrome
Benign cerebellar ataxia

KEY POINT

Pregnant women are at substantial risk for developing life-threatening varicella pneumonia.

KEY POINT

Herpes zoster rash does not cause transplacental transmission of varicella to a fetus.

Herpes zoster, or shingles, occurs by reactivation of latent VZV that, like other herpesviruses, becomes "dormant" within previously infected sensory neurons whose cell bodies reside within dorsal root ganglia. It is because of the dorsal root location of dormant virus that reactivation is manifest clinically as a painful vesicular rash located anatomically within a unilateral dermatomal distribution. This manifestation of VZV is commonly seen in the elderly and occasionally in individuals who have cell-mediated immunocompromise of various etiologies. Therefore, it is extremely uncommon in pregnant or other healthy women of reproductive age. Accordingly, pregnancy-associated zoster incidence is estimated at less than 0.5 in 10,000 pregnancies. Although direct contact with the dermatomally distributed, and often extremely painful, zoster rash can transmit chickenpox, there is no viremia in the affected individual (due to previous development of serologic immunity acquired during the previous primary infection) and, hence, no chance for respiratory droplet spread or transplacental transmission from affected women.[4]

Varicella in Pregnancy: Maternal Complications and Management

Chickenpox in adults is frequently a more severe disease, with markedly increased morbidity and mortality risks, than it is in children. Likewise, retrospective studies have suggested that life-threatening complications from varicella, although probably not more common, may be considerably more hazardous among pregnant women than among adults in general. By far the commonest, and obstetrically most relevant, of these complications is pneumonia (occurring in 20% of pregnancies complicated by varicella).[5]

Among pregnant woman, varicella pneumonia has a widely variable and unpredictable course. Typically it manifests as soon as 1 day and as late as 7 days after the first recognized features of the chickenpox rash. Presenting features range from subtle cough to full-blown features of pneumonitis including dyspnea, fever, pleuritic chest pain, and hemoptysis. Chest auscultation may be unremarkable at first despite, in some instances, worrisome complaints. The initial chest radiograph may even appear normal but more often is nonspecific, with findings ranging from a modest peribronchial nodular pattern to a diffuse miliary infiltrative pattern. Each of these initial chest radiographs may evolve over time into the diffuse "white out" pattern typical of the adult respiratory distress syndrome.

KEY POINT

Diagnosis and treatment of varicella pneumonia should be considered a medical emergency.

Unequivocally, varicella pneumonia diagnosed during any stage of pregnancy needs to be regarded as a medical emergency and, even if apparently very mild at initial presentation, demands immediate hospitalization with intensive maternal surveillance.[5] Therapy consists of *supportive care*, which may include supplemental oxygen only but, in women progressing toward respiratory failure, will require admission to the intensive care unit for supportive ventilation techniques such as bilevel positive airway pressure or, in most severe cases, intubation with mechanical ventilation. As important, and often life saving, is rapid institution of *antiviral therapy* that uses high-dose intravenous acyclovir (10 mg/kg every 8 hours) or its congener valacyclovir. Although most affected patients will have a mild course, those destined to progress rapidly toward respiratory failure cannot clearly be identified. Hence the recommendation of universal hospitalization for even mild respiratory symptoms.

Retrospective data, sometimes criticized for overestimating risk due to potential ascertainment bias, nonetheless should alarm the practicing obstetrician: These data predict mortality risks from VZV pneumonia in pregnancy of 40% in untreated mothers and as high as 14% even among those properly hospitalized and afforded acyclovir therapy.[5] Although outcomes appear to be considerably better in more recent series,[6,7] probably due to improved and more aggressive management, in view of the (1) still relevant maternal mortality risk, (2) high rate of pneumonia complicating varicella infection during pregnancy (20%), and (3) absence of any convincing evidence of embryo or fetal toxicity despite abundant and growing clinical experience with acyclovir during all trimesters of pregnancy, many experts including the American College of Obstetricians and Gynecologists currently recommend instituting oral acyclovir (800 mg five times daily) as soon as skin manifestations of chickenpox are identified in hopes of ameliorating the course of illness and minimizing risk for progression to pneumonia or other severe complications.[8]

KEY POINT

Consider oral acyclovir therapy at the onset of skin manifestations of chickenpox.

As with any life-threatening medical or surgical illness that complicates pregnancy, the fetal consequences of a profoundly altered maternal physiology need to be considered in pregnancies complicated by severe manifestations of varicella. Preterm labor and fetal distress are common in such cases, probably owing to the consequences of a combination of massive cytokine elaboration that is characteristic of the systemic inflammatory response syndrome, the attendant altered maternal hemodynamics, and ultimately tissue level hypoxia. Maternal and fetal risk benefit evaluation and management decisions under such circumstances are complex and deserve experienced, expert attention. Optimally, care for the sickest of such patients will involve multidisciplinary input including perinatologists, neonatologists, infectious disease specialists, intensivists, and/or anesthesiologists.

Direct Fetal and Neonatal Consequences of Maternal Varicella Infection

Aside from the various and potentially extensive fetal and neonatal harm that can occur as a consequence of premature delivery or hypoxia and asphyxia, each of which can occur secondary to the hostile uterine environment attendant with severe maternal infection (see above), varicella can also cause direct virus mediated fetal injury. That is, VZV is among several pathogens (classically grouped as the "TORCH" infections) that during maternal viremia can infect and traverse the placenta. Having thus gained access to the fetus, the virus can replicate and infect numerous developing organs, causing a variety of sequelae ranging from asymptomatic seroconversion to mild dermatomally distributed skin scarring or severe neurologic, visceral, dermatologic, and limb injuries (Table 22-2).[9]

Table 22-2. MANIFESTATIONS OF CONGENITAL VARICELLA SYNDROME

Central nervous system injury
Microcephaly
Cortical atrophy
Mental retardation
Neonatal seizures

Peripheral nervous system injury
Varying degrees and distribution of motor and/or sensory deficits
Bulbar palsy
Horner's syndrome
Optic atrophy

Eye injury
Chorioretinitis
Cataracts

Visceral injury
Focal necrosis and calcification within liver and bowel
Hydrops fetalis
Possibly, cardiac malformations

Limb injury
Skin contractures, usually localized to a peripheral nerves distribution
Postural abnormalities secondary to cicatricial (zig-zag) scarring skin changes
Limb or digit hypoplasia
Talipes

KEY POINT

The vast majority of cases of maternal infection with VZV result in no detectable fetal consequences.

At present, it is not completely clear how often fetal infection occurs, and among infected fetuses, how often recognizable features of the congenital varicella syndrome occur. However, it must be strongly emphasized that the vast majority of cases of maternal infection with VZV result in *no* detectable fetal sequellae.[10] In three recent prospective studies, fetal outcomes thought to be compatible with congenital varicella syndrome occurred in only 0.4–2.2% of infected pregnancies.[4,11,12] Most of the affected cases occurred among pregnancies in which maternal symptoms and seroconversion were documented at 8–20 weeks, although at least one affected infant's mother had onset of rash at 24 weeks. There have never been reports of congenital anomalies attributable to VZV occurring subsequent to a maternal outbreak of shingles (herpes zoster) during any trimester of pregnancy.[4] This is not surprising because there is no accompanying viremia in such cases.

Neonatal infection with VZV is, with the rare exception of nosocomial infections in the hospital nursery, transmitted vertically.[9] It is clinically most important in pregnancies in which the mother developed onset of chickenpox symptoms before, and still has active lesions during, delivery or rupture of membranes, or the mother has onset of rash within 48 hours after her delivery, indicating that she was very likely viremic during parturition. In cases in which maternal symptoms developed more than 5 days before delivery, maternal immunoglobulin (Ig) G antibodies have begun to elaborate. Like other IgG antibodies, these cross the placenta, where they confer sufficient passive immunity that the newborn is protected against severe sequelae, although mild infection may occur. In contrast, onset of symptoms less than 5 days before delivery or up to around 48 hours after delivery predict considerable risk for neonatal infection and, when infection occurs, potentially severe sequelae including disseminated disease eventuating in death (≤30%) or variably severe neurologic injury among survivors. Administration of varicella zoster immune globulin (VZIG) to newborns within 24 hours of birth appears to decrease the likelihood of clinical infection or severe sequelae when infection does occur.[9] Newborn VZIG should be administered even if the mother received VZIG before delivery.

> **KEY POINT**
>
> *Neonatal varicella is acquired vertically from an infected mother. The highest risk is when the clinical disease occurs less than 5 days and up to 48 hours after delivery.*

Diagnosis of Varicella During Pregnancy

Zoster and varicella are usually diagnosed clinically by their well-known and characteristic rashes. Occasionally, however, the rash may be subtle or atypical, in which case laboratory methods may be used to establish or confirm the diagnosis. Although culture of vesicular fluid is available, it is cumbersome and rarely used. More often, maternal serologic testing for IgM and IgG (evolving ≤3 days and as early as 5–7 days after onset of symptoms, respectively) is employed using an enzyme-linked immunosorbent assay. Documenting seroconversion is diagnostic. In asymptomatic, but ostensibly exposed, gravidas who are unsure of their chickenpox history, serologic testing can confirm susceptibility (absence of maternal VZV antibodies) or assure immunity (presence of VZV IgG). Other available methods include vesicular fluid sample evaluation by using serologic evaluation for VZV antigens by immunofluorescence or VZV DNA testing by molecular techniques based on polymerase chain reaction (PCR).

Prenatal diagnosis has been documented in numerous case reports and case series by using laboratory methodologies similar to those used in the mother. To prove fetal involvement, such testing demands that fetal tissue be obtained. For example, early efforts focused on serologic testing of fetal blood obtained by percutaneous umbilical blood sampling. However, this technique has yielded fairly poor sensitivity. More recently, PCR techniques seeking evidence of VZV DNA in amniotic fluid, fetal blood, or placental tissue have shown much higher sensitivity.[13] Unfortunately, however, although these methods can fairly reliably detect whether or not there has been fetal infection, they do not predict the presence or severity of fetal sequelae.[14] This is not a trivial matter because it is now clear that many *infected* fetuses are not detectably *affected* by the congenital syndrome. One partial solution to this dilemma, albeit imperfect, is using ultrasound assessment for features indicative of fetal injury concomitant with DNA evidence of fetal infection. Such manifestations may include variable combinations of growth restriction, microcephaly, intracranial or extensive intraabdominal calcifications, hydrops, characteristic limb deformities, or postural abnormalities. Most fetal medicine specialists agree that definitive ultrasound features of congenital varicella in this setting are a poor prognostic feature. In contrast, it must be acknowledged that the absence of ultrasonographically detectable features of congenital varicella does not guarantee a normal, unaffected neonatal outcome in a pregnancy with PCR confirmation of fetal infection. Accordingly, as with the management of severe maternal varicella, the complexity of the diagnostic evaluation and counseling of women faced with concerns about fetal involvement from VZV infection is such that the problem is ideally managed by a clinician or a multidisciplinary group of clinicians who have experience and specific expertise in this area of fetal medicine.

Prevention of Pregnancy Varicella and Its Maternal, Fetal, and Neonatal Consequences

Currently there are three methods to prevent varicella infection that complicates pregnancy or, in cases in which infection occurs, to decrease the attendant maternal and fetal risks.[15] The first and most effective method is to assure natural or vaccination-induced maternal immunity before pregnancy. A second approach is to counsel seronegative pregnant women to avoid exposure as much as possible. Third, there is the availability of VZIG that can be administered in hopes of decreasing maternal, fetal, and neonatal complications from the infection.

Serologic surveys have demonstrated that more than 95% of women who recall having had varicella as a child have confirmed positive IgG serology. Therefore, these women can be safely assumed to be at low, but not absent, risk for future VZV infection. Conversely, young women who do not recall or are unsure whether they had chickenpox are seropositive in fewer than 90% of cases. Hence, some authorities have recommended routine serologic testing of women for the purposes of future risk counseling and consideration of vaccination (although the cost effectiveness of such a strategy has been questioned). For women who are not pregnant (e.g., during preconception counseling or routine gynecologic encounters) and identified as seronegative (not immune), vaccination should be advised. Seroconversion will occur in 80–90% of healthy adolescents or adults after two doses given 4–8 weeks apart. However, because the vaccine, VIRIVAX, is a live, attenuated virus, it should not be given to pregnant women, and it is recommended to avoid pregnancy for a month after receiving it. Along these lines, one unexpected hazard that obstetricians should be aware of relates to several reports of pregnant women inadvertently given VIRIVAX when VZIG was intended.[16] Obviously one needs to be very clear about which agent is ordered and which their staff is giving to the patient. Nevertheless, it is somewhat reassuring that the VIRIVAX Pregnancy Registry (phone 1-800-986-8999), despite numerous early pregnancy exposures with close follow-up, have not yet identified a convincing case of VIRIVAX-related congenital varicella syndrome.[17]

In women known to be seronegative, a second "prevention" strategy is to use VZIG as soon as possible after a relevant exposure.[18] Household exposure causes the highest attack rate. Ideally, VZIG is given within the first 48 hours after exposure to an infectious source. However, it may be effective up to 96 hours after the exposure and should be given within that period. The main goal of the VZIG is to decrease the severity of, or possibly prevent, a maternal infection. Unfortunately, data are insufficient to determine whether VZIG affects the incidence or severity of congenital infection in treated but nevertheless infected pregnant women. The standard adult dose is 625 mg intramuscularly. The duration of VZIG benefit is 3 weeks. If exposure recurs after 3 weeks, VZIG should be given again. VZIG can prolong the incubation period of infection from the usual 10–21 days to longer than 28 days. VZIG results in false-positive findings of immunity for varicella for 2 months.

KEY POINT

VZIG should be given to seronegative women within 96 hours of an exposure and ideally within 48 hours.

A final and commonsense strategy for the prevention of pregnancy-associated varicella is to educate already pregnant but susceptible (seronegative) women about the hazards of chickenpox during pregnancy. Although it would not be possible to avoid all possible exposures to potentially infectious individuals (e.g., contact during the 48-hour prodromal period of secondary viremia before onset of diagnostic rash), the gravida could certainly limit or eliminate her exposure in social or occupational circumstances where there is a known or likely case. In addition, she would be aware of the importance of *immediately* reporting to her physician if she learns that she has had an inadvertent exposure. Importantly, this will allow that VZIG can be obtained and administered as quickly as possible.

Guiding Questions

For the pregnant woman exposed to chicken pox or shingles

- Does she have a history of infection or serologic testing?
- What was the setting of her exposure?
- At what stage of illness was the individual to whom she was exposed?
- How long ago was the exposure?

For the pregnant woman with chicken pox

- What is the gestational age?
- Does she have any chronic illness?
- Is she exposed to anyone else who is at risk of illness?
- Have you informed her about symptoms of varicella pneumonia?
- Does she have any symptoms of pneumonia or headache?
- If she is at term, have you notified the pediatricians?

What's the Evidence

The diagnostic and management issues of varicella have been extremely well studied, particularly in the pediatric population. The epidemiology of infection and immunity is well established.[1] The consequence of infection in pregnant women has been established by retrospective and prospective observational studies.[4] The use of oral antiviral medication has been studied in pediatric and adult populations and has demonstrated effectiveness in limiting the duration and severity of infection.[8] VZIG prophylaxis has been demonstrated to decrease the severity of maternal varicella infection.[18] Further research should target strategies to decrease the severity of neonatal varicella, including antiviral therapies for pregnant women with chickenpox.

Conclusion

Varicella infections are uncommon in pregnancy but pose particular maternal-fetal and neonatal risks. A key fact is that infectivity of chicken pox illness occurs from 48 hours prior to clinical evidence until all of the lesions have crusted over. The vast majority of pregnancies complicated by varicella infection have normal perinatal outcome. Pregnant women are at particular risk for serious infection including varicella pneumonia which should be considered a medical emergency. Acyclovir is beneficial in decreasing the severity of maternal illness. VZIG may be given to seronegative varicella- exposed women to decrease the severity of infection. VZIG given to a neonate whose mother had infection around the time of delivery can decrease the severity of neonatal illness. Serologic testing should be considered for women who do not have a history of chicken pox or shingles.

Discussion of Cases

CASE 1: EXPOSURE TO CHICKENPOX IN THE FIRST TRIMESTER

A young woman in her eighth week of pregnancy calls her obstetrician to report that her 6-year-old child, exposed more than 1 week ago to a child with chickenpox, has had a febrile illness for the past 2 days and now has vesicles.

What other history must you illicit?

Ask whether the mother has ever had chickenpox. If not, ask whether she has been previously serologically tested for immunity or received the VZV live attenuated vaccine.

She replies that she has never been vaccinated or tested, and she specifically recalls never having had chickenpox as a child, although she believes she may have been exposed.

What additional information or laboratory testing, if any, would you seek?

This situation is not an emergency but should be viewed as urgent. Most hospitals can arrange VZV serology testing with an expectation of results within 24 hours. Because as many as 90% of women who are unsure about their chickenpox history are found to be immune and VZIG is very expensive (>US $600 for the usual adult dosage), it is important to verify absence of immunity rather than treat empirically, if that is possible. Therefore, the patient is instructed to go directly to the hospital, where arrangements have been made for phlebotomy and VZV antibody testing.

The following day serologic results indicate absent VZV IgG, interpreted appropriately as absence of immunity.

Does this finding indicate medical intervention in this setting; if so, what is the currently recommended treatment?

VZIG, a pooled human immunoglobulin, is recommended to provide prophylaxis against or, more likely, decrease severity and morbidity of maternal infection. Although the VZIG can be given within 48 hours of relevant clinical exposure, it is probably effective (albeit to a lesser extent) up to 95 hours; Hence, the "urgency" of maternal evaluation and management.

Does the patient require any further testing, follow-up, or referral?

She remains at risk, despite the VZIG, for chickenpox and its potential for severe maternal and/or fetal sequelae. With this in mind, the patient is then referred to the local or regional perinatologist (or other fetal and maternal medicine specialist with expertise in fetal infections, prenatal diagnosis, and management of life-threatening maternal diseases). Under the care of a maternal-fetal medicine specialist, she can receive in-depth counseling with regard to fetal risks and prenatal diagnostic options and limitations should maternal seroconversion or clinical infection later occur. A maternal-fetal medicine specialist also can provide clinical care if the patient develops a clinically complicated VZV infection (high fever, extensive vesicular lesions, or respiratory symptoms) that requires hospitalization and expert care.

CASE 2: CHICKENPOX INFECTION AT 26 WEEKS' GESTATION

A women presents to the labor and delivery unit at 26 weeks of gestation with a history of low-grade fever and malaise of "a few days." This was followed the previous day by the onset of an initially mild pruritic rash that today has rapidly progressed so that it is now covering her face, trunk, limbs, and buttocks. Directed questioning uncovers a recent exposure to a child with a rash later diagnosed as chickenpox and an absence in the patient of childhood chickenpox or VZV vaccination. Review of symptoms is positive for dyspnea with even modest exertion, a "scratchy throat," and an occasional dry, nonproductive cough. Physical examination shows the classic early chickenpox exanthem with pruritic maculopapules and evolving vesicles. The patient is normotensive but mildly tachycardic and tachypneic (heart rate 114 beats/min and respiratory rate 30 breaths/min). Her temperature is 38.6°C. The uterus is soft, the fetus is active, and pelvic examination shows no vaginal or cervical vesicles and a closed, thick, cervix.

What tests, if any, are indicated at this time?

The rash and other clinical features are virtually diagnostic, especially in this clinical setting, of chickenpox. Accordingly, unless there is something atypical or unclear about the clinical findings, serology is probably not necessary. However, because of the vague respiratory complaints, a chest radiograph is indicated and, in this patient, shows a questionable reticular pattern centrally but is otherwise clear. Because the historical, clinical, and radiographic findings suggest VZV pulmonary involvement and the potential for fulminant progression to life-threatening pneumonitis, a baseline room air arterial blood gas should be considered and in this patient shows a pH of 7.48, partial pressure of oxygen of 90 mm Hg, partial pressure of carbon dioxide of 28 mm Hg, and saturated oxygen of 94%, indicating modest hyperventilation and a small, but clinically significant, alveolar-to-arterial oxygen gradient. In view of these findings, additional pregnancy-specific complications such as preterm labor and/or fetal compromise need consideration. Accordingly, fetal assessment (external fetal monitoring with backup of biophysical profile) and tocodynamometry are obtained and are reassuring.

What are the next steps in management of this patient?

She is given a diagnosis of acute, contagious chickenpox with a high suspicion of evolving VZV pneumonia. Because of the significant potential for the development of severe maternal (with attendant fetal) complications, a maternal-fetal medicine consultation should be obtained. If this is not available, consideration should be given to transferring the mother to a tertiary center that has expert perinatal and neonatal care. The patient should be isolated from other patients and cared for only by professionals with known VZV immunity. She should be placed immediately on high-dose (10 mg/kg every 8 hours) intravenous acyclovir therapy. She and her fetus then need close observation, which may include frequent clinical assessment, continuous or frequent pulse oximetry, and serial fetal assessment, particularly if maternal condition worsens or signs or symptoms of premature labor evolve. If pulmonary symptoms worsen, or oximetry demonstrates progressive hypoxia, this patient will need intensive care (preferably in a unit near the labor and delivery area but with full isolation capability) and possibly supplemental oxygen or ventilatory support.

REFERENCES

1 Centers for Disease Control and Prevention. Prevention of varicella: recommendations of the Advisory Committee on Immunization Practices (ACIP). *MMWR* 1996;45(RR-11):1–25.

2 Goldberg JM, Ziel HK, Burchette R. Evaluation of varicella immune status in an obstetrical population in relation to place of birth. *Am J Perinatol* 2002;19:387–394.

3 Haake DA, Zakowski PC, Haake DL, et al. Early treatment of varicella pneumonia in otherwise healthy adults. *Rev Infect Dis* 1990;12: 788–792.

4 Enders G, Miller E, Cradock-Watson J, et al. Consequences of varicella and herpes zoster in pregnancy. Prospective study of 1,739 cases. *Lancet* 1994;343:1547–1550.

5 Smego RA, Asperilla MO. Use of acyclovir for varicella pneumonia during pregnancy. *Obstet Gynecol* 1991;78:1112–1116.

6 Harger JH, Ernest JM, Thurnau GR, et al. Risk factors and outcome of varicella-zoster virus pneumonia in pregnant women. *J Infect Dis* 2002;185:422–427.

7 Jones AM, Thomas N, Wilkens EG. Outcome of varicella pneumonitis in immunocompetent adults requiring treatment in a high dependency unit. *J Infect Dis* 2001;43:135–139.

8 Ogilvie MM. Antiviral prophylaxis and treatment in chickenpox. A review prepared for the UK Advisory Group on Chickenpox on behalf of the British Society of Infection. *J Infect* 1998;36:31–38.

9 Nathwani D, Maclean A, Conway S, Carrington D. Varicella infections in pregnancy and the newborn. A review prepared for the UK Advisory Group on Chickenpox on behalf of the British Society of Infection. *J Infect* 1998 36:59–71.

10 Mattson SN, Jones KL, Gramling LJ, et al. Neurodevelopmental follow-up of children of women infected with varicella during pregnancy: a prospective study. *Pediatr Infect Dis J* 2003;22: 819–823.

11 Harger JH, Ernest JM, Thurnau GR, et al. Frequency of congenital varicella syndrome in a prospective cohort of 347 pregnant women. *Obstet Gynecol* 2002;100:260–265.

12 Pastuszak AL, Levy M, Schick B, et al. Outcome after maternal varicella infection in the first 20 weeks of pregnancy. *N Engl J Med* 1994;330:901–905.

13 Mouly F, Mirlesse V, Meritet JF, et al. Prenatal diagnosis of fetal varicella-zoster virus infection with polymerase chain reaction of amniotic fluid in 107 cases. *Am J Obstet Gynecol* 1997;177: 894–898.

14 Lecuru F, Taurelle R, Bernard JP, et al. Vericella zoster virus infection during pregnancy: the limits of prenatal diagnosis. *Eur J Obstet Gynecol Reprod Biol* 1994;56:67–68.

15 Perinatal viral and parasitic infections. *ACOG Pract Bull* 2000;20.

16 Wise RP, Braun MM. Seward JF, et al. Pharmacoepidemiologic implications of erroneous varicella vaccinations in pregnancy through

confusion with varicella immune globulin. *Pharmacoepidemiol Drug Saf* 2002;11:651–654.

17 Varicella vaccine exposure during pregnancy: data from the first 5 years of the pregnancy registry. *Obstet Gynecol* 2001;98:14–19.

18 Koren G, Money D, Boucher M, et al. Serum concentrations, efficacy, and safety of a new, intravenously administered varicella zoster immune globulin in pregnant women. *J Clin Pharmacol* 2002;42: 267–274.

Screening and Diagnosis of Tuberculosis During Pregnancy

**Purified protein derivative (PPD) skin testing offered
to all at risk pregnant women when they initiate prenatal care**

- High risk factors
  - HIV positive
  - Known recent contact with TB
  - Organ transplant recipient or
    other immunocompromised
    patient (receiving equivalent
    of >15 mg/d prednisone
    for >1 mo)

- Intermediate risk factors
  - Intravenous drug use
  - Immigration from high
    prevalence area (Asia,
    Africa, Latin America
    within 5 yrs)
  - Underserved population
  - Resident of long-term care
    facility, prison, or shelter
  - Certain medical conditions
    (Table 23-1)
  - Health care worker for above
    populations

Administer 0.1 mL PPD to raise 6–10 mm intradermal wheal and

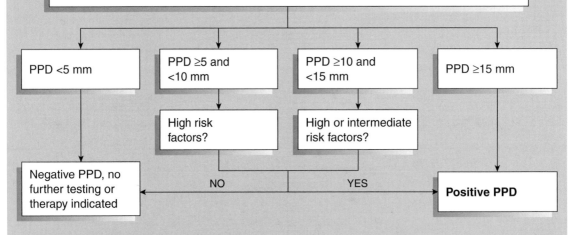

| PPD <5 mm | PPD ≥5 and <10 mm | PPD ≥10 and <15 mm | PPD ≥15 mm |

High risk factors?

High or intermediate risk factors?

Negative PPD, no further testing or therapy indicated

NO

YES

Positive PPD

23

Tuberculosis

Kim A. Boggess

Introduction

EPIDEMIOLOGY

Tuberculosis (TB) has reemerged as a serious health problem throughout the world. After years of decline after the introduction of effective chemotherapy, the incidence of TB in the United States increased significantly between 1985 and the early 1990s. In certain populations, up to 10% of women of childbearing age have positive findings on tuberculin skin test. From 1985 through 1992, reported cases of TB increased by 20%. Further, during that time, the number of TB cases in women of childbearing age increased by 40%.[1] In addition, multidrug-resistant TB is increasing, which can affect women of childbearing age.[2] The increase in TB can be attributed to a number of factors including the epidemic of human immunodeficiency virus infection (HIV), the increase in immigrants from endemic areas, and the lack of an adequate infrastructure to deal with the large increase in TB cases. Since 1992, the number of cases of TB has been decreasing. In 2001, 15,989 TB cases were reported throughout the United States. This represents a 2% decrease from 2000 and a 40% decrease from 1992. This decrease has been attributed to improvements in organized approaches to TB.

The primary strategy for preventing and controlling TB in the United States is to minimize the risk for transmission by the early identification and treatment of patients with active infectious TB.

KEY POINT

Clinicians should have a high index of suspicion for TB.

The second most important strategy is the identification of persons with latent tuberculous infection (LTI) and, if indicated, isoniazid (INH) chemoprophylaxis to prevent LTI from progressing to active infectious TB.

399

Evaluation of Positive PPD During Pregnancy

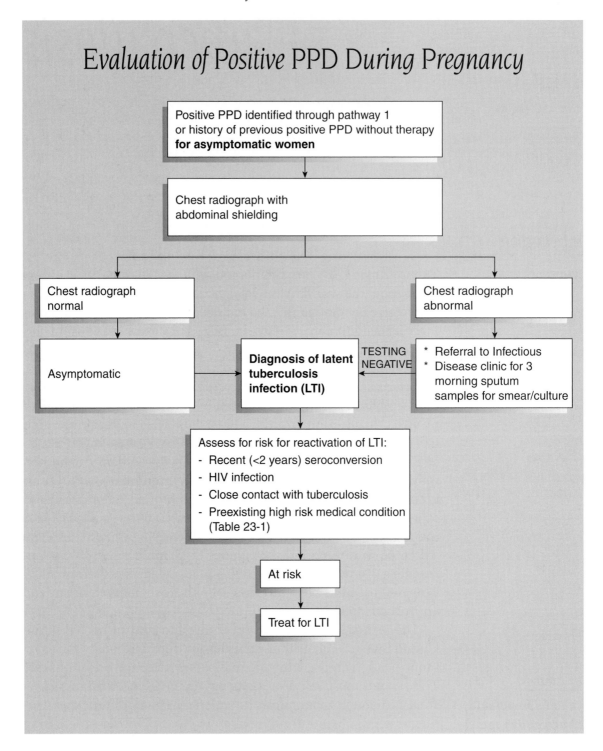

MICROBIOLOGY   TB is a chronic bacterial infection caused by *Mycobacterium tuberculosis* or *M. bovis*, which is transmitted by respiratory droplet and spread from person to person through the air. Transmission of TB is dependent on the number and/or viability of bacilli in expelled air, susceptible host factors, environment (shared air), and duration and/or frequency of exposure.[3] *Mycobacterium* possess surface lipids that render them acid fast. *Mycobacterium tuberculosis* has an immunoreactive surface that allows for survival within macrophages. Tubercular infection is characterized by primary infection in the lungs and the development of cell-mediated hypersensitivity and formation of granulomas. Extrapulmonary infection can and does occur. One of the striking characteristics of tubercular infection is the occurrence of a latency period that is followed by reactivation.[3]

CLINICAL SYMPTOMS   Primary tubercular infection may occur without symptoms and signs, may produce a typical primary complex, or may result in typical chronic pulmonary TB without a demonstrable primary complex. Early pulmonary TB is usually asymptomatic and does not produce symptoms until the bacillary population has reached a certain size. Symptoms at that point range from nonspecific constitutional symptoms such as anorexia, fatigue, weight loss, chills, afternoon fever, and, when these subside, night sweats. A productive cough is usually present, and hemoptysis can occur.[3]

Pregnancy and Tuberculosis

Before the introduction of effective treatment for pulmonary TB, there was little consensus on the potential health risk of pregnancy among infected women. Because of the prevalence and resurgence of TB, current recommendations state that all pregnant women who are at high risk for LTI or active TB should be offered purified protein derivative (PPD) skin testing. The prevalence of PPD positivity among pregnant women depends on risk factors of the population. Up to 21% of HIV-infected pregnant women have been reported to have positive results on PPD skin tests, and up to 1% have had active TB disease.[4] However, pregnancy does not appear to increase the risk for developing active TB in HIV-positive and HIV-negative women.[5]

Children born to women with active TB have increased risks of morbidity and mortality in the neonatal period, with an increase in prematurity, perinatal death, and low birth weight. Pulmonary TB and late onset of therapy increase these risks.[6]

TB can be difficult to diagnose during pregnancy. TB-related symptoms can mimic the physiologic changes that occur during pregnancy. As a consequence, pregnant women in high-risk groups and women from areas with high prevalences of HIV infection and TB should be routinely asked about contact with infectious TB patients, and tuberculin skin testing should always be considered for these women. Because prenatal or peripartum care is often the only contact many high-risk women have with the health care system, screening for TB and HIV counseling and testing should be offered at this time. Pregnancy can also delay diagnosis due to an increase in extrapulmonary presentation.[7]

Although women with TB have an excess of pregnancy complications such as miscarriage, when adequate therapy is initiated, TB appears to have no adverse effect on the pregnancy.[8] Transplacental passage of TB is extremely rare. Most perinatal infections occur when a mother with active TB handles her infant.[9] The risk of the child contracting TB from a mother with active disease during the first year of life may be as high as 50%.

KEY POINT

Screening of pregnant patients for TB should be based on consideration of risk factors.

Diagnosis

Screening for asymptomatic or symptomatic tubercular infection can be performed by administration of TB antigens and monitoring for a delayed, cell-mediated hypersensitivity response. The delayed hypersensitivity response can take up to 10 weeks after exposure to develop. Administration of PPD 0.1 mL to create a 6- to 10-mm subdermal wheal will result in different degrees of induration in an individual 48–72 hours after administration. Based on the sensitivity and specificity of PPD tuberculin skin testing and the prevalence of TB in different groups, three cutpoints have been recommended for defining a positive tuberculin skin reaction: at least 5 mm, at least 10 mm, and at least 15 mm of induration.[10,11] For persons at highest risk for developing active TB and infected with *M. tuberculosis*, induration of at least 5 mm is considered a positive result. For other persons with an increased probability of recent infection or with other clinical conditions that increase the risk for progression to active TB, induration of at least 10 mm is considered a positive result. For persons at low risk for TB, for whom tuberculin testing is not generally indicated, induration of at least 15 mm is considered a positive result (Table 23-1).

Table 23-1. **INTERPRETATION OF PURIFIED PROTEIN DERIVATIVE SKIN TEST**

REACTION ≥5 MM INDURATION	REACTION ≥10 MM INDURATION	REACTION ≥15 MM INDURATION
• HIV positive • Recent contacts of patients with TB • Fibrotic changes on chest radiograph consistent with previous TB • Patients with organ transplants and other immunosuppressed patients (receiving the equivalent of ≥15 mg/d of prednisone for ≥1 mo)	• Recent immigrants (i.e. ≤5 years) from high-prevalence countries • Intravenous drug use • Residents and employees of the following high-risk congregate settings: prisons and jails, nursing homes and other long-term care facilities, residential facilities for patients with AIDS, and homeless shelters • Mycobacteriology laboratory personnel • High-risk medical conditions: diabetes mellitus, silicosis, chronic renal failure, some hematologic disorders (e.g., leukemias and lymphomas), malignancies (lung or head and neck carcinoma), weight loss ≥10% ideal body weight, gastrectomy, and jejunoileal bypass	• Persons withno risk factor for TB

AIDS = acquired immunodeficiency syndrome; HIV = human immunodeficiency virus; TB = tuberculosis.

False-positive reactions can occur in individuals not infected with *M. tuberculosis*. These may be caused by:

1. Cross-reaction resulting from infection with mycobacteria other than TB.
2. History of bacilli Calmette-Guérin (BCG) vaccination.
3. Interpreting erythema rather than induration.

Most pregnant women diagnosed with TB are asymptomatic, and TB is detected only due to PPD screening,[12] thus emphasizing the importance of screening high-risk women. Pregnancy does not increase the risk for anergy, so an anergy panel is unnecessary in HIV-negative pregnant women.[13]

An individual may be infected with *M. tuberculosis* but have little or no reaction to skin testing. False-negative reactions in adults may be caused by:

1. Recent viral infections (rubella, mumps, influenza, measles, or chickenpox).
2. Overwhelming tubercular disease.
3. Immunosuppression due to advanced age, debility, malnutrition, or HIV infection.
4. Very recent tubercular infection.
5. Recent (≤4–6 weeks) immunization with certain live virus vaccination (measles, mumps, rubella, chickenpox, or smallpox).
6. High-dose steroids (prednisone ≥15 mg or equivalent daily for ≥1 month) and other immunosuppressive agents.
7. Improper antigen handling or storage, error in administration, or error in interpretation.

The definitive diagnosis of TB is based on identifying *M. tuberculosis* by culture or acid-fast stain of the sputum. First morning sputum specimens obtained on 3 consecutive days are usually the best source for detecting TB and should be undertaken in those at high risk for active disease; those with symptoms of active TB such as productive cough, weight loss, night sweats, fatigue, and malaise; and those with a positive PPD result and abnormal finding on chest radiograph[3] (Figure 23-1).

KEY POINT

Diagnostic criteria for latent and active TB vary with the risk factors of the individual.

TUBERCULOUS INFECTION VERSUS TUBERCULOUS DISEASE

A positive PPD result only means that the patient has been previously exposed to TB and that there are latent organisms present. Fewer than 10% of patients with a positive PPD result and an intact immune system will progress to active disease. However, targeted tuberculin skin testing for LTI is a strategic component of TB control that identifies persons at high risk for developing TB who would benefit by treatment of LTI. Persons with increased risk for developing active TB include those who have recent infection with *M. tuberculosis* and those who have clinical conditions that are associated with an increased risk for progression of LTI to active TB[14] (Table 23-2). Infected persons who are at high risk for developing active TB disease should be offered therapy for LTI irrespective of age.

Figure 23-1: Radiograph of an individual with cavitary tuberculosis (Courtesy of William C. Black, MD.).

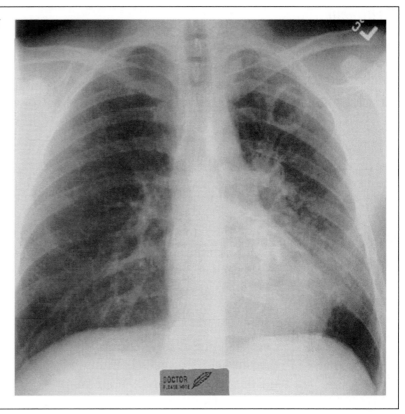

Table 23-2. TUBERCULOSIS CASE RATE BY RISK FACTOR

Risk Factor	*TB Cases/1000 Person-Years*
Recent TB infection	
Infection ≤1 year	12.9
Infection ≤1–7 years	1.6
HIV	35.0–162
Injection drug use	
HIV seropositive	76.0
HIV seronegative or unknown	10.0
Silicosis	68
Radiographic findings consistent with previous TB	2.0–13.6
Weight deviation from standard	
Underweight by ≥15%	2.6

HIV = human immunodeficiency virus; TB = tuberculosis.

Treatment

TUBERCULOUS DISEASE   Untreated TB in pregnancy poses a significant threat to the mother, fetus, and family. Adherence to therapy during pregnancy is difficult because of concern regarding fetal toxicity and pregnancy-related nausea. The Advisory Council for the Elimination of Tuberculosis recommends initial treatment for nonpregnant patients with four drugs: INH, rifampin, pyrazinamide, and ethambutol or streptomycin. All four first-line anti-TB drugs have an excellent safety record and are not believed to be associated with human fetal malformations. For pregnant women, streptomycin should be avoided because it may cause congenital ototoxicity.[11,15]

KEY POINT

Individuals with suspected active TB disease should be managed on a multidrug regimen with the guidance of a specialist in infectious diseases.

Toxicity to anti-TB medication is a concern. INH-induced hepatitis is a risk not limited to pregnancy but has been suggested as more prevalent among pregnant and immediately postpartum women.[16] Maternal side effects of anti-TB agents are listed in Table 23-3.[11]

The first 8 weeks of treatment of adults with pulmonary TB is intended to rapidly decrease the number of tubercle bacilli in the body and usually consists of four-drug therapy. The continuation phase of 16 weeks is intended to eliminate the smaller number of organisms that persist. If treatment is not continued long enough, some bacilli may survive and cause active disease later. In pregnant women, the preferred initial treatment is INH, rifampin, and ethambutol.

LATENT TUBERCULOUS INFECTION   Individuals with LTI who are at high risk for progression to TB disease should be given high priority for control of LTI regardless of age.[10] INH 300 mg daily for 9 months is the preferred regimen for

Table 23-3.   **SIDE EFFECTS OF ANTITUBERCULOUS AGENTS**

AGENT	MATERNAL SIDE EFFECTS
Isoniazid	Hepatitis, peripheral neuropathy (prevented with pyridoxine)
Ethambutol	Optic neuritis
Rifampin	Orange discoloration of body secretions, gastrointestinal upset, liver toxicity
Pyrazinamide	Hepatitis, hyperuricemia
Streptomycin	Cranial nerve VIII toxicity, nephrotoxicity

control of LTI. Nine months of therapy offers the highest degree of protection against the progression of LTI to TB disease. Approximately 90% of those who complete a full 9-month course of INH will be protected against progression compared with 70% who complete 6 months.[11] Preventive therapy with INH can be undertaken safely in pregnancy. INH for LTI is contraindicated for those with active hepatitis or end-stage liver disease. Rifampin plus pyrazinamide was previously recommended for management of LTI if an individual had close contact to INH-resistant, rifampin-sensitive TB, side effects to INH, or compliance with 6–9 months of therapy was unlikely. This drug combination is currently prohibited for management of LTI due to liver injury.[17] A 4-month course of daily rifampin is a reasonable alternative.[10] Before starting rifampin, baseline complete blood cell counts and liver function tests should be obtained and repeated if there is evidence of an adverse reaction.

KEY POINT

The decision to administer INH prophylaxis during pregnancy or the postpartum period should be made after careful consideration of the risks and benefits of such therapy.

Asymptomatic pregnant women with a negative finding on chest radiograph should start INH preventive therapy as soon as possible if they have one of the following factors:

1. HIV infection.
2. Close contact to infectious TB disease.
3. Recent (≤2 years) skin test conversion.
4. High-risk medical conditions.

Asymptomatic women with a negative finding on chest radiograph and no risk factors may elect to delay therapy until after delivery.

Pyridoxine (B$_6$) 50 mg daily should be administered with INH because of the increased risk of peripheral neuropathy in pregnancy. INH, although present in small amounts in the breast milk, is not contraindicated in women who breast feed. Breast-feeding infants whose mothers are taking INH should be given pyridoxine (1 mg/kg) daily as a supplement.

Before initiating INH prophylaxis, a baseline aspartate aminotransferase (AST) level should be obtained for pregnant women and women within 3 months of delivery. If the baseline AST level is at least three times the upper limit of normal, consideration of risk versus benefit to management of LTI should be made.[11] All pregnant and postpartum patients should be assessed monthly for adverse reactions to INH and have an AST performed.

Therapy should be stopped if signs and symptoms of hepato-toxicity are present or if AST is five times higher than the upper limit of normal.[11]

WHAT TO DO IF ...

1. A patient reports history of BCG vaccination.

Because most persons who have received BCG are from high-prevalence areas, and BCG vaccination protection is inconsistent and wanes with time, persons who test positive by skin testing should be evaluated and managed accordingly regardless of history of BCG vaccination.

2. A patient reports a previous positive finding with PPD (>2 years ago) but did not receive therapy.

Individuals with inadequate or untreated previous TB should have a chest radiograph performed. Those with chest radiographic findings suggestive of fibrotic lesions thought to represent previous TB should be treated for LTI after active TB has been ruled out. Treatment options during pregnancy include INH for 6–9 months. Those with chest radiographic findings suggestive of healed primary TB are not at increase risk for active TB disease.

3. A patient reports symptoms suggestive of TB (cough, fever, malaise, weight loss, night sweats, and hemoptysis).

Obtain chest radiograph and then refer the patient to an infectious disease clinic for three morning sputum samples for acid-fast smear, mycobacteria culture, and evaluation for extrapulmonary TB.

What's the Evidence

Most of the data about treatment of tuberculosis comes from studies in nonpregnant individuals. Retrospective data are used to evaluate the effect of the illness and treatment on maternal and perinatal outcomes. Some small studies address specific issues of treatment of pregnant women.[2,16]

Guiding Questions in Approaching the Patient

What is the patient's risk for active or latent TB?

- High-risk factors
  - Immigrant from a high-prevalence area

- Contact with an individual with known TB infection
- HIV positive
- Immunocompromised
- Intermediate-risk factors
  - Immigrant from a high-prevalence area
  - Underserved population
  - Resident of a prison or other long-term facility
  - Intravenous drug use
  - High-risk medical conditions
  - Health care worker for intermediate- and high-risk populations

How to determine who should receive therapy for LTI

- Assess risk for reactivation
  - Recent (<2 years) seroconversion
  - HIV positive
  - Close contact with a TB-infected individual
  - High-risk medical condition
- Assess risk for INH prophylaxis
  - Alcohol use, i.e., more than three drinks per day
  - Current hepatitis
  - High baseline levels of AST
  - Other comorbidities or contraindications to therapy
    - Active hepatitis
    - End-stage liver or kidney disease
    - Alcoholism
    - Potential adverse drug interactions
    - Peripheral neuropathy

Conclusion

Tuberculosis continues to be an international disease with prevalence determined by the impacts of immigration, HIV disease, adequacy of public health infrastructure and socioeconomic issues. Unfortunately, there is an increasing prevalence of multi-drug resistant tuberculosis complicating the success of treatment. All pregnant women at risk for latent or active tuberculosis should receive PPD skin testing. Pregnancy does not seem to increase the conversion to active tuberculosis, but women with active tuberculosis have a greater risk of adverse perinatal outcome. Without treatment children of women with tuberculosis are at great risk of developing tuberculosis. Individuals with latent tuberculosis infection at high risk for development of active disease should receive treatment. Treatment of women with active tuberculosis should be guided by an expert in Infectious Diseases.

Discussion of Cases

CASE 1: HEALTH RECENT IMMIGRANT WOMAN

A 30-year-old Hispanic women who immigrated to the United States 3 years previously presents for care at 14 weeks of gestation. A screening PPD at 48 hours shows 10-mm induration. She is otherwise healthy, with no contraindications to therapy and no reported recent exposure to an individual with TB. She also reports no previous knowledge of ever having a skin test performed.

What testing, if any, would you recommend at this point?

Chest radiograph with posteroanterior view and abdominal shielding.

If the chest radiograph is interpreted as negative for evidence of latent or active TB, does she require any further testing?

No, further testing is not recommended.

What is your recommendation for management of her LTI and when would you initiate therapy?

Prophylaxis with INH 300 mg/day for 9 months to be initiated during pregnancy if high risk for reactivation is present (<2 years for seroconversion, known exposure to TB, HIV positive, high-risk medical conditions) or postpartum if not at high risk for reactivation.

What are complications of INH therapy and how might they be avoided or managed?

Risk for INH-induced hepatotoxicity can be screened for by assessing this patient's risk of liver damage (alcohol use with more than three drinks per day, current hepatitis, or high baseline level of AST) and close surveillance for evidence of liver damage (AST determination monthly with discontinuation if levels are five times higher than the normal limit). INH-associated peripheral neuropathy in the mother and breast-feeding newborn can be avoided by supplementation with pyridoxine (B$_6$) 50 mg/day.

REFERENCES

1 Cantwell MF, Snider DE Jr, Cauthen GM, Onorato IM. Epidemiology of tuberculosis in the United States, 1985 through 1992. *JAMA* 1994; 272:535–539.

2 Shin S, Guerra D, Rich M, et al. Treatment of multidrug-resistant tuberculosis during pregnancy: a report of 7 cases. *Clin Infect Dis* 2003;36:996–1003.

3 Haas D, Des Prez R. Mycobacterium tuberculosis. In: Mandell G, Bennett J, Dolin R, eds. *Principles and Practices of Infectious Diseases, Volume 2.* New York: Churchill Livingstone, 1995.

4 Schulte JM, Bryan P, Dodds S, et al. Tuberculosis skin testing among HIV-infected pregnant women in Miami, 1995 to 1996. *J Perinatol* 2002;22:159–162.

5 Espinal MA, Reingold AL, Lavandera M. Effect of pregnancy on the risk of developing active tuberculosis. *J Infect Dis* 1996;173:488–491.

6 Figueroa-Damian R, Arredondo-Garcia JL. Neonatal outcome of children born to women with tuberculosis. *Arch Med Res* 2001;32:66–69.

7 Llewelyn M, Cropley I, Wilkinson RJ, Davidson RN. Tuberculosis diagnosed during pregnancy: a prospective study from London. *Thorax* 2000;55:129–132.

8 Maccato ML. Pneumonia and pulmonary tuberculosis in pregnancy. *Obstet Gynecol Clin North Am* 1989;16:417–430.

9 Perinatal prophylaxis of tuberculosis. *Lancet* 1990;336:1479–1480.

10 Jasmer RM, Nahid P, Hopewell PC. Latent tuberculosis infection. *N Eng J Med* 2002;347:1860–1866.

11 Centers for Disease Control. Treatment of tuberculosis. *MMWR* 2003;52(RR-11);1–77.

12 Carter EJ, Mates S. Tuberculosis during pregnancy. The Rhode Island experience, 1987 to 1991. *Chest* 1994;106:1466–1470.

13 Jackson TD, Murtha AP. Anergy during pregnancy. *Am J Obstet Gynecol* 2001;184:1090–1092.

14 Centers for Disease Control. Tuberculosis morbidity—United States, 1993. *MMWR* 1994;43:361–366.

15 Advisory Council for the Elimination of Tuberculosis. Tuberculosis elimination revisited: obstacles, opportunities, and a renewed commitment. *MMWR* 1999;48:1–13.

16 Franks AL, Binkin NJ, Snider DE Jr, et al. Isoniazid hepatitis among pregnant and postpartum Hispanic patients. *Public Health Reports* 1989;104:151–155.

17 Centers for Disease Control. Update: adverse event data and revised American Thoracic Society/CDC recommendations against the use of rifampin and pyrazinamide for treatment of latent tuberculosis infection—United States. *MMWR* 2003;52(31):735–739.

Gonorrhea Management in Pregnancy

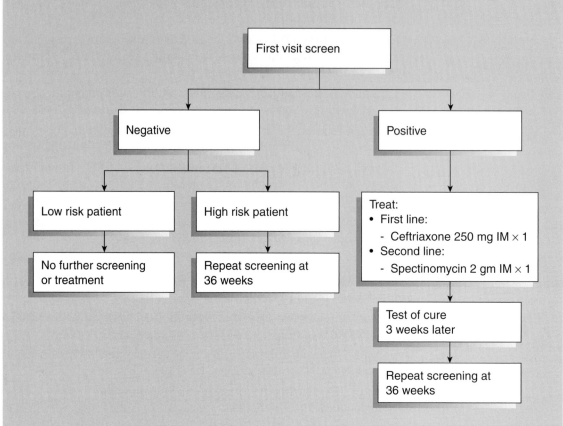

24 Gonorrhea and Chlamydia

David Chelmow

Introduction

INCIDENCE

KEY POINT

Gonorrhea and chlamydia are not uncommon.

Neisseria gonorrhea and *Chlamydia trachomatis* are sexually transmitted infections frequently encountered in pregnancy. In 2001, the Centers for Disease Control and Prevention (CDC) noted positive chlamydia assays in 7.4% (range 3.7–13.5%) of women ages 15–24 years prenatal clinics in 22 states in the United States.[1] Gonorrhea was less frequent, occurring in 0.9% (range 0.0–4.3%). These figures have been fairly stable, with a slight increase in chlamydia and slight decrease in gonorrhea since 1999.

MORBIDITY IN PREGNANCY

KEY POINT

Untreated gonorrhea and chlamydia can cause significant morbidity in pregnancy.

Gonorrhea and chlamydia are associated with significant maternal and neonatal morbidity. In early pregnancy, patients with a history of gonorrhea, chlamydia, or pelvic inflammatory disease are at greatly increased risk of ectopic pregnancy. Therefore, ectopic pregnancy must be ruled out in any patient with a history of these infections. Patients with gonorrheal or chlamydial cervicitis are also at increased risk for postabortal endometritis.

In later pregnancy, infection has the potential for maternal and neonatal morbidity. In the mother, untreated gonorrheal cervicitis has been associated with increased incidences of premature rupture of membranes (PROM), preterm delivery, chorioamnionitis, and postpartum endometritis.[2] Similarly, several studies have suggested that patients with chlamydia are at increased risk for PROM, preterm delivery, and intrauterine growth restriction. It has clearly been associated with postpartum endometritis.[2]

Chlamydia Management in Pregnancy

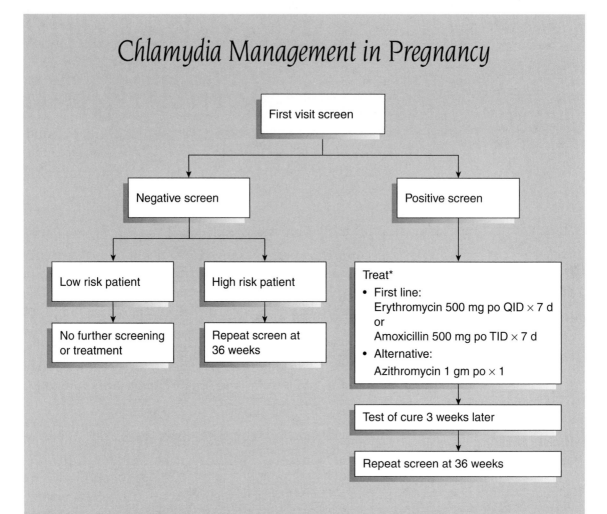

Both infections have the potential for significant neonatal morbidity. In addition to the consequences of prematurity related to the increased risk of PROM and preterm delivery, neonates born to mothers infected with gonorrhea are at increased risk of gonococcal ophthalmia neonatorum. They are also at risk for disseminated infection. Infants born to mothers with chlamydia are also at significant risk. Twenty percent to 50% will develop conjunctivitis in the first 2 weeks of life, and 10–20% will develop pneumonia in the first 3–4 months.[2]

WHAT'S THE EVIDENCE? Evidence for these morbidities comes from level 3 retrospective studies that have been well summarized by Sweet and Gibbs.[2] For gonorrhea, the evidence is from previous studies of women with untreated gonorrhea. Risk of preterm delivery and PROM persisted in one study despite treatment, suggesting that these risks may be associative and not causal. The link between untreated cervical gonorrhea and neonatal ocular infection is clearly causal. Because of the public health implications of these infections and the need to prevent neonatal ocular infection, there will never be randomized trials to adequately establish the benefit of gonorrheal management on other pregnancy outcomes.

For chlamydia, Sweet and Gibbs extensively reviewed a large number of retrospective studies that convincingly demonstrated the risks of neonatal infection and adverse pregnancy outcome in infected patients.[2] The causal relation is further strengthened by two previous nonrandomized studies. Cohen and coworkers compared women who had controlled chlamydia with patients whose treatment failed and patients who had negative cultures and noted that patients whose treatment failed had significantly higher risks of PROM and small-for-gestational-age infants, whereas the risk in the treated patients did not differ from that in uninfected patients.[3] Ryan and associates noted increased risks of PROM, low birth weight, and decreasing neonatal survival when untreated patients were compared with treated patients or uninfected controls.[4] Because of the proven links between gonorrheal and chlamydial cervicitis and neonatal infection, and the public health implications of these organisms, it is extremely unlikely that a randomized trial will ever be performed to fully delineate the role of screening and treatment in preventing adverse pregnancy outcome.

Screening

KEY POINT

Risk assessment is important in all pregnancies.

KEY POINT

All pregnancies should be routinely screened for gonorrhea and chlamydia.

KEY POINT

Screening for gonorrhea and chlamydia should be repeated in later pregnancy in high-risk patients.

The potential consequences of chlamydia and gonorrhea in pregnancy are significant enough that current recommendations address the screening of all women in pregnancy.[5] Particularly for chlamydia, even low-risk, nonpregnant populations of reproductive age often have low but not negligible (1–2%) rates of infection.

According to current (2002) recommendations by the CDC, all women should be screened for chlamydia at their first prenatal visit.[5] These same recommendations suggest that gonorrheal screening can be reserved for patients at risk (criteria not specified) or living in an area of high prevalence. Nonetheless, many providers routinely screen for both organisms at the first prenatal visit. Decisions about repeat screening are based on the provider's assessment of the patient's risk status. For low-risk patients whose screen at the first visit is negative, a single screen is adequate.

The 2002 guidelines of the CDC recommend screening for chlamydia and gonorrhea at the first prenatal visit, with a repeat screen in the third trimester.[5] Their rationale is to decrease the potential adverse sequelae of these organisms on the course of the pregnancy and to prevent maternal to neonatal transmission. The guidelines are vague about the optimal timing in the third trimester for repeat screening and criteria for defining high risk. Repeating the screening at 35–37 weeks of gestation seems a reasonable approach because it allows the results to be obtained before the onset of labor for most patients and allows minimal time after performing the assay for the acquisition of new infection. Further, it can be performed at the same time as the currently recommended culture for group B streptococcus.[6]

The CDC guidelines specifically state that women younger than 25 years or who have new or multiple sexual partners are at high risk for chlamydia and merit screening. The U.S. Preventative Services Task Force presents more detailed risk factors[7] (Table 24-1). However, it notes that an individual's risk depends on the number of risk factors and the local prevalence of infection. Clinics with high baseline prevalence of either infection can consider routine screening of all patients.

WHAT'S THE EVIDENCE?   Nelson and Helfand presented data on which the U.S. Preventative Services Task Force based their

Table 24-1. U.S. PREVENTATIVE SERVICES TASK FORCE RISK FACTORS FOR *CHLAMYDIA TRACHOMATIS*[a]

Woman with previous sexually transmitted diseases
New or multiple sex partners
Age ≤25 years
Inconsistent use of barrier contraceptives
Unmarried
African American
Cervical ectopy

[a]The task force has noted that age is the strongest predictor and that risk depends on the number of risk factors and the local prevalence of disease.
SOURCE: U.S. Preventive Services Task Force Screening for Chlamydial Infection. Recommendations and rationale. *Am J Prev Med* 2001;20(3S):90–94.

recommendations for chlamydial screening in pregnancy.[8] Their review included the reports by Ryan and colleagues[4] and Cohen and asssociates[3] that noted improved pregnancy outcomes after screening for and controlling chlamydia. No similar data exist for gonorrhea. The U.S. Preventative Services Task Force found no evidence for the appropriate screening period. First-trimester screening has theoretical advantages for improving pregnancy outcome, whereas third-trimester screening has theoretical advantages for decreasing neonatal infection. The rationale for the CDC recommendations, although not explicitly stated, likely derived from attempting to balance the clear advantages of treating chlamydia with the probable similar benefits of controlling gonorrhea. Their recommendations about timing of screening attempt to optimize prevention of adverse pregnancy outcome and neonatal infection and to minimize cost by avoiding repeat screening of low-risk women.

SCREENING METHODS   There are several screening methods for gonorrhea and chlamydia. For gonorrhea, culture on Thayer-Martin agar (predominantly lysed blood) is very reliable and has the benefit of allowing the monitoring of antibiotic resistance. Culture needs to be done in an appropriate carbon dioxide atmosphere, and the yield is improved by ensuring that specimens are transported in a high level of carbon dioxide.

Chlamydia testing is more problematic. It can be cultured, but testing requires tissue because *Chlamydia* is an intracellular organism. This is cumbersome, needs to be done in special laboratories, and is not the method of choice. Nonculture detection methods are normally used. This can be done by enzyme-linked immunosorbent assay, direct fluorescent antibody (DFA), or polymerase chain reaction. Early enzyme-linked immunosorbent assay and DFA, although moderately sensitive and specific (>95%), produced a significant number of false-positive results when low-risk populations were screened. The advent of polymerase chain reaction tests with improved specificity has minimized this problem. Similar tests are available for gonorrhea, and because they can be performed on the same swab as the chlamydial test, these swabs are often sent instead of culture for convenience. These tests are sensitive enough that, if repeat testing is performed, it should be delayed at least 3 weeks because residual DNA from the treated organisms can cause false-positive results.

WHAT'S THE EVIDENCE? Nelson and Helfand addressed screening techniques in their systemic review.[8] They reviewed 33 studies of nonpregnant patients and concluded that DNA amplification tests have better sensitivity and specificity than do antigen detection tests and have better sensitivity than does culture. They found no difference between DNA amplification urine tests and specimens obtained by endocervical swab. They also reviewed the much smaller group of studies (four in all) performed in pregnant women. These studies suggested that antigen detection and DNA amplification techniques have better sensitivity than do culture techniques. It seems reasonable to assume that the screening tests would behave similarly in pregnant and nonpregnant women, and that the results in nonpregnant women can be extended to those in pregnant women.

Treatment

GONORRHEA

Antibiotic resistance has become a major problem in the management of gonorrhea. Current recommendations balance cost, resistance patterns, ease of administration, and safety in pregnancy. Ceftriaxone, the first-line therapy for nonpregnant patients, is safe in pregnancy and is first-line therapy for pregnant patients. Cervicitis can be treated with a single injection of 125 mg intramuscularly. Larger doses are required for pharyngeal infection,

KEY POINT

Evidence-based treatment recommendations exist and should be followed for antibiotic therapy for gonorrhea and chlamydia in pregnancy.

proctitis, or disseminated gonorrhea. Quinolones, the other first-line therapy in nonpregnant patients, is discouraged in pregnancy because of concern regarding cartilage abnormalities when administered to pregnant canines. If a separate test for chlamydia was not performed at the time of the gonorrheal assay, consideration should be given to presumptive management of chlamydia because of a high incidence of coinfection. All infants should be administered silver nitrate or antibiotic ocular ointment to decrease the risk of gonococcal ophthalmia.

WHAT'S THE EVIDENCE? The use of ceftriaxone and spectinomycin to eradicate gonorrhea in nonpregnant men and women is well established.[9] Brocklehurst reviewed gonorrhea management in pregnancy and found two trials that compared antibiotic therapies in pregnancy.[10] These trials assessed 346 patients and noted nonsignificant differences in microbiologic cure rate between amoxicillin plus probenecid and ceftriaxone or spectinomycin or between ceftriaxone and cefixime.

CHLAMYDIA

Several agents effective against chlamydia are safe in pregnancy (Table 24-2). Of note, doxycycline and ofloxacin, two first-line agents for nonpregnant patients, should not be used in pregnancy.

Table 24-2. **RECOMMENDED REGIMENS FOR TREATMENT OF *CHLAMYDIA* IN PREGNANCY ACCORDING TO THE CENTERS FOR DISEASE CONTROL AND PREVENTION**

Erythromycin base 500 mg orally 4 times daily for 7 days
or
Amoxicillin 500 mg orally 3 times daily for 7 days

Alternative regimens
Erythromycin base 250 mg orally 4 times daily for 14 days
or
Erythromycin ethylsuccinate 800 mg orally 4 times daily for 7 days
or
Erythromycin ethylsuccinate 400 mg orally 4 times daily for 14 days
or
Azithromycin 1 g orally, single dose

SOURCE: Centers for Disease Control and Prevention. *Sexually Transmitted Disease Surveillance, 2001.* Atlanta: U.S. Department of Health and Human Services, 2002.

The CDC recommends erythromycin and amoxicillin as first-line agents during pregnancy.[5] Both require week-long courses and can cause extensive gastrointestinal upset in women already coping with morning sickness in pregnancy. A newer agent, azithromycin, is extremely effective against chlamydia, can be administered as a single oral dose, and has a growing body of trials supporting its safety and effectiveness in pregnancy.[11,12] Kacmar and colleagues compared azithromycin with amoxicillin and observed more gastrointestinal upset but better compliance with azithromycin.[13] Despite its higher costs, many providers use azithromycin as a first-line agent because of its greater effectiveness and higher rate of compliance.

What's the Evidence? Brocklehurst and Moody reviewed chlamydia management in pregnancy and concluded that amoxicillin has a cure rate similar to that of erythromycin and is better tolerated.[14] They also concluded that clindamycin and azithromycin appear to be effective, although the number of patients studied with these drugs was smaller.

OTHER CONSIDERATIONS

Sexual partners of all pregnant patients treated for gonorrhea or chlamydia should receive therapy. Treatment should be given according to CDC recommendations, and the obstetrician should consider administering the treatment to avoid the delay inherent in referring the partner (or partners) to a primary care provider. A careful history should be taken because more than one other partner may be involved and recurrence is likely if all partners are not treated.

Any patient treated for sexually transmitted disease (STD) needs education on the nature of STDs and protection against them. Patients may view condoms as protection against pregnancy and therefore unnecessary if already pregnant. Patients at risk should be counseled to be abstinent or to use condoms to prevent the acquisition of infection during pregnancy. Patients should be routinely screened for hepatitis B and syphilis and offered testing for the human immunodeficiency virus (HIV). Patients who previously declined HIV testing but are diagnosed with other STDs should be offered testing again.

The role of screening for hepatitis C in pregnant patients is not routinely recommended but is reasonable. Patients who acquire STDs in pregnancy should be rescreened for other STDs later in the pregnancy.

Patients diagnosed with gonorrhea or chlamydia in pregnancy should have a test of cure performed. This is particularly important in pregnancy because of the potential consequences of undiagnosed reinfection, the risk of reinfection, and the decreased effectiveness of some of the agents recommended in pregnancy, in particular erythromycin and amoxicillin for chlamydia. If ligase chain reaction testing is performed, the test of cure should be delayed at least 3 weeks after the completion of treatment to avoid false-positive results. Patients at high risk or whose chlamydia or gonorrhea was previously diagnosed in pregnancy should be rescreened at 35–37 weeks to diagnose reinfection in time to prevent neonatal infection at birth. High-risk patients should also be rescreened for syphilis and HIV.

As in nonpregnant patients, there are several instances when it would be reasonable to consider presumptive treatment in the absence of specific diagnostic test results. Patients with obvious mucopurulent cervicitis should be treated, particularly if they might not return for follow-up. Patients with a known exposure (i.e., a partner diagnosed and treated) should be similarly treated. Patients who are victims of sexual assault should receive postexposure prophylaxis to prevent infection.

Guiding Questions in Approaching the Patient

Screening

- Does the patient have a history of sexually transmitted disease?
- Does she have other risk factors?
- What is her gestational age?

Treatment

- Is the chlamydia or gonorrhea test positive?
- Does she have any drug allergies?
- Is there any question of poor compliance?
- Can her partner(s) be treated?

Discussion of Cases

A 26-year-old gravida 1 woman presents for her first prenatal visit 9 weeks after her last menstrual period. She has never had surgery and denies any medical problems. She takes only a prenatal vitamin and is allergic to penicillin. She is married and monogamous. She has had one previous sexual partner. She denies any vaginal discharge or bleeding. She denies any history of sexually transmitted infections. Her physical examination is unremarkable. Her pelvic examination shows no lesions on her vulva. Vaginal discharge is minimal and whitish but overall unremarkable. Her cervix is mildly purple and nulliparous. There is no evidence of mucopurulent cervicitis. The size of her uterus is consistent with her gestational age.

What screening for gonorrhea and chlamydia would you recommend at this time?

By age and history, she appears to be at quite low risk for sexually transmitted infection. According to current CDC guidelines, testing for chlamydia is recommended. Many providers also routinely test for gonorrhea.

You perform a ligase chain reaction test for chlamydia, which comes back positive. What other testing would you now recommend?

She should be screened for gonorrhea. Presumably, she was tested for syphilis, hepatitis B surface antigen, and offered HIV testing at her first prenatal visit. If she declined HIV testing, it should be offered again. Despite the high specificity of this test, false-positive results can occur, particularly in low-risk populations. You referred her partner to his primary care

physician who performed a urethral swab, which was also positive.

Her other test results are normal. What is the appropriate treatment?

The partner was treated with doxycycline 100 mg orally twice daily by his primary physician. You review the two CDC first-line options, amoxicillin and erythromycin. Because the patient is allergic to penicillin, you prescribe erythromycin 500 mg orally twice daily for 7 days.

You see her in the emergency room 2 days later. She has been trying to take the medicine as directed, but her morning sickness, previously tolerable, is now making it impossible for her to keep food or liquid down.

What alternatives are available?

You give her azithromycin 1 g orally as a single dose after successfully controlling her hyperemesis with intravenous hydration and antiemetics. Because of your concern about her hyperemesis, you give her a Compazine suppository 1 hour before the dose of antibiotic.

What counseling should be provided to the patient?

The patient and her partner need to be counseled on sexually transmitted infection and their prevention. If they are at continued risk, they should be counseled to use condoms. This couple had other partners before getting married but have been monogamous since their wedding. They feel certain that this infection

came from one of their previous partners, and they should not be further at risk.

What further testing should be performed?

You perform a test of cure 4 weeks after antibiotic administration. You deliberately wait at least 3 weeks to avoid false-positive results from residual DNA. The test comes back negative.

Is any further testing necessary?

She now has a history of sexually transmitted infection and should be followed as a high-risk patient. Because history may be unreliable, you are concerned about the possibility of reinfection and need to prevent the chance of maternal to fetal transmission. You repeat her gonorrhea and chlamydia assays at 36 weeks, when you also do her group B strep culture. Both come back negative.

CASE 2: TEEN WITH LATE PRENATAL CARE

A 17-year-old gravida 2, early abortion 1 woman presents for her first prenatal visit. She is unsure of the date of her last menstrual period. She came to your office 1 month after she noted fetal movement. She denies any medical problems and has never had surgery or been hospitalized. She is allergic to penicillin and is currently taking no medicines. She smokes one pack of cigarettes per day. She trades sex for cocaine and is unsure how many partners she has had. She denies a history of sexually transmitted infection but has never been tested. She uses condoms but irregularly.

Physical examination shows that she is healthy and visibly pregnant. No adenopathy is palpable. Fundal height is 24 cm, the vulva has no lesion, and the vagina is unremarkable. The cervix is nulliparous, is coated with purulent discharge, and bleeds easily when attempting to obtain a Papanicolaou's smear.

Specifically with regard to the risk of gonorrhea or chlamydia, what testing should be performed?

This patient is clearly at high risk for all sexually transmitted infections and should be screened for gonorrhea and chlamydia. She should also have a hepatitis B surface antigen, rapid plasma reagin (RPR), and have HIV testing recommended. Because the patient is at extremely high risk, her examination was consistent with mucopurulent cervicitis, and the significant risk that she may be difficult to contact with results or may not return, she should be presumptively treated for mucopurulent cervicitis. Because of concerns about compliance, your preference would be to give single-dose treatment. You give her azithromycin 1 g orally as a single dose to cover chlamydia. You question her about her penicillin allergy in an effort to determine whether you can give your preferred first-line gonorrhea therapy, intramuscular ceftriaxone. She has reported a history of "throat swelling" with ampicillin use, and you decide that spectinomycin, the second-line agent, would be more appropriate. Unfortunately, you use this rarely and must order it. Because of the many other issues that need to be addressed, you ask her to return in 48 hours, at which time you will have the results of her testing and the antibiotic to administer, if necessary.

Before she leaves your office, what risks of gonorrhea and cervicitis during pregnancy do you explain to her, and what other counseling do you provide?

You explain at length the nature of sexually transmitted infections. You strongly advocate condoms for protection because the patient is unlikely to be abstinent and her partners are unlikely to be treated. Specific to gonorrhea and chlamydia, you explain your concerns that active cervicitis may make her more likely to become infected with HIV. You explain that infection places the pregnancy at risk for preterm delivery, PROM, chorioamnionitis, and postpartum endometritis. You tell her the infant is more at risk for serious eye infection and pneumonia.

She returns as directed. Test results are positive for gonorrhea and chlamydia. Fortunately, the remainder of the STD screen was negative.

What treatment is appropriate at this point?

You have already provided therapy for chlamydia. You administer spectinomycin 2 g intramuscularly to treat the gonorrhea. You repeat your counseling regarding sexually transmitted infection and its prevention.

What further testing is necessary?

You schedule her to return in 3 weeks for a test of cure. Compliance should not be an issue because the medications were administered in your office, but you are very concerned about reinfection.

The test results were negative for gonorrhea and chlamydia assays were negative.

Is any further testing necessary?

This patient is at extraordinarily high risk. At the very least, you would like to rescreen her at 35–37 weeks. Because of her risk, you would like to do an additional screen between now and then.

Unfortunately, the patient is noncompliant with her prenatal care. You do not see her again until she presents at 34 weeks of gestation with ruptured membranes and fever.

How does her history of gonorrhea and chlamydia alter her management?

She clearly has chorioamnionitis and needs to be delivered. Assays for gonorrhea and chlamydia were performed at admission, but results will not be available until 2 days after delivery. Due to her fever, she needs antibiotic coverage for probable chorioamnionitis. Clindamycin and gentamicin intravenously would be a reasonable combination to provide coverage for group B *Streptococcus* in a penicillin-allergic patient, gram-negative neonatal pathogens, and gonorrhea and chlamydia (gentamicin in intravenous doses covers gonorrhea, and clindamycin is a useful second-line agent for chlamydia). These agents would also be excellent coverage for postpartum endometritis, for which this patient is at high risk. The infant should have antibiotic ocular ointment administered, and concerns regarding possible infection should be conveyed to the pediatrician.

REFERENCES

1 Centers for Disease Control and Prevention. *Sexually Transmitted Disease Surveillance, 2001*. Atlanta: U.S. Department of Health and Human Services, 2002.

2 Sweet RL, Gibbs RS. *Infectious Diseases of the Female Genital Tract*. Philadelphia: Lippincott Williams & Wilkins, 2002; p. 126.

3 Cohen I, Veille JC, Calkins BM. Improved pregnancy outcome following successful treatment of chlamydial infection. *JAMA* 1990; 263:3160–3168.

4 Ryan GM Jr, Abdella TN, McNeeley SG, et al. *Chlamydia trachomatis* infection in pregnancy and effect of treatment on outcome. *Am J Obstet Gynecol* 1990;162:34–39.

5 Centers for Disease Control and Prevention. Sexually transmitted diseases treatment guidelines 2002. *MMWR* 2002;51(RR-6).

6 ACOG Committee on Obstetric Practice. Prevention of early-onset group B streptococcal disease in newborns. ACOG Committee Opinion No. 279. American College of Obstetricians and Gynecologists. *Obstet Gynecol* 2002;100:1405–1412.

7 U.S. Preventive Services Task Force Screening for Chlamydial Infection. Recommendations and rationale. *Am J Prev Med* 2001; 20(3S):90–94.

8 Nelson HD, Helfand M. Screening for chlamydial infection. *Am J Prev Med* 2001;20(3S):95–107.

9 Moran JS, Levine WC. Drugs of choice for the treatment of uncomplicated gonococcal infections. *Clin Infect Dis* 1995;20(suppl 1): S47–S65.

10 Brocklehurst P. Antibiotics for gonorrhoea in pregnancy. Cochrane Database Syst Rev 2002;4.

11 Adair CD, Gunter M, Stovall TG, et al. *Chlamydia* in pregnancy: a randomized trial of azithromycin and erythromycin. *Obstet Gynecol* 1998;91:165–168.

12 Wehbeh HA, Ruggeirio RM, Shakem S, et al. Single dose azithromycin for *Chlamydia* in pregnant women. *J Reprod Med* 1998;43:509–514.

13 Kacmar J, Cheh E, Montagno A, Peipert JF. A randomized trial of azithromycin versus amoxicillin for the treatment of *Chlamydia trachomatis* in pregnancy. *Infect Dis Obstet Gynecol* 2001;9:297–303.

14 Brocklehurst P, Rooney G. Interventions for treating genital *Chlamydia trachomatis* infection in pregnancy. Cochrane Database Syst Rev 2002;4.

Approach to Hypertension in Pregnancy

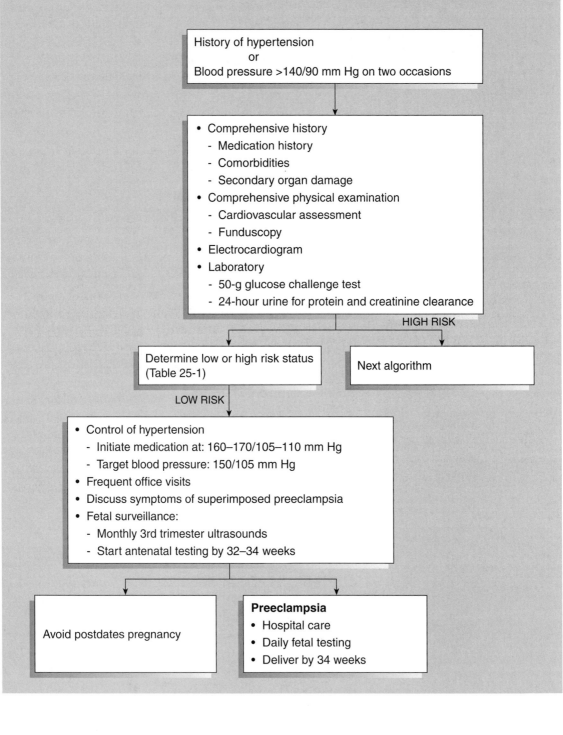

History of hypertension
or
Blood pressure >140/90 mm Hg on two occasions

- Comprehensive history
  - Medication history
  - Comorbidities
  - Secondary organ damage
- Comprehensive physical examination
  - Cardiovascular assessment
  - Funduscopy
- Electrocardiogram
- Laboratory
  - 50-g glucose challenge test
  - 24-hour urine for protein and creatinine clearance

HIGH RISK

Determine low or high risk status
(Table 25-1)

Next algorithm

LOW RISK

- Control of hypertension
  - Initiate medication at: 160–170/105–110 mm Hg
  - Target blood pressure: 150/105 mm Hg
- Frequent office visits
- Discuss symptoms of superimposed preeclampsia
- Fetal surveillance:
  - Monthly 3rd trimester ultrasounds
  - Start antenatal testing by 32–34 weeks

Avoid postdates pregnancy

Preeclampsia
- Hospital care
- Daily fetal testing
- Deliver by 34 weeks

25 Chronic Hypertension

Jeffiey C. Livingston
Hui Min Cheong

Introduction

Chronic hypertension is the most common maternal medical complication in pregnancy and varies with maternal age and ethnicity.[1] The prevalence of chronic hypertension in nonpregnant American women ages 20–29 years is about 1–1.5%. The prevalence approximately doubles with every decade of life during the reproductive years.[2] The incidence of chronic hypertension in pregnancy therefore is 1–5%. As women continue to delay childbearing, chronic hypertension in pregnancy will continue to be an increasing occurrence.

Definition and Diagnosis

KEY POINT

Diagnosis of chronic hypertension can be made by history or physical examination.

Diagnosis of chronic hypertension is made when a pregnant woman has blood pressures higher than 140 mm Hg systolic or 90 mm Hg diastolic on at least two occasions 4 hours apart before 20 weeks of gestation. A retrospective diagnosis can be made when hypertension persists beyond 6 weeks postpartum.[1] Severe hypertension is defined as blood pressure above 180 mm Hg systolic and/or 110 mm Hg diastolic.[3] Although diagnosis of chronic hypertension seems straightforward, diagnosing chronic hypertension in women whose blood pressure before pregnancy is unknown can be difficult. In a normal pregnancy complicated by chronic hypertension, there is a physiologic decrease in blood pressure, with a nadir early in the second trimester. Blood pressure returns to prepregnancy levels in the third trimester.[4] These physiologic

427

Approach to High Risk Hypertension

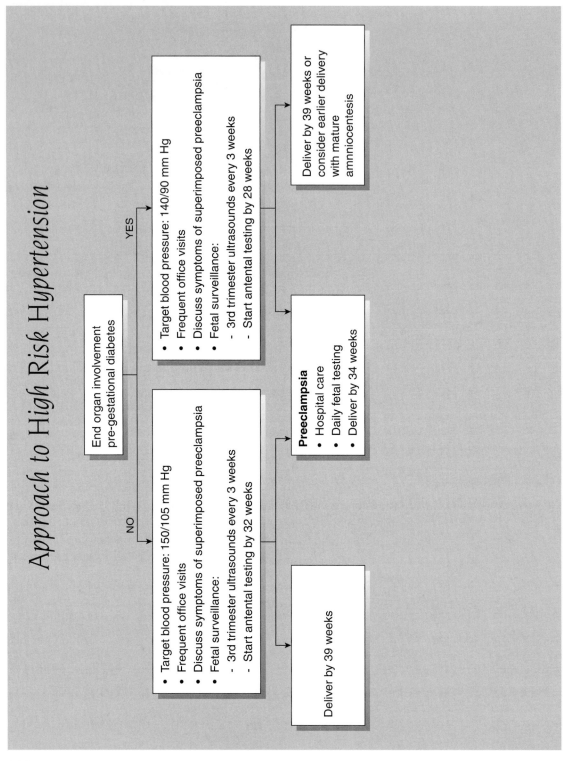

428

changes may result in a misdiagnosis of preeclampsia instead of chronic hypertension. Conversely, some women with chronic hypertension will be normotensive, especially in the midtrimester, secondary to this physiologic adaptation.

Etiology

Ninety percent of chronic hypertension is essential. The etiology of primary chronic hypertension is multifactorial. Secondary hypertension can result from underlying renal disorders (glomerulonephritis, interstitial nephritis, nephropathy, polycystic kidneys, or renal transplant), collagen vascular disorders (lupus erythematosus or scleroderma), endocrine diseases (diabetes mellitus with vascular involvement, pheochromocytoma, hyperaldosteronism, Cushing's disease, or thyrotoxicosis), or vascular disease (renal artery stenosis or aortic coarctation).

Morbidity Associated with Chronic Hypertension

MATERNAL RISK

Chronic hypertension increases maternal morbidity due primarily to superimposed preeclampsia or placental abruption.[5,6] There is a significant increase in the occurrence of preeclampsia. The incidence of superimposed preeclampsia is as high as 25% in women with chronic hypertension.[5] The risk of developing superimposed preeclampsia is highest in women who had chronic hypertension longer than 4 years, in those with severe range hypertension, and in those with a history of preeclampsia in a previous pregnancy. In women with chronic hypertension, the diagnosis of superimposed preeclampsia is often difficult to establish. There is no laboratory test that can be relied on, and clinical judgment is required to make the diagnosis. Hypertension associated with superimposed preeclampsia is often severe, labile, and difficult to control. Those with superimposed preeclampsia usually have new onset proteinuria (>300 mg/24 hour). If the patient has prepregnancy proteinuria, diagnosis can be made if there is a sudden increase in hypertension or worsening proteinuria. Superimposed preeclampsia is often associated with symptoms of end-organ involvement such as headaches, blurred vision, persistent nausea and vomiting, and epigastric or right upper quadrant pain. Women with superimposed preeclampsia may manifest changes associated with the HELLP (hemolysis, elevated liver enzymes, and low platelets) syndrome such as hemolysis (lactate dehydrogenase >600 U/L and total bilirubin >1.2 mg/dL), increases in liver enzymes (aspartate aminotransferase >70 U/L or lactate dehydrogenase >600 U/L), and a platelet count lower than 100,000/mm³. The risk of placental abruption in women with chronic hypertension is determined by degree of hypertension. The incidence of placental abruption is 1.5–2% in women with mild chronic hypertension and increases to 2.3–9.5% in women with severe hypertension.[5–9] Antihypertensive therapy does not decrease the risk of placental abruption.[10]

Women with chronic hypertension are also at an increased risk of life-threatening maternal complications such as acute pulmonary edema, hypertensive emergency, cerebral hemorrhage, or acute renal failure. These risks are greatly increased in women who have renal dysfunction or left heart failure before conception or in early pregnancy.

FETAL RISK

The risk of perinatal death increases three to four times in women who have chronic hypertension (on the order of 45 in 1000 women).[6,8,11] Major perinatal morbidities include small-for-gestational-age and low-birth-weight infants, especially in women who have severe hypertension. Because nearly 25% of women with chronic hypertension are delivered before 34 weeks, prematurity is the major contributor to poor perinatal outcomes in women with hypertensive disorders of pregnancy.[5] Superimposed preeclampsia is a leading cause of indicated preterm delivery. In a large observational report, nearly one of three pregnancies was delivered preterm and nearly one of four neonates spent time in an intensive care setting.[5]

KEY POINT

Surveillance for obstetric complications more common in women with hypertension is indicated.

Preconceptual Care and Initial Evaluation

The goal for the management of a pregnant woman with chronic hypertension is to maximize perinatal survival and decrease maternal and fetal morbidities. This can be achieved by careful surveillance during pregnancy, timely delivery, and careful postpartum management.

Management of chronic hypertension should begin before pregnancy. Maternal history should be reviewed to uncover any complications from the disease. Teratogenic drugs such as angiotensinogen-converting enzyme inhibitors should be discontinued. Physical examination should include a comprehensive cardiovascular assessment, funduscopy, and auscultation for abdominal bruits. An electrocardiogram should be performed. A 24-hour urine collection for total protein and creatinine clearance should also be obtained to assess for renal damage and to set a baseline for subsequent comparison. Because of the epidemiologic association between chronic hypertension and diabetes, an early glucose challenge test should be obtained. Based on history, physical examination, and laboratory assessments, women with chronic hypertension should be categorized into high-risk and low-risk groups. High-risk groups are those with the criteria in listed Table 25-1.

The effectiveness of antihypertensive medications in women with chronic hypertension to prevent adverse outcomes is unknown. There is conflicting literature regarding antihypertensive medications to prevent the incidence of superimposed preeclampsia.[10] The use of antihypertensive medications has not been shown to

Table 25-1. HIGH-RISK CRITERIA FOR WOMEN WITH CHRONIC HYPERTENSION IN PREGNANCY

Maternal History	*Physical Examination*	*Laboratory Evaluation*
Renal disease	Severe hypertension (>180/110 mm Hg)	Proteinuria, elevated creatinine
Cardiomyopathy		
Coarctation of the aorta	Retinopathy	Abnormal electrocardiogram
Retinopathy	Jugular venous distention	Abnormal glucose challenge test
Class B to F diabetes	Pulmonary edema	
Previous perinatal loss	Abnormal cardiac examination	
Collagen vascular disease	Discordant peripheral pulses	
Previous preeclampsia	Abdominal bruits	
Age >40 years		
Duration of hypertension >4 years		

affect perinatal survival, gestational age at delivery, or birth weight.

Low-Risk Chronic Hypertension

Women with mild chronic hypertension and no evidence of end-organ damage have a low-risk chronic hypertensive pregnancy. Because pregnancy outcome in these women is similar to that in the general population, antihypertensive medications should be discontinued in early pregnancy. However, careful management and observation are important. Frequency of clinic visits should be once every 4 weeks until 28 weeks, once every 2 weeks until 36 weeks, and then weekly thereafter. Patient should be observed for worsening hypertension or superimposed preeclampsia at each visit. It is important to monitor fetal growth because the majority of morbidity occurs with fetal growth restriction or superimposed preeclampsia. Ultrasound examinations should be done at 16–20 weeks of gestation, repeated at 26–28 weeks, and then monthly until delivery. First-line antihypertensive medications should be initiated if significant hypertension ensues (blood pressure >150–160 mm Hg systolic or 100–110 mm Hg diastolic). Although generally accepted in clinical practice, the usefulness of antenatal testing (nonstress test or biophysical profile) is supported by only level 3 evidence. Testing is indicated in the setting of fetal growth restriction or superimposed preeclampsia. In women with low-risk chronic hypertension, postdates should be avoided.

High-Risk Pregnancy

Women with any of the criteria for high-risk chronic hypertension pregnancy should have clinic visits tailored to clinical and laboratory findings (e.g., every 2–3 weeks in the first and second trimesters and then weekly). Ultrasound examinations should be obtained at 16–20 weeks, repeated at 24–26 weeks, and then every 3 weeks. Fetal surveillance with nonstress tests or biophysical profiles should begin at 32 weeks and then should be repeated twice weekly. In those with comorbidities (e.g., diabetes), testing should begin at 28 weeks.

Hospitalization is required if the patient develops hypertensive urgency or an emergency, superimposed preeclampsia, or nonreassuring fetal testing. The timing of delivery should be individualized. Delivery is recommended if any of the complications described above develop after 34 weeks. Women with high-risk chronic hypertension without any complications may continue the pregnancy until 39 weeks of gestation. Earlier delivery after demonstration of lung maturity by amniocentesis can be considered, especially if there is a history of previous fetal death or maternal comorbidities.

Pharmacologic Treatment for Chronic Hypertension

KEY POINT

Antepartum blood pressure targets depend on risk status.

Patients should be placed on antihypertensive medications to prevent severe hypertension and decrease maternal end-organ damage. In women who have low-risk chronic hypertensive pregnancy, hypertension should be treated if blood pressure exceeds 150–160 mm Hg systolic or 100–110 mm Hg diastolic. Control should be maintained at approximately 160 mm Hg systolic and 100 mm Hg diastolic. Women with high-risk hypertensive pregnancies should be placed on antihypertensive agents if their systolic blood pressure exceeds 150 mm Hg or diastolic blood pressure exceeds 100 mm Hg. In women with evidence of end-organ damage such as nephropathy or in those with pregestational diabetes, blood pressure should be treated when systolic blood pressure exceeds 140 mm Hg or diastolic blood pressure exceeds 90 mm Hg. Table 25-2 lists pharmacotherapeutic agents recommended for control of hypertension.

Hypertensive Emergency

Hypertensive emergency is defined as sustained hypertension with acute target organ involvement. The degree of hypertension is not important in separating hypertensive urgency from emergency. Acute target organ involvement is usually manifested by acute pulmonary edema, acute renal failure, or encephalopathy. Hypertensive emergencies may occur antepartum, intrapartum, or postpartum. Treatment mandates admission to a hospital unit experienced in the use of short trials of intravenous bolus medications or, preferably, continuous intravenous infusion of antihypertensive

***Table 25-2.* PHARMACOTHERAPY FOR PREGNANT WOMEN WITH CHRONIC HYPERTENSION**

Methyldopa	First line agent
	1–4 g/day in 4 divided doses
	Adverse effects: thirst, drowsiness, hemolysis, elevated liver enzymes
Labetalol	First-line agent
	100 mg twice daily to maximum of 2400 mg/day
	Adverse reactions: headache, tremulousness
Nifedipine	First-line agent
	Preferred in women with diabetes mellitus or vascular disease
	10–40 mg orally 3 times daily
	Adverse reactions: headache
Propranolol, atenolol	Second-line agent associated with lower birth weight
Clonidine	Third-line therapy
	0.1–03 mg/day in 2 divided doses to maximum of 1.2 mg/day
	Adverse reactions: rebound hypertension, rare at above doses
	Do not use with α-methyldopa
Diuretics	Second- or third-line therapy
	First-line therapy in women with congestive heart failure
	Furosemide preferred to thiazides
	Adverse reaction: decreased plasma volume
Angiotensin-converting enzyme inhibitors	Contraindicated during pregnancy
	First-line therapy in postpartum women with diabetes, nephropathy, or heart failure
	Adverse reactions: neonatal renal failure, renal dysgenesis, pulmonary hypoplasia
Hydralazine	Second- or third-line therapy
	Adverse reactions: lupus-like syndrome

KEY POINT

Hypertensive emergencies require prompt treatment.

medication. Pharmacologic agents commonly used are listed in Table 25-3. The goal of therapy should be a decrease in blood pressure by 25% during the first hour of therapy. Continuous fetal heart rate monitoring should modify therapy if the fetus is viable and of an appropriate gestational age. A comprehensive evaluation for an etiology of the hypertensive crisis is mandatory.

Table 25-3. HYPERTENSIVE EMERGENCY PHARMACOTHERAPY DURING PREGNANCY

Labetalol	20 mg IV bolus, then 40 mg 10 min later, then 80 mg every 10 min for 3 doses until blood pressure is controlled or maximum of 300 mg/24 h Contraindications: asthma or congestive heart failure
Hydralazine	5 mg IV or 10 mg IM; repeat at 20-min intervals; if not successful by 20 mg IV or 30 mg IM, consider another drug
Sodium nitroprusside	Use in intensive care setting; start at 0.3 µg/(kg · min) with maximum of 10 µg/(kg · min) Concern for fetal toxicity from cyanide metabolite Maximum duration not well established but likely safe for 1–2 h
Nitroglycerin	Potent short-acting vasodilator Use in patients with pulmonary edema Start at 10–20 µg/min, titrate until maximum of 10–20 µg/min if needed
Nicardipine	Short-acting calcium channel blocker Hypotension when used with $MgSO_4$ IV dose: 5 mg/h, titrate until effective or maximum of 15 mg/h

IM = intramuscularly; IV = intravenously.

Intrapartum Management

Intrapartum management of women with chronic hypertension is characterized by blood pressure control and observation for associated obstetric conditions. Women with sustained hypertension (>30 minutes) should be treated with intravenous bolus medications to obtain blood pressures of 160/105–110 mm Hg. However, blood pressures should not be lowered by more than 25% per hour because of the potential for fetal decompensation. Careful epidural anesthesia is ideal for most women with chronic hypertension because it is associated with a decrease of approximately 15% in blood pressure. Care should be taken not to administer antihypertensive medications immediately before epidural dosing. Conversely, general anesthesia with endotracheal intubation is associated with an acute increase in blood pressure during intubation, and care should be taken to control hypertension before elective intubation. Close surveillance for the common complications of superimposed preeclampsia and placental abruption should continue during the intrapartum period.

Postpartum Management

Postpartum management includes tighter control of blood pressure with a goal of 140/90 mm Hg because fetal concerns no longer exist. Moreover, because of the increase in systemic vascular resistance immediately postpartum and, often, excessive intrapartum intravenous fluid administration, the risk is highest for pulmonary edema during the postpartum period. Afterload reduction can help prevent postpartum pulmonary edema. Postpartum oral pharmacologic therapy should be tailored to individual non–pregnancy-related risk factors. For those with heart failure, diabetes, or nephropathy, angiotensin-converting enzyme inhibitors are first-line therapy. Dosage adjustment can often be accomplished as an outpatient.

KEY POINT

Postpartum pharmacotherapy should be individualized.

What's is the Evidence

Considerable retrospective data exist with regard to the incidence of the disease and the maternal and fetal outcomes.[5] Well-designed studies demonstrate that antihypertensive therapy does not impact on the risk of abruption, perinatal outcome, prematurity, or birthweight.[3,10] Based on the preponderance of data the use of angiotensin-converting enzyme inhibitors in the second and third trimesters causes fetal and neonatal renal failure and death.

Guiding Questions in Approaching the Patient

Diagnosing chronic hypertension

- What is the antepartum intake blood pressure? At what gestational age is the pregnancy?
- Is this chronic hypertension or preeclampsia?
- Is there a secondary cause of hypertension?

Management

- Is the patient high or low risk? Are there any comorbidities that make the pregnancy high risk?
- Are appropriate medications being used to achieve antepartum, intrapartum, and postpartum target blood pressures?

Conclusion

Chronic hypertension is the most common medical illness complicating pregnancy. Chronic hypertension needs to be distinguished from preeclampsia and from superimposed preeclampsia. The bulk of maternal and perinatal morbidity is seen in the setting of preeclampsia and severe hypertension. Determining which patients have co-morbidities such as renal failure and heart disease is critical to improving outcomes. Medical therapy should be selected to prevent severe hypertension and to protect against end organ damage.

Discussion of Cases

CASE 1: YOUNG WOMAN WITH MILD HYPERTENSION

A 27-year-old gravida 1 at 13 weeks of gestation presents for her first pregnancy visit. She is otherwise healthy. She weighs 95 kg and has a blood pressure of 148/92 mm Hg. Physical examination is normal. Ultrasound demonstrated an intrauterine pregnancy consistent with the determined gestational age. The patient was brought back to the clinic the following day with a blood pressure of 150/96 mm Hg.

What testing would you recommend at this point?

A 24-hour urine for protein and creatinine clearance, electrocardiogram, and a 50-g glucose challenge test.

How would you plan to manage her pregnancy if these tests show no abnormalities?

The patient should be followed every 4 weeks until 28 weeks, every 2 weeks until 36 weeks, and then weekly. The patient should be educated about proper nutrition, weight gain, and symptoms of superimposed preeclampsia. Serial fundal heights and monthly ultrasound examinations should be done from 26 weeks to delivery. If hypertension continues to be well controlled and uncomplicated, delivery should be considered at 39 weeks of gestation.

The patient continues to be compliant with follow-up. However, at 24 weeks, her blood pressure increases to 175/108 mm Hg with no proteinuria.

What classes of medication could be used to control her blood pressure?

A central acting agent such as α-methyldopa, an α or β blocker such as the commonly used labetalol, and a calcium channel blocker such as the commonly used nifedipine.

What other investigations should you obtain at this point?

Liver function tests and serum creatinine level, a complete blood count (platelets and hematocrit), a 24-hour urine for protein and creatinine clearance, and possibly toxicologic screening, including cocaine metabolites.

CASE 2: MULTIPARA WITH CHRONIC HYPERTENSION

A 37-year-old gravida 2, para 0100 at 29 weeks of gestation presents with a 6-year history of chronic hypertension. She has no symptoms of preeclampsia. She has been on labetalol with good blood pressure control until today. She also has a history of previable induction at 22 weeks of gestation due to severe preeclampsia. Her blood pressure today is 190/115 mm Hg. On examination, there is no papilledema, and her abdomen is soft and nontender. Her extremities show 3+ pitting edema with brisk deep tendon reflexes. There are no other abnormal findings. Fetal monitoring is reassuring. She is hospitalized for observation. She receives steroids for fetal lung maturity in case of need for premature delivery.

What investigations would you perform to evaluate for superimposed preeclampsia?

Liver function tests and serum creatinine, a complete blood count (platelets and hematocrit), a 24-hour urine for protein and creatinine clearance, and possibly toxicologic screening, including cocaine metabolites.

What medications, if any, would you use to gain control of her blood pressure in a hypertensive urgency situation?

Consider intravenous labetalol or hydralazine; if blood pressure remains uncontrolled, consider nicardipine or nitroglycerin. Once blood pressure is controlled and headache resolves, she may continue with labetalol or add methyldopa or nifedipine.

Results of the laboratory tests were normal. The patient's headache and epigastric pain increases even after institution of these thera-

pies. Blood pressures are now 210/150 mm Hg. The patient is now incoherent.

What would be the management of an emergency hypertensive situation?

The patient needs to be transferred to an intensive care unit and continue intravenous antihypertensive medications, preferably with a continuous infusion. A sodium nitroprusside infusion could be used temporarily, if necessary. The goal is to decrease blood pressure by 25% or to 160/110 mm Hg, whichever is the least decrease. Intake and output should be carefully recorded to prevent fluid overload and monitor for renal failure. Fetal heart rate should be monitored continuously.

The patient's blood pressure is now controlled at 145/95 mm Hg. Her symptoms have completely resolved.

What would be the management of this patient now?

Blood pressure should be controlled with oral medication, and the patient should be observed closely for preeclampsia.

What would indicate the need for delivery?

Maternal characteristics are a platelet count below 100,000 cells/mm^3; deterioration of hepatic or renal function including oliguria (<500 mL/24 hours); persistent severe headache, visual changes, epigastric pain, nausea or vomiting; proteinuria higher than 5 g/day; and suspected placental abruption. Fetal characteristics are severe fetal growth restriction, nonreassuring fetal surveillance, and oligohydramnios.

REFERENCES

1 Report of the National High Blood Pressure Education Program Working Group on High Blood Pressure in Pregnancy. *Am J Obstet Gynecol* 2000;183:s1–s22.

2 Burt VL, Whelton P, Roccella E, et al. Prevalence of hypertension in the US adult population. Results from the Third National Health and Nutrition Examination Survey, 1988–1991. *Hypertension* 1995;25: 305–313.

3 American College of Obstetricians and Gynecologists. Chronic hypertension in pregnancy. ACOG Practice Bulletin no 29. *Obstet Gynecol* 2001;98:177–185.

4 Benetto C, Zonca M, Marozio L, et al. Blood pressure patterns in normal pregnancy and in pregnancy-induced hypertension, pre-eclampsia, and chronic hypertension. *Obstet Gynecol* 1996;88: 503–510.

5 Sibai BM, Lindheimer M, Hauth J, et al. Risk factors for pre-eclampsia, abruptio placenta, and adverse neonatal outcomes among women with chronic hypertension. *N Engl J Med* 1998;339:667–671.

6 Rey E, Couturier A. The prognosis of pregnancy in women with chronic hypertension. *Am J Obstet Gynecol* 1994;171:410–416.

7 Sibai BM. Chronic hypertension in pregnancy. *Obstet Gynecol* 2002;100:369–377.

8 Ferrer RL, Sibai BM, Murlow CD, et al. Management of mild chronic hypertension during pregnancy: a review. *Obstet Gynecol* 2000;96: 849–860.

9 Ananth CV, Smulian JC, Demissie K, et al. Placental abruption among singleton and twin births in the United States: risk factor profiles. *Am J Epidemiol* 2001;153:771–778.

10 Sibai BM, Mabie WC, Shamsa F, et al. A comparison of no medication versus methyldopa or labetalol in chronic hypertension during pregnancy. *Am J Obstet Gynecol* 1990;162:960–966.

11 Montan S, Ingemarsson I, Marsal K, et al. Randomized controlled trial of atenolol and pindolol in human pregnancy: effect on fetal haemodynamics. *BMJ* 1992;304:946–949.

Evaluation for Pulmonary Embolism during Pregnancy

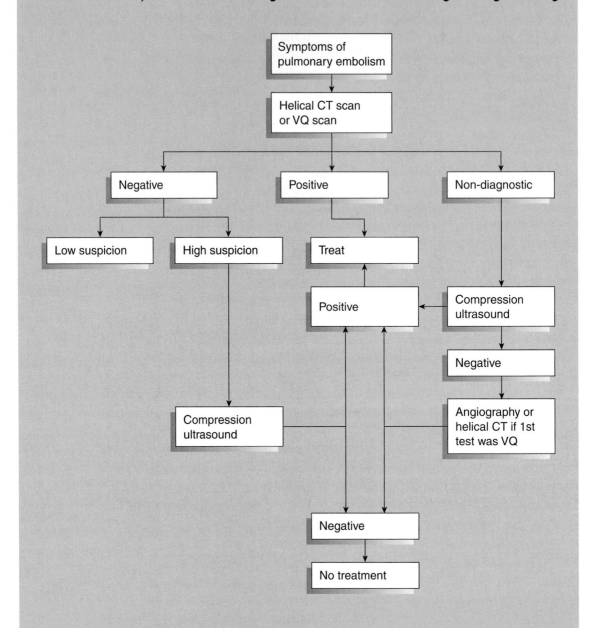

26 *Thromboembolism*

Tanya K. Sorensen

Introduction

KEY POINT

Venous thromboembolism is a leading cause of maternal mortality.

Venous thromboembolism (VTE) is among the most common serious complications of pregnancy. A leading contributor to perinatal mortality, pulmonary embolism often kills within minutes of occurrence.[1] Ideally, obstetric practitioners strive to identify at-risk patients and treat to prevent thrombosis. Short of that, our goal must be to recognize promptly and manage acute thrombotic events in pregnancy. We have derived many of our strategies for prevention, diagnosis, and management of VTE from studies of nonpregnant patients. An evidence-based approach for the gravid patient awaits large trials. In the meantime, synthesis of data from all specialties must suffice.

Determining Risk and Diagnosing Thromboembolism in Pregnancy

RISKS FOR THROMBOEMBOLISM IN PREGNANCY

Thromboembolism occurs in all trimesters of pregnancy and postpartum.[2] This is due in part to pregnancy-related alterations in the coagulation and fibrinolytic systems that promote blood clotting. There are several risk factors specific to pregnancy. Procoagulant factors II, VII, VIII, X, and XII increase, and the anticoagulant protein S decreases. Venous stasis in the legs, exacerbated by uterine compression, contributes to clotting tendency. Surgery is a common risk factor for thrombosis, and thrombosis occurs more often after cesarean section than after vaginal delivery.[3]

Women who previously had thrombosis during or outside pregnancy are at particular risk for recurrence. Among patients with a previous thrombosis, recurrence during a subsequent untreated pregnancy was 10.9% in one retrospective study compared with

441

Management of Women with Prior Deep Venous Thrombosis

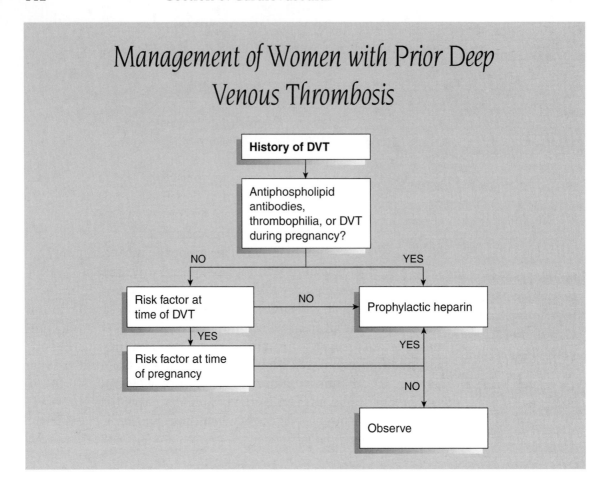

3.7% recurrence in nonpregnant patients with a similar history (RR 3.5, CI 1.6–7.8).[4] Significant family history of clotting may also predispose an individual to VTE. It is important to elicit a detailed history at the first prenatal visit. Elicited information should include timing of the event in the patient or her family, age at occurrence, risk factors such as surgery, oral contraceptive use, or prolonged immobilization when the thrombosis occurred, and results of any evaluation that was completed.

Evaluation of a patient or her family may include testing for a thrombophilia. Ample data implicate heritable and acquired abnormalities of hemostasis in the etiology of VTE.[5] Approximately 50% of women with VTE during pregnancy will have a thrombophilia. Issues related to thrombophilias are discussed in detail in Chap. 27. Inherited disorders include mutations in factor V and prothrombin (factor II), deficiencies of protein S, protein C, and antithrombin III, and hyperhomocysteinemia due to abnormality of the methylenetetrahydrofolate reductase gene. The antiphospholipid antibody syndrome is an acquired thrombophilia associated with risk for VTE in pregnancy.

Pregnant women may be subject to additional risk factors for thrombosis. For instance, obesity, multiple gestations, chorioamnionitis, pregnancy-induced hypertension, smoking, and cesarean section may increase rates of abnormal clotting.[3,4] A study of prescribed bedrest during pregnancy noted an incidence of 15.6 thromboembolic events in 1000 women using bedrest for preterm labor or preterm premature rupture of membranes compared with 0.8 in 1000 among pregnant women who did not use bedrest.[6] Prolonged airplane or car travel also imposes a common risk.

KEY POINT

Maintain a high index of suspicion to detect thromboembolism in pregnancy.

Careful evaluation for risk factors is essential. Evidence is accumulating that risk factors can guide diagnosis and treatment strategies. The pretest probability of thrombosis in a case of suspected pulmonary embolism may determine the extent and exhaustiveness of a diagnostic evaluation. The presence of risk factors may also influence the length and intensity of therapy. Most importantly, decisions regarding prophylaxis for thrombosis are currently based entirely on assessment of risk. Nevertheless, it is clear that universal screening for thrombophilia is not warranted.

DIAGNOSIS OF THROMBOEMBOLISM IN PREGNANCY

The most important aspect of diagnosis of VTE in pregnancy is to maintain a high index of suspicion. Presenting complaints of deep venous thrombosis or pulmonary embolus can be subtle and may mimic normal physiologic changes of pregnancy. Due to the potential deadly nature of the disease, clinicians should investigate symptoms liberally.

Deep venous thrombosis is most common in the left leg in pregnancy. Symptoms include pain or tenderness in 90% of patients and swelling in 80%. Redness and warmth are less common. On examination, an enlarged leg (75%) and tenderness (70%) are the most common signs. Less frequent findings are Homan's sign, redness, palpable cord, and warmth.[7] Clinical signs are not sufficient to institute therapy. Most patients with symptoms will have negative imaging studies for thrombosis. Because anticoagulation may have serious side effects, definitive diagnosis is required.

Initial testing for deep venous thrombosis should include compression ultrasound, a technique that uses the ultrasound probe to apply pressure to the vein to detect a filling defect in the vessel. This is a highly sensitive and specific method. However, if compression ultrasound is negative or indeterminate and clinical suspicion remains high, contrast venography may safely be used in pregnancy for definitive diagnosis.

Pulmonary embolism most often occurs postpartum but may be seen at any time during pregnancy. Sixty-three percent of patients will have dyspnea, and 55% will have pleuritic chest pain. Fewer than 50% will have cough, sweating, hemoptysis, or syncope. Physical examination often demonstrates tachycardia (65%) and tachypnea (58%).[7] Rales, cyanosis, and heart murmurs are seen late in the clinical course.

The long-accepted standard for initial evaluation of pulmonary embolus has been the ventilation perfusion (VQ) scan. Using technetium, radiation exposure to the fetus is very low at 100–370 μGy. The VQ scan may be read as negative, low probability, moderate probability, high probability, or indeterminate. A negative scan can be relied upon to rule out pulmonary embolus as can a low-probability scan in a low-risk patient. A high-probability result can be considered diagnostic of pulmonary embolus. Unfortunately, as many as 40–50% of VQ scans are moderate probability or indeterminate, necessitating further evaluation.[8] In a case of high clinical suspicion or a high-risk patient, further evaluation should also be considered when there is a low-probability result. A low-risk next step is lower extremity compression ultrasound. If positive, the clinician may proceed to treat. However, if negative, pulmonary angiography is warranted.

Helical or spiral chest computed tomography (CT) may be a reliable alternative to a VQ scan for initial evaluation. It may also be an alternative to angiography in the case of a nondiagnostic VQ result.[2] Radiation exposure to the fetus is lower than that for a VQ scan.[9] Helical CT is highly sensitive and specific for detecting pulmonary embolism in main, lobar, and segmental pulmonary arteries (Figure 26-1). It is less effective in detecting subsegmental thromboses. Nondiagnostic tests occur in fewer than 10% of cases. Helical CT has replaced VQ scanning in many centers. The main drawback to use in pregnancy is the paucity of data in gravid patients. The safest and most cost-effective use of helical CT in the diagnostic

Figure 26-1: Helical computed tomogram of a massive pulmonary embolism (Courtesy of William C. Black, MD.).

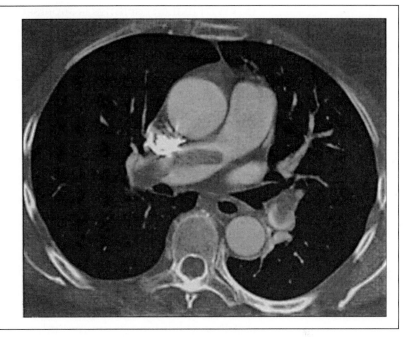

algorithm for pulmonary embolism is controversial. Questions remain as to whether helical CT should replace VQ, and, if so, whether follow-up compression ultrasound is required. Alternative proposals suggest helical CT replace angiography when other tests are nondiagnostic.

The standard of care for diagnosing a pulmonary embolus in pregnancy is evolving. A suggested approach is as follows. When pulmonary embolus is suspected, a VQ scan or helical CT should be ordered. If high probability or positive, therapy should be started. If negative or low probability in a low-risk patient, then therapy can be withheld. High-risk patients who do not have high-probability VQ results or positive helical CT results should have further testing. Follow-up testing should first include compression ultrasound. If positive, therapy should begin. If negative, pulmonary angiography, or in cases where the initial test was a VQ scan, helical CT should be performed.

Prophylaxis and Therapy for Thromboembolism in Pregnancy

The mainstay of therapy for clots in pregnancy for decades has been unfractionated heparin. Use of low-molecular-weight heparin

(LMWH) in many settings is superseding the use of unfractionated heparin, and LMWH is currently commonly used in obstetrics.[10] Neither heparin preparation crosses the placenta, but warfarin sodium does and is contraindicated during pregnancy except in rare circumstances, such as patients with mechanical heart valves. Each LMWH preparation has its own pharmacokinetic characteristics. The clinician should become familiar with the specific dosing and administration for the drug being used. LMWH is partly degraded in the liver and excreted by the kidney. There are several advantages to this more expensive drug. LMWH is more bioavailable, has greater dose-independent clearance, and has a longer half-life than does unfractionated heparin. Therefore, LMWH has a more predictable dose-response anticoagulant effect, thus decreasing the need to monitor blood levels, and can be given once daily. When monitoring is undertaken, however, activated partial thromboplastin time (APTT) is not accurate as it is for unfractionated heparin, and anti–factor Xa levels are used. The results are laboratory dependent, and consistency in laboratory use is important for accurate comparisons of serial results.[11]

Risks of heparin use in pregnancy include bleeding, heparin-induced thrombocytopenia, and adverse effects on bone density. All of these complications may be less with LMWH than with unfractionated heparin. However, with either form of heparin, supplemental calcium is recommended, and the maternal platelet count should be assessed 1–2 weeks after instituting therapy.

Management of acute VTE in pregnancy consists of initial intravenous infusion of unfractionated heparin for 5–7 days followed by subcutaneous injections of LMWH or unfractionated heparin. The subcutaneous dose of unfractionated heparin can be estimated by the total 24-hour intravenous dose. Initial use of subcutaneous injections of LMWH may be an acceptable alternative. For unfractionated heparin, monitoring includes APTT measurements on a regular basis with a goal of prolongation to 1.5–2.5 times normal. For LMWH, weight-based dosing is indicated. Because of the physiologic changes in pregnancy and increasing maternal weight, monitoring of anti–factor Xa levels should be considered. The therapeutic range for twice-daily LMWH is a peak (4 hours after dose) anti–factor Xa level of 0.5–1.2 U/mL.[11,12] Generally accepted, specific recommendations are not available for timing and frequency of anti–factor Xa levels. For treatment of

VTE it is reasonable initially to obtain levels weekly and for prophylaxis to obtain levels monthly. Recommendations for duration of therapy vary, but conservatively, full anticoagulation should continue for at least 6 months and to at least 6 weeks postpartum.

In the postpartum period warfarin sodium is an alternative to heparin and is often preferred by patients due to its oral administration. It can be safely used in breast feeding. However, warfarin sodium requires ongoing monitoring of prothrombin time and therefore may be less convenient than LMWH. If LMWH is continued postpartum, there is some evidence that dosing should be decreased. Anti–factor Xa levels may be used to determine the correct dose.

KEY POINT

It is essential to assess patients for risk factors for thrombosis before initiating therapy.

Preventative use of heparin for VTE in pregnancy is subject to many opinions and little objective data. In cases in which there is a history of thrombosis associated with a known situational risk factor not related to pregnancy, heparin may be withheld. Issues of prophylaxis in the setting of a thrombophilia are discussed in detail in Chap. 27.

Prophylactic-dose heparin is associated with fewer side effects and complications than is full-dose heparin. Nevertheless, it is prudent to obtain a maternal platelet count after instituting therapy and to provide supplemental calcium. For most patients, heparin should be started in the first trimester and continued through 6 weeks after delivery. An exception might be an otherwise low-risk patient who is not on prophylaxis but subsequently develops a risk factor such as requiring bedrest or a cesarean section. It is reasonable to institute prophylactic therapy at the time this new risk factor occurs. All patients who receive prophylaxis during pregnancy should receive anticoagulation for 6 weeks postpartum. Some clinicians recommend preventative therapy only peripartum or postpartum, but in light of many recent studies indicating that thromboses occur at a high rate throughout pregnancy and the puerperium, this seems an outdated approach.

KEY POINT

The choice, dose, and duration of therapy for patients with, or at risk for, thromboembolism must be individualized.

HEPARIN DOSING RECOMMENDATIONS

Recommendations for dosing of heparin for VTE are derived mainly from the nonobstetric literature. These are summarized in Table 26-1 and are based in part on current guidelines from the American College of Obstetrics and Gynecology and national clinical practice guidelines (www.guideline.gov).[11-13] Adjusted-dose heparin is given to patients at highest risk, including those with

***Table 26-1.*   HEPARIN IN PREGNANCY—RECOMMENDATIONS**

Low (prophylactic)-dose regimen
Use for
Thrombophilia disorder without history of thrombosis but with strong
  family history of thrombosis
Previous thrombosis without thrombophilia
Dosing
Unfractionated heparin 5000–10,000 U every 12 h
LMWH (peak anti–factor Xa 0.2–0.6 U/mL)
  Dalteparin 5000 U/day
  Enoxaparin 40 mg/day

Adjusted-dose regimen
Use for
Antithrombin deficiency
Combined heritable thrombophilias
Antiphospholipid antibodies or thrombophilia and history of
  thrombosis
Valvular heart disease and atrial fibrillation
Thromboembolism in current pregnancy (dalteparin is not approved
  for this indication)
Dosing
Unfractionated heparin (APTT 1.5–2.5 times normal)
  ≥10,000 U 2–3 times daily
LMWH (peak anti–factor Xa 0.2–0.6 U/mL)
  Dalteparin 200 U/kg every 12 h
  Enoxaparin 1 mg/kg every 12 h

APTT = activated partial thromboplastin time; LMWH = low-molecular-weight heparin.

artificial heart valves, atrial fibrillation due to abnormal heart
valves, antithrombin deficiency, combined thrombophilias,
antiphospholipid antibody syndrome with a history of thrombosis, recurrent thromboembolism, and homozygous factor II or V
deficiency with a history of clotting.

Guiding Question in Approaching the Patient

- Are there additional current risk factors that increase the
  possibility of thromboembolism?

  Low-dose heparin can be used for patients with other thrombophilias or patients with current situational risk factors and other
  lower risk situations. Data to support these recommendations are
  sparse.

Management of anticoagulation around the time of delivery can be logistically difficult. Ideally, LMWH should be discontinued 24 hours before delivery. Specifically, the American Society of Regional Anesthesia has recommended against epidural or spinal anesthesia within 24 hours of adjusted-dose enoxaparin dose (1 mg/kg) and within 12 hours after low-dose LMWH. Unfractionated heparin can be restarted 6–8 hours after an uncomplicated delivery and 12–24 hours after a complicated delivery including cesarean section. If adjusted-dose LMWH is restarted, the first dose can be given 24 hours after surgery. If an indwelling catheter is used, an additional 2 hours should pass before the next LMWH dose. If low-dose LMWH is used, the first dose after delivery can be given 8 hours postoperatively. The next dose can be given 24 hours later. If an indwelling catheter is used, the catheter can be removed a minimum of 12 hours after the last dose, and the next dose can be given 2 hours later.

Discontinuing anticoagulation could be orchestrated around the time of a planned delivery. Alternatively, patients can be switched from LMWH to unfractionated heparin at 36 weeks of gestation to allow shorter duration of anticoagulation effect and the ability for an APTT to assess degree of anticoagulation. Postpartum, patients can choose whether to restart LMWH or initiate warfarin.

Another special case is septic pelvic thrombophlebitis. This has long been a diagnosis of exclusion in the febrile postpartum patient who does not respond to antibiotic therapy. This situation usually occurs after operative delivery, and therapy consists of adding heparin to the therapeutic regimen. Current evidence suggests that patients with CT evidence of pelvic thrombosis do not benefit from heparin and that prolonged antibiotic therapy alone is sufficient.[14]

What's the Evidence?

Although there is a substantial body of knowledge about VTE in the general population, very little of it has addressed pregnancy. Specific concerns that need to be addressed in large trials include optimal and cost-effective diagnosis for pulmonary embolism, optimal duration of treatment after VTE in pregnancy, accurate identification of patients who would benefit from prophylaxis, and timing and duration of prophylactic therapy.

Progress has been made in some areas, notably in confirming safety and effectiveness of LMWH in pregnancy and in delineating relative risks of various conditions for VTE in pregnancy. Several studies have investigated the use of LMWH in pregnancy. A 2001 retrospective case review of 624 pregnancies, including 49 cases of treatment and 574 of prophylaxis. One case of LMWH-associated hemorrhage was reported, with no other complications noted. Eight patients in the prevention group, or 1.3%, had thrombotic events. The reasons for treatment in these patients were not delineated.[15]

Another 36 pregnancies were observed prospectively after diagnosis of acute VTE and treatment with the LMWH enoxaparin 1 mg/kg twice daily. In 33 cases, anti–factor Xa activity was sufficient, and LMWH therapy was continued. Three patients required lower doses. No patients had hemorrhage, thrombocytopenia, or further thrombosis.[16] A similar study of the LMWH dalteparin in 20 patients with acute VTE found that standard dosing of 100 IU/kg twice daily was insufficient in most patients and that 105–118 IU/kg was adequate. No patients developed hemorrhage or recurrent thrombosis. There was no comment on thrombocytopenia.[17]

Another retrospective study reviewed cases in which enoxaparin had been used solely for prevention of clot in high-risk pregnancies. A dose of 40 mg/day resulted in a mean anti–factor Xa level of 0.235 U/mL. There were two cases of hemorrhage due to vaginal lacerations at delivery, but no report of increased blood loss at cesarean section. Heparin-induced thrombocytopenia did not occur. No patient had VTE while on LMWH. Epidural or spinal anesthesia was safely used in 22 patients. There were no vertebral or hip fractures.[18]

One further study regarding safety of LMWH use in pregnancy is important. Forty-four patients with confirmed previous or current VTE were randomly assigned to receive LMWH or unfractionated heparin during pregnancy and postpartum. The outcome variable was bone mineral density measured by dual x-ray absorptiometry of the lumbar spine postpartum, and measurements were also compared with those of postpartum patients who were not exposed to heparin. Use of unfractionated heparin was significantly associated with lower bone density than in untreated or LMWH-treated patients.[19]

Based on the studies reviewed thus far, it appears that the recurrence risk of thrombosis in gravid patients treated with prophylactic heparin is considerably lower than the 10.9% expected rate in high-risk patients. However, risk factors that warrant therapy remain unclear.

Guiding Question in Approaching the Patient

- If the patient previously had thromboembolism, were temporary risk factors present?

One prospective study of 125 pregnant patients with a single previous episode of thrombosis withheld heparin until postpartum. Of 44 women who had no thrombophilia and a temporary risk factor at the time of their previous episode, none had VTE. Conversely, three (5.9%) of the remaining patients with thrombophilia or a history of idiopathic thrombosis had recurrence. The investigators concluded that therapy is unnecessary in the first group. Confirmation of these findings is called for.[20]

Conclusion

Because thromboembolic disease is such a major threat to pregnant women, ongoing attention to new data regarding risk identification, diagnosis, and treatment is essential. Trials specifically addressing the care of gravidas will be most helpful and may lead to modifications of recommendations presented in this chapter. Current best practice takes in to account risk factors of the individual balanced with potential side effects and inconvenience of treatment and includes frank discussion with the patient regarding available evidence before establishing a therapeutic plan.

Discussion of Cases

CASE 1: HEALTHY WOMAN WITH DYSPNEA AFTER AN AIRPLANE TRIP

A 32-year-old gravida 1, para 0 patient presents to the emergency room at 29 weeks of gestation with shortness of breath. She describes difficulty catching her breath while unpacking this afternoon after a business trip to Hawaii. This has worsened over the past several hours. She has also had chills and a nonproductive cough.

Initial examination shows a blood pressure of 156/96 mm Hg, pulse of 112 beats/min, a temperature of 100.0°F, and an oxygen saturation by pulse oximeter of 88% on room air. She is alert and oriented but appears uncomfortable. Lung fields have diffuse wheezes, and cardiac examination is significant for a class II/VI systolic murmur. Fetal heart tones are present. There is moderate bilateral lower extremity edema.

What is your differential diagnosis?

Pulmonary embolus, pneumonia, severe pre-eclampsia, and cardiomyopathy or undiagnosed valvular disease.

What is your next step?

After administering oxygen and initiating fetal monitoring, an arterial blood gas is drawn, which shows a partial pressure of oxygen of 92 mm Hg, and partial pressure of carbon dioxide of 32 mm Hg, and pH of 7.27. Laboratory analysis shows a serum creatinine level of 0.8 mg/dL, a platelet count of 180,000/mm^3, normal levels of hepatic transaminases, hematocrit value of 34%, and normal electrolytes. White blood cell count is 14,000/mm^3. Coagulation panel including prothrombin time, PTT, fibrinogen, and fibrin split products in yielded values in the normal range. Maternal electrocardiogram shows sinus tachycardia. The fetal heart rate monitor shows a flat baseline without accelerations or decelerations and a rate of 160 beats/min. Tocometry indicates infrequent irregular contractions, but examination shows the cervix to be long and closed.

What imaging studies should you order?

Chest radiograph shows a small pleural effusion on the left with an area possibly indicating atelectasis in the left lower lobe. The cardiac silhouette is mildly enlarged. VQ scan is indeterminate.

How will you proceed?

Compression ultrasound of the lower extremities is negative. Due to a high level of suspicion, a helical CT is performed and indicates a thrombus in the left pulmonary circulation at the segmental level in the lower lobe.

What therapy is indicated?

Intravenous unfractionated heparin is administered with an APTT 2.5 times the normal level for 5–7 days. LMWH is then started based on body weight calculations. Levels of anti–factor Xa are monitored to confirm adequate dosing. Duration of therapy will be 6 months. After delivery, the patient is given the option of switching to warfarin sodium.

What further workup is needed?

Anticardiolipin antibodies are negative. Thrombophilia workup shows that the level of protein S is 38% of normal. The patient is heterozygous for the factor V Leiden mutation. Maternal echocardiogram is normal.

Do these findings modify your recommendations?

Level of protein S is affected by pregnancy and is not an accurate reflection of protein S deficiency. In pregnancy a level of protein S below 35% is considered abnormal. If protein S levels are obtained during pregnancy, they should be repeated postpartum. Prophylactic heparin is recommended in future pregnancies.

CASE 2: YOUNG WOMAN WITH EXTENSIVE FAMILY HISTORY OF THROMBOTIC DISEASE

A 19-year-old primigravida presents to your office for a new prenatal visit at 12 weeks of gestation. She reports a completely uncomplicated medical history. She has had no arterial or venous thrombosis, miscarriages, or thrombocytopenia. However, she does provide a family history of blood clot in the leg in her sister and maternal aunt. Her maternal grandmother died of a pulmonary embolism. Her father had a myocardial infarction at age 50 years.

What evaluation would you like to do?

She should have a thrombophilia panel study done. This includes antithrombin III deficiency, prothrombin gene mutation, factor V gene mutation, deficiency of protein S, deficiency of protein C, and hyperhomocysteinemia due to abnormality of the methylenetetrahydrofolate reductase gene mutation.

Her studies indicate a prothrombin gene mutation that is heterozygous for methylenetetrahydrofolate reductase gene mutation.

What implication does this have for her pregnancy?

Because of the strong family history and her prothrombin gene mutation, you recommend that she take low-dose heparin prophylaxis for the duration of the pregnancy and 6 weeks postpartum. The methylenetetrahydrofolate reductase gene abnormality is very common in the general population and will not alter your management plans. She should consider informing her family members of her gene abnormality.

Are there any other ongoing pregnancy management issues?

She will need to have a platelet count assessed 1–2 weeks after initiating heparin. She should be encouraged to consume calcium and vitamin D. It is not necessary to follow anti–factor Xa levels. She is not at risk for uteroplacental insufficiency. She will need to stop her heparin early when she goes into labor.

REFERENCES

1 Berg CJ, Chang J, Callaghan WM, Whitehead SJ. Pregnancy-related mortality in the United States, 1991–1997. *Obstet Gynecol* 2003;101: 289–296.

2 Dizon-Townson D. Pregnancy-related venous thromboembolism. *Clin Obstet Gynecol* 2002;45:363–368.

3 Ros HS, Lichtenstein P, Bellocco R, et al. Pulmonary embolism and stroke in relation to pregnancy: how can high-risk women be identified? *Am J Obstet Gynecol* 2002;186:198–203.

4 Pabinger I, Grafenhofer H, Kyrle PA, et al. Temporary increase in the risk for recurrence during pregnancy in women with a history of venous thromboembolism. *Blood* 2002;100:1060–1062.

5 Lockwood CJ. Inherited thrombophilias in pregnant patients: detection and treatment paradigm. *Obstet Gynecol* 2002;99:333–341.

6 Kovacevich GJ, Gaich SA, Lavin JP, et al. The prevalence of thromboembolic events among women with extended bedrest prescribed

as part of the treatment for premature labor or preterm premature rupture of membranes. *Am J Obstet Gynecol* 2000;182:1089–1092.

7 Gherman RB, Goodwin TM, Leung B, et al. Incidence, clinical characteristics, and timing of objectively diagnosed venous thromboembolism during pregnancy. *Obstet Gynecol* 1999;94:730–734.

8 Barbour LA. ACOG Committee on Practice Bulletins—Obstetrics. ACOG practice bulletin. Thrombembolism in pregnancy. *Int J Gynaecol Obstet* 2001;75:203–212.

9 Winer-Muram HT, Boone JM, Brown HL, et al. Pulmonary embolism in pregnant patients: fetal radiation dose with helical CT. *Radiology* 2002;224:487–492.

10 American College of Obstetricians and Gynecologists. American College of Obstetrics and Gynecology Committee Opinion: safety of Lovenox in pregnancy. *Obstet Gynecol* 2002;100:845–846.

11 Duplaga BA, Rivers CW, Nutescu E. Dosing and monitoring of low molecular weight heparin in special populations. *Pharmacotherapy* 2001;21:218–234.

12 Institute for Clinical Systems Improvement. *Venous Thromboembolism.* Bloomington, MN: Institute for Clinical Systems Improvement, 2003.

13 Ginsberg JS, Greer I, Hirsch J. Use of antithrombotic agents during pregnancy. *Chest* 2001;119(suppl):122S–131S.

14 Brown CE, Stettler RW, Twickler D, Cunningham FG. Puerperal septic thrombophlebitis: incidence and response to heparin therapy. *Am J Obstet Gynecol* 1999;181:143–148.

15 Lepercq J, Conard J, Borel-Derlon A, et al. Venous thromboembolism during pregnancy: a retrospective study of enoxaparin safety in 624 pregnancies. *Br J Obstet Gynaecol* 2001;108:1134–1140.

16 Rodie VA, Thomson AJ, Stewart FM, et al. Low molecular weight heparin for the treatment of venous thromboembolism in pregnancy: a case series. *Br J Obstet Gynaecol* 2002;109:1020–1024.

17 Jacobsen AF, Qvigstad E, Sandset PM. Low molecular weight heparin (dalteparin) for the treatment of venous thromboembolism in pregnancy. *Br J Obstet Gynaecol* 2003;110:139–144.

18 Ellison J, Walker ID, Greer IA. Antenatal use of enoxaparin fo prevention and treatment of thromboembolism in pregnancy. *Br J Obstet Gynaecol* 2000;107:1116–1121.

19 Pettila V, Leinonen P, Markkola A, et al. Postpartum bone mineral density in women treated for thromboprophylaxis with unfractionated heparin or LMW heparin. *Thromb Haemost* 2002;87:182–186.

20 Brill-Edwards P, Ginsberg JS, Gent M, et al. Safety of withholding heparin in pregnant women with a history of venous thromboembolism. *N Engl J Med* 2000;343:1439–1474.

Approach to Diagnosis and Management of Thrombophilia Disorders

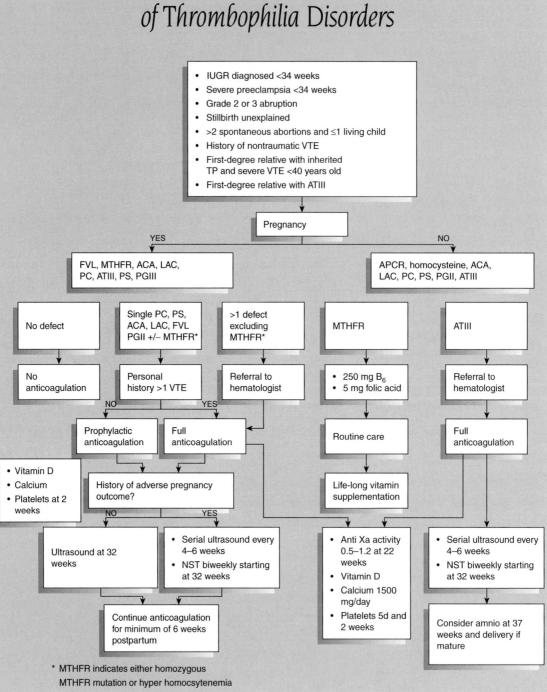

27 Thrombophilia in Pregnancy

Michele R. Lauria

Introduction

Thrombophilic disorders are a group of acquired and inherited conditions that cause increased blood clotting tendency. In non-pregnant individuals, they manifest as thromboembolic phenomenon. In pregnancy, they may increase the risk of thromboembolism and are associated with different conditions related to abnormal placentation. Pregnancy conditions associated with thrombophilic disorders include recurrent miscarriage, placental abruption, early onset severe preeclampsia, early onset severe fetal growth restriction, severe placental abruption, and fetal death. Up to 65% of women who develop one of these complications will have a thrombophilia. The most common thrombophilias are antiphospholipid antibody (APA) syndrome; activated protein C resistance, most commonly factor V Leiden mutation (FVL), prothrombin gene mutation (PGII), protein S deficiency (PS), protein C deficiency (PC), antithrombin III deficiency (ATIII), and hyperhomocysteinemia; and most commonly homozygous methylenetetrahydrofolate reductase deficiency (MTHFR). Table 27-1 lists the inheritance and testing of these most common disorders.

Etiology of Thrombophilia and Prevalence in the General Population

Many of the thrombophilias are inherited. Numerous gene defects have been described for PS, PC, and ATIII. These defects variably affect the quantity or quality of the protein produced. Activated protein C resistance is predominantly caused by FVL. FVL, PGII, and MTHFR are due to single base-pair substitutions. FVL is the

Table 27-1. COMMON THROMBOPHILIAS IN PREGNANCY

TYPE	ETIOLOGY	DIAGNOSIS
APA syndrome: classic	Acquired	Personal history of 1 of the following: Recurrent pregnancy loss: >2 SAB with <1 live birth Unexplained second- or third-trimester fetal death Unexplained venous or arterial thrombosis Autoimmune thrombocytopenia, hemolytic anemia Stroke, transient ischemic attack, amaurosis fugax, *Livedo reticularis* *and* Laboratory testing: lupus anticoagulant (LAC) *or* ACA IgG >15–20 GPL units
Protein C deficiency	Acquired or inherited	Protein C activity <67%; pregnancy has little effect on testing, but low levels may be found in response to infection or stress
Protein S deficiency	Acquired or inherited	During pregnancy protein S activity <35% is abnormal; in nonpregnant individuals, abnormal is <65% for women; abnormal test results in pregnancy should be verified postpartum off all exogenous hormones
Antithrombin III deficiency	Acquired or inherited	Antithrombin III activity <80%; abnormal results should prompt testing outside pregnancy to determine whether the deficiency is functional or quantitative
Factor V Leiden		In pregnancy use PCR testing for gene mutation Outside pregnancy, determine activated protein C resistance; a normalized ratio >0.85 is normal
Prothrombin gene mutation		PCR testing only
Methylenetetrahydrofolate reductase deficiency		In pregnancy, use PCR testing; positive results are homozygous for the mutation; ~50% of the population is heterozygous Outside pregnancy, random plasma homocysteine >15 μmol/L

ACA = anticardiolipin antibody; GPL = IgG anti-phospholipid antibody; IgG = immunoglobulin G; PCR = polymerase chain reaction; SAB = spontaneous abortion.

most common inherited thrombophilia and is found in 20% of individuals with a first thrombosis episode and in up to 50% of individuals with a recurrence.[1] PGII is the next most common thrombophilia, occurring in 2% of the general population and in 6% of individuals with a first-time thrombosis.[2] APA syndrome is an acquired autoimmune disorder. The frequencies of APAs are 1–2% in the general population and 5–15% among those with a history of venous thromboembolism.

Who Should Be Tested?

KEY POINT

The prevalence of an inherited thrombophilia in persons of European descent is estimated to be up to 20%. Further, 10–12% of women with an inherited thrombophilia and thrombosis will have more than one thrombophilia present.

Clinicians must be cautious about whom they choose to test for thrombophilia. Approximately 5% of the population is positive for FVL and 2% for PGII. The APAs may be present as a transitory response to infection or for no clear reason. Except for ATIII, it is unclear whether there is any clinical significance to the presence of a thrombophilia in the absence of a personal history of adverse pregnancy outcome or thromboembolic event. This suggests that there are determinants other than the abnormal gene that affect pregnancy outcome. One factor may be age. Most individuals with inherited thrombophilias do not develop an adverse event until their 40s or later, with the exception of persons with ATIII. Prospective studies of women with negative histories of thrombosis or adverse pregnancy outcome but with thrombophilia have not shown an increased risk of pregnancy complications, except for a slight increased incidence of thrombosis.[3] Some clinicians recommend testing and treatment if there is a strong family history of severe thromboembolic events early in life (younger than 50 years). Because there are so many different gene defects that cause the deficiencies and because we do not understand how other biologic and environmental factors interact to cause thrombosis, it seems reasonable that women with family members who had early and severe thrombosis are at higher risk of thrombosis during pregnancy than are their counterparts with the same thrombophilia but a less severe family history. Because of the exceptionally high risk of thrombosis caused by ATIII deficiency, ATIII status should be determined in any individual who has a first-degree relative with proved ATIII, and treatment during pregnancy should be offered regardless of personal history.

The following characteristics should prompt screening:

- More than two miscarriages with no more than one living child
- Unexplained second- or third-trimester fetal demise
- Severe preeclampsia with onset before 34 weeks of gestation
- Severe unexplained growth restriction in the late second or early third trimester
- Nontraumatic arterial or venous thrombosis (superficial thrombosis does not qualify)
- Stroke or transient ischemic attack
- History of early onset severe thromboembolism in a first-degree relative who has an inherited thrombophilia
- First-degree relative with ATIII
- Unexplained autoimmune thrombocytopenia

Treatment and Pregnancy Management

Treatment is best understood in terms of patient categories.

- *Women with thrombophilia and adverse pregnancy outcome, as defined above, but no history of venous thromboembolism (VTE):* Aside from APA syndrome, there are no prospective randomized studies of treatment versus observation for pregnant women with thrombophilia. However, most will treat all thrombophilia as APA syndrome is treated, assuming a similar disease pathogenesis. Women with APA syndrome should take low-dose aspirin (81 mg) daily and start prophylactic doses of heparin once fetal cardiac activity is established, usually at approximately 6 weeks. Some patients may wish to start heparin with a missed menses. Because only prophylactic doses are used, this is unlikely to cause complications should miscarriage occur. Recommendations for management of other thrombophilias generally do not include use of low-dose aspirin.
- Serial ultrasound examinations for growth, every 4–6 weeks, should be considered, starting at 24 weeks. Nonstress tests (NSTs) or other antenatal testing regimen should be started by 32 weeks. If the previous adverse event was fetal death,

early delivery should be considered. If elective delivery based on history is planned before 39 weeks of gestation, fetal lung maturity should be established. Delivery should not be undertaken electively before 37 weeks without full consideration of the implications of iatrogenic prematurity.

- *Women with thrombophilia and history of VTE without adverse pregnancy outcome:* If there was a single VTE episode and full treatment has been completed, then prophylactic heparin should be adequate except for APA syndrome. Women with APA syndrome and a history of thrombosis are at exceptionally increased risk of thrombosis during pregnancy. The American College of Obstetricians and Gynecologists recommends full anticoagulation.[4] An ultrasound examination should be obtained at 32–34 weeks for fetal growth. It is not clear that prenatal testing or early delivery is necessary, especially if the patient has had other normal pregnancies.

- *Women with thrombophilia, history of VTE, and adverse pregnancy outcome:* These women should have full anticoagulation and undergo fetal testing as outlined for patients with thrombophilia and adverse pregnancy outcomes.

- *Women with APA syndrome and VTE:* These women should have full anticoagulation and undergo fetal testing as outlined for patients with thrombophilia and adverse pregnancy outcomes, regardless of their pregnancy history.

- *ATIII deficiency regardless of personal pregnancy or VTE history:* These women should have full anticoagulation. Serial ultrasound examinations for fetal growth and NSTs beginning at 32 weeks should also be obtained. Elective delivery by 37 weeks should be considered because these patients may be at increased risk for severe placental abruption.

- *Women with adverse pregnancy outcomes not severe enough to fulfill the criteria for testing and a thrombophilia:* There is no evidence that treatment will improve outcome in this group. Studies of the incidence of thrombophilia in individuals with less severe pregnancy complications have not shown an increased incidence of thrombophilia. Therefore, these individuals may just coincidentally have a thrombophilia. The exception is ATIII *deficiency.* If the woman has a first-degree family member who has the same thrombophilia and developed early onset severe thrombosis, prophylactic doses of heparin should be considered.[5]

- *Women with thrombophilia diagnosed based on a family member with VTE but no personal history of adverse pregnancy outcome or VTE:* Most of these individuals do not need special treatment in pregnancy. The exception is those with first-degree family members who have severe and early onset thrombophilia. These individuals may benefit from prophylactic-dose heparin.

- *Homozygous MTHFR:* The effects of this defect can be overcome with folic acid (5 mg/day) and vitamin B_6 (100 mg/day) supplementation that starts before conception.[6] Aspirin has also been included in studies of this regime.[7] Other interventions should be based on routine care guidelines or the presence of other thrombophilias.

Low-Molecular-Weight Heparin Versus Unfractionated Heparin

Low-molecular-weight heparin (LMWH) is considered the standard of care by many practitioners due to decreased frequency of dosing, lower incidence of thrombocytopenia, and decreased bone loss. It is significantly more expensive than unfractionated heparin. For women who are at high risk of osteoporosis and who will need prolonged anticoagulation, LMWH should be used.

HEPARIN DOSING AND OTHER CONSIDERATIONS

Heparin undergoes renal excretion. Increased glomerular filtration rate, weight gain, and increased volume of distribution during pregnancy results in larger dosage requirements that increase as pregnancy progresses.

Prophylactic dose

- Enoxaparin (Lovenox) 40 mg/day subcutaneoulsy
- Dalteparin (Fragmin) 5000 IU/day subcutaneously
- Unfractionated heparin 5,000–10,000 U subcutaneously every 12 hours. Extremely thin patients should start at 5000 U and obese (body mass index $\geq$30 kg/m^2) patients should start at 10,000 U. Increasing the dose in the mid second trimester to account for increased renal clearance should be considered.

Full anticoagulation (adjusted dose)

- Enoxaparin 1 mg/kg subcutaneously every 12 hours
- Dalteparin 200 IU/kg subcutaneously daily
- Unfractionated heparin: There are several ways to initiate the dose. One is to hospitalize the woman and start intravenous heparin. Once a stable and therapeutic partial thromboplastin time (PTT) has been obtained (two times the patient's normal PTT), then the total daily dose of intravenous heparin can divided into three doses of subcutaneous heparin and injected every 8 hours. The use of a pharmacy algorithm for intravenous dosing can greatly decrease the time needed to reach a therapeutic dose. The other method is to calculate a dose based on the patient's weight and start with subcutaneous dosing, with daily adjustments to reach a therapeutic PTT that is checked 3–5 hours after injection. I have found no algorithms to assist in this process. However, it seems reasonable that an intravenous algorithm could be modified to guide subcutaneous dosing. In general, most patients will need 35,000–40,000 U total, divided into 8-hour dosing.

What about steroids? Heparin should not be used with high-dose prednisone due to the increased risk of osteoporosis and fractures, the lack of evidence that combination therapy improves pregnancy outcomes, and the increase in preterm premature rupture of membranes (PPROM) and preeclampsia.[8]

CHECKING LEVELS

PROPHYLACTIC It is probably not necessary to check levels. Some recommend a peak anti–factor Xa level of 0.2–0.6 U/mL. This is obtained 4 hours after injection.[9]

FULL ANTICOAGULATION (ADJUSTED DOSE) Patients with artificial heart valves and some with histories of severe thrombosis may require different therapeutic levels. It may be helpful to seek the assistance of a hematologist.

- *Unfractionated:* Activated PTT drawn 3 hours after the dose should be 1.5–2.0 times normal. PTT should be checked every week due to variability of absorption and availability.
- *LMWH:* Peak levels using an assay appropriate for the type of heparin should be checked in the mid second trimester or every trimester. Test results can vary between laboratories.

Most recommend anti–factor Xa levels of 0.5–1.2 U/mL 4 hours after injection.[9] In some institutions, this is referred to as a heparin assay. Activated PTT does not reflect the activity of LMWH and should not be used.

OSTEOPOROSIS

KEY POINT

All women on heparin should take supplemental calcium and vitamin D.

The average bone loss from unfractionated heparin therapy is 5%, and one third of patients will lose at least 10% or more.[10] Bone density imaging postpartum should be considered for women who smoke or have a strong family history of osteoporosis. Whenever either type of heparin is given, vitamin D and calcium supplementation (calcium carbonate 1500 mg/day) and weight-bearing exercise should also be performed.

SKIN REACTIONS

Skin reactions occur in approximately 1% of patients. If they are mild, a different type of LMWH may be tried. However, if they progress, then heparin of all types should be avoided due to the risk of anaphylaxis. The newer heparinoids such as lepirudin could be considered.[11]

THROMBOCYTOPENIA

There are two types of heparin-induced thrombocytopenia. The immediate type is reversible and does not require discontinuation of therapy. The later onset immune type can result in severe thrombocytopenia and typically occurs at 5–14 days. Therefore, for patients on unfractionated heparin, platelet counts should be checked on day 5 and then periodically during the first 2 weeks of therapy.[10] For patients taking LMWH, a reasonable alternative is to test platelets 1–2 weeks after initiation of treatment. Danaparoid should be considered for further anticoagulation for women who develop heparin-induced thrombocytopenia.[9]

REGIONAL ANESTHESIA

There are case reports of epidural hematomas in elderly women receiving LMWH, although most had other risk factors. The American Society of Regional Anesthesia has recommended against epidural or spinal anesthesia within 12 hours of prophylactic-dose LMWH or 24 hours of adjusted-dose (twice daily) LMWH.[12] Unfractionated heparin can be restarted 6–8 hours after an uncomplicated delivery and 12–24 hours after a complicated delivery including cesarean section.

If adjusted-dose LMWH is restarted, the first dose can be given 24 hours after surgery. If an indwelling catheter is used, an additional 2 hours should pass before the next LMWH dose. If low-dose LMWH is used, the first dose after delivery can be given 8 hours postoperatively. The next dose can be given 24 hours later. If an indwelling catheter is used, the catheter can be removed a minimum of 12 hours after the last dose, and the next dose can be given 2 hours later.

DELIVERY

Because of the risks of epidural hematomas, patients receiving LMWH should be switched to unfractionated heparin at about 37 weeks of gestation. Patients should discontinue heparin with onset of labor. An alternative is be to continue LMWH until a scheduled delivery.[9] If the patient is at exceptionally high risk of thrombosis (i.e., proximal deep vein thrombosis ≤2 weeks), the patient is administered intravenous unfractionated heparin that is discontinued 4–6 hours before expected delivery time.

POSTPARTUM CARE
KEY POINT

Women who receive heparin therapy during pregnancy should receive warfarin or heparin for 6 weeks postpartum.

Patients remain at increased risk of thrombosis for a minimum of 6 weeks after pregnancy. Anticoagulation should be continued throughout this period. Guidelines recommend that warfarin be given for 4–6 weeks after delivery with a target INR of 2–3.[9] Warfarin is safe for breast feeding and is less expensive than LMWH; however, initially levels need to be obtained frequently until a therapeutic dose is reached and then every week. Continuing subcutaneous heparin is also an option.

NONOBSTETRIC CARE

The inherited thrombophilias are acquired in an autosomal dominant pattern. Depending on the specific defect, testing of other family members may be useful. If the patient has a newly diagnosed thrombophilia and a history of VTE, referral to a hematologist for long-term management is appropriate. All women with thrombophilia are at life-long increased risk of thromboembolism. They should also have thromboembolism precautions for any surgery or period of immobilization. Women with MTHFR should have folic acid supplementation (5 mg/day). In addition to the risk of venous thrombosis, there is a high rate of medical complications in the 5 years after pregnancy in women with APA syndrome. These complications include stroke, transient ischemic attacks, amaurosis fugax, new onset systemic lupus, or new onset autoimmune thrombocytopenia.

What's the Evidence

PATHOPHYSIOLOGY	The common pathway to pathology in pregnancy is through the placenta. Infarction, necrosis, and thrombosis are lesions that have been described in placentas of women with thrombophilia and adverse pregnancy outcomes. Vascular disease has been found on maternal and fetal surfaces. Infarcts on the fetal side are probably due to fetal thromboembolic events and may reflect fetal inheritance of a thrombophilia. Gris and coworkers described placentas of women who had stillbirths at more than 22 weeks of gestation.[13] The placentas from women who had thrombophilia always had evidence of maternal vascular disease, more so if they had a combined deficiency that included MTHFR. In a referral series of women with adverse pregnancy outcome and thrombotic lesions of the placenta, 10 of 13 women had a thrombophilia.[14] Five of the infants had neurologic lesions, and all had thrombotic lesions in the fetal circulation. These and other studies have emphasized the importance of thorough histologic examination of the placenta when there is a poor pregnancy outcome.[15] However, placental lesions do not universally indicate thrombophilia. Sikkema and associates found no difference in the placentas of women with thrombophilia and preeclampsia or intrauterine growth retardation compared with those without thrombophilia who also had pregnancies complicated by these conditions.[16]

ROLE OF THE FETUS The role of the fetus is unclear in pregnancy complications related to thrombophilia. Severe inherited thrombophilia, such as homozygous PC or PS, or combined thrombophilia is rare and has been described in early neonatal demise. Infarcts on the fetal surface of the placenta are probably due to fetal thromboembolism and are associated with an increased incidence of cerebral palsy and neurologic impairment. The infarcts may be the results of fetal thrombophilia.[14] One study of FVL deficiency and miscarriage found that the fetuses with FVL were more likely to undergo miscarriage. In addition, there was a 10-fold increase in the carrier frequency of FVL in fetuses whose placentas had greater than 10% infarction.[17]

PREGNANCY ***RECURRENT MISCARRIAGE*** APA syndrome is the most well-known cause of recurrent pregnancy loss. There is substantial controversy regarding the role of the other thrombophilias, in particular FVL, MTHFR, and PTII. This controversy most likely arises from the different study designs. A recent meta-analysis found that carriers of FVL or PGII have double the risk of recurrent pregnancy loss.[18]

STILLBIRTH Although the gestational age definition for stillbirth versus miscarriage varies across studies, there is a consistent association of stillbirth with an increased incidence of thrombophilia. In one study, 232 consecutive women without a history of thrombosis who had fetal loss after 22 weeks were compared with 464 controls matched by maternal age at first pregnancy and number of pregnancies.[13] They found an increased incidence of FVL, LAC, and ACA immunoglobulin G, with 21.1% of women who had stillbirths and a thrombophilia versus only 3.9% of controls. Women with two stillbirths were even more likely to carry a thrombophilia than were those with only one. Overall, although there was no significant association of MTHFR with stillbirth, the risk of stillbirth was significantly greater if MTHFR was present with another thrombophilia and especially if folic acid supplementation did not occur. Other researchers have described an increased incidence of thrombophilia among women with stillbirth.[19]

EARLY ONSET SEVERE PREECLAMPSIA Several studies have reported an increased incidence of thrombophilia among women with severe preeclampsia before 34 weeks. The reported incidence of thrombophilia is 5–79%.[6,20] PS and ACA are the most commonly described. Hyperhomocysteinemia has also been implicated. In contrast to the studies discussed above, Paternoster and associates observed no difference in the frequency of FVL among women with preeclampsia compared with controls but did find a significantly lower activated protein C sensitivity ratio than in controls.[21] In summary, it appears that there is an increased incidence of thrombophilia among women with severe, early onset preeclampsia and testing of this group is warranted.

ABRUPTION Abruption can be classified into grades based on clinical criteria. Grades 2 and 3 are associated with vaginal bleeding or concealed hemorrhage; uterine tenderness; and one of the following: fetal distress, maternal shock, or maternal coagulopathy.

The incidence of thrombophilia is 20–60% in women with high-grade abruption.[22]

INTRAUTERINE GROWTH RETARDATION Most studies have reported an increased incidence of thrombophilia among women with severely growth restricted children, especially if onset was in the late second or early third trimester.[22,23] Not all studies have confirmed this association. A recent study reported a 69% prevalence of thrombophilia in mothers of growth restricted infants, with 33% of mothers with severe second-trimester fetal growth restriction (22–26 weeks of gestation) and multiple thrombophilia defects.[24]

THROMBOPHILIAS AND RISK OF THROMBOSIS

There have been several large European studies of the effect of inherited thrombophilias. In one study, carriers were categorized as symptomatic or nonsymptomatic based on their personal history of thromboembolism.[25] The investigators interviewed 793 relatives of 145 symptomatic carriers of thrombophilia. Carriers of PC, PS, and ATIII had an aggregate baseline risk of 10% per year for VTE, whereas noncarriers had a risk of 0.1%/year. Pregnancy was associated with an increase in risk from 0.5% without thrombophilia to 4.1% with thrombophilia. With oral contraceptives, the risk of VTE increased from 0.7% without a thrombophilia to 4.3%, and the risk of thrombophilia with surgery was 8.1%. When FVL was evaluated separately, there was no increased risk of VTE with surgery, hormonal contraceptives or pregnancy, while the increased risk was maintained for ATIII, PC and PS. Other studies have confirmed these findings.

TREATMENT

For women identified as having a thrombophilia based on adverse pregnancy outcome alone, the only randomized controlled treatment trials are for APA syndrome. One may argue that treatment should be withheld until such studies are performed; however, several studies have pointed to an increased risk of VTE in thrombophilia carriers during pregnancy. Because most poor pregnancy outcomes are due to placental thrombosis, it seems logical to offer treatment to women diagnosed with thrombophilia based on pregnancy history alone.[26] The standard treatment is prophylactic doses of heparin. One could consider the addition of aspirin 81 mg/day, as is used commonly in therapy for APA syndrome. Treatment of APA syndrome with heparin and low-dose aspirin improves pregnancy outcome.[27] In women with only immunoglobulin M ACAs or low titers of immunoglobulin G ACAs, randomized trials did not show improved outcome.

Treatment of other thrombophilia disorders has been evaluated mostly with historical controls.[28,29] Riyazi and colleagues performed a retrospective study of 26 treated persons with thrombophilia and compared their outcomes with subsequent pregnancies in women with thrombophilia who did not receive LMWH or aspirin but had similar poor pregnancy histories. Women with a single thrombophilia who underwent treatment had children with significantly higher birth weights.[30] In a study of 207 consecutive patients with preeclampsia or fetal growth restriction, Leeda and associates found that treatment of women with hyperhomocysteinemia increased birth weight by 1000 g and prolonged pregnancy by 6 weeks compared with historical controls.[6]

Population screening studies of FVL mutation have shown that, overall, these women do not appear to be at increased risk for adverse pregnancy outcomes, but they are at an eightfold increased risk of VTE in pregnancy. Similar studies have not been done for other thrombophilias. However, it seems reasonable that factors other than thrombophilia interact to cause adverse pregnancy outcomes, and that treatment solely for the benefit of the fetus without a poor pregnancy history is unwarranted. Treatment to prevent VTE during pregnancy may be beneficial.

Guiding Questions in Approaching the Patient

- Does the patient have a personal history of thrombosis or thrombophilia-related adverse pregnancy outcome?
- Was complete testing performed? Was the presence of antibodies for APA syndrome confirmed on two occasions at least 8 weeks apart? Was abnormal PC, PS, and ATIII testing confirmed outside of pregnancy and without the use of hormonal contraception and anticoagulants?
- What type of postpartum anticoagulation is indicated?
- Are there long-term health issues that need to be addressed outside of pregnancy?
- Are there implications for the woman's children and other family members?

Conclusion

The thrombophilias pose a risk for thromboembolism and adverse pregnancy outcomes. Treatment with heparin can decrease the risk of these adverse outcomes. Criteria exist to determine which individuals should be tested for the inherited and acquired thombophilias (see clinical pathway). The use of prophylactic or therapeutic heparin depends on the clinical circumstance as does the need for fetal testing. Any woman who receives heparin during pregnancy should receive anticoagulation for 6–8 weeks after delivery.

Discussion of Cases

CASE 1: PATIENT WITH HISTORY OF SEVERE, EARLY ONSET PREECLAMPSIA

Ms. Smith is a 21-year-old gravida 2, para 0101 who presents for initiation of care at 8 weeks of gestation. Her first pregnancy was complicated by early onset severe preeclampsia that necessitated delivery at 26 weeks. This child is doing well and has no major complications of prematurity.

What historical questions are pertinent?

Was Ms. Smith screened for a clotting disorder in her previous pregnancy? Has Ms. Smith ever had a blood clot? Have any of her family members had blood clots, early heart attacks, or early strokes? If they have, were they tested for a thrombophilia?

Ms. Smith does not recall being screened for clotting disorders during or after her previous pregnancy. She has never had a blood clot. Her father had several blood clots in his legs at age 45 years. He is on long-term anticoagulation. She states that he has a clotting disorder but does not know what the name of it is. She has minimal contact with him.

What tests should you order?

You should obtain the following tests: ACAs, LAC, FVL, MTHFR, PC activity, PS activity, ATIII activity, and MTHFR.

Ms. Smith had an ATIII activity of 40.

How do you counsel Ms. Smith?

Ms. Smith has a rare clotting disorder that is one of the most severe. She is at increased risk for blood clots during pregnancy, surgery, or any period of inactivity. She should receive anticoagulation medication for life. She is also at increased risk for recurrent preeclampsia, growth restriction, and placental abruption. Heparin will improve her outcome but cannot guarantee a normal delivery.

How do you treat Ms. Smith?

Ms. Smith should receive full-dose anticoagulation with enoxaparin or unfractionated heparin. Because enoxaparin is easier to use

and associated with less bone loss, enoxaparin is the more reasonable choice.

Ms. Smith is started on enoxaparin 1 mg/kg twice daily by subcutaneous injection.

How do you monitor the Lovenox therapy?

Heparin levels or anti–factor Xa activity should be checked at 22 weeks or every 4–6 weeks. Therapeutic peak levels are 0.5–1.2 at 4 hours after injection. A platelet count should be obtained at initiation of therapy and in 1–2 weeks.

What additional supplementation should you give?

She should receive calcium carbonate 1500 mg and vitamin D supplementation. Serial ultrasounds for fetal growth should be obtained every 4–6 weeks due to the increased risk of intrauterine growth retardation. NSTs should be started at 32 weeks.

Because of the increased risk of placental abruption and other pregnancy complications, amniocentesis for fetal lung maturity should be considered at 37 weeks. Ms. Smith should be switched to unfractionated heparin if she wishes to use regional anesthesia. This should occur at 36 weeks of gestation. Activated PTT should be checked weekly, 4–6 hours after injection. Vaginal delivery should be attempted, but continuous fetal heart rate monitoring should be performed.

Ms. Smith should be referred to a hematologist and should undergo further testing to determine wether she has a functional rather than a qualitative defect. This should be performed 8 weeks after pregnancy. She should not receive hormonal contraception. She should have long-term anticoagulation therapy with warfarin. Her siblings should be tested for ATIII deficiency because it is inherited as autosomal dominant. In addition, her children are at 50% risk and should undergo testing at puberty. There is very little risk of abnormal clotting before puberty.

CASE 2: NULLIPARA WITH A FAMILY HISTORY OF FACTOR V LEIDEN

Ms. Jones is a 35-year-old gravida 1, para 0 who presents at 18 weeks of gestation. Her sister was recently diagnosed with FVL mutation due to a stillbirth at 14 weeks. Ms. Jones underwent testing and also has the mutation.

What historical questions are pertinent?

Did Ms. Jones' sister have a full thrombophilia evaluation and were any other factors positive? Has Ms. Jones ever had a blood clot? Have any of her family members had blood clots, early heart attacks, or early strokes? If they have, were they tested for a thrombophilia?

Ms. Jones states that her sister had a full screen for thrombophilia, but that Ms. Jones was tested only for FVL. Ms. Jones had a blood clot in her leg when she was 18 years old. It occurred 2 months after starting birth control pills. Her father died of a myocardial infarction at age 47 years. He has a sister who had a stroke at age 49 years. However, they were all obese and smoked heavily. These events occurred many years ago, and she is not sure that any testing for thrombophilia was done.

What tests should you order?

You should complete the thrombophilia screen because 12% of patients with a thrombophilia and a history of thrombosis will have a combined defect.

Ms. Jones is also homozygous for MTHFR.

How do you counsel Ms. Smith?

Ms. Jones has two clotting disorders, FVL and MTHFR. Combined with her history of venous thrombosis, these disorders place her at increased risk of a blood clot during pregnancy. She may also be at increased risk for still-birth, placental abruption, and preeclampsia. However, this is debatable.

How do you treat Ms. Smith?

Ms. Jones should receive prophylactic anti-coagulation and folic acid supplementation.

Ms. Smith is started on enoxaparin 40 mg/day.

How do you monitor the enoxaparin therapy?

Heparin levels are not necessary with pro-phylactic anticoagulation. She remains at risk of heparin-induced thrombocytopenia. A platelet count should be obtained at initiation of therapy and at 1–2 weeks.

What additional supplementation should you give?

She should receive calcium carbonate 1500 mg/day and vitamin D supplementation. An ultra-sound for fetal growth should be obtained at 32 weeks. If growth and fluid are normal, it is unclear whether NSTs are needed.

Because of the increased incidence of epidural hematomas in women receiving LMWH, she should be switched to unfraction-ated heparin at 37 weeks. Depending on her size, her dose should be 7500 or 10,000 U twice daily. There is no need for labor induction before term.

Ms. Jones should be told that she is at increased risk for blood clots during high-risk situations such as prolonged inactivity or surgery. Prophylaxis for deep vein thrombosis should be provided. She should also use hor-monal contraception. If she has daughters, their health care providers may wish to test them for FVL before starting them on hor-monal contraception because they are at a 50% risk of inheriting FVL. She should take a mul-tivitamin with folic acid for life. She should be urged to find a primary care physician and share with that person her personal and family history and her thrombophilia test results.

REFERENCES

1 McColl MD, Ramsay JE, Tait RC, et al. Risk factors for pregnancy asso-ciated venous thromboembolism. *Thromb Haemost* 1997;78: 1183–1188.

2 Walker ID. Thrombophilia in pregnancy. *J Clin Pathol* 2000;53: 573–580.

3 Lindqvist P, Dahlback B, Marsal K. Thrombotic risk during preg-nancy: a population study. *Obstet Gynecol* 1996;335:108–114.

4 ACOG Educational Bulletin. Antiphospholipid syndrome. Number 244, February 1998. American College of Obstetricians and Gynecologists. *Int J Gynaecol Obstet* 1998;61:193–202.

5 ACOG Educational Bulletin. Thromboembolism in pregnancy. Number 234, March 1997. American College of Obstetricians and Gynecologists. *Int J Gynaecol Obstet* 1997;57:209–218.

6 Leeda M, Riyazi N, de Vries JI, et al. Effects of folic acid and vitamin B_6 supplementation on women with hyperhomocysteinemia and a history of preeclampsia or fetal growth restriction. *Am J Obstet Gynecol* 179(1):135–9, 1998 Jul.

7 Riyazi N, Leeda M, de Vries JI, Ituijens PC, van Geijn, Dekker GA. Low-molecular-weight heparin combined with aspirin in pregnant women with thrombophilia and a history of preeclampsia or fetal growth restriction: a preliminary study. *Eur J Obstet Gynecol Reprod Biol* 1998;80:49–54.

8 Cowchock FS, Reece EA, Balaban D, et al. Repeated fetal losses associated with antiphospholipid antibodies: a collaborative randomized trial comparing prednisone with low-dose heparin treatment. *Am J Obstet Gynecol* 1992;166:1318–1323.

9 Ginsberg JS, Greer I, Hirsch J. Use of antithrombotic agents during pregnancy. *Chest* 2001;119(suppl):122S–131S.

10 Barbour LA. ACOG Committee on Practice Bulletins—obstetrics. ACOG practice bulletin. Thrombembolism in pregnancy. *Int J Gynaecol Obstet* 2001;75:203–212.

11 Koch P, Munssinger T, Rupp-John C, Uhl K. Delayed-type hypersensitivity skin reactions caused by subcutaneous unfractionated and low-molecular-weight heparins: tolerance of a new recombinant hirudin. *J Am Acad Dermatol* 2000;42:612–619.

12 Horlocker T, Wedel D, Benzon H, et al. Regional anesthesia in the anticoagulated patient: defining the risks (the Second ASRA Consensus Conference on Neuraxial Anesthesia and Anticoagulation). *Reg Anesth Pain Med* 2003;28:172–197.

13 Gris JC, Quere I, Monpeyroux F, et al. Case-control study of the frequency of thrombophilic disorders in couples with late foetal loss and no thrombotic antecedent—the Nimes Obstetricians and Haematologists Study5 (NOHA5). *Thromb Haemost* 1999;81: 891–899.

14 Arias RW, O'Riordan MA. Placental lesions associated with cerebral palsy and neurologic impairment following term birth. *Arch Pathol Lab Med* 2000;124:1785–1791.

15 Roberts D, Schwartz RS. Clotting and hemorrhage in the placenta—a delicate balance. *N Engl J Med* 2002;347:57–59.

16 Sikkema JM, Franx A, Bruinse HW, et al. Placental pathology in early onset pre-eclampsia and intra-uterine growth restriction in women with and without thrombophilia. *Placenta* 2002;23: 337–342.

17 Dizon-Townson DS, Nelsen LM, Jang H, et al. The incidence of factor V Leiden mutation in an obstetric population and its relationship to deep vein thrombosis. *Am J Obstet Gynecol* 1997;176: 883–886.

18 Kovalevsky G, Gracia CR, Berlin JA, et al. Evaluation of the association between hereditary thrombophilias and recurrent pregnancy loss: a meta-analysis. *Arch Intern Med* 2004;164:558–563.

19 Many A, Elad R, Yaron Y, et al. Third-trimester unexplained intrauterine fetal death is associated with inherited thrombophilia. *Obstet Gynecol* 2002;99(5 pt 1):684–687.

20 Kupferminc MJ, Fait G, Many A, et al. Severe preeclampsia and high frequency of genetic thrombophilic mutations. *Obstet Gynecol* 2000; 96:45–49.

21 Paternoster DM, Stella A, Simioni P, et al. Activated protein C resistance in normal and pre-eclamptic pregnancies. *Gynecol Obstet Invest* 2002;54:145–149.

22 Kupferminc MJ, Eldor A, Steinman N, et al. Increased frequency of genetic thrombophilia in women with complications of pregnancy. *N Engl J Med* 1999;340:9–13.

23 Infante-Rivard C, Rivard G-E, Yotov WV, et al. Absence of association of thrombophilia polymorphisms with intrauterine growth restriction. *N Engl J Med* 2002;347:19–25.

24 Kupferminc MJ, Many A, Bar-Am A, et al. Mid-trimester severe intrauterine growth restriction is associated with a high prevalence of thrombophilia. *BJOG* 2002;109:1373–1376.

25 Simioni P, Tormene D, Prandoni P, et al. Incidence of venous thromboembolism in asymptomatic family members who are carriers of factor V Leiden: a prospective cohort study. *Blood* 2002;99: 1938–1942.

26 Kearon C, Crowther M, Hirsh J. Management of Patients with hereditary hypercoagulable disorders. *Annu Rev Med* 2000;51: 169–185.

27 Levine JS, Branch DW, Rauch J. The antiphospholipid syndrome. *N Engl J Med* 2002;346:752–763.

28 Nelson-Piercy C, Letsky EA, de Swiet M. Low-molecular-weight heparin for obstetric thromboprophylaxis: experience of sixty-nine pregnancies in sixty-one women at risk. *Am J Obstet Gynecol* 1997; 176:1062–1068.

29 Dulitzki M, Pauzner R, Langevitz P, et al. Low-molecular-weight heparin during pregnancy and delivery: preliminary experience with 41 pregnancies. *Obstet Gynecol* 1996;87:380–383.

30 Riyazi N, Leeda M, de Vries JI, et al. Low-molecular-weight heparin combined with aspirin in pregnant women with thrombophilia and a history of preeclampsia or fetal growth restriction: a preliminary study. *Eur J Obstet Gynecol Reprod Biol* 1998;80:49–54.

Arrhythmia Assessment and Management

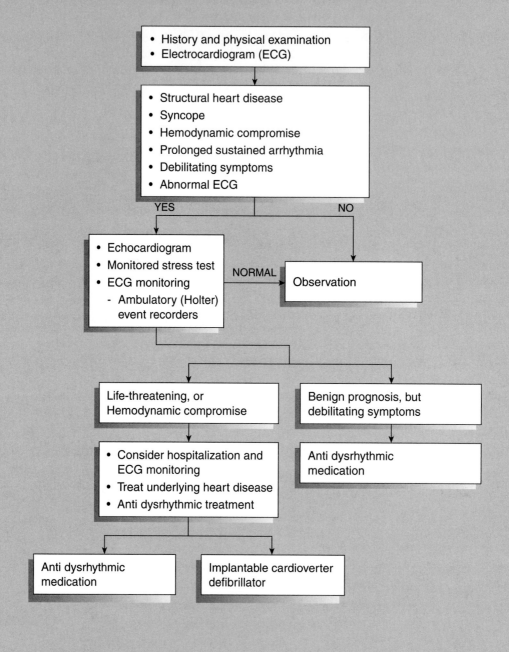

28 Arrhythmias During Pregnancy

Barbara Rackow Gerling

Introduction

Symptoms that may be attributable to cardiac arrhythmias are common during pregnancy. The symptoms and the actual occurrence of arrhythmia may be alarming to the patient and the providers of medical and obstetric care. Fortunately, the vast majority of patients do not have a life-threatening arrhythmia, and most can be treated successfully with minimal therapeutic interventions. Patients with significant heart rhythm disturbances or the potential for a life-threatening arrhythmia or underlying structural heart disease should be cared for by an experienced cardiologist in conjunction with a high-risk obstetric team. The most appropriate term for a cardiac rhythm disturbance is *dysrhythmia*, but the term *arrhythmia* is used most commonly in practice and is used in this chapter.

Implications of Heart Rhythm Disturbances During Pregnancy

KEY POINT

There is no role for empiric treatment. Complete and accurate arrhythmia documentation, diagnosis, and prognostic assessment are mandatory.

Arrhythmias are common in nonpregnant women without heart disease. In a study of 24-hour ambulatory electrocardiographic (ECG) monitoring of 50 healthy women, 88% had atrial or ventricular premature beats.[1] Data regarding the incidence of cardiac arrhythmias during pregnancy are mixed. Some studies have suggested an increased risk, whereas others have not. The prevalence of arrhythmia is higher in women with underlying structural heart disease. Arrhythmia symptoms tend to be more severe during pregnancy.

When evaluating a pregnant woman for real or potential arrhythmias, the health care provider must make a careful assessment of maternal and fetal risks and of maternal symptoms. Most arrhythmias that occur in patients with structurally normal hearts are prognostically benign, although they may be quite bothersome. The most common arrhythmias that occur during pregnancy are atrial or ventricular premature beats and paroxysmal supraventricular tachycardia (SVT). Short runs of nonsustained SVT without symptoms of hemodynamic compromise (e.g., syncope or lightheadedness) or a structurally abnormal heart are unlikely to lead to significant maternal or placental hypoperfusion and fetal compromise. These patients can often be treated with reassurance and instruction in the use of vagal maneuvers to terminate the sustained tachycardias. Treatment is indicated only for the amelioration of symptoms.

Some arrhythmias are directly life threatening or are markers of increased risk of mortality and syncope. In general, high-risk arrhythmias occur in patients with underlying structural heart disease. Sustained tachycardia or syncope in the setting of structural heart disease is more likely to be ventricular tachycardia, atrial fibrillation, or atrial flutter, which requires intervention. Patients with a severe cardiomyopathy or congenital heart disease with decreased ventricular function are at highest risk for sudden cardiac death and syncope when ventricular arrhythmias are present. Electrophysiologic substrates that are associated with an increased risk of sudden death without structural heart disease include the long QT syndrome (LQTS), Brugada's syndrome, and Wolff-Parkinson-White (WPW) syndrome, which is rare. Identification of patients with high-risk arrhythmias is important, and treatment of these women is essential.

Data obtained from a comprehensive history (Table 28-1) can elucidate the mechanism of the heart rhythm disturbance and the prognosis associated with the arrhythmia. Palpitations that are described as skipped beats without sustained rapid heart rhythms are often premature atrial or ventricular beats and are unlikely to be worrisome. Irregular rapid palpitations are often associated with atrial fibrillation. Sustained tachycardia is usually a supraventricular arrhythmia but may be found to be a more serious ventricular arrhythmia or atrial fibrillation. A careful cardiac history including the potential for structural heart disease is critical. A family history of sudden death may indicate an increased risk of inherited disorders that predispose to life-threatening ventricular arrhythmias.

Careful objective evaluation is also necessary (Table 28-2). A complete physical examination to ascertain the presence of

Table 28-1. HISTORY

Skipped beats
Sustained rapid heart rate
Duration of symptoms
Syncope history
Associated symptoms such a lightheadedness, shortness of breath,
  exercise intolerance
Initiating triggers and terminating influences
Character of the onset and termination of the palpitations or
  arrhythmia: sudden or gradual
History of structural heart disease: congenital heart disease,
  valvular heart disease, cardiomyopathies, coronary heart disease
Symptoms suggestive of structural heart disease: dyspnea,
  orthopnea, paroxysmal nocturnal dyspnea, edema, exercise
  intolerance, chest discomfort
Family history of heart disease, arrhythmia, sudden cardiac death
Previous arrhythmia and assessments

structural heart disease and a 12-lead electrocardiogram at rest to identify potential arrhythmia substrates are required for all patients with syncope or arrhythmia symptoms. Further testing with prolonged ECG monitoring, echocardiography, and even stress testing should be used for any patient with significant or sustained symptoms or examination findings suggestive of cardiopulmonary limitation or disease. Specific arrhythmia identification can be accomplished by outpatient 24- or 48-hour ambulatory ECG monitoring (Holter monitor), month-long transient-event monitors or loop recorders for less frequent symptoms, and inpatient telemetric monitoring.

Table 28-2. OBJECTIVE ASSESSMENT

Physical examination
Resting heart rate and blood pressure, oxygen saturation
Jugular venous pressure
Pulmonary rales
Heart murmur, gallops, rubs, thrills, heaves
Edema
Peripheral pulses

Diagnostic testing
Electrocardiogram
Echocardiogram
Stress testing
Ambulatory electrocardiographic monitoring (Holter monitoring,
  event recorder, inpatient telemetry monitoring)

Arrhythmias may have unfavorable maternal and fetal prognostic implications, and treatment may result in adverse outcomes. As a consequence, empiric arrhythmia therapy has no role in pregnant patients. However, when necessary, there should be no hesitation in initiating antiarrhythmic therapy with knowledge of the specific arrhythmia substrate and which drugs or interventions are appropriate.

Specific Arrhythmia and Treatment Strategies

ARRHYTHMIA MECHANISMS

The metabolic, hormonal, and hemodynamic changes that occur during pregnancy can lead to aggravation of preexisting structural heart disease and alterations of the electrophysiologic substrate. These alterations can result in the new appearance or exacerbation of previous arrhythmias.

Arrhythmias are most commonly classified by the chamber of origin, ventricular or supraventricular, which is often identified by the appearance of the electrocardiogram. A narrow QRS complex generally originates in the atrium or atrioventricular junction. A wide QRS complex may originate in the ventricle or may be an aberrantly conducted or preexcited supraventricular beat. Arrhythmias may arise from an irritable focus or be the result of one or more circular loops of electrical activity (reentrant).

SPECIFIC ARRHYTHMIA AND SYMPTOM COMPLEXES

PALPITATIONS

KEY POINT

The need for therapy should be strong. The decision to treat should be guided by the maternal and fetal consequences of the arrhythmia and the severity of symptoms.

Palpitations may be described as an awareness of an abnormal beating of the heart and are a common cause for concern among patients. In a controlled study of symptomatic pregnant women compared with asymptomatic controls, there was no difference in arrhythmia occurrence between groups (56% vs. 58%).[2] In addition only 10% of the reported symptoms were associated with the presence of any arrhythmia. The majority of the ectopy was ventricular and supraventricular premature beats that, in structurally normal hearts, are benign. Therefore, the primary goal for management of these patients with palpitations and atrial or ventricular premature beats is reassurance and avoidance of triggers such as caffeine, smoking, and alcohol. If the ectopy is associated with an arrhythmia and is bothersome enough to warrant treatment, β-adrenergic antagonists may be helpful. However, it is worth noting that it is often difficult to eradicate all atrial or ventricular premature beats and render these patients entirely asymptomatic.

SYNCOPE

Syncope and presyncope (lightheadedness) are common reasons for referral of pregnant patients to a cardiologist. Different physiologic changes during a normal pregnancy contribute to an increased risk of syncope. Although the most likely cause of syncope during pregnancy is postural or neurocardiogenic syncope, the potential for life-threatening conditions is a real concern. LQTS, Brugada's syndrome, arrhythmogenic right ventricular dysplasia (ARVD), and ventricular arrhythmias associated with structural heart disease are potential mechanisms of syncope that may be life threatening. Structural heart disease without arrhythmia may also cause syncope. Aortic stenosis, pulmonary hypertension, and pulmonary emboli are dangerous and should be considered. As a consequence, all pregnant patients with syncope require a complete history, physical examination, and evaluation for underlying structural heart disease or high-risk electrophysiologic substrates (Table 28-3).

SUPRAVENTRICULAR TACHYCARDIA

SVTs are rarely associated with an increased risk of cardiac arrest or syncope. Prolonged periods of a rapid rhythm of any mechanism may lead to a tachycardia-induced cardiomyopathy and subsequent congestive heart failure. Fortunately, the left ventricular dysfunction associated with this cardiomyopathy is often reversible simply by controlling the heart rate, whether or not the tachycardia is terminated. SVT may be a trigger for syncope in women prone to neurocardiogenic syncope but is rarely the sole cause of syncope. A small percentage of patients with WPW syndrome have a rapidly conducting accessory pathway that may increase the risk of ventricular fibrillation in the setting of concomitant atrial fibrillation or flutter. Paroxysmal SVTs are the most common sustained arrhythmia in pregnant patients with normal hearts, followed by focal atrial tachycardias. Atrial fibrillation and flutter are quite uncommon in the absence of structural heart disease.

ATRIOVENTRICULAR NODAL REENTRANT TACHYCARDIA AND ATRIOVENTRICULAR RECIPROCATING TACHYCARDIA The most common SVTs are caused by reentry (or circular conduction of the electrical impulse) involving the normal atrioventricular (AV) node. AV nodal reentrant tachycardia (AVNRT) is characterized by conduction down one pathway and return by another pathway within or near the AV node. The electrocardiogram in the absence of SVT is generally normal. The tachycardia is characterized by

Table 28-3. **EVALUATION OF THE PATIENT WITH SYNCOPE**

SYMPTOM/SIGN	DIAGNOSTIC CONSIDERATIONS	FURTHER TESTING
Triggers		
Stress	Neurocardiogenic	
Standing	syncope	
Exercise recovery	Orthostatic syncope	
Fear/pain		
Family history		
Syncope	Brugada's syndrome	Electrocardiogram
Sudden death	Long QT syndrome	Echocardiogram
	Cardiomyopathy	Ambulatory electrocardio-
	ARVD	graphic monitoring
		Cardiology consultation
Structural heart disease		
Heart failure	Valvular heart	Electrocardiogram
Exercise	disease	Echocardiogram
intolerance	Cardiomyopathy	Ambulatory electrocardio-
Murmur	Congenital heart	graphic monitoring
	disease	Cardiology consultation
	Life-threatening	Stress testing
	arrhythmia	
	Coronary heart	
	disease	
Palpitations		
Prolonged	Structural heart	Electrocardiogram
Irregular	disease	Echocardiogram
	Long QT syndrome	Ambulatory electrocardio-
	Brugada's syndrome	graphic monitoring
	Cardiomyopathy	Cardiology consultation
	ARVD	
Neurologic signs		
Postictal phase	Seizure	Neurologic consultation
Focal neurologic	Eclampsia	Electroencephalogram
Findings	Cerebrovascular	Magnetic resonance
	disease	imaging/computed
		tomogram

sudden onset and termination of palpitations, with heart rates in the range of 150–250 beats/min. The electrocardiogram during SVT displays a narrow QRS complex often without a discernible P wave because atrial and ventricular activations occur nearly simultaneously.

AV reciprocating tachycardia (AVRT) is usually characterized by antegrade conduction down the normal AV node and retrograde conduction up an accessory pathway. This extra pathway is composed of specialized conduction tissue that connects the atrium and ventricle most commonly on the left side of the heart but has been reported to occur at any site along the AV groove. AVRT also starts and stops suddenly and cannot be distinguished from AVNRT based on symptoms. The ECG in sinus rhythm may be normal (the pathway is concealed) or may show the delta wave characteristic of WPW syndrome (the pathway is overt).

ECG findings for WPW syndrome is notable for a PR interval shorter than 120 ms, the presence of a delta wave (a slurred, slowly rising onset of the QRS complex), and a QRS duration longer than 120 ms. During AVRT the P wave is often inverted in the inferior leads (II, III, aVF) and located beyond the end of the QRS. The accessory pathway, when overt, may conduct rapidly and result in a very rapid ventricular response to atrial fibrillation or flutter with a wide and alarming QRS complex. This wide QRS complex is termed *preexcited* because the ventricles are activated early by the pathway before normal AV nodal conduction can occur. In addition, in rare instances, the accessory pathway may participate in AVRT as the antegrade limb conducting to the ventricles with the normal AV node functioning as the retrograde limb conducting back to the atria. In this instance, the ECG will demonstrate a wide complex QRS tachycardia that may be difficult to distinguish from ventricular tachycardia.

ATRIAL TACHYCARDIA Atrial tachycardia is uncommon in pregnant and nonpregnant women. It is a regular tachycardia that originates in the right or left atrium with an atrial activation sequence that is different from normal, resulting in a P-wave morphology that is different from the P wave of normal sinus rhythm. Onset and termination may be gradual or sudden, with a heart rate of 100–250 beats/min. During the tachycardia, P waves are usually distinctly noted. In nonpregnant women, atrial tachycardia is often associated with structural heart disease; however, in pregnant patients, it seems to occur without cardiac pathology.[3] It may be persistent and refractory to medical treatment. In reported cases, the arrhythmia has not been associated with significant adverse maternal or fetal outcomes, and most tachycardias disappeared after delivery.

ACUTE TREATMENT OF SUPRAVENTRICULAR TACHYCARDIA   Acute episodes of paroxysmal SVT are generally well tolerated by the mother and fetus and are approached in the same manner as for nonpregnant patients (Table 28-4). Vagal maneuvers (carotid sinus massage, Valsalva) should be attempted first because these interventions slow AV nodal conduction and may terminate tachycardias that include the AV node as part of the reentrant pathway. If vagal maneuvers are unsuccessful, the first drug of choice is adenosine, a purine-based nucleoside that decreases sinus node automaticity and slows AV nodal conduction. Adenosine is preferred to β-adrenergic blockers or verapamil because it has a rapid onset of action with a very short half-life (<10 seconds). If adenosine fails to terminate the arrhythmia but AV block occurs, then the mechanism is most likely atrial tachycardia, atrial fibrillation, or atrial flutter that does not require conduction through the AV node for continuation of the tachycardia. Atrial tachyarrhythmias are often unresponsive to β-adrenergic blockade, verapamil, and digoxin, and more potent antiarrhythmic agents are often required. Because atrial tachyarrhythmias rarely cause hemodynamic compromise, intravenous antiarrhythmic agents are not recommended. In the rare instance when hemodynamic compromise is present, rapid termination of the arrhythmia is mandatory with adenosine or sedation and electrical cardioversion. The tachyarrhythmia may lead not only to maternal compromise but also to fetal distress.

LONG-TERM TREATMENT OF SUPRAVENTRICULAR TACHYCARDIA   Patients with paroxysmal SVT caused by reentry usually have normal hearts and tolerate occasional short episodes of tachycardia without

Table 28-4.   **ACUTE TREATMENT OF SUPRAVENTRICULAR TACHYCARDIA**

General approach is similar to usual guidelines outside pregnancy
For a well-tolerated regular supraventricular tachycardia
Vagal maneuvers (Valsalva, carotid sinus massage)
Adenosine 6 mg intravenously followed by 12–18 mg intravenously if
  no response given near central circulation with a rapid fluid bolus
Intravenous β-adrenergic blockers, verapamil, digoxin
For hemodynamically significant supraventricular tachycardia
Sedation and direct-current cardioversion

---

maternal or fetal consequences. Hence, long-term suppressive drug therapy is not recommended, and reassurance is offered instead. In the rare patient with frequent, prolonged, or poorly tolerated SVT, long-term suppressive therapy should be considered. In the pregnant patient, β-adrenergic blockade, verapamil, or digoxin are recommended as first-line intervention. If arrhythmia continues postpartum, and certainly if future pregnancies are considered, then curative therapy with catheter ablation should be considered.

ATRIAL FIBRILLATION AND FLUTTER Atrial fibrillation and flutter in the absence of structural heart disease or endocrine abnormalities are rare in a young population. Therefore, all patients should have a complete evaluation with not only a comprehensive history and physical examination but also a full laboratory examination looking for thyroid and lung diseases and cardiac imaging with echocardiography to evaluate unrecognized cardiac pathology. Typical atrial flutter is characterized by an organized, rapid, atrial activation that has a sawtooth pattern on the ECG. The atrial rate is usually 250–350 beats/min with 2:1 AV conduction resulting in a ventricular response of 150 beats/min. Atrial fibrillation is marked by chaotic and disorganized atrial activation at 350–600 beats/min that results in the absence of clear P waves on the ECG and a characteristic rapid, "irregularly irregular" ventricular activation. The ventricular response to atrial fibrillation is often slower than the heart rate with atrial flutter.

The clinical presentation of atrial fibrillation and flutter depends on the presence or absence of underlying heart disease. Patients without heart disease are often bothered by palpitations and, occasionally, chest discomfort and dyspnea. Atrial fibrillation or flutter may lead to congestive heart failure and significant hemodynamic compromise in patients with structural heart disease, especially those patients who have mitral or aortic stenosis or ventricular hypertrophy and are dependent on the contribution of atrial contraction to ventricular filling and cardiac output. Although not associated with an increased risk of cardiac arrest, persistent atrial fibrillation and flutter (>48 hours in duration) are associated with an increased risk of stroke in patients with concomitant diabetes, structural heart disease, or hypertension.

ACUTE TREATMENT OF ATRIAL FIBRILLATION OR FLUTTER   The immediate goal in the acute intervention of atrial fibrillation or flutter is
slowing of the ventricular response. This is most rapidly accomplished by cautious intravenous administration of β-adrenergic
blockers. Verapamil may be considered, although it is a potent
vasodilator and negative inotropic agent and may precipitate
hypotension and heart failure in patients with structural heart disease. Intravenous digoxin may also be considered; however, the
onset of action is hours, which is often too long to be practical. If
the duration of atrial fibrillation or flutter has been shorter than 48
hours, the risk of stroke is low, and cardioversion should be considered to avoid the need for long-term anticoagulation. For atrial
fibrillation or flutter longer than 48 hours in duration in the absence
of anticoagulation, the risk of stroke is 5% with cardioversion.
Acute rate control is indicated, followed by a decision to accept the
arrhythmia and anticoagulate patients with risk factors for stroke
or attempt cardioversion after appropriate anticoagulation to prevent stroke. Current guidelines[4] for all patients with atrial fibrillation or flutter suggest at least 3 weeks of fully therapeutic
anticoagulation or cardioversion under transesophageal guidance
to assess the left atrium for thrombus.[4] Anticoagulation is continued for at least 1 month after cardioversion in all patients. There
are no data to support the use of unfractionated heparin or other
anticoagulants other than warfarin in the prevention of stroke associated with atrial fibrillation or flutter. The use of warfarin during
pregnancy is associated not only with an increased risk of bleeding but also with fetal coagulopathy and embryopathy, especially
when used during the first trimester. As a consequence, the best
approach is rapid cardioversion. If hemodynamic compromise is
present, cardioversion is indicated regardless of the duration of
atrial fibrillation.

LONG-TERM TREATMENT OF ATRIAL FIBRILLATION OR FLUTTER   Because
of the uncertainties of anticoagulation in the pregnant patient,
suppression of atrial fibrillation and flutter should be strongly
considered, although the strategy of rhythm control has never been
shown to decrease the risk of stroke. Maintenance of sinus rhythm
can be accomplished by repeated cardioversions, as needed. β-
Adrenergic blockers and verapamil are not likely to be successful

but can be tried to avoid the small but potential side effect of inducing undesirable arrhythmias with antiarrhythmic medications. Often more potent antiarrhythmic agents such as quinidine or flecainide are necessary. Aggressive therapy for any underlying medical or cardiopulmonary disease is mandatory. Postpartum, ablation may be considered, but the success rate for cure is less than that achieved with AVNRT or AV reciprocating tachycardias.

VENTRICULAR TACHYCARDIA

Ventricular tachycardia originates below the AV node and the His bundle in the specialized conduction system of the ventricles or in the ventricular myocardium itself. It is manifested as a sequence of three or more wide QRS complexes at a rate of at least 120 beats/min. The arrhythmia may be regular or irregular, and the QRS morphology may be monomorphic or polymorphic. Although ventricular tachycardia may be benign in young individuals without heart disease, the presence of even nonsustained short runs of ventricular tachycardia may be a marker of an increased risk of maternal mortality, especially in the presence of structural heart disease or cardiomyopathy.

LONG QT SYNDROME LQTS is a congenital and often familial condition with multiple, recently defined, genetic markers. It is notable for prolonged myocardial repolarization that is often manifested on the resting sinus rhythm ECG as a long QT interval. The ventricular tachycardia is polymorphic with changing heart rate and QRS morphologies and is traditionally labeled *torsades de pointes*. There are specific criteria that are used to make the diagnosis of LQTS.[5] Of note, cardiac function is often normal. Despite normal cardiac function, these patients are at increased risk for sudden cardiac death and require careful evaluation. One study found that cardiac events, defined as the combined incidence of LQTS related death, aborted cardiac arrest, and syncope, were significantly increased in LQTS pregnancies, especially in the 40-week postpartum period, with an event rate of 23.4%.[6] The investigators also reported that β-adrenergic blockade significantly decreases this risk.

IDIOPATHIC VENTRICULAR TACHYCARDIA Fortunately, the most common cause of ventricular arrhythmias in pregnant patients is idiopathic ventricular tachycardia, which is not associated with underlying structural heart disease. These ventricular arrhythmias are often discovered incidentally during evaluations for other issues but may be associated with palpitations and, occasionally, intermittent lightheadedness. Idiopathic ventricular tachycardia is a benign condition that may be associated with syncope in rare instances but is unlikely to lead to cardiac arrest and death.

ACUTE TREATMENT OF VENTRICULAR TACHYCARDIA Although sudden death is, fortunately, rare, patients with ventricular tachycardia require emergent evaluation and treatment. Hospital admission and maternal and fetal monitoring are mandatory. In patients with hemodynamic compromise and sustained ventricular tachycardia, cardiopulmonary resuscitation as needed and sedation and electrical cardioversion should be rapidly employed. When maternal compromise is not a concern, more leisurely termination of sustained tachycardias may be accomplished with intravenous β blockers, lidocaine, procainamide, quinidine, or amiodarone administered in the same doses used in nonpregnant patients. Acute administration of verapamil should be avoided because it has been associated with hemodynamic collapse and cardiac arrest in nonpregnant patients, likely due in part to its vasodilatory effects.

LONG-TERM TREATMENT OF VENTRICULAR TACHYCARDIA Treatment is determined by maternal prognosis and the presence of underlying heart disease. Ventricular arrhythmias may be associated with significant risk independent of pregnancy or may be exacerbated by pregnancy, and therapy may adversely affect the fetus. The long-term maternal prognosis should be carefully considered in the decision to become pregnant and the decision to terminate pregnancy. However, if high-risk ventricular arrhythmias are identified during the pregnancy, there should be no hesitation to initiate aggressive treatment.

Antiarrhythmic therapy should be considered in patients with significant symptoms or sustained ventricular arrhythmias with or without structural heart disease. Patients with significant cardiac pathology should have their underlying heart disease aggressively optimized. Implantable cardioverter-defibrillators (ICDs) may be implanted under echocardiographic guidance in pregnant patients.

ICDs have been shown to decrease mortality in nonpregnant patients with ischemic cardiomyopathies and low ejection fractions, although the benefit in nonischemic substrates is less clear. Assessment of arrhythmia substrate and treatment success may be guided by prolonged ECG monitoring (in-hospital telemetry and subsequent outpatient Holter monitoring) and stress testing. Women with LQTS should be aggressively treated with β-adrenergic blockade at the maximally tolerated dose with consideration for ICD implantation. Patients with idiopathic ventricular arrhythmias often are successfully treated with β-adrenergic blockers, verapamil, and, occasionally, more potent antiarrhythmic agents such as quinidine or flecainide.

BRADYCARDIA AND CONGENITAL AV BLOCK

Symptomatic bradyarrhythmias in pregnancy are uncommon because the heart rate normally increases by 10–20 beats/min during pregnancy. Most often, bradycardia during pregnancy is related to congenital complete heart block. Patients with symptomatic congenital complete heart block, a prolonged QT interval, or a wide complex escape rhythm usually have already received a pacemaker. Pregnancy is generally well tolerated in patients who have asymptomatic or previously undiagnosed complete heart block. Labor and delivery may be associated with increased vagal tone and slowing of the heart rate during Valsalva. Temporary transvenous or external pacing has been employed successfully. Successful pacemaker implants during pregnancy using electrocardiographic or echocardiographic guidance have been described.

Treatment Modalities

All therapeutic interventions have the potential for adverse outcomes. When intervening in a pregnant woman, the potential complications affect not only the mother but also the fetus. However, it is essential to administer necessary drugs or use required interventions in the pregnant woman to protect the mother and optimize fetal outcome. No woman should receive suboptimal medical care simply because she is pregnant.

MEDICATIONS

Most antiarrhythmic agents are considered category C, which denotes the absence of controlled studies in animals or humans, or animal studies that suggest potential risk, but no confirmation in human studies. Amiodarone and atenolol are exceptions and are labeled category D. Experience with the different antiarrhythmic agents varies widely. In general, the agents that have been available the longest, digoxin and quinidine, have the best safety data. When considering use of medications, it is also important to consider the metabolic and hemodynamic changes associated with pregnancy because these alterations may affect the dosing of medications. Dosing must be titrated to not only drug levels but also the desired clinical therapeutic effect. Due to potential changes in maternal pharmacokinetics, maternal complications, and adverse fetal effects, it is recommended to use the fewest drugs at the lowest effective dose. However, there should be no hesitation to intervene with pharmacologic therapy when needed. Clearly, the successful outcome of pregnancy is dependent on the use of necessary therapy to protect the mother.

β BLOCKERS

In general, β blockers are easy to titrate and have a wide safety margin. The likelihood of inducing undesirable arrhythmias is exceedingly low. The main side effects associated with β blockers are bradycardia, hypotension, and bronchospasm. β Blockers are negative inotropic drugs and may worsen cardiac function in patients with already compromised ventricular function. β-Adrenergic blockers are classified as category C, with the exception of atenolol, which has been associated with growth retardation in babies when exposed to atenolol even during the first trimester[7] and is a category D agent. The main adverse fetal effect associated with β-blocker use has been intrauterine growth restriction. Neonatal manifestations include delayed onset of spontaneous respiration, hypoglycemia, hypotonia, and bradycardia.[8] Use of cardioselective $β_1$ antagonists, such as metoprolol, is recommended because they are less likely to interfere with $β_2$-mediated uterine relaxation and peripheral vasodilatation. In general, administration of metoprolol and other β-adrenergic antagonists is considered safe in pregnancy.

CALCIUM CHANNEL BLOCKERS

Verapamil and diltiazem block the calcium channel in cardiac tissue and slow or block conduction through the AV node. They are primarily used in the management of supraventricular arrhythmia but are occasionally used in the management of idiopathic ventricular tachycardia. Verapamil has been used to control arrhythmias and hypertension in pregnant women and has not been associated with significant fetal abnormalities. In general, calcium blockers appear safe in the management of arrhythmia during pregnancy; however, due to limited data on calcium antagonists, β blockers are preferred as first-line therapy.

DIGOXIN

Digoxin has long been safely used in the management of supraventricular arrhythmias. It is less effective than β blockade or calcium blockade and as a consequence is not considered the first choice in nonpregnant women. Due to increased renal digoxin excretion during pregnancy, drug levels may decrease by as much as half. During the later stages of pregnancy, the measured digoxin levels may be falsely high due to circulating digoxin-like substances.[8] Digoxin dose requirement is generally increased during pregnancy.

ADENOSINE

Adenosine is an endogenous purine nucleoside that has an extremely short half-life (<10 seconds). It is a potent blocker of AV conduction and is used in the acute termination of SVT and the rare idiopathic ventricular tachycardia. It may cause minor maternal bradycardia and dyspnea that are short-lived. It may also induce maternal bronchospasm, particularly patients with asthma. There have been no reports of teratogenicity or fetal toxicity when used during pregnancy, although the data are limited. Because of its extremely short half-life, toxicity is unlikely, and it is considered the drug of first choice for terminating supraventricular arrhythmias that include the AV node when vagal maneuvers have failed.

ATROPINE

Atropine is a potent vagolytic agent and has been used in the acute management of bradycardia and vagal reflex activation. It rapidly crosses the placenta and may result in transient fetal tachycardia and loss of beat-to-beat variation.[9]

ANTIARRHYTHMIC DRUGS

More potent antiarrhythmic drugs with direct cardiac ion channel effects are also used in the management of maternal arrhythmia. Because they are also associated with a small but present risk of promoting an arrhythmia (proarrhythmia), their use is generally restricted to patients with life-threatening arrhythmias or patients whose therapy with simpler medications such as β-adrenergic blockers, calcium blockers, or digoxin has failed. Initiation of these drugs should be performed in the hospital with continuous ECG monitoring.

LIDOCAINE   Lidocaine is available only in the intravenous form and is used only for short-term termination and prevention of ventricular arrhythmias, in addition to its use as an anesthetic agent. It is not known to have teratogenic effects, but it may increase myometrial tone, decrease placental blood flow, and cause fetal bradycardia.[8] It is recommended to avoid lidocaine during prolonged labor or fetal distress because fetal acidosis can lead to higher free drug concentrations and fetal neurologic or cardiac toxicity.

QUINIDINE   Quinidine has the longest history of safety during pregnancy. It may be used to control refractory supraventricular arrhythmias but is used less often to manage ventricular arrhythmias due to the development of newer agents. Although rare reports of fetal thrombocytopenia, crania nerve VIII palsy, and potentiation of uterine contractions have been published, quinidine is considered safe for use during pregnancy. Its use must be carefully monitored with trough plasma levels and periodic electrocardiography.

AMIODARONE   Amiodarone is often considered the most efficacious antiarrhythmic drug and one of the drugs least likely to promote undesirable arrhythmias. Amiodarone has cardiac and noncardiac side effects, making it a drug that requires careful monitoring by experienced physicians. Amiodarone has a high iodine content that crosses the placenta and has a high affinity for the neonatal thyroid. It has resulted in neonatal goiter and hypo- and hyperthyroidism.[10] In addition, neonatal bradycardia and QT prolongation, low birth weight, premature birth, and death, and mildly impaired cognitive development have been reported. As a consequence, amiodarone has been classified as category D, and its use should be reserved for life-threatening arrhythmia therapy without alternatives.

OTHER ANTIARRHYTHMIC DRUGS   Limited data exist about the use in pregnancy of other much less commonly used antiarrhythmic drugs. These agents include procainamide, flecainide, propafenone, sotalol, dofetilide, and ibutilide. Decisions about their use should take into consideration any evidence that exists about safety in pregnancy and the potential use of effective medications that have been on the market a relatively long time.

CARDIOVERSION

Electrical cardioversion has been performed successfully and repeatedly during all stages of pregnancy, with no evidence of fetal compromise.[11] It is important to monitor the mother and fetus for adverse effects. Initiation of arrhythmias is a known risk of cardioversion. The risk of inducing fetal arrhythmia is small because the current density reaching the fetus is insignificant, and the fetus has a high fibrillation threshold.

PACEMAKERS AND IMPLANTABLE CARDIOVERTER-DEFIBRILLATORS

When indicated, devices have been successfully implanted under echocardiographic or ECG guidance. The outcomes of pregnancies in patients with previously implanted pacemakers or defibrillators depend on the underlying heart disease and not the presence of the device. Patients without structural heart disease do well. A multicenter retrospective analysis of 44 pregnant patients who had a previously implanted defibrillator found that pregnancy did not increase the number of ICD-related complications or result in a large number of ICD discharges.[12]

ABLATION

Radiofrequency catheter ablation has become first-line management for many supraventricular arrhythmias. It is generally performed under fluoroscopic guidance to position catheters and guide the ablation and, hence, should be considered only for the extremely rare, hemodynamically significant arrhythmias that are not controlled pharmacologically during pregnancy. Women who have symptomatic arrhythmias may consider ablation before pregnancy to decrease the chance that pharmacologic therapy might be necessary.

CARDIOPULMONARY RESUSCITATION

Cardiac arrest is rare during pregnancy and occurs in 1 in 30,000 births.[11] A cardiovascular emergency in a pregnant woman is marked by a special situation, i.e., the presence of the fetus. Emergency cesarean section has the best chance of improving outcome for mother and fetus and should be considered early in the management of cardiovascular collapse.[13] The gravid uterus may result in compression of the iliac and abdominal vessels when the mother is in the supine position, resulting in decreased venous return to the heart, decreased cardiac output, and hypotension.

Guidelines outlining issues associated with pregnancy have been published recently.[13] In essence, the approach to a pregnant woman in cardiac arrest is unchanged from standard Basic and Advanced Life Support guidelines, except to consider the effect of the gravid uterus and the need to resuscitate the fetus. Aortocaval compression should be relieved by manually displacing the gravid uterus or by using wedge-shaped cushions, overturned chairs, a rescuer's thighs, or commercially available foam-cushion wedges to accomplish left lateral tilt. Chest compressions should be performed higher on the sternum to adjust for the upward displacement of pelvic and abdominal contents. There are no modifications to the standard Advanced Life Support algorithms for medications, intubation, and defibrillation. The decision to perform emergency cesarean section should be considered early in the course of the cardiac arrest intervention. The goal is to deliver the fetus within 4–5 minutes after onset of arrest. Clearly, the decision to perform a cesarean section is a difficult one. Cesarean section removes a significant hemodynamic burden on the mother and allows direct resuscitation on the newborn. The timing of cesarean section is guided by the likelihood of rapid and successful maternal resuscitation with "simple" interventions such as direct cardioversion balanced against the need to begin measures to resuscitate the infant. The longer maternal resuscitative efforts fail, the less likely resuscitation will result in maternal or fetal survival without any long-term sequelae. The best chance for the unborn child lies in successful resuscitation of the mother. Resuscitation may depend on emergency cesarean section. In the setting of cardiac arrest, anesthesia is not required, and minimal preparation is necessary. There will not be blood loss. Clinicians—who are not surgeons have no obligation to perform this procedure.

What's the Evidence?

There are no specific controlled trials of management of heart rate abnormalities in pregnant women. Retrospective studies have provided some insight into the prevalence, type, and severity of rhythm disorders in pregnant women. Choices of medications are based on combinations of those used by the general population and known or presumed adverse effects in pregnancy.

Guiding Questions in Approaching the Patient

Assessing the arrhythmia

- Is structural heart disease present?
- Is a high-risk electrophysiologic substrate present?
- How bothersome are the symptoms?
- What are the maternal and fetal consequences of the arrhythmia?
- What is the arrhythmia burden, i.e., how often does the arrhythmia occur and how long does it last?
- How can the arrhythmia mechanism be determined?

Treating the arrhythmia

- What is the risk of the arrhythmia to the mother and fetus?
- How severe are the symptoms?
- What are the risks of the therapeutic options to the mother and fetus?
- What is the least invasive intervention?
- What therapy should be offered after delivery in anticipation of future pregnancies?

Conclusion

While cardiac symptoms are common in pregnancy, arrhythmias are not. Those arrhythmias with poor prognosis and those which are difficult to manage are quite uncommon. An accurate diagnosis is needed before any therapy is initiated. Patients with significant arrhythmias, especially if seen in conjunction with structural heart disease, should be managed with the assistance of a cardiologist. Many medications are acceptable during pregnancy, but therapeutic choices will need to be made on an individual basis taking into consideration the gestational age, severity of symptoms, and risks of specific medications.

Discussion of Cases

CASE 1: PATIENT WITH A PAST HISTORY OF INTERMITTENT DYSRHYTHMIA

A 29-year-old woman was previously seen for evaluation of frequent fast heart rhythms during her first pregnancy. She had a nearly life-long history of an intermittent rapid heart rhythm. Previous evaluation included a normal resting electrocardiogram and a 24-hour ambulatory ECG monitor that showed occasional episodes of non-sustained (5–30 beats) atrial tachycardia at 130–150 beats/min. She was aware of palpitations but was not particularly bothered by the arrhythmia, so treatment was never undertaken. At 18 weeks of gestation, she was referred for very frequent and short runs of a rapid pulse leading to an average heart rate of 120 beats/min discovered on physical examination.

What data would you obtain at this time?

A comprehensive history and physical examination should look for evidence of structural heart disease or hemodynamic compromise potentially related to the arrhythmia.

Her history elicited decreasing exercise tolerance, dyspnea on exertion, orthopnea, nocturia, and occasional lightheadedness, all of which she attributed to her pregnancy. She had no history of syncope. She was taking only prenatal vitamins. Physical examination was notable for a blood pressure of 86/50 mm Hg, an irregular heart rate of 115 beats/min, and very frequent short runs of a rapid rhythm spaced by only a few beats at a normal heart rate. Jugular venous pressure was high. Her carotid and peripheral pulse amplitudes were normal. Lung examination showed dullness at both bases, with occasional inspiratory crackles. Cardiac examination was notable for normal S_1 and S_2 heart sounds, but she had a soft S_3 gallop and a soft systolic murmur at the left sternal border and apex. She had significant ankle edema.

What laboratory evaluation would you order?

Complete blood cell count, chemistries, and thyroid function; electrocardiogram; echocardiogram; and 24-hour ambulatory ECG monitor.

Laboratory evaluation showed a hemoglobin level of 9.8 g/dL, sodium level of 133 mmol/L, and potassium level of 3.9 mmol/L. Her renal, liver, and thyroid test results were normal. Electrocardiogram displayed rare normal sinus beats with frequent runs of an irregular atrial tachycardia at 130 beats/min. She had nonspecific ST and T wave abnormalities. The 24-hour ambulatory ECG monitoring disclosed an average heart rate of 123 beats/min with rare normal beats separating frequent runs of atrial tachycardia lasting 5–84 beats at 130–160 beats/min. Echocardiography showed four-chamber dilatation, poor left ventricular function, and a left ventricular ejection fraction of 20% (normal >55%). All four valves were anatomically normal, but she had moderately severe mitral regurgitation, likely related to the left ventricular dilatation.

What are the implications of the atrial tachycardia and cardiomyopathy?

The patient clearly has congestive heart failure with an associated SVT. It is possible that she had a preexisting cardiomyopathy that was exacerbated by her pregnancy and resulted in stimulation of atrial tachycardia. Conversely, it is possible that she had a chronic atrial tachycardia substrate that was exacerbated by her pregnancy, leading to a tachycardia-induced cardiomyopathy. The implications are important because the short- and long-term maternal prognoses are limited if she had a primary cardiomyopathy. In contrast, if she had a tachycardia-induced cardiomyopathy, her heart failure may be reversible and her prognosis good. The distinction was important because termination of pregnancy was being considered.

What is the recommendation for initial management?

Rapid control of heart rate with pharmacologic therapy and reassessment of ventricular function to distinguish tachycardia-induced cardiomyopathy from a primary cardiomyopathy. Repeat 24-hour ambulatory ECG monitoring to assess efficacy of therapy.

Combination therapy with digoxin 0.375 mg/day and metoprolol 75 mg/day was started. Two weeks later, her exercise limitations, dyspnea, and edema had decreased. The palpitations continued but were less frequent. Echocardiography showed a significant increase in the patient's ventricular function, with a left ventricular ejection fraction of 45%. Holter monitoring showed an average 24-hour heart rate of 89 beats/min, with a 75% decrease in atrial tachycardia burden. The digoxin level was within the therapeutic range. Repeat Holter monitoring demonstrated an average daily heart rate of 83 beats/min. Given the increase in ventricular function, the most likely diagnosis is frequent atrial tachycardia leading to a tachycardia-induced cardiomyopathy. The decision was made to continue her medications with careful and frequent maternal and fetal monitoring. The remainder of her pregnancy was uncomplicated. Repeat echocardiography just before delivery showed a left ventricular ejection fraction of 50%. She delivered a healthy daughter at term without complications during labor and delivery.

What diagnostic and therapeutic interventions should be taken postpartum?

Decrease the digoxin dose, repeat 24-hour ambulatory ECG monitoring, obtain follow-up echocardiogram, and discuss long-term antiarrhythmic therapy.

Due to decreasing renal clearance and volume of distribution of digoxin postpartum, the dose was decreased and eventually stopped 7 weeks postpartum. Metoprolol 100 mg/day was continued. Holter monitoring 8 weeks postpartum showed normal sinus rhythm throughout, with rare episodes of short, nonsustained atrial tachycardia. Her average heart rate over that 24-hour period was 72 beats/min. Echocardiography showed normalization of left ventricular function. Radiofrequency ablation was successfully performed at 6 months postpartum, and metoprolol was discontinued.

CASE 2: PATIENT WITH NEW-ONSET PALPITATIONS AT 20 WEEKS'

A 35-year-old woman presented for evaluation of palpitations during her 20th week of pregnancy. She had no history of palpitations preceding her pregnancy and had two previous uncomplicated pregnancies at ages 27 and 32 years.

What data would you obtain at this time?

A comprehensive history and physical examination and an electrocardiogram.

She described the palpitations as occasional "flip flops" of her heart that occurred irregularly 10 or 20 times a day. She had no sustained rapid heart beating. There were no clear triggering factors, including time of day or activity. She had eliminated caffeine and alcohol during her pregnancy. She denied orthopnea, paroxysmal nocturnal dyspnea, dyspnea on exertion, exercise limitation, edema, chest discomfort, fatigue, lightheadedness, or loss of consciousness. She had no family history of sudden death, congenital heart disease, or coronary artery disease. She was taking only prenatal vitamins. Her physical examination was entirely normal. Electrocardiogram was normal. She had a single atrial premature beat during the rhythm strip that reproduced her symptoms.

What would you do next?

Provide reassurance and clinical follow-up.

Single atrial premature beats are common during pregnancy and are often present without underlying cardiac pathology. In the absence of clinical suspicion of structural heart disease, maternal and fetal prognoses are excellent and no further intervention is needed. With reassurance, palpitations often become less worrisome to the patient, thus obviating potentially toxic pharmacologic therapy.

REFERENCES

1 Sobotka PA, Mayer JH, Bauernfeind RA, et al. Arrhythmias documented by 24-hour continuous ambulatory electrocardiographic monitoring in young women without apparent heart disease. *Am Heart J* 1981;101:573–579.

2 Shotan A, Ostrzega E, Mehra A, et al. Incidence of Arrhythmias in normal pregnancy and relation to palpitations, dizziness, and syncope. *Am J Cardiol* 1997;79:1061–1064.

3 Doig JC, McComb JM, Reid DSA. Incessant atrial tachycardia accelerated by pregnancy. *Br Heart J* 1992;67:266–268.

4 Albers GW, Dalen JE, Laupacis A. Antithrombotic therapy in atrial fibrillation. *Chest* 2001;119:194S–206S.

5 Schwartz PJ, Moss AJ, Vincent GM, et al. Diagnostic criteria for the long QT syndrome. *Circulation* 1993;88:782–784.

6 Rashba EJ, Wojciech A, Moss AJ, et al. Influence of pregnancy on the risk for cardiac events in patients with hereditary long QT syndrome. *Circulation* 1998;97:451–456.

7 Lip GY, Beevers M, Churchill D, et al. Effect of atenolol on birth weight. *Am J Cardiol* 1997;79:1436–1438.

8 Page RL. Treatment of arrhythmias during pregnancy. *Am Heart J* 1995;130:871–876.

9 James PR. Cardiovascular disease. *Best Pract Res Clin Obstet Gynaecol* 2001;15:903–911.

10 Widerhorn J, Bhandari AK, Bughi S, et al. Fetal and neonatal adverse affects profile of amiodarone treatment during pregnancy. *Am Heart J* 1991;122:1162–1166.

11 Page RL, Hamdan MH, Joglar JA. Arrhythmias occurring during pregnancy. *Card Electrophysiol Rev* 2002;6:136–139.

12 Natale A, Davidson T, Geiger MJ, et al. Implantable cardioverter-defibrillators and pregnancy. A safe combination? *Circulation* 1997; 96:2808–2812.

13 *Guidelines 2000 for cardiopulmonary resuscitation and emergency cardiovascular care.* Part 8: advanced challenges in resuscitation: section 3: special challenges in ECC. The American Heart Association in collaboration with the International Liaison Committee on Resuscitation. *Circulation* 2000;102(8 suppl):I 229–252.

Approach to Structural Heart Disease in Pregnancy

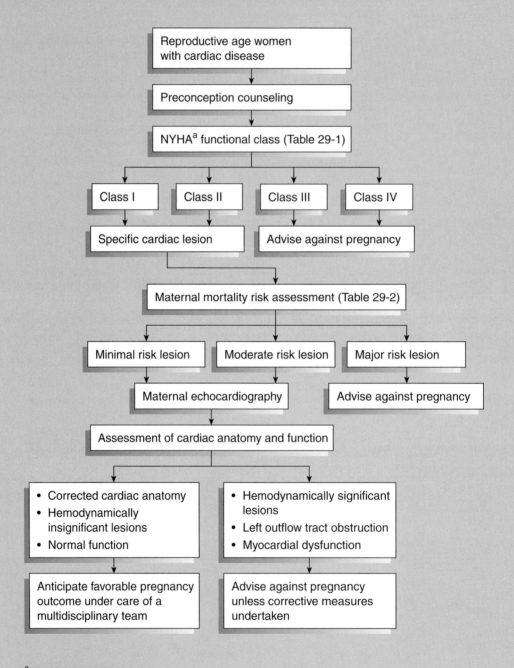

Reproductive age women with cardiac disease → Preconception counseling → NYHA[a] functional class (Table 29-1)

Class I, Class II → Specific cardiac lesion

Class III, Class IV → Advise against pregnancy

Specific cardiac lesion → Maternal mortality risk assessment (Table 29-2)

Minimal risk lesion, Moderate risk lesion → Maternal echocardiography

Major risk lesion → Advise against pregnancy

Maternal echocardiography → Assessment of cardiac anatomy and function

- Corrected cardiac anatomy
- Hemodynamically insignificant lesions
- Normal function

→ Anticipate favorable pregnancy outcome under care of a multidisciplinary team

- Hemodynamically significant lesions
- Left outflow tract obstruction
- Myocardial dysfunction

→ Advise against pregnancy unless corrective measures undertaken

[a]New York Heart Association

29 Structural Heart Disease

Annette Perez-Delboy
Lynn L. Simpson

Introduction

Despite advances in medical and surgical care, cardiac disease remains a significant cause of maternal mortality that is responsible for an estimated 10–15% of maternal deaths. More than 50% of current cases of heart disease encountered in pregnancy are related to congenital cardiac defects, and this is expected to increase because nearly 90% of women born with congenital heart disease are surviving to adulthood.[1]

Normal Physiologic Changes of Pregnancy

Pregnancy causes substantial changes in the maternal cardiovascular system, including an increase in cardiac output and blood volume and a decrease in systemic vascular resistance and arterial pressure.[2] Cardiac output begins to increase by the 10th week of pregnancy and plateaus at 20 weeks of gestation at about 40% above prepregnancy values. There is an additional 20% increase in cardiac output in the second stage of labor, with marked fluctuations in the immediate postpartum period secondary to autotransfusion from the contracted uterus. Blood volume begins to increase early in the first trimester and plateaus at 30–32 weeks of gestation at about 50% above baseline. A decrease in systemic vascular resistance helps to counterbalance the increase in cardiac output and blood volume in pregnancy. Overall, systolic and diastolic blood pressures decrease by 5–15 mm Hg and reach a nadir at

24–32 weeks of gestation. It can take months for these normal physiologic changes of pregnancy to completely return to baseline values.

Management of Cardiac Disease

PRECONCEPTION COUNSELING

To counsel women well about their risks, assessments need to be made of their cardiac condition, maternal functional status, need for further palliative or corrective surgery, additional risk factors, maternal life expectancy, support systems, expected perinatal outcomes, ability to care for a child, and recurrence risk of congenital heart disease. Unfortunately, there are limited contemporary data on pregnancy outcomes in women with heart disease.

The New York Heart Association (NYHA) classification is used to define functional status (Table 29-1). Patients with NYHA classes I and II tend to tolerate the physiologic changes of pregnancy without major complications and can anticipate favorable maternal and perinatal outcomes. The most common complication in these women is the development of pulmonary edema. Adverse maternal and fetal outcomes are associated with NYHA class III and IV manifestations including cyanosis, left outflow tract obstruction, and myocardial dysfunction. Women with cyanotic heart disease have increased risks of spontaneous abortion, preterm delivery, and stillbirth.[3] Overall, fetal wastage with cyanotic heart disease is 35% and increases to virtually 100% when maternal hematocrit levels increase above 65%. Patients with left heart obstruction, defined as mitral valve area smaller than 2 cm^2, aortic valve area smaller than 1.5 cm^2, or peak left ventricular outflow gradient

Table 29-1. **NEW YORK HEART ASSOCIATION FUNCTIONAL CLASSIFICATION SYSTEM**

Class I	Uncompromised; ordinary physical activity does not precipitate dyspnea, angina, fatigue, or palpitations; no limitations of physical activity
Class II	Slightly compromised; ordinary physical activity will precipitate symptoms; slight limitation of physical activity
Class III	Markedly compromised; less than ordinary physical activity precipitates symptoms; comfortable at rest but marked limitation of physical activity
Class IV	Severely compromised; inability to perform any physical activity without discomfort; symptoms present at rest

KEY POINT

A critical aspect to preconception counseling is to determine the maternal functional status as defined by the NYHA classification.

above 30 mm Hg by echocardiography, or decreased ventricular systolic function defined as an ejection fraction lower than 40%, are also at high risk for pregnancy-related complications.

Patients with congenital shunts have been reported to have favorable outcomes if their functional class and ventricular function are good.[4] Such patients include those with atrial septal defect (ASD), ventricular septal defect (VSD), patent ductus arteriosus (PDA), atrioventricular septal defect, tetralogy of Fallot, and complex cardiac lesions. However, women with complex lesions are often more symptomatic, which may reflect their more complex cardiac anatomy and residual hemodynamic abnormalities. Although successful cardiac surgery has been reported in pregnancy, recent reviews have suggested that maternal mortality is higher than in nonpregnant patients and that the perinatal mortality is increased.[5] As a result, cardiovascular surgery and corrective repairs of hemodynamically significant defects should be completed before conception whenever possible to avoid these procedures during pregnancy.

The presence of an arrhythmia, ventricular dysfunction, a mechanical heart valve, or a prosthetic conduit increases a woman's risk during pregnancy. Although tissue valves are preferred to mechanical valves for women in their reproductive years to obviate anticoagulation during pregnancy, these valves are prone to rapid deterioration that requires early reoperation and replacement. The presence and severity of pulmonary hypertension, cyanosis, and congestive heart failure will influence preconception counseling because functional deterioration and maternal mortality are significant risks. Chronic hypoxemia is associated with decreased fetal growth and poor perinatal outcomes. There is a 50% probability of fetal death if maternal arterial oxygen saturation is less than 85%. In general, patients can expect a decrease of one NYHA class in functional status during pregnancy. As a result, women with NYHA class III or IV symptoms should avoid pregnancy or be advised to terminate pregnancy if it occurs. Although sporadic successful pregnancies have been reported, pregnancy is not advised in women with severe pulmonary hypertension, Eisenmenger syndrome, Marfan syndrome with aortic root dilation, severe aortic stenosis, and severe left ventricular dysfunction. Maternal mortality risks associated with various conditions can be used to guide preconception counseling[6] (Table 29-2).

Table 29-2.   CARDIAC DISEASE AND RISK OF MATERNAL DEATH

CARDIAC DISORDER	MORTALITY RISK
Group 1: minimal risk ASD VSD PDA Pulmonic or tricuspid disease Tetralogy of Fallot, corrected Tissue valve Mitral stenosis, NYHA classes I and II	1%
Group 2: moderate risk Mitral stenosis, NYHA classes III and IV Aortic stenosis Coarctation without valvular involvement Tetralogy of Fallot, uncorrected Previous myocardial infarction Marfan syndrome, normal aorta Mitral stenosis with atrial fibrillation Artificial valve	5–15%
Group 3: major risk Pulmonary hypertension Coarctation with valvular involvement Marfan syndrome with aortic involvement	25–50%

ASD = atrial septal defects; NYHA = New York Heart Association; PDA = patent ductus arteriosus; VSD = ventricular septal defects.
Source: Hung L, Rahimtoola SH. Prosthetic heart valves and pregnancy. *Circulation* 2003;107:1240.

Patients with congenital heart disease need to understand the risk of recurrence in their offspring. Although the prevalence of major congenital heart disease in the population is 4 in 1000, the risk increases 10-fold in first-degree relatives (2–4%). There is an approximately 10% incidence of fetal congenital heart disease in women born with cardiac anomalies. About half of the fetal defects observed in women with congenital heart disease are concordant with the defect found in the mother. Left heart obstructive lesions are reported to have a higher recurrence rate, and some autosomal disorders such as Marfan syndrome and 22q11 deletion conditions have a 50% recurrence risk.

ANTEPARTUM CARE   A multidisciplinary team including specialists in cardiology, anesthesiology, and maternal fetal medicine needs to design early in pregnancy a well-documented plan of care for each patient. The clinical team must clearly document delivery instructions and contingency plans should complications arise.

General measures include decreasing anxiety, restricting sodium intake, increasing periods of rest, limiting weight gain, and decreasing exposure to heat and humidity. Potential adverse events include development of congestive heart failure, arrhythmias, thromboembolism, complications from anticoagulation, or consequences of pulmonary vascular disease. A limitation of physical activity is recommended when ventricular dysfunction is present, and in some cases, prolonged hospitalization may be required. Early identification and control of hypertension, infection, hyperthyroidism, and anemia can decrease demands on the heart.

A common problem in patients who have undergone surgery for congenital heart disease is the occurrence of arrhythmias during pregnancy. These arrhythmias can be life threatening, particularly in the presence of ventricular hypertrophy, ventricular dysfunction, and conditions in which the right ventricle serves as the systemic ventricle. Sustained supraventricular tachycardias including atrial flutter and fibrillation should be managed promptly. Cardioversion can be safely used in pregnancy if medical therapy is unsuccessful.

Anticoagulation will be necessary in some cardiac patients. Warfarin is a known teratogen whose manifestations include nasal hypoplasia, optic atrophy, digital abnormalities, and mental impairment. Warfarin exposure in any trimester may result in central nervous system defects. Overall, teratogenic effects are estimated to occur in about 10% of exposed fetuses. Uteroplacental bleeding and fetal hemorrhage during delivery are potential risks if warfarin is not discontinued at least 2 weeks before birth.

Heparin has been a common anticoagulant used in pregnancy because it does not cross the placenta and poses no teratogenic or hemorrhagic risk to the fetus. Low-molecular-weight heparin has some advantages over unfractionated heparin including greater bioavailability and lower incidence of maternal adverse effects such as thrombocytopenia and osteoporosis. Although low-molecular-weight heparins are a promising alternative to unfractionated heparin, recommendations for their use in pregnancy have been limited to prophylaxis in the second and third trimesters of pregnancy. Despite the increasing use of low-molecular-weight heparins for therapeutic anticoagulation in pregnancy, there are few studies demonstrating its effectiveness in pregnant women.

In addition, it has been recommended that low-molecular-weight heparins not be used in patients with prosthetic heart valves due to reports of thrombosis and death.[7] There are also recent concerns about the effectiveness of subcutaneous unfractionated heparin in cases of mechanical valves.[8] As a result, anticoagulation in pregnant women with mechanical heart valves is problematic. Different approaches have been proposed. One compromise of risks and benefits may be to substitute warfarin with intravenous unfractionated heparin in the first trimester and the last few weeks of pregnancy to decrease the risk of warfarin embryopathy and bleeding complications in the mother and infant. After delivery, warfarin is restarted with concurrent use of intravenous heparin until therapeutic anticoagulation on oral therapy is achieved.

Prevention and early recognition of congestive heart failure are important aspects of antenatal care. Pneumococcal and influenza vaccines are recommended because infections can precipitate heart failure. Onset of congestive heart failure is often gradual and insidious, so frequent prenatal visits and evaluations are necessary. In some cases, hospitalization for closer observation may be necessary.

> **KEY POINT**
>
> *The optimal approach to anticoagulation in pregnancy remains controversial, particularly in women with mechanical heart valves.*

INTRAPARTUM CARE

The management of labor and delivery must be carefully planned in women with cardiac disease. Attention to volume and blood loss replacement, pharmacologic support, endocarditis prophylaxis, and the need for anticoagulation are primary concerns. Efforts to preserve ventricular function, maintain adequate preload, and avoid undesirable decreases in afterload are warranted. Decreases in systemic vascular resistance are especially dangerous if there is right-to-left shunting in the presence of pulmonary hypertension. Maternal anxiety and tachycardia should be avoided. Medical treatment should be optimized before labor to avoid rapid or wide fluctuations in preload, cardiac output, and heart rate. Epidural anesthesia can be provided safely in most cardiac cases if the block is produced in gradual increments with sufficient volume preloading and judicious use of vasopressors to minimize the risks of vasodilation and hypotension associated with sympathetic blockade.

Delivery in a tertiary care center with an experienced multidisciplinary team is recommended for patients with major congenital heart disease. Women with minor conditions such as repaired or small ASDs and VSDs, repaired tetralogy of Fallot without residual cardiac disease, and mild valvular stenosis or regurgitation may deliver in other settings. Although delivery at a regional referral center may not be warranted, consultation before delivery can be useful to confirm an appropriate management strategy for these patients.

Patients with stenotic lesions may not tolerate the hemodynamic changes associated with pregnancy and labor and delivery. The fixed cardiac output of aortic and mitral stenosis can be difficult to manage. Although invasive cardiovascular monitoring may be useful in these patients, it may be a technical challenge if there has been previous cannulation of central arteries and veins. In cases of pulmonary hypertension or when the systemic ventricle is the right ventricle, central venous pressure monitoring can be used to detect changes in preload and guide fluid replacement.

For patients who require anticoagulation, heparin should be discontinued 4–6 hours before induction and resumed 6–12 hours postpartum. Some clinicians recommend continuing anticoagulation throughout delivery for women with mechanical heart valves.

Although the American Heart Association supports endocarditis prophylaxis only for high-risk patients before complicated vaginal deliveries, many centers apply broader indications for prophylactic antibiotics by initiating therapy in all high- and moderate-risk cases.[9] Conditions considered to define a woman at high risk include prosthetic cardiac valves, previous bacterial endocarditis, complex congenital cyanotic heart disease, or surgically constructed shunts or patches. Moderate-risk cases include other congenital heart malformations, valvular heart disease, hypertrophic cardiomyopathy, and mitral valve prolapse with regurgitation. Chemoprophylaxis is not recommended for isolated mitral valve prolapse, ASDs, pacemakers, and surgically corrected lesions without prosthetic material. Risks associated with intrapartum antibiotics are acceptable to many physicians and patients after considering the 1–5% incidence of transient bacteremia associated with delivery and the life-threatening potential of bacterial endocarditis. The current antibiotic recommendations for endocarditis prophylaxis are listed in Table 29-3.[10]

Table 29-3. ANTIBIOTIC RECOMMENDATIONS FOR BACTERIAL ENDOCARDITIS PROPHYLAXIS

Standard regimen

Ampicillin 2 g and gentamicin 1.5 mg/kg (maximum 120 mg) IV/IM with completion of infusions 30 min before delivery; 6 h later: ampicillin 1 g IM/IV or amoxicillin 1 g PO

Penicillin-allergic regimen

Vancomycin 1 g IV over 1–2 h and gentamicin 1.5 mg/kg IV (maximum 120 mg) with completion of infusions 30 min before delivery

IM = intramuscularly; IV = intravenously; PO = orally.

KEY POINT

Liberal use of peripartum antibiotics for endocarditis prophylaxis is reasonable in most cases of cardiac disease.

Vaginal delivery is recommended for most women with structural heart disease, with cesarean section reserved for standard obstetric indications. Left lateral decubitus positioning of the woman can decrease the hemodynamic fluctuations that accompany uterine contractions. Voluntary pushing during the second stage of labor is minimized to avoid effects on venous return. An operative vaginal delivery with forceps or vacuum may be used to shorten the second stage. Cesarean section should be considered for delivery if warfarin anticoagulation has not been discontinued for at least 2 weeks because of the risk of fetal intracranial bleeding. Some clinicians recommend cesarean section before labor in cases of Marfan syndrome with a dilated aortic root.

POSTPARTUM CARE

Increases in cardiac output are observed immediately postpartum and do not return to baseline levels for many days. Monitoring of cardiac patients for a minimum of 3 days postpartum is recommended, with an increase to 7 days for patients with Eisenmenger syndrome. There are rapid intravascular volume shifts in the first 2 weeks after delivery, and most maternal deaths related to cardiac disease occur postpartum. An early postpartum evaluation in addition to the standard 6-week visit should be considered in cases of major cardiac disease.

Congenital Cardiac Defects

Structural heart disease can be congenital or acquired. Maternal and fetal risks depend on the specific lesion and its severity. Unrepaired ASD, VSD, and PDA are associated with a risk for

KEY POINT

> *More than half of cases of heart disease encountered in pregnancy are related to congenital cardiac defects.*

Eisenmenger physiology and paradoxical embolism. The development of Eisenmenger physiology is extremely serious and is discussed in detail below. ASDs and VSDs strain right-sided heart function and PDAs strain left-sided heart function. Serial echocardiography is recommended to assess ventricular function, pulmonary arterial pressure, and valvular sufficiency in pregnant women with unrepaired lesions.

ATRIAL SEPTAL DEFECT

ASDs are one of the most common forms of congenital heart disease found in pregnant women and comprise up to 25% of all cardiac defects.[10] The vast majority are detected and repaired in childhood. Under these circumstances, there are usually no long-term sequelae and the prognosis is excellent. Although patients with unrepaired ASDs are usually asymptomatic, they may present with increasing shortness of breath and easy fatigability in pregnancy. Palpitations are common. Closure of an ASD, surgically or in the catheterization laboratory, does not eliminate the possibility of arrhythmias. Late complications of ASDs include paroxysmal atrial flutter, persistent atrial fibrillation, sick sinus syndrome, tricuspid and mitral regurgitations, and right ventricular dysfunction. It is estimated that up to 15% of patients with an ASD will have preconceptual pulmonary vascular disease. In the absence of pulmonary hypertension, a favorable outcome can be expected. The risks are greatest when repairs are performed after childhood.

VENTRICULAR SEPTAL DEFECT

VSDs account for about 25% of cardiac defects. Overall, 80% of childhood VSDs close spontaneously, and the majority that do not close are repaired. Most small VSDs are asymptomatic, but dyspnea on exertion, exercise intolerance, and shortness of breath may develop in pregnancy. Persistent small defects carry a risk of endocarditis and paradoxical embolism. Women with repaired VSDs or small unrepaired muscular VSDs usually tolerate pregnancy without significant complications.

VSDs may be closed surgically with a patch or nonsurgically in the catheterization laboratory. Conduction abnormalities and arrhythmias are more common after closure with a right ventriculotomy. Unrepaired defects may be associated with the development of aortic regurgitation, arrhythmias, congestive heart failure, pulmonary valvular disease, pulmonary hypertension, right-to-left shunting, and Eisenmenger physiology. Aortic regurgitation occurs in 5–10% of patients, and up to 10% may develop congestive heart failure. Large, untreated membranous VSDs are most commonly associated with the development of pulmonary hypertension and subsequent pulmonary vascular disease. Cardiomegaly at the time of diagnosis is associated with a poor prognosis for long-term survival.

PATENT DUCTUS ARTERIOSUS

The ductus arteriosus connects the aorta to the main pulmonary trunk and persists when the normal postnatal closure fails to occur. Fortunately, most PDAs are detected and repaired in infancy. A history of ligation of a patent ductus arteriosus in infancy does not pose any problems for a pregnant woman. However, patients with unrepaired PDAs may present with exercise intolerance, dyspnea, and shortness of breath. Left ventricular and atrial enlargement may result from the increased volume load on the left side of the heart. Unrepaired PDAs are also prone to bacterial endocarditis. Treatment options in the adult include surgical ligation with suture closure or coil balloon embolization in the catheterization laboratory. Women with uncomplicated closed defects tend to have favorable pregnancy outcomes; therefore, PDAs should be closed before conception whenever possible. Pulmonary hypertension may still develop after successful ligations, particularly when these repairs are performed after childhood.

In left-to-right shunt lesions such as PDAs, the effect of the increase in cardiac output during pregnancy is counterbalanced by the decrease in peripheral vascular resistance. Large, unrepaired PDAs pose a risk for arrhythmias, ventricular dysfunction, pulmonary hypertension, and Eisenmenger physiology. Prophylaxis for bacterial endocarditis is recommended for unrepaired or complicated PDAs during the intrapartum period.

AORTIC STENOSIS

Congenital aortic stenosis can lead to severe left ventricular hypertrophy that may be unable to respond to the normal hemodynamic changes of pregnancy. Additional cardiac defects such as coarctation are found in 5% of patients with congenital aortic stenosis.[11] Women with mild aortic stenosis are advised to complete their childbearing before aortic valve replacement, if possible, to avoid the need for anticoagulation in pregnancy. Women with symptomatic or severe aortic stenosis should undergo surgical correction before pregnancy. Balloon valvuloplasty may be indicated as a temporizing measure for symptomatic patients during gestation.

The ability of pregnant women with aortic stenosis to increase stroke volume and cardiac output can be limited, which may result in increased left ventricular pressures, dysfunction, and ischemia. Although the left ventricle becomes hypertrophied and noncompliant, it usually does not dilate until it begins to fail. Patients with aortic stenosis tend not to become symptomatic until the valve opening narrows by at least one-third. Mild aortic stenosis, defined as a valve area of 1.5–2.5 cm^2 with a peak gradient lower than 50 mm Hg (normal valve area 2.5–3.5 cm^2), is well tolerated in pregnancy. Moderate aortic stenosis is defined as a valve area of 1.0–1.5 cm^2 and a peak gradient of 50–75 mm Hg. With progressive stenosis, cardiac output becomes fixed and the maintenance of coronary and cerebral perfusion can become problematic. Angina, myocardial infarction, transient ischemic attacks, stroke, and sudden death may occur. The volume load associated with pregnancy is not well tolerated if the valve area is smaller than 1.0 cm^2 and patients with gradients higher than 100 mm Hg are at greatest risk.

The intrapartum period is dangerous for patients with a fixed cardiac output. Decreased venous return to the heart through blood loss, hypotension, inferior vena caval compression, and regional analgesia must be avoided to decrease maternal risks. Generous preloading provides a margin of safety for preserved cardiac output. Invasive hemodynamic monitoring is useful for cases of moderate to severe aortic stenosis to maintain pulmonary capillary wedge pressures at 16–18 mm Hg. Endocarditis prophylaxis is indicated for aortic stenosis of any etiology.

Idiopathic hypertropic subaortic stenosis, an autosomal dominant disorder with a variable penetrance, has the same prognosis as aortic stenosis. Both are associated with sudden death due to left ventricular hypertrophy and decreased venous return. Similar to aortic stenosis, symptomatic patients with should be treated with propanolol. Hypotension and tachycardia should be avoided in pregnancy.

COARCTATION OF THE AORTA

Coarctation of the aorta comprises 8% of cardiac defects seen in adults. Coarctation may be isolated or complex, associated with PDA, aortic stenosis, aortic regurgitation, or monosomy X. About 10% have cerebral artery aneurysms and 25% have a bicuspid aortic valve. Life expectancy is markedly decreased if coarctation is not corrected due to complications of hypertension, left ventricular outflow obstruction, congestive heart failure, aortic rupture, intracranial hemorrhage, and infective endocarditis. Patients with longstanding, uncorrected coarctation may present with systolic pressures over 250 mm Hg and marked left ventricular hypertrophy. There is a high incidence of hypertension, premature coronary artery disease, recoarctation, and aortic valve disease after repair. The persistence of hypertension after surgical correction may lead to aneurysm formation and dissection of the aorta and frequently involves the ascending segment rather than the site of the initial coarctation. Rupture of the aorta is a potential risk late in pregnancy or during labor and delivery. Maternal deaths may also result from associated congestive heart failure, intracranial hemorrhage, and bacterial endocarditis. Hypotension below the level of uncorrected coarctation may result in uteroplacental insufficiency and intrauterine fetal growth restriction. β Blockers used to decrease the risk of aortic dissection in high-risk women can also contribute to poor fetal growth.

PULMONIC STENOSIS

Women with mild or moderate pulmonic stenosis tend to have favorable pregnancy outcomes. Although the gradients across the valve can be overestimated in pregnancy due to increases in cardiac output, stenosis of the pulmonary valve is classified as mild (<49 mm Hg), moderate (50–79 mm Hg), and severe (>80 mm Hg). Fortunately, most cases of pulmonic stenosis are detected and corrected before childbearing. In uncorrected pulmonic stenosis, hemodynamic changes of pregnancy may precipitate right heart failure, tricuspid regurgitation, and atrial arrhythmias. Right ventricular enlargement and poststenotic dilation of the pulmonary artery may occur. Irrespective of symptoms, a patient with severe pulmonic stenosis should undergo surgical correction before pregnancy. When indicated, balloon valvuloplasty may be used during pregnancy.

EBSTEIN ANOMALY

Ebstein anomaly consists of a dysplastic tricuspid valve in which the posterior and septal leaflets are tethered into the right ventricle. This results in atrialization of a portion of the right ventricle with different degrees of tricuspid regurgitation. In mild cases, women tend to be asymptomatic and pregnancy is well tolerated. In symptomatic patients, easy fatigability and dyspnea on exertion are common complaints. Severe tricuspid regurgitation can lead to right ventricular dysfunction, decreased pulmonary artery blood flow, and arrhythmias. Ebstein anomaly is often associated with preexcitation or Wolfe-Parkinson-White syndrome. A patent foramen ovale or ASD is present in about half of patients with Ebstein anomaly.[1] In these cases, flow to the pulmonary artery can be obstructed and right-to-left shunting across the interatrial connection can result in cyanosis. Replacement of the tricuspid valve and surgical repair of the right atrium may be necessary in extreme cases. However, the current intervention of choice is the surgical reconstruction of the tricuspid valve whenever possible.

Patients with Ebstein anomaly often reach childbearing age. Fetal risks include prematurity, intrauterine growth restriction, and death, particularly in patients with cyanosis. The incidence of congenital heart disease in the offspring of women with Ebstein anomaly is 6%.[11] Overall, favorable maternal and fetal outcomes can be expected in most cases of Ebstein anomaly.

TETRALOGY OF FALLOT

Tetralogy of Fallot is the most common form of cyanotic heart disease in adults. Long-term survival is rare without surgical correction. Tetralogy of Fallot consists of severe valvular or subvalvular pulmonary stenosis, a large VSD, right ventricular hypertrophy, and an overriding aorta. Before surgical repair, cyanosis and dyspnea on exertion are common clinical features. Pregnancy with uncorrected tetralogy of Fallot is not advised. The decrease in systemic vascular resistance and the increase in cardiac output that occur in normal pregnancy increase right-to-left shunting. Uncorrected tetralogy of Fallot has a maternal mortality rate as high as 15% with a 30% fetal loss rate.[1] Poor prognostic signs include a maternal hematocrit value higher than 60, oxygen saturations less than 80%, and right ventricular hypertension with pressures above 120 mm Hg.

Most women with tetralogy of Fallot currently entering their reproductive years have had surgical correction. Ectopic ventricular contractions are common after repair, and right bundle branch block occurs in more than 90% of patients. Ventricular arrhythmias, syncope, and sudden death are late complications in 1–3% of patients. Residual pulmonary regurgitation, right ventricular outflow obstruction, and right ventricular dilation and dysfunction with tricuspid regurgitation may also follow successful repairs. A residual shunt after repair can lead to the development of pulmonary hypertension and bacterial endocarditis. Left ventricular dysfunction may be present from previous volume overload, thus increasing the likelihood of complications during pregnancy.

Women who have undergone palliative rather than corrective repairs are at considerably higher risk during pregnancy. Pregnancy is also not well tolerated by patients who have undergone repair of complex pulmonary atresia. Overall, women who have undergone corrective surgery early in life can anticipate favorable pregnancy outcomes.

COMPLETE TRANSPOSITION OF THE GREAT ARTERIES

In complete transposition of the great arteries, the aorta arises from the right ventricle and the pulmonary artery arises from the left ventricle. As a result, blood flow within the heart is in parallel rather than in series, and survival is dependent on the presence of additional lesions to allow for the mixing of venous and arterial blood. A large VSD may provide a natural shunt, or a balloon atrial septostomy may be needed in the newborn period. Surgical approaches aim to improve the mix of oxygenated with unoxygenated blood. Many women currently in their reproductive years will have undergone an interatrial repair such as the Mustard procedure, which redirects systemic venous return to the left ventricle and pulmonary venous return to the right ventricle. In this type of repair, the morphologic right ventricle supports the systemic circulation. The arterial switch operation has recently become the standard surgical approach for complete transposition of the great arteries. This anatomic repair establishes the left ventricle as the systemic ventricle. The long-term effects of the arterial switch operation are unknown, but it is anticipated that there will be fewer complications and, to date there seems to be fewer life-threatening arrhythmias.

Successful pregnancies have been reported after interatrial repair for transposition of the great arteries. Patients with normal exercise tolerance and good functional status before pregnancy tend to have favorable maternal and fetal outcomes.[12] However, the systemic right ventricle may fail in pregnancy due to the increase in volume loading. In addition, supraventricular tachycardias may occur in women with Mustard-type repairs. Overall, these complications are most common in the third trimester and postpartum period.

CONGENITAL CORRECTED TRANSPOSITION OF THE GREAT ARTERIES

In corrected transposition of the great arteries, blood travels from the morphologic right atrium across the mitral valve into a morphologic left ventricle, which is connected to the pulmonary artery. The pulmonary venous blood travels back into a morphologic left atrium, across the tricuspid valve into a morphologic right ventricle, and into the aorta. As a result, the morphologic right ventricle functions as the systemic ventricle. VSDs, pulmonary valve stenosis, and Ebstein anomaly with tricuspid regurgitation may be found in cases of corrected transposition of the great vessels. Complete heart block develops in 1% of patients per year as a result of an abnormal conduction system.

Many women with corrected transposition are asymptomatic during their reproductive years. Pregnancy is usually well tolerated, with a live-birth rate higher than 80%.[13] Potential complications include dysfunction of the systemic right ventricle, worsening atrioventricular regurgitation, and congestive heart failure. Atrial arrhythmias and atrioventricular heart blocks may also occur. Surgical intervention may involve closing associated VSDs or relieving associated pulmonary stenosis. Permanent pacing may be necessary in up to 40% of cases because of the development of complete heart block. Maternal outcomes are dependent on the function of the systemic right ventricle, degree of atrioventricular valve regurgitation, severity of left ventricular outflow obstruction, and the presence of heart block.

SINGLE VENTRICLE HEARTS

There is a wide spectrum of anatomic abnormalities in patients who do not have suitable anatomy to allow for a two-ventricle repair. In such instances, the volume of the single ventricle is chronically overloaded, which is problematic for the patient who desires pregnancy. Various procedures have been developed to direct systemic venous blood to the pulmonary circulation by bypassing the single ventricle. Patients with univentricular repairs continue to have a limited ability to increase cardiac output. Overall, the 10-year survival rate after a Fontan palliation is about 60–80%.[1] Although pregnancy poses significant risks, favorable outcomes can be achieved after Fontan operation. Complete atrioventricular septal defects, comprised of an ostium primum ASD, a membranous VSD, and a single atrioventricular valve, function like a univentricular heart with systemic pressures in both ventricles. Although the data are limited, it is expected that women undergoing early definitive repair will have improved pregnancy outcomes.

EISENMENGER SYNDROME

Eisenmenger syndrome develops when pulmonary pressures with preexisting left-to-right shunts increase to systemic levels followed by bidirectional or right-to-left shunting. This results in decreased pulmonary perfusion, hypoxemia, and cyanosis. Systemic hypotension in patients with Eisenmenger syndrome can result in sudden death. Unrepaired VSDs, ASDs, and PDA may result in the development of Eisenmenger physiology. Maternal risks associated with pregnancy are prohibitive when the pulmonary vascular resistance reaches systemic levels.

In the past, pulmonary hypertension and Eisenmenger syndrome had up to a 50% risk of maternal mortality. Contemporary data show that Eisenmenger syndrome carries a 30% risk of maternal death and a deterioration of physical status during gestation.[14] Fetal outcome is also poor, with a 35% incidence of spontaneous abortion, 50% prevalence of intrauterine growth restriction, and an increase in preterm birth. Despite recent reports of improved maternal survival, significant morbidity and mortality exist, and pregnancy should be strongly discouraged in women with Eisenmenger syndrome. Termination of pregnancy is recommended if early in gestation.

For patients who elect to conceive and continue a pregnancy, early hospitalization, supplemental oxygen, maintenance of systemic vascular resistance, and anticoagulation should be considered. Inhaled nitric oxide and prostacyclin are effective pulmonary vasodilators and have been used in pregnancy to decrease pulmonary arterial pressures. Maternal deaths may result from right

KEY POINT

Eisenmenger syndrome may be due to an unrepaired VSD, ASD, or PDA and carries a significant risk of maternal mortality.

heart failure, pulmonary hypertension, or pulmonary hemorrhage. Although sudden death can occur at any time, the risk is greatest in the intrapartum and early postpartum periods. A major goal during this critical time is to maintain pulmonary blood flow. Right heart preload is vital for pulmonary artery perfusion, which can be decreased by blood loss, supine hypotension, and conduction anesthesia. Women with pulmonary hypertension should be given oxygen intrapartum, adequate preloading with preparations for possible blood loss, and induction of labor in a controlled setting. Delayed deterioration and postpartum deaths may also occur, so these patients should remain in hospital for at least 1 week for observation after delivery.

Marfan Syndrome
Marfan syndrome is an inheritable connective tissue disorder. Although Marfan syndrome is a multisystem disorder, the most clinically significant manifestation is the presence of cardiovascular disease. Individuals with Marfan syndrome are predisposed to the development of aortic root dilation and valvular insufficiency. Mitral valve prolapse with regurgitation is common and can result in endocarditis or lead to congestive heart failure. The natural history of the disease includes a substantial risk of sudden and premature death from aortic dissection and rupture. Life expectancy is significantly decreased in Marfan syndrome, with a mean age of death of 28 years. Cardiovascular complications are responsible for nearly all early deaths. There are two primary issues concerning pregnancy in patients with Marfan syndrome: maternal risk of aortic dissection and fetal risk of being affected with the disease.

In the past, women with Marfan syndrome were advised against pregnancy based on a reported 50% chance of death from aortic dissection. However, most maternal deaths reported with Marfan syndrome occur in patients with preexisting cardiovascular disease.[15] Contemporary estimates of maternal mortality rates appear to be low, particularly if cardiovascular involvement is minimal before conception.[14] It has been recommended that women with evidence of hemodynamic compromise or aortic dilation wider than 40 mm be counseled against pregnancy. However, aortic dissection has been reported to occur with aortic root dilation narrower than 40 mm. Patients planning pregnancy need to be aware of the low but potential risk for this serious complication. Patients with significant aortic dilation, aortic regurgitation, or marked mitral valve dysfunction should be advised against pregnancy because of the significant risk of aortic dissection. In addition to risks to her own health, a woman with Marfan syndrome must consider the 50% risk of transmitting the autosomal dominant disease to her offspring. Although there appears to be a high degree of penetrance, there is a wide variability in the expression of the disease. Genetic linkage analysis and fetal echocardiography may be used for prenatal diagnosis.

In ongoing pregnancies, serial echocardiography should be carried out to evaluate aortic root size and cardiac valvular function. The rate of aortic root dilation in patients with Marfan syndrome can be decreased by long-term administration of β blockers. Twenty percent of all aortic dissections that occur in women with Marfan syndrome are associated with pregnancy. Surgical repair should be considered if the aortic root measures larger than 55 mm, although corrective surgery may prove to be beneficial at an earlier stage of aortic enlargement in women planning pregnancy. The optimal time to perform a prophylactic repair is before conception. However, surgery for aortic dilation and dissection has been accomplished during pregnancy.

The primary goal of intrapartum management is to decrease the cardiovascular stress involved in labor and delivery. Regional anesthesia with an early epidural should be considered to minimize the pain and stress of labor. Most patients with minimal cardiac abnormalities are able to tolerate bearing down in the second stage without adverse effects. Endocarditis prophylaxis should be administered to women with Marfan syndrome because virtually all will have abnormalities of the cardiac valves.

MITRAL VALVE PROLAPSE AND REGURGITATION

Mitral valve prolapse is very common and affects up to 15% of women at reproductive age. Most patients are asymptomatic, but anxiety, palpitations, dyspnea, and syncope can occur. β Blockers are considered for symptomatic patients. Most women with mitral valve prolapse tolerate pregnancy well. Endocarditis prophylaxis is recommended when mitral regurgitation complicates mitral valve prolapse. Significant mitral regurgitation can lead to left ventricular dysfunction, and women with significant ventricular dysfunction should be strongly advised to avoid pregnancy. Severe mitral regurgitation should prompt surgical repair or replacement of the valve before conception.

Acquired Heart Disease

MITRAL STENOSIS

Rheumatic heart disease is currently uncommon in the United States, but, when it occurs, the characteristic cardiac lesion is mitral stenosis with or without aortic regurgitation. Symptoms usually do not develop until the valve area is smaller than 2.5 cm^2. As the valve area decreases, diastolic filling of the left ventricle is decreased, resulting in a relatively fixed cardiac output. The left atrium can become overdistended and enlarged, thus increasing the risk of atrial fibrillation and subsequent thrombus formation. Pulmonary edema and hypertension are additional risks with severe mitral stenosis. The volume load of pregnancy is not well tolerated if the valve area is smaller than 1.0 cm^2. The maintenance of left ventricular preload is essential in pregnant women with mitral stenosis.

Patients with this degree of mitral stenosis should undergo surgical correction before conception. Management of mitral stenosis includes valvotomy or mitral valve replacement. Although these procedures are best accomplished in the nonpregnant state, they have been performed successfully during gestation. Heart failure is a common complication in pregnancies after mitral valvotomy due to the development of mitral regurgitation. Valve replacement is considered first-line therapy in most cases.

KEY POINT

Rheumatic heart disease is decreasing in frequency, but mitral stenosis and replacement mechanical valves pose significant management issues during pregnancy.

Medical management of mitral stenosis may include administration of antiarrhythmic agents, β blockers to control heart rate, and careful use of diuretics. The critical aspects of intrapartum care include preserving adequate diastolic filling time and sufficient preload to the left ventricle. In cases of severe stenosis, this can be achieved by maintaining maternal heart rates of 70–90 beats/min and pulmonary capillary wedge pressures of 14–16 mm Hg. Relief of pain is another important aspect of intrapartum care, and a carefully administered epidural is often the optimal method of analgesia. In the postpartum period, autotransfusion from the contracted uterus must be anticipated as well as prompt recognition and management of postpartum hemorrhage.

Women with mechanical heart valves will require therapeutic anticoagulation during gestation. There is some controversy over the optimal anticoagulation regimen for these patients. Tissue valves have been considered safer in pregnancy because anticoagulation is not required. However, these valves have a finite life and usually require reoperation with insertion of a mechanical valve once childbearing is complete. Although anticoagulation is not required, prophylaxis for endocarditis is recommended intrapartum for women with tissue valves.

PULMONIC AND TRICUSPID INSUFFICIENCY

Fortunately, right-sided valvular lesions are rare and pregnancy tends to be well tolerated in women who have pulmonic or tricuspid insufficiency. Most patients with these lesions are asymptomatic. Although cautious fluid administration is recommended during labor and delivery, invasive hemodynamic monitoring is rarely indicated. Most clinicians will administer intrapartum antibiotics for bacterial endocarditis prophylaxis.

MITRAL AND AORTIC INSUFFICIENCY

Mitral regurgitation is usually well tolerated in pregnancy. Atrial enlargement can lead to the development of atrial fibrillation in patients with longstanding mitral insufficiency. Although aortic regurgitation imposes a volume load on the heart, women with aortic insufficiency generally have favorable pregnancy outcomes. Treatment is often delayed until symptoms of left ventricular dysfunction appear. It is advised that childbearing be completed before valve replacement to avoid the need for anticoagulation during pregnancy. Endocarditis prophylaxis is recommended for all regurgitant valvular disease.

MYOCARDIAL INFARCTION

Myocardial infarction in pregnancy is rare. The prognosis for women who develop a myocardial infarction during pregnancy worsens with advancing gestational age. Overall, the mortality risk associated with a myocardial infarction in pregnancy is 20–30%, but this risk may be as high as 50% in the third trimester.[16] Whenever possible, delivery should be delayed at least 2 weeks after a myocardial infarction to allow the damaged myocardium to begin healing. Invasive hemodynamic monitoring should be considered intrapartum if there is evidence of ventricular dysfunction. The optimal route of delivery is controversial, but cesarean section has traditionally been reserved for standard obstetric indications. Induction of labor is best accomplished in a controlled setting with epidural anesthesia and shortening of the second stage by an operative vaginal delivery. Methylergonovine should not be used in these patients for the management of postpartum hemorrhage because of its potential to cause coronary vasospasm. For women with previous myocardial infarction, the presence of significant left ventricular dysfunction, congestive heart failure, or NYHA class III or IV symptoms are contraindications to pregnancy. For asymptomatic patients with a remote myocardial infarction and no significant ventricular dysfunction, pregnancy is a possibility. However, clinical deterioration and congestive heart failure are potential complications. In general, it is recommended that women delay childbearing for at least 1 year after a myocardial infarction.

PERIPARTUM CARDIOMYOPATHY

Peripartum cardiomyopathy is defined as heart failure that develops in the last month of pregnancy or within 5 months of delivery in the absence of an identifiable cause or preexisting heart disease. Left ventricular systolic dysfunction, recognized on echocardiogram as an ejection fraction lower than 45% and a shortening fraction lower than 30%, is the classic finding in peripartum cardiomyopathy. Peripartum cardiomyopathy occurs in 1 in 3000–4000 live births, with maternal mortality risks of 10–50%.[17] Risk factors include multiparity, advanced maternal age, multifetal gestation, preeclampsia, hypertension, and African American race. Most cases present within 1 month of delivery. Other preexisting or coincidental conditions must be excluded, such as congenital heart disease, rheumatic heart disease, infective endocarditis, viral myocarditis, hypertension, thyrotoxicosis, diabetes, and obesity. Overall, identifiable underlying disease is found in 75% of cases of peripartum heart failure.

The primary treatment includes decreasing preload with diuretics, decreasing afterload with vasodilators, and increasing contractility with inotropic medications. About half of all patients go on to have a dilated cardiomyopathy, whereas the remaining patients have a full recovery after delivery. Overall prognosis is poor if left ventricular function and cardiac size do not normalize within 6 months. Cardiac transplantation is an option for patients who do not recover because it provides them with the potential for future childbearing.

Among pregnancies in women with heart transplants, hypertension occurs in 44%, preeclampsia in 22%, preterm labor in 30%, and organ rejection in 20%.[18] Women should delay childbearing for at least 1 year after transplantation, at which time acute rejection and need for immunosuppressive therapy have lessened. Although immunosuppression remains a risk for infection and possibly decreased fetal growth, in utero exposure often occurs without significant sequelae to the fetus. Overall, the 3-year survival rate after transplantation is 75%. Recurrent peripartum cardiomyopathy has been described; therefore, the risks and benefits of future childbearing must be carefully considered in these patients. Women at highest risk of clinical deterioration and death in subsequent pregnancies are those with persistent left ventricular dysfunction.

What's the Evidence

Currently, cardiac disease complicates about 1% of pregnancies and comprises a very heterogeneous group of lesions. As a result, major clinical trials on cardiac disease in pregnancy are lacking, and management must be based on small case series and the collective experience of a multidisciplinary team. Although there is widespread expertise in the management of rheumatic heart disease, there is a relative lack of experience in caring for pregnant women with congenital heart defects. As with many medical problems in pregnancy, pregnancy-specific controlled trials are unlikely. The best information that we can gather at present consists of descriptions of experience at individual institutions with substantial experience with these patients. Comparisons of cohorts with and without specific interventions will be of some use.

Guiding Questions in Approaching the Patient

- What is her functional status?
- What is the maternal mortality risk associated with her specific cardiac defect?
- What is her current cardiac anatomy and recent hemodynamic evaluation?
- Are there additional maternal and fetal risks associated with her specific cardiac defect?

Conclusion

Congenital heart disease is currently the most common type of heart disease observed in women of reproductive age. Most patients with congenital cardiac defects will have undergone corrective or palliative surgery before pregnancy. Fortunately, most young women with heart disease do well during pregnancy. Despite recent advances, women with severe left ventricular outflow obstruction, pulmonary hypertension, Eisenmenger syndrome, and Marfan syndrome with an enlarged aortic root should avoid pregnancy. Women with left-to-right shunts, right outflow tract obstruction, or surgical correction of cardiac defects usually have successful pregnancies, although medical interventions for the management of arrhythmias and heart failure may be necessary. Because more women with congenital heart disease are reaching childbearing age, it is important for obstetricians to become familiar with various cardiac defects and their implications in pregnancy. A multidisciplinary approach involving the specialties of maternal fetal medicine, cardiology, anesthesiology, and clinical genetics is important for optimal care.

Discussion of Cases

CASE 1: MULTIPARA WITH UNCORRECTED TETRALOGY OF FALLOT

A 37-year-old gravida 3, para 2 woman presents at 18 weeks for a fetal echocardiogram for the indication of a family history of congenital heart disease. The fetal echocardiogram is normal, but on further questioning, it is determined that the woman has uncorrected tetralogy of Fallot. In addition, she reports that she has had several episodes of supraventricular tachycardia that has required medical therapy over the past 2 years. A maternal echocardiogram is performed, which confirms uncorrected tetralogy of Fallot with a right ventricular ejection fraction of 20% and systemic pressures in the pulmonary arteries. The maternal oxygen saturation is 72%.

Is the appropriate next step in the management of this patient referral to a cardiac surgeon, termination of the pregnancy, genetics consultation, or disability for the duration of the pregnancy?

The pregnancy should be terminated. There is a 5–15% risk of maternal mortality associated with uncorrected tetralogy of Fallot. This risk increases to 25–50% with the coexistence of pulmonary hypertension. Cyanotic heart disease is also associated with poor perinatal outcomes. Although the overall fetal loss rate with uncorrected tetralogy of Fallot is about 30%, it may be even higher in this particular

case because of the state of her oxygenation. Pregnancy with uncorrected tetralogy of Fallot is risky and not advised. Although consultation with members of the multidisciplinary team caring for women with cardiac disease will be necessary, including preoperative assessments by cardiology and anesthesiology, termination of pregnancy is an appropriate next step in this case due to the significant risk of maternal death.

CASE 2: POSTPARTUM CARDIOVASCULAR COLLAPSE

A 42-year-old gravida 2, para 1 woman with a twin gestation presents at 32 weeks of gestation in active preterm labor. Her previous pregnancy was complicated by preeclampsia and resulted in a cesarean delivery at 30 weeks of gestation. A repeat cesarean section is performed for a non-vertex presenting twin. Postoperatively, she has significant uterine atony and is taken back to the operating room, where a total abdominal hysterectomy is performed. Within 1 hour of the second procedure, her oxygen saturation is difficult to maintain. She is reintubated and transferred to the intensive care unit. An echocardiogram shows mitral valve prolapse, but otherwise the cardiac anatomy is normal. Left ventricular ejection fraction is estimated to be 15%. On further questioning of her family, she had complained of a persistent cough and shortness of breath on minimal exertion for several weeks.

Which condition is most likely responsible for her postoperative low oxygen saturation: myocardial infarction, preeclampsia, mitral valve prolapse, or peripartum cardiomyopathy?

Peripartum cardiomyopathy is the likely cause. Peripartum cardiomyopathy presents as heart failure late in gestation or within 5 months of delivery in the absence of an identifiable cause. Maternal symptoms such as chronic cough, fatigue, or dyspnea are often attributed to the effects of pregnancy. The classic echocardiographic finding is left ventricular systolic dysfunction with an ejection fraction below 45%. This patient has several risk factors for peripartum cardiomyopathy including multiparity, advanced maternal age, and a twin gestation. Medical therapy includes decreasing preload with diuretics, decreasing afterload with vasodilators, and increasing contractility with an inotrope. Overall, about half of patients will have a full recovery, whereas the remaining patients will develop dilated cardiomyopathy. Women with persistent left ventricular dysfunction are advised against future pregnancies due to significant risks of clinical deterioration and death.

REFERENCES

1 Colman JM, Sermer, M, Seaward PGR, et al. Congenital heart disease in pregnancy. *Cardiol Rev* 2000;8:166–173.

2 Clark SL, Cotton DB, Lee W, et al. Central hemodynamic assessment of normal term pregnancy. *Am J Obstet Gynecol* 1989;161:1439–1442.

3 Sawhney H, Suri V, Vasishta K, et al. Pregnancy and congenital heart disease—maternal and fetal outcome. *Aust N Z J Obstet Gynaecol* 1998;38:266–271.

4 Zuber M, Gautschi N, Oechslin E, et al. Outcome of pregnancy in women with congenital shunt lesions. *Heart* 1999;81:271–275.

5 Weiss BM, von Segesser LK, Alon E, et al. Outcome of cardiovascular surgery and pregnancy: a systematic review of the period 1984–1996. *Am J Obstet Gynecol* 1998;179:1643–1653.

6 American College of Obstetricians and Gynecologists. Cardiac disease in pregnancy. *ACOG Tech Bull* 1992;168.

7 Ginsberg JS, Chan WS, Bates SM, et al. Anticoagulation of pregnant women with mechanical heart valves. *Arch Intern Med* 2003;163:694–698.

8 Hung L, Rahimtoola SH. Prosthetic heart valves and pregnancy. *Circulation* 2003;107:1240–1246.

9 Dajani AS, Taubert KA, Wilson W, et al. Prevention of bacterial endocarditis. Recommendations by the American Heart Association. *JAMA* 1997;277:1781–1794.

10 Findlow D, Doyle E. Congenital disease in adults. *Br J Anaesth* 1997;78:416–430.

11 Connolly HM, Warnes CA. Ebstein's anomaly: outcome of pregnancy. *J Am Coll Cardiol* 1994;23:1194–1198.

12 Lao TT, Sermer M, Colman JM. Pregnancy following surgical correction for transposition of the great arteries. *Obstet Gynecol* 1994;83:665–668.

13 Connolly HM, Grogan M, Warnes CA. Pregnancy among women with congenitally corrected transposition of great arteries. *J Am Coll Cardiol* 1999;33:1692–1695.

14 Daliento L, Somerville J, Presbitero P, et al. Eisenmenger syndrome. Factors relating to deterioration and death. *Eur Heart J* 1998;19:1845–1855.

15 Simpson LL, Athanassiou AM, D'Alton ME. Marfan syndrome in pregnancy. *Curr Opin Obstet Gynecol* 1997;9:337–341.

16 Hands ME, Johnson MD, Saltzman DH, et al. The cardiac, obstetric, and anesthetic management of pregnancy complicated by acute myocardial infarction. *J Clin Anesth* 1990;2:258–268.

17 Lupton M, Oteng-Ntim E, Ayida G, et al. Cardiac disease in pregnancy. *Curr Opin Obstet Gynecol* 2002;14:137–143.

18 Scott JR, Wagoner LE, Olsen SL, et al. Pregnancy in heart transplant recipients: management and outcome. *Obstet Gynecol* 1993;82:324–327.

Pathway for Management of Chronic Asthma

Mild intermittent asthma
Short-acting β_2 agonist as
needed for symptoms

REQUIRING SHORT-ACTING β_2 AGONIST
>2x/WEEK OR HAVING NIGHTTIME
SYMPTOMS >2x/MONTH?

Mild persistent asthma
- Add long-term treatment with anti-inflammatory agent
- Inhaled corticosteroids (low dose)–1st choice
- Cromolyn-alternative

SYMPTOMS NOT ADEQUATELY CONTROLLED*?

Moderate persistent asthma
Increase dose of the inhaled corticosteroid (medium dose)
or
Add long-acting β_2 agonist (1st choice)
Add theophylline (alternative)

SYMPTOMS NOT ADEQUATELY CONTROLLED*?

Severe persistent asthma
Increase dose of the inhaled corticosteroid (high dose) (1st choice)
and/or
Add long-acting β_2 agonist
and/or
Periodic use of systemic corticosteriods
and/or
Add sustained theophylline
and/or
Add leukotriene receptor antagonist (consider risk/benefit)

*Goals of asthma control: Minimal or no chronic symptoms day or night, Minimal or no
exacerbations, no limitations on activities; no school/work missed, minimal use of short-
acting β_2 agonists, and minimal or no adverse effects from medications. (NAEPP guidelines)

30 Asthma in Pregnancy

Theresa L. Stewart

Introduction

Asthma is a chronic inflammatory disorder of the airways that has been studied extensively, but its etiology remains unknown. By definition, the airway changes seen during its acute attacks are often at least partly reversible spontaneously or with the use of medications. Histopathologically, the key components of the disease process include numerous inflammatory cells with their secretory products, airway edema, bronchial smooth muscle hyperplasia, and an altered, thickened basement membrane. The clinical diagnosis is considered in patients with a history of episodic symptoms of airway obstruction that include cough, shortness of breath, and wheezing. Spirometry that demonstrates the reversibility of the airway obstruction strongly supports the diagnosis, and the diagnosis can only be established after other causes of airway obstruction have been considered and ruled out.

According to the National Institutes of Health (NIH), the prevalence of asthma has trended upward over the past 20 years. Compared with men, women are more commonly affected and are responsible for more hospitalizations and more emergency room visits. In 1995 the prevalence of asthma among females was 61 in 1000 individuals, thus ranking among the most common chronic conditions in the United States.[1] Because obstetricians and gynecologists are the primary care physicians for many of these women, especially during pregnancy, it is important to be current in the most recent asthma management recommendations. Research on pregnancy has shown that outcome is directly related to the control of asthma, with those patients

Pathway for Management of Acute Asthma Exacerbation

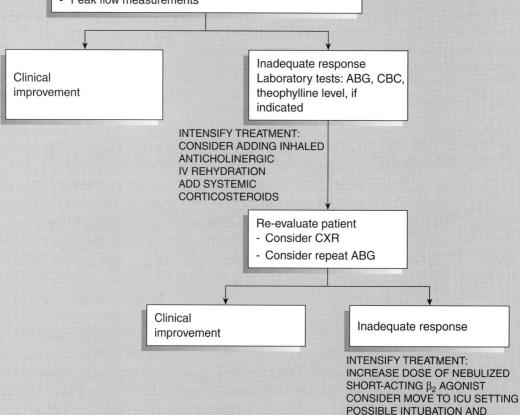

- Brief history and physical examination
- Peak flow and consider ABG
- Start initial treatment promptly:
  - Supplemental oxygen
  - Short-acting inhaled β_2 agonist (nebulizer or MDI with spacer)-treatments every 20–30 minutes $\times$ 3
  - Fetal monitoring (in the 3rd trimester)

- Re-evaluate patient (symptoms, auscultation, pulse, respiratory rate)
- O_2 saturation (goal $\geq$95%)
- Peak flow measurements

Clinical improvement

Inadequate response
Laboratory tests: ABG, CBC, theophylline level, if indicated

INTENSIFY TREATMENT:
CONSIDER ADDING INHALED ANTICHOLINERGIC
IV REHYDRATION
ADD SYSTEMIC CORTICOSTEROIDS

Re-evaluate patient
- Consider CXR
- Consider repeat ABG

Clinical improvement

Inadequate response

INTENSIFY TREATMENT:
INCREASE DOSE OF NEBULIZED SHORT-ACTING β_2 AGONIST
CONSIDER MOVE TO ICU SETTING
POSSIBLE INTUBATION AND MECHANICAL VENTILATION

achieving appropriate control having outcomes similar to those of nonasthmatic pregnant patients.[2]

Fortunately, asthma is an illness whose severity can often be controlled. The frequency of acute exacerbations can be markedly decreased with proper management and patient education. This chapter covers some of the general management recommendations for the pregnant patient with asthma and recommendations for treatment during acute asthma exacerbations.

Classification of Asthma

In a patient with an existing diagnosis of asthma, the first step in management is defining the severity of disease. The NIH has published two excellent references for the management of asthma. The first, which is specifically targeted for obstetric patients, is the report of the Working Group on Asthma and Pregnancy of the National Asthma Education and Prevention Program (NAEPP)[3] and the other is the NAEPP Expert Panel's guidelines for the diagnosis and management of asthma.[4] These can be accessed through the NIH's Web site (http://www.nhlbi.nih.gov/guidelines/asthma/asthgdln.htm). Many of the recommendations in this chapter are taken from these two guidelines.

The classification of asthma severity is based on the patient's medical history and lung function assessment. Assessment of lung function can be performed by spirometry with a forced expiratory volume in 1 second (FEV_1) or by a more easily obtainable, peak expiratory flow rate (PEFR). The next step in evaluating the underlying severity includes obtaining a detailed description of the patient's symptoms. The frequency, type, and timing of symptoms the patient is experiencing should be obtained. Any activity or exposures that trigger symptoms and frequency of medication use should also be documented. Based on this information, the severity of asthma is divided into four categories: mild intermittent, mild persistent, moderate persistent, and severe persistent.[4]

Management of Chronic Asthma

The guidelines for the management of asthma follow a stepwise approach to medications. The recommended management depends on the severity of the underlying asthma and the severity of the individual exacerbation. For long-term symptoms of asthma, a "step-up" approach is used in which medications are started at lower doses and increased gradually until symptoms are adequately controlled. Additional drugs are added sequentially after an individual response has been evaluated and found to be inadequate. During acute exacerbations, a higher dose of medication is often started and, once control is achieved, the dose is gradually decreased until the lowest dose required to maintain control of symptoms is reached ("step-down" method).[4] Most pharmacologic therapies for asthma focus on decreasing the inflammatory response or reversing the bronchoconstriction seen in acute episodes.

All patients, regardless of asthmatic severity, should have available a short-acting, inhaled β_2 agonist for quick relief of bronchoconstrictive symptoms. Albuterol is the most widely used medication in this class. Albuterol can be given as a metered dose inhaler (MDI), a dry powered inhaler, or as a nebulized solution. The use of a spacer or holding chamber can often improve the delivery of the medication into the lungs, especially during a severe exacerbation or in those patients who have difficulty with coordination of breathing (slow inhalation followed by 10 seconds of holding) that is required for the use of the MDI. The usual dose varies with the clinical indications: two puffs 5 minutes before exercise or exposure or two puffs every 4–8 hours for up to 24 hours during an exacerbation. Each puff contains albuterol 90 µg. The use of short-acting inhaled β_2 agonists is not generally recommended for long-term or routine daily use.[5] The amount of albuterol should be monitored because escalating doses may indicate worsening asthma control and the need to start the patient on a long-term medication. Once a patient's asthma progresses from mild intermittent to mild persistent, the use of a daily medication is indicated.

Studies have shown that therapy for asthma, in terms of long-term outcome, should be aimed at the prevention and/or decrease in the inflammatory response. Inhaled steroids are the most effective long-term therapy and the treatment of choice for all persistent asthma.[4] Corticosteroids improve peak expiratory flow and clinical symptoms and decrease airway hyperresponsiveness and the frequency of exacerbations. There are different inhaled steroids available. All can be used as low, medium, or high doses. If starting inhaled steroids in a patient with mild persistent asthmatic symptoms, the usual approach is to begin with a low dose and increase the dosage until symptoms are controlled. Goals for asthma therapy include no limitations on activities, no missed workdays, minimal use of short-acting β agonists, minimal or no side effects from medications, and minimal to no symptoms throughout the day and night.[4] During an acute exacerbation, a higher dose may be used initially and then gradually titrated down after the acute episode has resolved. Beclomethasone has the most information available concerning its use in pregnancy and therefore is often the drug of choice when treatment is initiated during pregnancy. At similar doses, there is no reason to believe that the other inhaled steroids are less safe than beclomethasone. Therefore, when a patient whose asthma is controlled with another inhaled steroid becomes pregnant, there is no obstetric reason to change her steroid inhaler. Another drug that aims at decreasing the inflammatory response is inhaled cromolyn. This agent is an alternative therapy for patients with mild persistent asthma and can be used safely in pregnancy.

For patients with moderate persistent symptoms, the dose of the inhaled steroid can be increased (medium dose) or consideration can be given to adding a long-acting β agonist as the next step. The long-acting β agonists have been shown to improve lung function, decrease asthma symptoms, and improve quality of life. These agents are particularly helpful for patients with night-time symptoms.[6]

Patients with severe persistent symptoms usually require multiple medications to control their symptoms. Usually a combination of large-dose inhaled corticosteroids, a long-acting bronchodilator such as a long-acting β agonist or sustained released theophylline, and the periodic use of systemic corticosteroids is needed.

The leukotriene modifiers montelukast, zafirlukast, and zileuton are the newest class of drugs used to control asthma. The specific clinical indication for these drugs is still being explored. They are usually considered an alternative for patients with mild persistent symptoms or as part of a combination regimen for patients with more severe symptoms. The leukotriene modifiers have the least amount of pregnancy safety data and therefore are not considered first-line treatment in pregnant asthmatic patients. In patients whose asthma has been difficult to control before pregnancy without the use of montelukast or zafirlukast, one could consider continuing these medications because preliminary studies have been reassuring. However, some animal studies have demonstrated adverse effects with zileuton, so this drug should be avoided in pregnancy.[7]

One of the most important aspects of asthma management is patient education. The patient's self-management is often the key to controlling disease. Patients must be educated about asthma. They should be aware of situations and conditions that precipitate exacerbations so that they can be avoided. They should be able to assess the severity of their symptoms and initiate therapy and, most importantly, they need to know when to seek medical care. Regular use of home monitoring with a hand-held peak flow meter is usually recommended for patients with moderate to severe asthma, and all asthmatic patients should have a rescue/action plan that has been explained and discussed with them. Patient education and early treatment allow better control of symptoms and can prevent a severe exacerbation.

Management of Acute Asthma

When an asthmatic patient presents with an exacerbation, a brief history and physical examination should be performed, with the goal to start therapy very early in the presentation. Some measurement of expiratory flow (PEFR or FEV_1) should be performed as part of the initial evaluation. This initial evaluation will give the provider some insight into the severity of the exacerbation and the possibility of impending respiratory failure. Arterial blood gas assessment should be used liberally in the management of pregnant women presenting with an acute exacerbation of asthma. Guidance from the NAEPP Working Group suggests that arterial blood gases must be assessed when patients present with obvious hypoventilation, cyanosis, or severe distress after initial therapy, or if the PEFR is less than 200 L/min or the FEV_1 remains less than 40% of the predicted value.[3] Importantly, initiation of therapy for acute asthma in pregnancy should not be delayed while performing or awaiting the results of pulmonary function tests or arterial blood gas analysis. A normal maternal arterial partial pressure of oxygen (PaO_2) is 101–108 mm Hg early in pregnancy and decreases to 90–100 mm Hg near term. There is a widened

KEY POINT

Physiologic changes associated with normal pregnancy make the pregnant asthmatic patient more susceptible to the effects of hypoxia.

KEY POINT

Due to maternofetal physiology, the fetus may show signs of hypoxia before the mother does.

alveolar-arterial oxygen gradient [$P(A − a)O_2$] that averages 20 mm Hg in the third trimester.[8] The normal physiologic increase in minute ventilation during pregnancy is reflected by an arterial partial pressure of carbon dioxide ($Paco_2$) of 27–32 mm Hg and an increase in pH from 7.40 to 7.45.[9] As a result of these physiologic changes, a $Paco_2$ higher than 35 mm Hg, with a pH below 7.35 in the presence of a decreasing Pao_2, should be considered respiratory failure in a pregnant asthmatic patient.

The patient should be placed in a near-sitting position, with a leftward tilt, especially if in the third trimester. Supplemental oxygen should be given to the mother to maintain a Pao_2 higher than 65 mm Hg or an oxygen saturation of 95% on oxygen (fraction of inspired oxygen) of 35–60% without causing hypercarbia. Therapy should be directed toward correcting maternal hypoxia, rapidly reversing airflow obstruction, and optimizing uteroplacental function. Maternal Pao_2 should be monitored closely because fetal oxygen saturation can decrease profoundly, with maternal values below 60 mm Hg. Monitoring and resuscitative equipment should be readily available (including electronic fetal heart rate monitoring, if appropriate for gestational age). If a severe exacerbation or life-threatening asthma is suspected, provisions for intubation and ventilation should be accessible, preferably in an intensive care unit. Intravenous access should be started for administration of medications and for careful rehydration because, during an exacerbation, patients are frequently volume depleted secondary to decreased oral intake and high respiratory insensible losses.

The last component of the primary therapy of an acute asthma exacerbation includes the use of short-acting β_2 agonists and systemic corticosteriods.[4] Initial treatment starts with a short-acting β_2 agonist by MDI every 20 minutes or by nebulizer. The patient should then be reevaluated to ensure response to the therapy. If the immediate response is inadequate or the patient has recently discontinued oral systemic steroids, oral steroids should be added at this point. Anticholinergic therapy can be added to the β agonist if the exacerbation is severe or response is inadequate. The frequency and duration of the therapies depend on the patient's response. Inhaled β-agonist therapy can be spread out to every hour and then every 4–6 hours as the patient continues to improve.

KEY POINT

The threshold for when to hospitalize a patient for asthma exacerbations should be lower in the pregnant than in the nonpregnant population.

After initial stabilization of the patient has occurred, a workup for a possible cause of the asthma exacerbation should be considered. The workup should be guided by the patient's history of present illness and usually includes a chest radiograph to rule out other pulmonary disease. The decision of whether to admit for hospitalization should be based on the severity of the exacerbation and the severity of the underlying disease. It is recommended that admission for asthma be more liberal in pregnant patients secondary to the physiologic changes in pregnancy that make them more susceptible to the development of hypoxia.

What's the Evidence?

In previous studies, investigators noted significant increases in rates of abortion, preterm labor, low birth weight, and neonatal hypoxia in pregnant asthmatic patients.[10–12] Reporting on 277 patients with asthma in the Collaborative Study of Cerebral Palsy, Mental Retardation, and Other Allied Neurological Diseases, Gordon and coworkers found a perinatal mortality rate double that of controls without asthma.[13] In the subgroup of patients with severe asthma (repetitive attacks, persistent symptoms, or status asthmaticus), the perinatal mortality rate was 28%. Greenberger and colleagues demonstrated that, among women with asthma, those whose pregnancy is complicated by status asthmaticus have significantly smaller infants and a greater frequency of intrauterine growth retardation.[14] However, many of the studies that addressed pregnancy outcome have not controlled for the level of asthma control during the pregnancy and this may have played a significant role in determining outcome. This concept is supported by data from Schatz and colleagues[2] that showed, when asthma during pregnancy is controlled with step therapy, as currently recommended,[4] adverse perinatal outcomes are not increased over those in the general population.

In terms of the safety of asthma medications during pregnancy, there is a significant amount of data available. The value of inhaled steroids in pregnant asthmatic patients has been documented in a number of studies. In a prospective study by Stenius-Aarniala and associates, 504 patients with asthma were followed to assess the effects of regularly used inhaled steroids in pregnancy.[15] They compared the frequency of acute asthma attacks, length of gestation, length of the third stage of labor, amount of hemorrhage, and neonatal complications after delivery in women who routinely used inhaled steroids versus women who did not. The risk of having an acute asthma attack was significantly decreased in those women who regularly used inhaled steroids (RR 0.22, 95% CI 0.11–0.44). There were no significant differences in any of the other outcomes they examined. In addition, Wendel and coworkers reported that, in pregnant women who were admitted to the hospital for an asthma exacerbation, the readmission rate was decreased by 55% in women who had inhaled steroids (beclomethasone) added to the treatment regimen compared with women who were discharged home with only a steroid taper and a β_2 agonist.[16]

Short-acting β agonists have been used for many years in the pregnant population and have not been shown to have any adverse maternal or fetal effects.[17] The safety of long-acting inhaled β agonists has been evaluated but only in small studies. There have not been reports of adverse outcomes associated with their use, and, depending on the clinical scenario, the benefits may outweigh any theoretical risks.[7]

Guiding Questions in Approaching the Patient

The pregnant asthmatic patient

- What is the severity of the underlying illness?
- Is the patient being optimally treated for her disease level?
- Is the patient able to self-assess and monitor her disease severity?
- Is she able to maintain nearly normal activity levels and lung function?
- Is the patient educated regarding her illness and actively involved in avoiding exacerbations?
- Does the patient have a written action or rescue plan?

The pregnant asthmatic during an acute attack

- How severe is the exacerbation?
- Is the patient responding to the initial treatment?
- Is there a treatable cause for the acute exacerbation?
- Is electronic fetal monitoring indicated (dependent on gestational age)?

- Does the patient require inpatient hospitalization for this episode?
- What can be done to prevent recurrence of the exacerbation?

Conclusion

Optimization of asthma control can significantly decrease adverse outcomes in pregnant patients so that their risk closely approximates the risk of the uncomplicated pregnancy. Although the physiologic changes that accompany normal pregnancy need to be kept in mind while caring for these patients, their asthma management is not substantially different from that in the nonpregnant patient. As with any chronic maternal illness, fetal exposure to minimally studied drugs is a recurring problem in obstetrics. Fetal outcome can be assured only when maternal health is optimized. Risk-versus-benefit considerations need to be individualized, and the importance of maintaining asthma control cannot be underestimated.

Discussion of Cases

CASE 1: ASTHMA EXACERBATION

A 31-year-old gravida 1, para 0 at almost 32 weeks presents with complaints of worsening asthma symptoms despite increased use of albuterol inhaler for 2 days. She has had asthma for 6 years. She was previously hospitalized for asthma and that was at the time of her original asthma diagnosis. Her usual PEFR is 400 L/min. She takes inhaled beclomethasone daily and usually uses her albuterol inhaler two to three times a week. She also has seasonal allergies and takes an antihistamine as needed. She has had increasing symptoms of allergies over the past 5 days. On physical examination, minimal expiratory wheezing is heard on auscultation. Her PEFR is 150 L/min. Her initial treatment consisted of an inhaled, short-acting β_2-agonist nebulizer every 20 minutes three times daily. Upon reevaluation her PEFR is 170 L/min and she states she is feeling minimally improved.

What is the next step for her management?

Because her PEFR is still below 50% of her baseline level and has improved only by approximately 10%, further evaluation and an increase in her therapy is indicated. An arterial blood gas should be obtained and electronic fetal monitoring started. A pulse oximeter should be placed for continuous maternal assessment, nebulized treatment should be continued, and the addition of systemic steroids would be indicated.

After her next treatment, the patient states she is beginning to notice some improvement and her repeat PEFR is 240 L/min. Her oxygen saturation is 96% on oxygen 4 L. Chest radiograph shows no infiltrate. The fetal heart rate monitoring is reassuring. Clinically, she is volume depleted and intravenous hydration is initiated. Her nebulizer treatments are spread out to every 2–4 hours. She is admitted for observation and continues to gradually improve over the next 24 hours. On her third day of admission, her oxygen saturation is 98–100% on room air. She is discharged home on systemic corticosteroids for 5 days and inhaled steroid is restarted at a higher dose. The patient has an action and rescue plan and a follow-up appointment in 3 days.

CASE 2: ASTHMA AND FEBRILE ILLNESS

The same patient as described for case 1 presents in a similar manner except that, approximately 12 hours after admission, she complains of worsening symptoms and her oxygen saturation shows a decrease to 91%. Her PEFR is now 170 L/min. Her cough has worsened, and her temperature is 101.8°F. Auscultation demonstrates expiratory wheezing and decreased breath sounds.

What is the next step in her management?

Increase her oxygen supplementation and β₂-agonist nebulized treatments again. Addition of anticholinergics may be considered. Because she has a change in her symptoms and a new fever, a repeat chest radiograph should be obtained.

Repeat chest radiograph shows a right lower lobe infiltrate that had not been noted the previous day.

What is the most likely diagnosis and is this a complication of the asthma exacerbation?

Community-acquired pneumonia is the most likely diagnosis. The pneumonia is most likely the etiology rather than a complication of the asthma exacerbation. When a patient presents with volume depletion and early in the infectious process, the infiltrate can be difficult to visualize on radiograph. After hydration and progression of the infection, the infiltrate is more easily identified. The only addition to this patient's asthma management would be antibiotics. This patient needs to have frequent reevaluation to ensure improvement in respiratory status. She is at an increased risk for respiratory failure and the need for intubation and mechanical ventilation.

REFERENCES

1 National Institutes of Health, National Heart, Lung and Blood Institute. Asthma statistics. Data Fact Sheet January 1999.

2 Schatz M, Zeiger RS, Hoffman CP, et al. Perinatal outcomes in the pregnancies of asthmatic women; a prospective controlled analysis. *Am J Respir Crit Care Med* 1995;151:1170–1174.

3 National Institutes of Health, National Heart, Lung, and Blood Institute. *Management of Asthma During Pregnancy: Report of the Working Group on Asthma and Pregnancy.* National Asthma Education Program, NIH Publication No. 93-3279. Washington, DC: Public Health Service, US Department of Health and Human Services, 1993.

4 National Institutes of Health, National Heart, Lung and Blood Institute. *National Asthma Education and Prevention Program Expert Panel Summary Report: Guidelines for the Diagnosis and Treatment of Asthma—Update on Selected Topics.* NIH Publication No. 02-5075. Washington, DC: Public Health Service, US Department of Health and Human Services; 2002.

5 Drazen JM, Israel E, Boushey HA, et al. Comparison of regularly scheduled with as-needed use of albuterol in mild asthma. *N Engl J Med* 1996;335:841–847.

6 Moore RH, Khan A, Dickey BF. Long-acting inhaled beta2-agonists in asthma therapy. *Chest* 1998;113:1095–1108.

7 American College of Obstetricians and Gynecologists/American College of Allergy, Asthma and Immunology. The use of newer asthma and allergy medications during pregnancy. *Ann Allerg Asthma Immunol* 2000;84:475–480.

8 Awe RJ, Nicotra MB, Newsom TD, Viles R. Arterial oxygenation and aveolar-arterial gradients in term pregnancy. *Obstet Gynecol* 1979;53:182–186.

9 Hankins GD, Clark SL, Harvey CJ, et al. Third-trimester arterial blood gas and acid base values in normal pregnancy at moderate altitude. *Obstet Gynecol* 1996;88:347–350.

10 Schaefer G, Silverman F. Pregnancy complicated by asthma. *Am J Obstet Gynecol* 1961;82:182–191.

11 Bahna SL, Bjerkedal T. The course and outcome of pregnancy in women with bronchial asthma. *Acta Allerg* 1972;27:397–406.

12 Sims CD, Chamberlain GVP, De Swret M. Lung function tests in bronchial asthma during and after pregnancy. *Br J Obstet Gynaecol* 1976;83:434–437.

13 Gordon M, Niswander KR, Berendes H, Kantor AG. Fetal morbidity following potentially anxiogenic obstetric conditions: bronchial asthma. *Am J Obstet Gynecol* 1970;106:421–429.

14 Greenberger PA, Patterson R. The outcome of pregnancy complicated by severe asthma. Allergy Proc 1988;9:539–543.

15 Stenius-Aarniala BS, Hedman J. Acute asthma during pregnancy. *Thorax* 1996;51:411–414.

16 Wendel PJ, Ramin SM, Barnett-Hamm C, et al. Asthma treatment in pregnancy: a randomized controlled study. *Am J Obstet Gynecol* 1996;175:150–154.

17 Schatz M, Zeiger RS, Harden KM, et al. The safety of inhaled beta-agonist bronchodilators during pregnancy. *J Allergy Clin Immunol* 1988;82:686–695.

Pathway to Management of Pneumonia

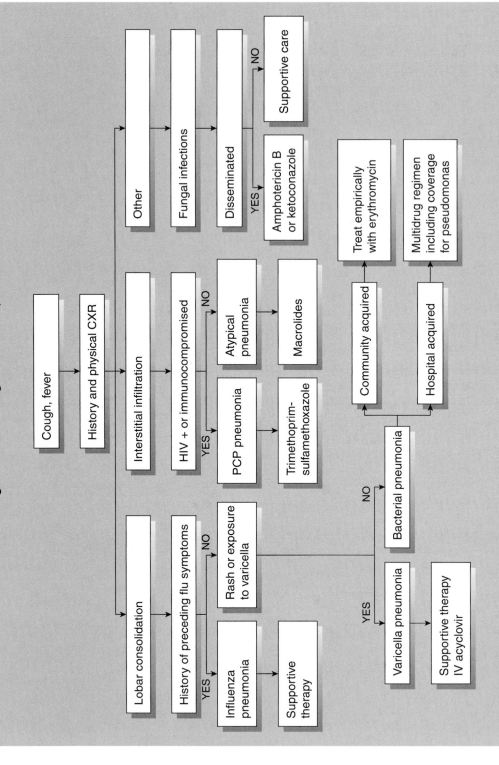

31

Pneumonia

Erika Peterson

Introduction

Pneumonia is an infection of the lung parenchyma including alveolar spaces and interstitial tissue. The pathogen usually reaches the lungs by inhalation or aspiration from the upper respiratory tract. It then reaches the bronchioles, proliferates, and causes an inflammatory reaction. This causes a congestion of fluid into the alveolar spaces. Pneumonia can be classified into three types: lobar pneumonia, which affects an entire lobe; bronchopneumonia, which affects the alveoli contiguous to the bronchi; and interstitial pneumonia, which affects the interstitial tissue. Pneumonia is a fairly rare complication of pregnancy that occurs in fewer than 1% of pregnancies.[1] However, pregnancy has many effects on the pulmonary system such as increased cardiac load and decreased ventilatory reserve that can lead to difficulty in combating respiratory infections. Pneumonia is one of the leading causes of maternal death related to nonobstetric infection.[1]

Etiologies

BACTERIAL PNEUMONIA

KEY POINT

Streptococcus pneumoniae *is the most common bacterial pathogen in community-acquired pneumonia in the general population.*

Streptococcus pneumoniae is the most common bacterial pathogen in community-acquired pneumonia in the general population. Gram stains of a sputum sample show gram-positive diplococci. *Haemophilus influenza* is the second most common pathogen in pneumonia in the pregnant population. It is a pleomorphic gram-negative coccobacillus, but Gram stains are often inconclusive and, hence, not ideal for diagnosis. Other rare causes of community-acquired pneumonia are *Klebsiella pneumoniae*, a gram-negative rod, and *Staphylococcus aureus*, a gram-positive coccus usually

541

seen in clusters. *Mycoplasma* and *Chlamydia pneumoniae* usually cause a more mild atypical pneumonia.

VIRAL PNEUMONIA

Pneumonia related to a viral infection is usually a complication of an upper respiratory viral infection. The two most common causes of viral pneumonia are influenza and varicella zoster. The influenza virus is an RNA virus that usually causes a self-limiting upper respiratory infection. It has three different strains: influenza A, influenza B, and influenza C. Influenza A is responsible for most of the endemic outbreaks and is usually a more severe infection. Influenza B is less common and has a milder course. Influenza C is the least clinically significant. The varicella virus is a DNA herpesvirus. It is characteristically a very contagious virus that presents with a pustular rash that is most common in children. Fewer than 2% of adults acquire or contract a primary infection.[2] Viral pneumonia can occur with any of these infections and significantly increases their morbidity and mortality. Secondary bacterial pneumonia can also occur with influenza or varicella pneumonia.

FUNGAL AND PARASITIC PNEUMONIAS

KEY POINT

Prevention of aspiration pneumonia in the postpartum period includes the use of antacids before anesthesia, the preferential use of regional anesthesia, and the use of rapid sequence induction.

Fungal and parasitic infections are rare in the healthy patient. Both are more common in the immunocompromised patient. *Pneumocystis carinii* is a parasitic infection that has gained prevalence with the increased number of patients who are infected with the human immunodeficiency virus (HIV). It is seen almost exclusively in immunocompromised hosts and causes an interstitial pneumonia that is often life threatening.

Many fungi can cause pneumonia, including histoplasmosis, blastomycosis, coccidioidomycosis, and cryptococcosis. Spores are present in soil and cause infection after inhalation. Most infections are self-limiting and usually mild. In some studies, coccidioidomycosis manifested as a more severe disseminated infection during pregnancy.[3] However, studies done in endemic areas have not shown this increased risk of dissemination and have noted that maternal mortality is rare.[4]

ASPIRATION PNEUMONIA

Aspiration of gastric contents was previously associated with high morbidity and mortality rates during labor and delivery. Gastric contents in the lung cause an immediate chemical pneumonitis followed by a secondary bacterial pneumonia. Pregnant women are at increased risk of aspiration due to delayed gastric emptying, relaxation of the gastroesophageal sphincter, and increased intra-abdominal pressure secondary to the gravid uterus. Prevention of aspiration pneumonia in the postpartum period includes the use of antacids before anesthesia, the preferential use of regional anesthesia, and the use of rapid sequence induction.

Diagnosis

KEY POINT

The common symptoms of pneumonia include dyspnea, chest pain, fever, malaise, and productive cough.

The common symptoms of pneumonia include dyspnea, chest pain, fever, malaise, and productive cough. The diagnosis of pneumonia in the nonpregnant population is usually straightforward, but misdiagnosis is not uncommon in the pregnant patient. Yost and coworkers found a 10% rate of misdiagnosis in their series.[5] The diagnosis is complicated by confusion of symptoms with normal physiologic changes in pregnancy. Dyspnea is a common physiologic symptom in normal pregnant women, especially in the second and third trimesters. Other diagnoses in the differential include asthma (Chap. 30), tuberculosis (Chap. 23), and pulmonary embolism (Chap 26). Clinical signs include decreased breath sounds, rales, and dullness to percussion. Mild leukocytosis is common. The diagnosis is confirmed by chest radiograph, but this does not confirm the etiology. Chest radiography with two views exposes the fetus to approximately 0.02–0.07 mrad of radiation.[6] This small dose is not associated with an adverse outcome, and chest radiographs should not be avoided in pregnancy when indicated. Sputum culture is diagnostic in fewer than 50% of cases. Serology may be helpful in the diagnosis of viral etiologies, but in most cases of viral pneumonia the precedent clinical presentation is usually diagnostic. Clinical presentation of aspiration pneumonia usually involves respiratory distress or cough, fever, and decreased oxygen saturation. Aspiration pneumonia should always be considered if symptomatology begins 24–48 hours after delivery, especially after cesarean section or general anesthesia.

Management

The treatment of choice will depend on the suspected etiology. In the case of community-acquired bacterial pneumonia, antimicrobial therapy must be focused on the most common pathogens. Because identification of a specific pathogen is usually difficult and requires days to confirm, the initial choice of antibiotics is usually empiric. Erythromycin therapy is recommended in an uncomplicated case of community-acquired pneumonia.[7] The usual dose is 500–1000 mg every 6 hours, orally or intravenously. The newer erythromycin analogs are also acceptable. Azithromycin is commonly used for outpatient therapy secondary to once-a-day dosing. Penicillins and cephalosporins have also been shown to be safe in pregnancy and provide good coverage if *Staphylococcus* or *Haemophilus* is suspected. The American Thoracic Society has established guidelines for hospitalization of community-acquired pneumonia in the nonpregnant population (Table 31-1).[7] These factors have been associated with an increased risk of respiratory distress. Although studies have shown that pneumonia in pregnancy can be managed on an outpatient basis,[5] patients are often initially treated as inpatients to assess for possible deterioration.

Viral pneumonia is usually associated with a more serious course. Influenza pneumonia may run a self-limiting course of 3–5 days and may not require any treatment other than supportive measures. If symptoms persist or worsen, then broad-spectrum antibiotics such as cephalosporin are usually necessary to cover a potential superimposed bacterial infection. Viral agents such as amantadine can be used to help decrease the length and severity of the course. Amantadine is a category C drug, which has been shown to be teratogenic in large doses in animals. There is no clear evidence of teratogenicity in humans. Varicella pneumonia has been associated with a mortality rate of 10–35% in the pregnant patient.[8] Hospitalization is usually necessary. Treatment is supportive with fluids, oxygen, and bedrest. Intravenous acyclovir 10 mg/kg every 8 hours is considered by most the therapy of

Table 31-1. **AMERICAN THORACIC SOCIETY GUIDELINES FOR HOSPITALIZATION OF PATIENTS WITH COMMUNITY-ACQUIRED PNEUMONIA**

Coexisting illness
Altered mental status
Respirations >30 breaths/min
Temperature >38.3°C
White blood cell count <4,000 cells/mm^3 or >30,000 cells/mm^3

Source: American Thoracic Society. Guidelines for the management of adults with community-acquired pneumonia. *Am J Respir Crit Care Med 2001*;163:1730–1754.

choice. If a pregnant woman has been exposed to varicella, administration of varicella zoster immunoglobin within 96 hours of exposure may help to prevent or attenuate infection.

Pneumocystis pneumonia has a maternal mortality rate that has been noted to be extremely high, at 50–60%.[9] Respiratory failure that requires intubation is common. Therapy involves hospitalization, with administration of trimethoprim-sulfamethoxazole, or pentamidine. Both drugs are category C, but secondary to the severity of the infection, the benefits largely outweigh the potential risks. The Center for Disease Control and Prevention has recommended prophylaxis for pneumocystic infection in patients with HIV and severe compromise, including women with a CD4 count lower than 200/μL, a history of oral candidiasis, or if CD4 cells constitute fewer than 20% of lymphocytes.[10] Prophylaxis is oral double-strength trimethoprim-sulfamethoxazole once daily. Treatment of disseminated fungal infections, such as coccidioidomycosis, usually involves amphotericin B or ketoconazole. Both drugs are pregnancy category C. Amphotericin B data are limited, but no adverse outcomes have been reported. Ketoconazole has been shown to have teratogenic effects in large doses in animals. No human data are available.

Management of aspiration pneumonia involves broad-spectrum antibiotics including coverage for gram-negative and anaerobic organisms. Supportive therapy is important until antibiotics can be administered and be effective.

Maternal and Fetal Complications

Pneumonia has been reported in all stages of pregnancy. Patients with pneumonia during the antepartum period are more likely to receive tocolytics and steroids for fetal lung maturity.[11] Compared with controls, patients with pneumonia were more likely to deliver more small-for-gestational-aage infants and more likely to deliver before 34 weeks of gestation.[11] In the setting of varicella pneumonia, fetal varicella syndrome complicates 2% of cases. *Pneumocystis carinii* pneumonia associated with HIV has been shown to have a very high mortality rate in pregnant women. Thus, fetal mortality is also high, and many surviving infants have an added morbidity secondary to preterm delivery.[12]

What's the Evidence?

ANTIBIOTIC REGIMENS Therapeutic guidelines published by the American Thoracic Society involve the use of cefuroxime plus erythromycin for uncomplicated community-acquired pneumonia. This regimen has shown to give a clinical cure rate of 91%.[13] Two separate randomized trials performed in nonpregnant patients have shown that azithromycin is as effective as cefuroxime plus erythromycin, with fewer adverse effects.[13,14] The guidelines on treatment based on coverage of the most common organisms are generally accepted in the pregnant woman, despite a lack of any randomized trials in this population.

RISK FACTORS Munn and associates showed that pregnant women with pneumonia are more likely to have asthma and anemia, receive tocolytics and steroids, and deliver at a mean earlier gestational age than pregnant controls.[11]

NEED FOR HOSPITALIZATION Guidelines for hospitalization in the non-pregnant state proposed by the American Thoracic Society were studied during pregnancy by Yost and colleagues.[5] These investigators found that pregnant women who did not meet these guidelines for hospitalization did not have a complicated course of the disease. Conversely, 96% of women who had a complicated course would have met guidelines for hospitalization. They showed that, by using the American Thoracic Society guidelines for hospitalization, they would have decreased the number of patients admitted by 25%.[5]

Guiding Questions in Approaching the Patient

- Has the patient had any preceding flu-like symptoms?
- Does the patient have a rash?
- Has the patient been in any areas endemic to fungal pathogens?
- Is the patient immunocompromised?
- Does the patient have a risk factor for aspiration pneumonia?

Conclusion

Although pneumonia rarely occurs during pregnancy, it can cause many complications including preterm delivery or death. The diagnosis of pneumonia is clinical, and the etiology is often suspected by exposure history. Hospitalization is usually necessary in the initial period to decrease the risk of complications. Bacterial pneumonia requires antibiotic therapy, whereas other forms of pneumonia usually involve only supportive therapy.

Discussion of Cases

CASE 1: COMMUNITY-ACQUIRED PNEUMONIA

A 30-year-old gravida 1, para 0 at 30 weeks of gestation is hospitalized with preterm labor, and she received betamethasone and intravenous magnesium sulfate. She was otherwise healthy before admission to the hospital. About 24 hours after admission the patient develops a productive cough, dyspnea, and a fever of 101.5°F. She had a mildly increased leukocyte count of 13,000 and chest radiography showed a right lower lobe infiltrate.

What organism is most likely responsible for this presentation?

Streptococcus pneumonia, Mycoplasma pneumonia, or Haemophilus influenza.

Does she require any further testing for diagnosis?

The use of sputum Gram stain and culture for diagnosis are somewhat controversial. The American Thoracic Society recommends sputum culture if drug resistance or an unusual organism is suspected. Therapy should not be withheld while awaiting these results.

What is the best initial management?

Empiric therapy should cover the most frequent organisms that cause community-acquired pneumonia. Erythromycin is usually the initial therapy. Alternatives include other macrolides or cephalosporins.

CASE 2: PNEUMONIA IN AN IMMUNOCOMPROMISED PATIENT

A 27-year-old gravida 4, para 2012 at 37 weeks of gestation has HIV that was diagnosed 2 years previously. The patient's disease has not been well controlled and she has a CD4 count of 112. She presents with complaints of contractions every 7 minutes. Her cervix is 1 centimeter dilated, 50% effaced, and −2 status. In response to questioning, the patient reports a dry cough during the past 2 weeks. She has been becoming increasingly dyspneic over the past week. Her blood pressure is 110/72 mm Hg, her respiratory rate is 30 breaths/min, and her temperature is 100.7°F. Chest radiography shows diffuse patchy infiltrates.

What organisms is most likely responsible for this presentation?

Pneumocystis carinii.

Does she require further testing for diagnosis?

Bronchial biopsy can be obtained for definitive diagnosis but is not necessary before beginning therapy.

What is the best initial management?

Trimethoprim-sulfamethoxazole.

Will her labor have any effect on her respiratory status?

Studies have shown no adverse effects related to labor during the course of pneumonia. There is no evidence suggesting delay of delivery in a term pregnancy based on respiratory status.

What is the mortality rate of this in pregnancy?

The mortality rate with *P. carinii* pneumonia is as high as 50%.

REFERENCES

1 Kaunitz AM, Hughes JM, Grimes DA, et al. Causes of maternal mortality in the United States. *Obstet Gynecol* 1985;65:605–612.

2 Preblud SR. Age specific risk of varicella complications. *Pediatrics* 1981;68:14–17.

3 Peterson CM, Schuppert PC, Pappagianis D. Coccidioidomycosis and pregnancy. *Obstet Gynecol Surv* 1993;48:149–156.

4 Caldwell JW, Arsura EL, Kilgore WB, et al. Coccidioidomycosis in pregnancy during an epidemic in California. *Obstet Gynecol* 2000;95:236–239.

5 Yost NP, Bloom SL, Richey SD, et al. An appraisal of treatment guidelines for antepartum community-acquired pneumonia. *Am J Obstet Gynecol* 2000;183:131–135.

6 American College of Obstetricians and Gynecologists Committee Opinion #158, "Guidelines for Diagnostic Imaging in Pregnancy." September, 1995.

7 American Thoracic Society. Guidelines for the management of adults with community-acquired pneumonia. *Am J Respir Crit Care Med* 2001;163:1730–1754.

8 American College of Obstetrics and Gynecology. Pulmonary disease in pregnancy. *ACOG Tech Bull* 1996.

9 Saade GR. Human immunodeficiency virus (HIV) related pulmonary complications in pregnancy. *Semin Perinatol* 1997;21:336.

10 Center for Disease Control and Prevention. USPHS/IDSA guidelines for the prevention of opportunistic infections in persons infected with human immunodeficiency virus. *MMWR* 1999;48:(RR-10):1.

11 Munn MB, Groome LJ, Atterbury JL, et al. Pneumonia as a complication of pregnancy. *J Matern Fetal Med* 1999;8:151–154.

12 Ahmad H, Mehta NJ, Manikal VM, et al. *Pneumocystis carinii* pneumonia in pregnancy. *Chest* 2001;120:666–671.

13 Vergis EN, Indorf A, File TM Jr, et al. Azithromycin vs. cefuroxime plus erythromycin for empirical treatment of community-acquired pneumonia in hospitalized patients: a prospective, randomized multicenter trial. *Arch Intern Med* 2000;160:1294–1300.

14 Plouffe J, Schwartz DB, Koloksthis A, et al. Clinical Efficacy of intravenous followed by oral azithromycin monotherapy in hospitalized patients with community-acquired pneumonia. *Antimicrob Agents Chemother* 2000;44:1796–1802.

Evaluation for Carpal Tunnel Syndrome

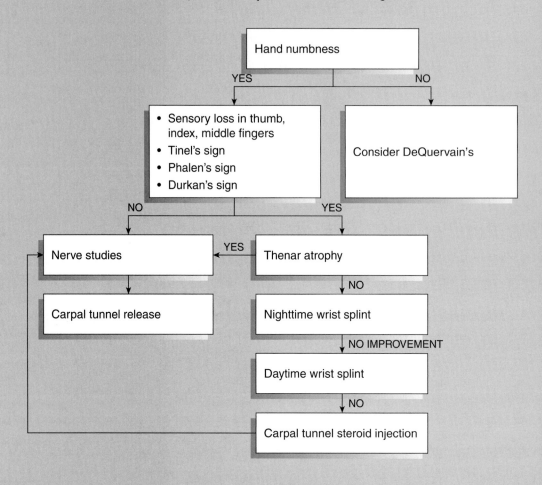

32 Carpal Tunnel Syndrome

Charles Cassidy
Johnny Chang

Introduction

During pregnancy, hormonal and anatomic changes contribute to a host of musculoskeletal complaints. Of these complaints, hand and wrist pain comprise the second largest proportion after low back pain.[1] Carpal tunnel syndrome (CTS) affecting the flexor compartment of the wrist is the most commonly encountered disorder that affects the hand and wrist in pregnancy. Although patients typically expect some degree of musculoskeletal discomfort in pregnancy, it is critical that these conditions be diagnosed and followed to alleviate potentially debilitating symptoms and to prevent permanent damage.

Anatomy and Pathophysiology

BORDERS OF THE CARPAL CANAL

The carpal tunnel is a passageway in the wrist bounded posteriorly by the arch of the carpal bones and anteriorly by the transverse carpal ligament (flexor retinaculum), a thickening of the deep fascia of the forearm at the wrist. The contents of the carpal tunnel include the median nerve ands nine flexor tendons: four flexor digitorum superificialis, four flexor digitorum profundus, and the flexor pollicis longus. During hand and wrist movements such as wrist flexion and extension, the tendons glide significantly. The tendon lining, or tenosynovium, provides lubrication and nutrition for the tendons as they slide against the osteofibrous walls of the carpal tunnel.

The median nerve occupies a superficial position in the carpal tunnel and imposes on the deep surface of the transverse carpal ligament. During flexion and extension of the wrist, the position and morphology of the median nerve can change significantly; the nerve can shift anteroposteriorly and can assume a circular or elliptical shape as it is relaxed or stretched.

DISTRIBUTION OF THE MEDIAN NERVE

Proximal to the carpal tunnel, the median nerve innervates most of the flexor muscles of the forearm and of the elbow joint, anterior wrist joint, and distal radioulnar joint. Before reaching the carpal tunnel, the median nerve gives off a palmar cutaneous branch that provides cutaneous sensory innervation to the radial palmar surface including the thenar eminence. After passing through the carpal tunnel, the median nerve first provides a recurrent branch, which supplies motor innervation to the thenar muscles: opponens pollicis, abductor pollicis brevis, and flexor pollicis brevis. Together the thenar muscles coordinate to oppose the thumb against the other digits. The median nerve then gives off branches that provide motor innervation to the first two lumbrical muscles and the critical sensory branches to the palmar surface of the radial three and a half digits. On the dorsum of the hand, the median nerve provides sensory innervation to the distal half of the thumb, index finger, middle finger, and the radial half of the ring finger.

PATHOPHYSIOLOGY

There is some dispute over the precise etiology and pathophysiology of CTS, although various studies have provided insights. Ultimately, CTS is a neuropathy in which the median nerve is compressed as it passes through the carpal tunnel. The increased pressure, which can be duplicated by the physician using direct digital compression, leads to epineurial ischemia, decreased axonal transport, and intraneural ischemia. It is these conditions, and not direct mechanical damage, that adversely affect the median nerve and result in the clinical presentation of CTS. Although these vascular conditions are reversible, prolonged compression can eventually lead to neuronal fibrosis and persistent motor and sensory deficits.[2,3]

Etiologically, idiopathic and pregnancy-related CTS are different, and, as a consequence, somewhat different diagnostic and treatment philosophies apply. It is theorized that, in idiopathic CTS, repetitive insults to the flexor tenosynovium leads to necrosis, fragmentation, edema, and fibrosis. The edema and fibrous hypertrophy contribute to further injury and the progression of

CTS symptoms. Although CTS has been publicized in recent years as an occupation-related disorder, such correlations have not been supported by scientific studies.[2] Repetitive motions during work may be the eventual cause of median nerve injury, but more significant correlations have been found between median nerve slowing and predisposing factors such as increased body mass index, age, wrist depth-to-width ratio ("square wrist"), and female sex. In addition, associations have been made between CTS and systemic conditions including diabetes mellitus, rheumatoid arthritis, hypothyroidism, and pregnancy. Nonetheless, the importance of systemic factors in predisposing patients to CTS cannot be disregarded; this systemic influence is supported by the tendency of CTS to present bilaterally in patients.[2]

EFFECTS OF PREGNANCY

In light of the importance of systemic conditions in the genesis of CTS, it is hardly surprising that CTS commonly presents during pregnancy. Various studies have estimated the incidence of pregnancy-related CTS (PRCTS) as 1–50%, depending greatly on study design, diagnostic criteria, and diagnostic methods. The incidence of PRCTS is 1–50%. However, there is general consensus that hormonal changes and decreased venous return during pregnancy lead to generalized edema, which in turn compresses the median nerve in the carpal tunnel.[4] Increases in serum estrogen, aldosterone, cortisol, and prolactin in the puerperium, have been implicated. This hormonal etiology is supported by the increased incidence of CTS in women who use oral contraceptives.[1,4]

In addition, various studies have noted a possible association between preeclampsia and PRCTS, estimating that 9.3% of patients with PRCTS had preeclampsia,[4] and, conversely, that 63% of patients with preeclampsia complained of some type of hand symptoms.[5] Patients with preeclampsia are especially at risk for developing CTS. Some investigators have also suggested that the increase in the hormone relaxin during pregnancy could be an etiologic factor in the development of PRCTS. Relaxin might lead to relaxation of the transverse carpal ligament, thus allowing excessive deformation of the median nerve.

CTS can occur de novo in the puerperium and is most likely associated with breast feeding and the accompanying increase in serum prolactin, which promotes fluid retention. Symptoms develop soon after the start of lactation and resolve for almost all patients soon after weaning, although positive signs and symptoms may persist, suggesting permanent damage from median nerve compression.[6] Although postpartum CTS of lactation is similar in most ways to PRCTS, it is important to recognize the difference between newly developed CTS in the puerperium and persistent signs and symptoms due to PRCTS, which may indicate a progression of the condition or permanent median nerve lesions.

Diagnosis

HISTORY

The diagnosis of PRCTS is based largely on the report of symptoms and presence of signs from the patient's history and physical examination. Frequently, patients will not volunteer symptoms because of a common expectation that various discomforts are normal in pregnancy; thus, the physician must take the initiative to discover relevant symptoms. Patients tend to be older primigravidas in the third trimester of pregnancy. The presentation of symptoms is bilateral in about three of four patients and constitutes a triad of symptoms: paresthesia, numbness, and pain in the median nerve distribution.[7] Pain is particularly pronounced at night, possibly due to nocturnal peripheral vasodilation exacerbating edema in the carpal tunnel and the tendency to flex the wrist during sleep. Night pain and tingling in all of the fingers are common complaints. To establish the distribution of symptoms, the physician may ask the patient to choose between clearly marked sensory distribution diagrams of the hand[5,8] or ask the patient to mark the locations of sensory symptoms on a blank diagram. Although the median nerve innervates only the radial three and a half digits, most patients with CTS complain of tingling in all fingers. Although spread of symptoms in the hand beyond the median nerve distribution is suggestive of other neuropathies, radiation of pain or discomfort proximally as far as the shoulder is not uncommon in CTS. Motor symptoms such as grip weakness, loss of dexterity, or general complaints of "clumsiness" may accompany or follow these sensory symptoms and are indicative of more advanced median nerve lesions. Specifically, the patient may have difficulty opposing the thumb against the other digits.

PHYSICAL EXAMINATION

In addition to symptoms, physical examination may disclose various signs and observations to support the diagnosis. Dry skin in the median nerve distributions is a sign of autonomic nerve involvement. Visible thenar atrophy, a late finding, can be observed by comparing the thenar eminences of both hands. Thenar weakness can serve as a more objective indicator of recurrent median nerve deficits and can be assessed by holding the dorsum of the hand against the tabletop and asking the patient to point the thumb upward against resistance. Another way to assess thenar strength is to ask the patient to oppose the thumb to the ring finger against resistance.

Several provocative tests are commonly used clinically in the diagnosis of CTS, including Tinel's test, Phalen's test, and the carpal compression (or Durkan's) test (Figures 32-1 to 32-3). Tinel's sign is a quick and simple indicator of CTS. It is elicited by percussion of the median nerve at the carpal tunnel and is considered positive if the patient experiences paresthesias, or "electric shocks," along the median nerve distribution as a result. Tinel's sign tends to have low sensitivity for detecting CTS, possibly due to variability in the performance of the test, but it possesses higher specificity. In contrast, Phalen's test has higher specificity and good sensitivity and is considered a more reliable test for CTS. Phalen's sign is elicited by gravity-assisted flexion of the wrists, which is accomplished by

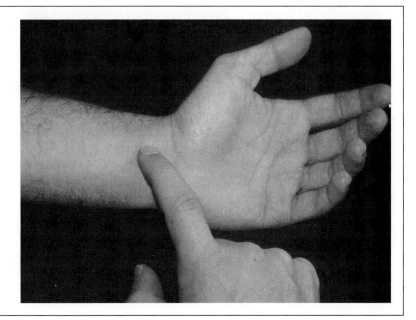

Figure 32-1: Tinel's sign is performed by percussing directly over the median nerve at the wrist crease. Paresthesias in the median nerve distribution is a positive sign.

Figure 32-2: Phalen's sign is performed by having the patient place her wrists in flexion. A positive test result reproduces the symptoms of numbness.

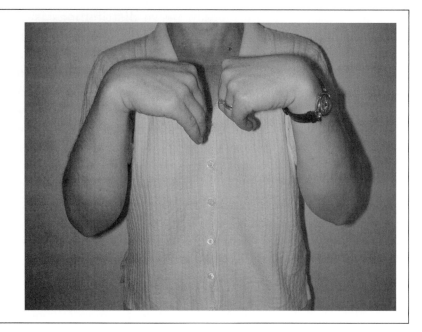

Figure 32-3: In Durkan's sign, the examiner applies direct pressure over the median nerve at the wrist. A positive test result reproduces the symptoms of numbness.

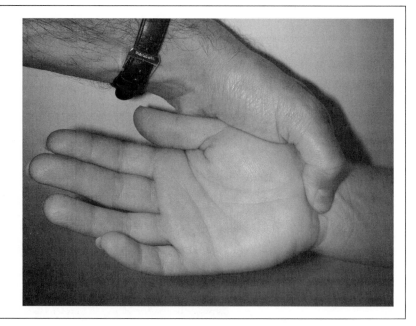

placing the elbows on a table with the forearms perpendicular to it and letting the hands drop. Phalen's sign is considered present if paresthesias and numbness occur along the median nerve distribution within 60 seconds. Provocative tests (Tinel's, Phalen's, and Durkan's) are confirmatory.

Because CTS results from compression of the median nerve, direct digital compression can be used to reproduce the symptoms of CTS. In the carpal compression test, or Durkan's test, moderate pressure is applied with both thumbs over the transverse carpal ligament.[9] A positive result with the carpal compression test is defined as paresthesia or numbness within 30 seconds over the median nerve distribution. To improve the objectivity of these provocative tests, Durkan constructed an instrument that provides a precise amount of pressure on the median nerve by using a calibrated piston. Durkan's test provides a measure of objectivity to the standard provocative tests for CTS.

In addition to these provocative tests, which aim to reproduce the sensory symptoms of median nerve compression, direct sensory examinations can be used to help gauge the presence and progression of CTS. The static two-point discrimination test is commonly performed by the application of two dull points separated by a known distance. The failure to distinguish a separation of 6 mm or more is considered a positive finding. A better sensory test for CTS is the Semmes-Weinstein monofilament, which can detect a progressive decline in the number of functioning nerve fibers. Monofilaments of increasing calibrated diameters are pressed perpendicularly into the palmar surfaces of each digit until the monofilament bends, thus applying a known force on the skin. The threshold is reached with the first monofilament that the patient detects; a value of 2.83 or higher is considered a positive finding.[2] The common and simple pinprick test can serve as a rough threshold test to help guide clinical diagnosis, although it is crude and will only detect more advanced cases of CTS.

NERVE STUDIES

Although clinical diagnosis of CTS is typically based on signs and symptoms elicited through the history and physical examination, electrodiagnostic nerve conduction studies and electromyogram serve as objective gold standards for the detection and measurement of median nerve compression neuropathy. In cases where objective evidence of CTS is required, such as in legal actions and clinical studies, nerve conduction studies are invaluable. Other effective uses include localizing a nerve lesion, tracking the progress of CTS or recovery from it, and aiding in differential diagnosis between CTS and other conditions with similar presentations.[2]

Although electrodiagnostic studies serve these purposes well and provide an important, direct look at nerve condition, it is arguable as to whether they should be a part of the typical clinical diagnostic evaluation. Some studies have touted the ability of nerve conduction studies to detect subclinical CTS and developing median nerve lesions due to its increased sensitivity to nerve conduction disturbances.[3,10] However, it is unclear whether patient outcomes are improved by nerve conduction studies when compared with a combination of symptoms and signs.[11]

CLINICAL DIAGNOSIS It is clear that no single symptom, test, or study can be used to definitively diagnose CTS. Thus, a combination of signs and symptoms should be used. Phalen's and Tinel's tests are simple to perform and, with a carefully constructed history, constitute an effective clinical picture. A diagram of the hand can help the layperson to describe the distribution of symptoms. In addition, the Semmes-Weinstein monofilament and Durkan's test can provide reasonably objective findings. In cases of more advanced CTS, thenar atrophy may be apparent, and even a pinprick test may indicate prolonged nerve compression and significant neuropathy. Electrodiagnostic studies can be used when necessary to supplement inconclusive signs and symptoms, aid in differential diagnosis, or track the progress of the neuropathy and guide treatment decisions and planning.

It is important to recognize conditions that are similar to CTS in presentation. The differential diagnosis of CTS includes more proximal nerve compression resulting from cervical disk herniation (in particular C_5 and C_6), cervical ribs, or other abnormal or anomalous structures in the forearm and arm. Conditions affecting the brachial plexus and its nerve roots may also present with signs and symptoms suggestive of CTS. It is particularly important to recognize these potentially severe conditions. Osteoarthritis of the finger joints can result in pain similar to that encountered in CTS, whereas stenosing tenosynovitis of the tendons in the hand ("trigger finger") and de Quervain's tenosynovitis may produce symptoms that confound the diagnosis of CTS.

Treatment

PRCTS is generally considered a self-limiting disorder, with symptoms beginning to resolve spontaneously and dramatically in patients after delivery. Turgut and associates reported complete resolution of symptoms in 60% of patients within 1 month and in 95% of patients within 1 year.[7] Because of this characteristic, which is compounded by the special considerations of maternal and fetal safety in pregnancy, conservative management is generally advocated before invasive treatments are considered. However, in some cases, the severity of symptoms and resulting debility may dictate more aggressive treatment. PRCTS is usually a self-limiting disorder.

SPLINTS

The first management of choice for PRCTS is splinting. A volar wrist splint that maintains the wrist in a neutral or slightly extended position is preferred. Wrist splints are the mainstay of treatment. The splint is worn mainly at night but may also be worn during the day as symptoms dictate. Patient education on CTS and the importance of wrist positioning also can be helpful. It has been suggested that proper splinting may work by increasing blood flow to the median nerve and preventing prolonged provocative positioning of the wrist during sleep. Although some studies have disputed the efficacy of splinting as a management for PRCTS, most have reported significant symptomatic relief for the vast majority of patients.[12] A good part of this discrepancy may be due to differences in the severity of cases, the use of different diagnostic criteria, and variations in splinting technique.

The variability in success rates underscores the importance of proper splinting, appropriate patient education, and diligent tracking of patient progress. In addition to splinting, it is important to understand the underlying neuropathy and the potential for permanent median nerve lesions. It is also important to recognize any underlying systemic factors and conditions.

STEROID INJECTION

Another nonsurgical management option for PRCTS is injection, in which a corticosteroid such as betamethasone is injected directly into the carpal tunnel. Its success rate in eliminating the symptoms of PRCTS has been documented at higher than 60% and was largely dependent on the severity of the neuropathy at time of treatment.[2] In general, patients with night symptoms refractory to splinting are delighted by the relief from injection. Although the beneficial effects of steroid injections in controlling idiopathic CTS rarely last longer than 1 year,[2] this time span is more than sufficient for the brief natural history of PRCTS. In mild or moderate cases, steroid injections can dramatically improve the condition of the median nerve as determined by electromyographic tests and thus improve the patient's long-term prognosis.[10] We use a combination of betamethasone 6 mg and 1% Xylocaine 2 mL injected under sterile conditions 1 cm proximal to the wrist crease by using a 25-gauge needle.

SURGICAL DECOMPRESSION

Surgical decompression of the median nerve during pregnancy is rarely necessary. Indications for surgery include incapacitating symptoms refractory to splinting and injection and advanced median nerve lesions as demonstrated by thenar atrophy or nerve studies.[1] Persistence or progression of PRCTS symptoms postpartum may be another indication for surgery.[13] In a carpal tunnel release, the surgeon decompresses the median nerve by incising the transverse carpal ligament.[2] Postoperative management typically includes the use of a wrist splint for 1–2 weeks. Major complications are uncommon. Symptomatic relief due to surgical release is generally dramatic, although permanent motor deficits and slow neurologic recovery are not uncommon, most likely due to the greater severity of the cases selected for surgical management.[10,13]

TREATMENT SELECTION

Together, splinting, steroid injections, and surgical release constitute the primary management modalities for PRCTS. In mild to moderate cases, night splinting is indicated in addition to patient education and close follow-up of symptom progression. Injections can provide significant relief when the condition fails to respond to splinting. Long-term follow-up should continue into the postpartum period because of potentially persistent median nerve lesions and muscle atrophy and because women with PRCTS may be at greater risk of CTS recurrence postpartum and in subsequent pregnancies.[1,13] Administration of a diuretic such as hydrochlorothiazide can provide an additional nonsurgical measure that may help to relieve edematous pressure on the median nerve, especially for CTS of lacation,[1] although its efficacy is still largely unproved for PRCTS.[7] In more severe cases or when the patient does not respond to conservative management, surgical release of the transverse carpal ligament may be required.

What's the Evidence?

The information published about PRCTS is essentially limited to retrospective and prospective population studies describing natural history and response to standard treatment. Evaluation and management of PRCTS is limited to extrapolation from the general population.

Guiding Questions in Approaching the Patient

Confirming the diagnosis

- Does the woman have numbness and tingling?
- Where is the numbness?
- Are the symptoms intermittent or constant?
- Does she have night pain?
- Are there any associated medical conditions (diabetes, hypothyroidism, or inflammatory arthritis)?

Evaluating response to treatment

- Has the night pain stopped?
- Are the symptoms no longer constant?

Conclusion

At present, there are many differing views on the pathophysiology, diagnosis, and management of idiopathic CTS and PRCTS. Simple, effective, and inexpensive tools to deal with the condition are available. Perhaps the most significant obstacle to proper diagnosis and management of PRCTS is simply the patient's assumption that its symptoms are a normal, expected part of pregnancy and that they do not warrant attention. Patient education and early detection of PRCTS is important, not only to alleviate the patient's symptoms but also to guard against potential permanent neuromuscular consequences.

Although there is a good amount of disagreement over diagnostic methods, a careful history and a combination of simple tests can prove to be very effective. A clinical examination should include a careful history to discover potential signs of PRCTS. For quick and easy tests, Phalen's and Tinel's signs provide very reasonable sensitivity and specificity when used in conjunction. The Semmes-Weinstein monofilament test provides a more quantitative picture of nerve status, although a simple pinprick test may suffice in some cases. In more advanced cases, thenar atrophy may be apparent. Electrodiagnostic testing should be reserved for situations in which the results may affect management decisions or when objective or progressive data are required.

Once PRCTS is diagnosed, conservative management is usually effective at minimizing symptoms. Proper splinting and patient compliance are critical to treatment success. In refractory cases, carpal tunnel steroid injections are often successful in alleviating symptoms for the remainder of pregnancy. Rarely is surgical decompression necessary during pregnancy.

Postpartum follow-up should be the rule for all patients. Although PRCTS is generally considered self-limiting and believed to resolve spontaneously after delivery, some cases do persist and some electrodiagnostic studies have found residual electrophysiologic deficiencies in many patients.[10,14] In addition, women with PRCTS should be informed that carpal tunnel symptoms may persist or recur if they choose to breast feed. PRCTS tends to recur in subsequent pregnancies, and patients may be at higher risk for CTS in later life.[1] For patients who do not develop CTS during pregnancy, it is not uncommon for CTS to develop de novo during lactation. The physician should be guided by the philosophy of early detection and long-term follow-up for all patients in the management of PRCTS.

Discussion of Cases

CASE 1: BILATERAL HAND PAIN AND NUMBNESS IN THE THIRD TRIMESTER

A 37-year-old woman at 32 weeks of gestation presents with a 2-week history of intermittent bilateral hand pain and numbness. All fingertips are involved. She occasionally awakens with hand pain that resolves after getting up and shaking her hands. She is otherwise healthy.

What should you look for on examination?

Dry skin in the thumb, index, and middle fingers; thenar weakness and/or atrophy; and Tinel's, Phalen's and Durkan's signs.

Is any further testing recommended?

No. Further testing is not necessary unless the provocative test results are negative or the patient has thenar atrophy, in which case a nerve study should be obtained.

Her condition fails to improve after 2 weeks of night splinting.

What should you do?

Advise her to also use the wrist splints during the day. Depending on the degree of her discomfort, she may benefit from a carpal tunnel steroid injection.

She chooses to continue with the splints. Her symptoms persist several weeks after delivery.

Does she require further testing?

No. Explain to her that her carpal tunnel symptoms will most likely continue until she stops breast feeding.

Her symptoms persist several months after she discontinues breast feeding.

Is a nerve study necessary?

If the clinical picture is consistent with CTS, she does not necessarily require nerve studies. A carpal tunnel steroid injection would be a reasonable next step. If she obtains significant, temporary relief from the injection, she would be a good candidate for carpal tunnel release. Nerve studies would be obtained if the steroid injection fails to provide any relief, if her symptoms are constant, and/or she has developed thenar atrophy.

CASE 2: UNILATERAL HAND PAIN AT 28 WEEKS

A 27-year-old woman at 28 weeks of gestation presents with a several-week history of dominant right hand pain. The pain is located on the radial aspect of the hand and wrist and is aggravated by gripping or pinching. She has some vague tingling on the dorsum of her hand.

How should you direct the history and examination?

Ask her whether the problem is primarily pain or numbness and tingling. Help her to localize the area of altered sensation. Perform the carpal tunnel provocative tests.

Her primary problem is pain. The carpal tunnel provocative test results are negative.

What is the diagnosis?

The most likely diagnosis is DeQuervain's tenosynovitis. This is a form of tendonitis

involving the first extensor compartment. There may be associated swelling in the region of the radial styloid. The confirmatory test is Finkelstein's test, in which the patient places her thumb in the palm, wraps her fingers around it, and deviates the wrist ulnarward. A positive test reproduces the pain. Patients with DeQuervain's tenosynovitis occasionally complain of tingling on the dorsum of the hand. This sensory distribution is distinctly different from the median nerve distribution of CTS and is the result of irritation of the radial sensory nerve.

What is the management of DeQuervain's tenosynovitis?

A custom-molded thermoplastic radial gutter splint made by the hand therapist is the initial therapy. If symptoms fail to improve, a steroid injection into the first extensor compartment will usually solve the problem.

REFERENCES

1 Heckman JD, Sassard R. Musculoskeletal considerations in pregnancy. *J Bone Joint Surg* 1994;76:1720–1730.

2 Szabo RM. Entrapment and compression neuropathies. In: Green DP, ed. *Green's Operative Hand Surgery,* 4th ed. Philadelphia: Churchill Livingstone, 1999; p. 1404–1447.

3 Padua L, Aprile I, Caliandro P, et al. Symptoms and neurophysiological picture of carpal tunnel syndrome in pregnancy. *Clin Neurophysiol* 2001;112:1946–1951.

4 Eckman-Ordeberg G, Salgeback S, Ordeberg G. Carpal tunnel syndrome in pregnancy: a prospective study. *Acta Obstet Gynecol Scand* 1987;66:233–235.

5 McLennan HG, Oats JN, Walstab JE. Survey of hand symptoms in pregnancy. *Med J Aust* 1987;147:542–544.

6 Weimer LH, Yin J, Lovelace RE, et al. Serial studies of carpal tunnel syndrome during and after pregnancy. *Muscle Nerve* 2002;25: 914–917.

7 Turgut F, Cetinsahin M, Turgut M, et al. The management of carpal tunnel syndrome in pregnancy. *J Clin Neurosci* 2001;8:332–334.

8 Katz JN, Stirrat CR, Larson MG, et al. A self-administered hand symptom diagram for the diagnosis and epidemiologic study of carpal tunnel syndrome. *J Rheumatol* 1990;17:1495–1497.

9 Wainner RS, Boninger ML, Balu G, et al. Durkan gauge and carpal compression test: accuracy and diagnostic test properties. *J Orthop Sports Phys Ther* 2000;30:676–682.

10 Seror P. Pregnancy-related carpal tunnel syndrome. *J Hand Surg* 1998;23:98–101.

11 Szabo RM, Slater RR Jr, Farver TB, et al. The value of diagnostic testing in carpal tunnel syndrome. *J Hand Surg Am* 1999;24:704–714.

12 Courts RB. Splinting for symptoms of carpal tunnel syndrome during pregnancy. *J Hand Ther* 1995;8:31–34.

13 al Qattan MM, Manktelow RT, Bowen CV. Pregnancy-induced carpal tunnel syndrome requiring surgical release longer than 2 years after delivery. *Obstet Gynecol* 1994;84:249–251.

14 Padua L, Aprile I, Caliandro P, et al. Carpal tunnel syndrome in pregnancy: multiperspective follow-up of untreated cases. *Neurology* 2002;59:1643–1646.

Management of Pregnancy Related Back Pain

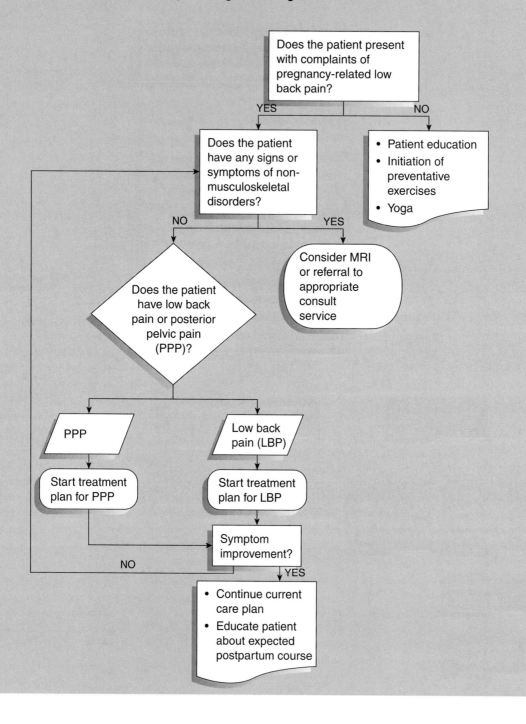

33 Back Pain

Curtis L. Cetrulo
Kristine M. King

Introduction

KEY POINT

Up to 80% of women will experience some form of back pain during pregnancy.

Back pain is one of the most common complaints of pregnancy. Most pregnant patients will experience some degree of back pain during their pregnancy. Prospective studies have shown that 50–80% of women report some form of back pain during pregnancy.[1,2] In addition, one third of pregnant women have described their back pain as "severe," i.e., interfering with their normal daily life and well-being.[1] Physiologically, back pain in pregnancy can be partly explained by the pressure that the growing uterus places on the muscles of the back, specifically the paraspinal muscles. Hormonal mechanisms have also been implicated.

The high prevalence of back pain in pregnancy could lead to dismissal of complaints of back pain as normal or expected. It takes considerable medical judgment to discern the "normal" or expected amount of physiologic back pain from pathologic back pain. Our two case discussions at the end of the chapter illustrate this point.

Risk Factors

It is difficult to define risk factors for a condition that nearly 80% of pregnant patients will develop. Multiple prospective studies have attempted to elucidate risk factors but without much reproducibility. Various factors that have been proposed include multiparity, younger age, older age, high body mass index, large weight gain during pregnancy, male sex of fetus, smoking, previous back pain, posterior or fundal placenta, larger fetus, strenuous work, and an inability to rest

567

frequently at work. The only factor that seems to be significant in several studies is a history of low back pain before pregnancy or in a previous pregnancy. Smoking may also be a significant risk factor for back pain in pregnancy. In nonpregnant patients, smoking is thought to be a risk factor for a prolapsed disc.

Physiologic Mechanisms

KEY POINT

Biomechanical factors (such as postural changes) alone cannot explain back pain of pregnancy.

The physiologic changes of pregnancy largely contribute to gestational back pain. Factors related to posture and weight gain during pregnancy in addition to hormonal and endocrine changes have been implicated. Normal postural alterations include a lordotic posture due to weight gain concentrated low in the pelvis. This leads to a feeling of falling forward, so women tend to shift the upper body back over the pelvis to restore the center of gravity (Figure 33-1). The actual degree of spinal lordosis is controversial, with studies suggesting increased and decreased lumbar lordosis during pregnancy. When directly measured in one study, lumbar lordosis was not shown to change significantly from 12 weeks to 36 weeks of gestation. However, patients with a naturally large lumbar lordosis were particularly susceptible to back pain.[3] It is likely that the exaggerated lordotic posture places mechanical stresses on the back muscles and contributes to pain.

Non–posture-related factors also play a role in the back pain of pregnancy. If the gravid uterus were the only contributing factor, back pain would be expected to increase throughout the gestation, with a sharp increase in the third trimester, when growth is fastest. Instead, it has been demonstrated that the incidence of pregnancy-related back pain increases most in the first and second trimesters and tends to level off after 22 weeks.[2]

Hormonal and endocrine changes during pregnancy have been postulated to contribute to joint laxity and make the spine and sacroiliac joints "less stable." Mean total body water increases during pregnancy, and it has been shown that there is fluid retention in the connective tissue ground substance. Using magnetic resonance imaging (MRI), higher signal intensity (corresponding to high water content) is seen in the cervixes of pregnant women with back pain compared with pregnant women without back pain.[4] Joint laxity appears to increase in pregnant patients, especially during a second pregnancy. This increased laxity returns to

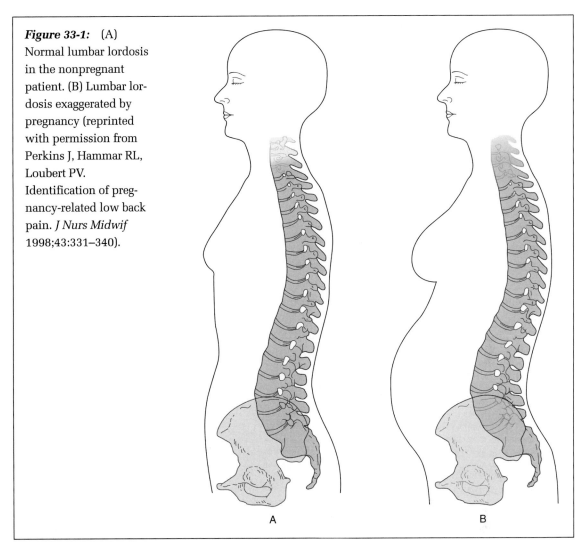

Figure 33-1: (A) Normal lumbar lordosis in the nonpregnant patient. (B) Lumbar lordosis exaggerated by pregnancy (reprinted with permission from Perkins J, Hammar RL, Loubert PV. Identification of pregnancy-related low back pain. *J Nurs Midwif* 1998;43:331–340).

A

B

baseline levels postpartum.[5] The joint laxity during pregnancy is postulated to be due to increased serum levels of relaxin. Relaxin is a peptide hormone of the insulin-like growth factor family that is produced by the corpus luteum and placenta. It remodels pelvic connective tissue in several mammalian species during pregnancy. In pregnant humans, the peak levels of relaxin appear to occur around 12 weeks of gestation, decrease until 17 weeks, and then remain stable throughout pregnancy.[6] Higher serum levels of relaxin have been found in patients with severe pelvic joint pain compared with pregnant patients without back pain. These high levels return to normal in the immediate postpartum period.[7]

Diagnosis

Any pregnant patient who complains of significant back pain needs to undergo a thorough history and physical examination. Pain drawings and pain assessment scales are used commonly in assessment of back pain in nonpregnant patients and can be useful in pregnant patients to elucidate the exact location and severity of their pain. Patients may complain of "back pain" and mean anything from shoulder and neck pain to sacroiliac and hip pain. Most pregnant patients localize their pain to low lumbar or sacroiliac areas. Pain in either area also may be associated with symphysis pubis pain.[1] The two types of pain are distinct in cause, clinical presentation, and management. Therefore, it is imperative to correctly define the type of back pain that the patient is feeling.

Pain severity and its radiation, if any, should be assessed. Associated symptoms should be explored. Decreased strength and loss of control over bladder or bowel function are symptoms of a potential medical emergency.

A complete physical examination, including pelvic examination, should be the next step. Palpation of the spine and paraspinal muscles and assessment for costovertebral angle tenderness should be done. Attention should be given to neurologic examination of the lower extremities and perineum.

Spinal configuration and mobility tests and an ability to reproduce the pain can be used to refine the diagnosis. Scoliosis should be assessed by inspection of the spine with the woman standing and bending forward. Mobility is assessed by range-of-motion examinations at various joints. In general, tests of pain provocation have better reproducibility than do tests of configuration or mobility. Pain provocation tests have been shown to have better sensitivity the lower they are in the spine.[8] Pain provocation tests are considered positive if they provoke or release pain in a location related to the test procedure. Sciatic nerve compression is evaluated by the straight-leg raise test. The straight-leg raise test should be applied to both legs with the patient in the supine position. The test is considered positive when back pain of any degree occurs when the leg is less than 70 degrees from the table. Pain may be provoked in the sacral area by pressure over the

KEY POINT

Lumbar disc herniation is a serious condition that must not be overlooked in the evaluation of a pregnant patient with back pain.

posterior superior iliac spine in the standing position. Sacroiliac joint instability in pregnant patients is evaluated by the posterior pelvic pain provocation test. This is performed with the patient supine, with the hip flexed 90 degrees. Pressure is applied to the knee in a downward fashion. The test is considered positive if pain occurs in the sacral or buttock area[9] (Figure 33-2). Direct pressure should also be applied to the symphysis pubis to determine the presence of pain.

Radiologic studies should be reserved for patients with signs and/or symptoms of neurologic disease or fracture. MRI is the radiologic study of choice for the spine during pregnancy. No ionizing radiation is required to obtain an MRI; instead, radiofrequency waves emitted by different tissues when influenced by a powerful magnet are analyzed. MRI is generally considered safe in pregnancy after the first trimester. Any radiologic abnormality should be considered in light of clinical findings. Disc bulge or prolapse have been associated with back pain in pregnancy.[4] However, more than 50% of asymptomatic women of childbearing age may have disc herniation or bulging, whether or not they are pregnant.[10]

Clinical Syndromes

The back pain of pregnancy cannot be assigned a single diagnosis. It is not the same clinical entity as low back pain in a nonpregnant patient. Complaints of back pain in pregnancy generally fall into two typical types of pain: lumbar, or low back, pain, and posterior pelvic, or sacroiliac joint, pain.

Muscular insufficiency is another term for mild musculoskeletal low back pain. These patients complain of tiredness and stiffness that is worse at the end of the day. They may have tenderness over the paravertebral muscles, but range of motion is normal. The pain is similar to the lumbar pain experienced by nonpregnant women. It tends to be aggravated by activities such as prolonged standing or sitting.

Pelvic or sacroiliac joint instability, also known as posterior pelvic pain, is much more prevalent than lumbar pain during pregnancy. It is defined as deep pain at the sacroiliac joint that develops in relation to pregnancy or delivery and is felt distal and lateral to the L_5/S_1 vertebrae. It may be unilateral or bilateral and may radiate to the posterior thigh or knee. It is postulated to

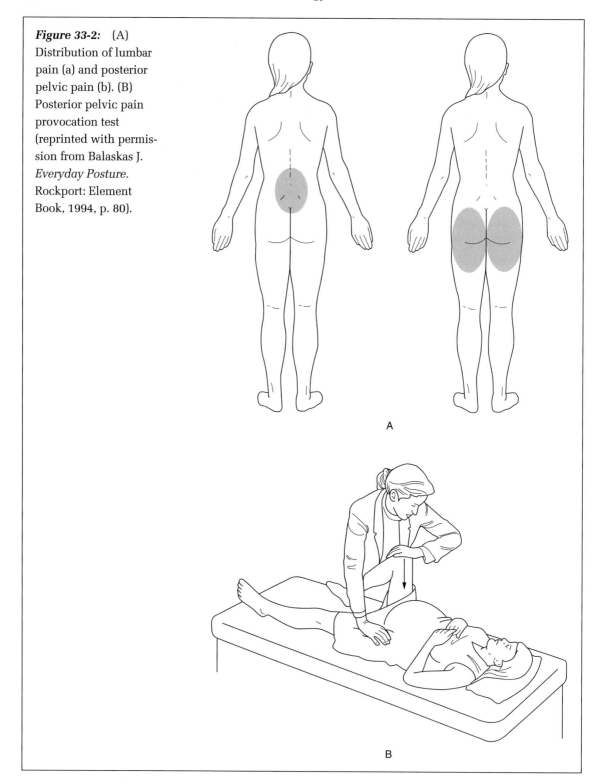

Figure 33-2: (A) Distribution of lumbar pain (a) and posterior pelvic pain (b). (B) Posterior pelvic pain provocation test (reprinted with permission from Balaskas J. *Everyday Posture.* Rockport: Element Book, 1994, p. 80).

A

B

result from joint laxity at the sacroiliac joint. On examination, patients have a positive result on a posterior pelvic pain provocation test, pain located in the deep pelvis and gluteal area and over the symphysis pubis, and a waddling gait. The pain is aggravated by prolonged postures, extreme flexion or extension of the hip or sacroiliac joint, and asymmetric loading of the pelvis, which leads to difficulty with walking, prolonged sitting, climbing stairs, and turning at night.[11]

Sciatica commonly occurs in association with sacroiliac joint dysfunction. The L_4–L_5 component of the sciatic nerve courses anteriorly to the sacroiliac joint, so relaxation of the joint may affect the nerve. The pain of sciatica is characteristically located in the buttock, with radiation down the back of the leg.

Pubic symphysis separation or symphysiolysis is a condition that is overdiagnosed in many patients who complain of back or pelvic pain in pregnancy. The diagnosis should be made in a patient who has difficulty walking, has pain over the symphysis pubis, but does not have symptoms of the other clinical syndromes described above.

Lumbosacral disc disease has an incidence of 2.5 in 1000 live births and may be worsened by pregnancy. Patients may present with pain alone or with more serious neurologic signs such as loss of sensation or loss of bowel and bladder function.

Other, more rarely seen conditions include spondylolisthesis and coccydynia.

It should always be kept in mind that the differential diagnosis of back pain in pregnancy extends beyond musculoskeletal disorders. The patient with new onset back pain should be evaluated for evidence of preterm labor or abruption, urinary tract infection, pyelonephritis, or nephrolithiasis. Rarely, back pain in pregnancy is the presenting symptom for spinal tumors, metabolic bone disease, or rheumatologic diseases such as rheumatoid arthritis (Table 33-1).

Treatment

The management of the back pain of pregnancy can be challenging for the physician and the patient. Multiple treatment modalities have been described (Table 33-2). All therapies have been shown to be less effective during pregnancy than after delivery.[12] However, most pregnant patients are able to find some relief or at least stop the progression of their pain.

Table 33-1. **DIFFERENTIAL DIAGNOSIS OF BACK PAIN IN PREGNANCY**

Musculoskeletal disorders
Obstetric complications
Preterm labor or spontaneous miscarriage
Abruption

Genitourinary system disorders
Urinary tract infection
Pyelonephritis
Renal calculi

Inflammatory disorders
Osteoarthritis
Rheumatoid arthritis
Ankylosing spondylitis

Hematologic or neoplastic disorders
Sickle cell crisis
Lymphoma
Metastatic bone lesions
Multiple myeloma

Metabolic bone disease
Hypoparathyroidism
Osteoporosis
Osteomalacia

Source: Adapted from MacEvilly M, Buggy D. Back pain and pregnancy: a review. *Pain* 1996;64:405–414.

Table 33-2. **MANAGEMENT OF BACK PAIN IN PREGNANCY**

Management of low back pain in pregnancy
Using back support such as a small pillow while sitting
Postural correction to a "neutral spine"
Avoiding prolonged sitting or standing
Taking a midday rest to relieve tired muscles
Using a small footstool for one foot for sitting or standing, alternate feet
Yoga and pelvic tilting exercises

Management of posterior pelvic pain in pregnancy
Minimizing activities that exacerbate the pain, e.g., high-impact exercise or asymmetric loading
Using a sacral belt for support
Decreasing overflexion of the hips and lower spine when sitting and exercising
Brief periods of bedrest may be indicated for acute episodes of pain

Source: Adapted from Perkins J, Hammer R, Loubert P. Identification and management of pregnancy-related low back pain. *J Nurs Midwif* 1998;43:331–340.

The most important factor in successful management of back pain is patient education. Patients who receive advice about back care early in pregnancy tend to report less low back pain and less intense pain when it does occur.[13,14] Patients should be counseled early in the first trimester about the effects of pregnancy on their posture and informed of interventions that may be helpful if they begin to experience back discomfort. Attempting to maintain a neutral posture will decrease mechanical strain on the lower back. Smoking cessation should be encouraged.

Many patients report alleviation of their pain when lying down. Massage and heat applied to the back muscles are helpful for many women. External supports, such as binders or support belts, are a common intervention recommended for back pain in pregnancy and provide relief to many patients. The common lumbar belt is difficult to use due to the growing abdomen, but a low sacroiliac belt may be helpful. Brief (1–2 week) periods of bedrest appear to be very helpful in some patients, especially when combined with exercises.[12]

Acupuncture, physical therapy, and water aerobics are among the few interventions that have been scientifically studied. In a randomized, prospective trial, pregnant patients with low back pain received acupuncture or physical therapy, consisting of water therapy and individual exercises, for 1 month. Acupuncture was shown to significantly relieve pain and disability from low back pain compared with pretreatment levels and compared with physical therapy. Physical therapy did not relieve pain but was shown to halt the expected worsening of pain.[15] Water aerobics decreased pain 1 week postpartum and significantly decreased work time missed due to back pain in a small cohort of women.[16]

Exercise would seem to be a logical intervention if muscular weakness is assumed to be the cause of back pain. One study showed exercise to benefit women with low back pain but showed little benefit for pelvic pain.[14] Another study of an exercise program for pregnant women showed relief from low back pain. Rather, the exercise group reported more pain compared with controls.[17]

Yoga postures are an ideal form of exercise for the pregnant patient at risk for, or suffering from, back pain. However, some modification needs to be clear when recommending yoga. No inverted postures (head or shoulder stands) should be performed because of the possible effect on uterine blood flow. After 20 weeks of gestation, the pregnant woman should avoid postures that require her to lie on her back to avoid supine hypotension. Recommended postures include pelvic tilt early in pregnancy, cat and cow poses, child pose, camel, upward-facing dog, and the mirror pose (see Figs. 33-1 and 33-2). Abdominal or "belly-breathing" is an important part of relaxation and meditation that should be included in the practice of yoga during pregnancy. There are many excellent texts and videos on the subject of prenatal yoga.[18–20]

At times, it is necessary to use pharmacotherapy to control the back pain of pregnancy. For new mild lumbar or posterior pelvic pain, acetaminophen can be safely used for short periods while other therapeutic measures are taking effect. The total daily dose of acetaminophen should not exceed 4 g. In patients who develop acute back pain secondary to muscle spasm or trauma, muscle relaxants such as Flexeril can be used for short periods. If a patient with ongoing back pain is not responding to the measures outlined above and is developing progressive worsening pain, a small dose of narcotic pain medicine may be used. As always, patients with pain unresponsive to management should first be evaluated for any neurologic cause for their pain. If narcotics are indicated, a short-acting narcotic should be used first. If longer-term narcotic therapy seems to be required, the equivalent dose of a long-acting narcotic can be substituted. The patient should be educated about the potential for tolerance and increasing narcotic requirement. Patients with a history of narcotic dependence or those who appear to be getting pain medicine from multiple physicians should be limited to a small number of pills at a time. If large doses of narcotics are being used by the patient to control pain, the risk of fetal narcotic dependence after birth should be addressed.

Pregnancy Outcome and Follow-up

Many patients who have had significant back pain during pregnancy will experience worsening of the pain during labor and delivery. An upright posture during the early part of the first stage of labor may help relieve pain for some patients. Ambulating during labor is also helpful in decreasing back pain. Back pain does not seem to be correlated with increased length of labor or increased operative delivery rates.[21] The risk factors identified for new onset back pain after pregnancy include a history of back pain (before or during pregnancy), heavier weight, and advanced age.[22]

Postpartum, back pain generally resolves within 6 weeks. However, some patients complain of pain longer than 3 years postpartum.[23,24] Persistent postpartum back pain occurs more commonly in patients with the most disabling back pain during pregnancy, but any back pain during pregnancy carries a 40% risk of postpartum back pain. Typically the pain is in the low back, as opposed to the pelvic pain of pregnancy. The causes of postpartum back pain are the same as those for back pain during pregnancy. Muscle endurance is decreased in the large pelvic and dorsal muscles of patients with persistent low back pain postpartum.[24] In addition, women experiencing back pain during pregnancy may complain of back pain in relation to menstruation or oral contraceptive use, suggesting a role for hormonal factors.

The long-term effect of low back pain during pregnancy should not be underestimated. Some patients with severe low back pain during pregnancy have changed occupation due to persistent back pain, and a small percentage report having decided to refrain from future pregnancy for fear of recurrent low back pain.[25] Patients with back pain in pregnancy are at risk for back pain in subsequent pregnancies. In two studies, 85–94% of patients with significant back pain during pregnancy reported recurrent low back pain in their next pregnancy.[12,25]

Epidural-Related Backache

The role of epidural anesthesia in postpartum chronic back pain is controversial. Many patients will relate the onset of postpartum back pain to epidural anesthesia. Retrospective studies have shown evidence in support of and against a causal relation between epidurals and subsequent back pain. Recent studies have shown no difference in the incidence of immediate or chronic back pain after pregnancy in patients who did or did not receive an epidural.[22] Two prospective cohort studies that compared patients receiving epidural anesthesia with those not receiving epidural anesthesia found no significant difference in reported back pain at 6 weeks and at 1 year after delivery.[26,27] These studies did find an increase in back pain on the first postpartum day in patients who had received epidurals and ascribed this finding to local trauma to the spinal ligaments and muscles from epidural placement. Another mechanism that has been postulated to cause the pain is the motor blockade resulting in immobility for hours during labor. More recently, the increased use of combined spinal and epidural anesthesia, or "walking epidural," has provided an alternative with much less motor blockade. Patients have reported a higher degree of satisfaction with this technique compared with patients confined to bed, and a trend toward less back pain has been shown. The type of anesthetic used in the epidural infusion is generally not implicated in low back pain that occurs after an epidural. Chloroprocaine, a local anesthetic that is rarely used in general obstetric practice, can cause direct neural irritation and back pain when used in large doses.

It is important to realize that new onset low back pain may be a symptom of a more serious condition. Back pain after epidural anesthesia is the presenting symptom for epidural hematoma and epidural abscess. Care should be taken to exclude these conditions before discharge of a patient with new onset postpartum back pain.

Guiding Questions in Approaching the Patient

Assessing risk factors for back pain during this pregnancy

- Does she have a history of back pain?
- Is this her first pregnancy; if not, did she have back pain in her previous pregnancies?
- What is her current body mass index, and how much weight has she gained during the pregnancy?
- What kind of physical work or exercise does she do?
- Does she smoke?

Assessing the pain and level of acuity

- Where is the pain located? Is it lumbar or posterior pelvic pain?
- How severe is the pain?
- Has she noticed any loss of strength?
- Has she noted any change in sensation in her perineum or lower extremities?
- Has she experienced urinary retention or incontinence of urine or stool?

Assessing possible therapeutic options

- Is the patient motivated to seek therapy?
- What are her expectations from treatment, i.e., resolution or nonprogression of pain?
- Does the patient have any secondary gain from the diagnosis of "back pain"?

Conclusion

Back pain during pregnancy is a common complaint and is often dismissed by the obstetric health care provider, even though pregnancy-related back pain can have a significant detrimental effect during the pregnancy and afterward. It is important to pay attention to the complaint of back pain in pregnancy and to properly assess it to ensure a woman's well-being during the childbearing years. A systematic approach to the identification and management of back pain in pregnancy is suggested to prevent it when possible, decrease or ameliorate it at times, and actively detect acute, potentially serious problems.

Discussion of Cases

CASE 1: LUMBAR DISC HERNIATION

A 24-year-old primigravida presented at 26 weeks of of gestation with a triplet pregnancy and complaining of low back pain. She had not had back pain before pregnancy, and this pain was new within the past 2 weeks. On initial examination, the patient had pain localized to the lumbar area. She had an intact neurologic examination. The straight-leg raise test was positive, consistent with a suspected diagnosis of sciatica. There was no evidence of preterm labor, urinary tract infection, or kidney stones.

What is your recommendation for initial management?

The patient was counseled about the causes of back pain in pregnancy and the effect of the multiple gestations on her posture. The patient was told to use acetaminophen and hot packs as needed. A physical therapy consultation was obtained and the patient was provided with a walker and taught range-of-motion exercises. She was also counseled to remain on modified bedrest for 1–2 weeks.

Shortly thereafter, the patient presented to a local emergency room complaining of difficulty urinating, loss of sensation in the vagina, and numbness and tingling of the buttocks, perineum, and left leg.

What other testing, if any, would you recommend at this point?

Thorough neurologic examination showed sensory loss over the S_1–S_4 dermatomes, greater on the left than the right, and a decreased ankle jerk reflex. Postvoid residual measurement was 200 mL, thus confirming urinary retention.

Your examination is concerning for disc herniation, and you are aware that this can be a medical emergency. You plan to obtain an MRI, but the patient is hesitant to undergo imaging in pregnancy.

How would you counsel her?

An MRI is the ideal test for imaging the spine. MRI is considered safe in pregnancy after 12 weeks of gestation because it does not use ionizing radiation to obtain the image. Before 12 weeks of gestation, safety is unknown because studies are limited.

MRI showed a disc herniation at L_5–S_1. The patient was then seen by the neurosurgical consultant who confirmed the emergent nature of the problem, and the patient was immediately taken to the operating room for L_5–S_1 diskectomy. The patient went home on postoperative day 3 after an uneventful postoperative course. She returned at 35 weeks to deliver three healthy infants by cesarean section.

CASE 2: FRACTURED VERTEBRAE

A 29-year-old gravida 1, para 1 was seen in consultation 6 weeks postpartum with a complaint of new onset low back pain. She had a normal vaginal delivery of a 7 lb 6 oz infant under epidural anesthesia. The second stage of labor lasted 2 hours 30 minutes. She first noted the pain in the first few days after delivery over the site of her epidural insertion. She feels that the pain has gotten significantly worse over the subsequent weeks and was interfering with her ability to care for her baby.

The patient noted pain in the mid-lumbar region on a pain drawing, with no radiation. On examination, the epidural puncture site was not visible, but there was tenderness to palpation in the midback. Pain provocation tests including straight-leg raise did not elicit pain. She had an intact neurologic examination.

What is your differential diagnosis?

Postpartum lumbar pain or epidural-related pain. Pain that develops in the postpartum period generally follows a characteristic pattern. The pain usually develops during labor or within the first few days postpartum but tends to improve by 6 weeks postpartum. It is unlikely that a patient who did not have back pain during pregnancy would have persistent back pain after pregnancy. Back pain related to epidural anesthesia is a controversial issue. Many patients will identify epidural anesthesia as the source of their postpartum back pain, but several studies have not supported the association. It is common to have pain immediately after delivery at the point of epidural catheter insertion due to trauma to the spinal ligaments; however, this pain should not persist longer than a few days. In a patient with persistent pain and point tenderness,

epidural hematoma and epidural abscess should be considered in the differential.

What other testing, if any, would you recommend at this point?

No further testing is recommended at this time.

What is your recommendation for initial management?

The patient was initially treated with conservative management including oral analgesics, local heat, and gentle exercises.

The pain persisted despite compliance with this plan. She was reexamined and seemed to be more tender in the midback. Her history was reviewed, which disclosed a medical history significant for valvular heart disease, and the patient takes Coumadin for anticoagulation when not pregnant. She was currently on heparin, which was begun 6 months before her pregnancy. She had continued the heparin because she was told not to breast feed while taking Coumadin.

What further testing would you recommend at this time?

Spinal radiography or MRI. Spine radiographs showed vertebral compression fractures of two vertebrae, felt to be secondary to long-term heparin exposure and inadequate calcium supplementation.

REFERENCES

1 Ostgaard HC, Andersson GBJ, Karlsson K. Prevalence of back pain in pregnancy. *Spine* 1991;16:549–552.

2 Kristiansson P, Svardsudd K, von Schoultz B. Back pain during pregnancy: a prospective study. *Spine* 1996;21:702–709.

3 Ostgaard HC, Andersson GBJ, Schultz AB, et al. Influence of some biomechanical factors on low-back pain in pregnancy. *Spine* 1993;18:61–65.

4 Chan YL, Lam WW, Lau TK, et al. Back pain in pregnancy—magnetic resonance imaging correlation. *Clin Radiol* 2002;57:1109–1112.

5 Calguneri M, Bird HA, Wright V. Changes in joint laxity occurring during pregnancy. *Ann Rheum Dis* 1982; 41:126–128.

6 Kristiansson P, Svardsudd K, von Schoultz B. Serum relaxin, symphyseal pain, and back pain during pregnancy. *Am J Obstet Gynecol* 1996;175:1342–1347.

7 MacLennan AH, Nicolson R, Green R, et al. Serum relaxin and pelvic pain of pregnancy. *Lancet* 1986;II:243–244.

8 Kristiansson P, Svardsudd K. Discriminatory power of tests applied in back pain during pregnancy. *Spine* 1996;21:2337–2344.

9 Ostgaard HC, Zetherstrom G, Roos-Hansson E. The posterior pelvic pain provocation test in pregnant women. *Eur Spine J* 1994;3:258–260.

10 Weinreb JC, Wolbarsht LB, Cohen JM, et al. Prevalence of lumbosacral intervertebral disc abnormalities on MR images in pregnant and asymptomatic nonpregnant women. *Radiology* 1989;170:125–128.

11 Perkins J, Hammer R, Loubert P. Identification and management of pregnancy-related low back pain. *J Nurs Midwif* 1998;43:331–340.

12 Mens JMA, Vleeming A, Stoeckart R, et al. Understanding peripartum pelvic pain: implications of a patient survey. *Spine* 1996;21:-1363–1370.

13 Orvieto R, Achiron A, Ben-Rafael Z, et al. Low-back pain of pregnancy. *Acta Obstet Gynecol Scand* 1994;73:209–214.

14 Ostgaard HC, Zetherstrom G, Roos-Hansson E, et al. Reduction of back and posterior pelvic pain in pregnancy. *Spine* 1994;19:894–900.

15 Wedenberg K, Moen B, Norling A. A prospective randomized study comparing acupuncture with physiotherapy for low-back and pelvic pain in pregnancy. *Acta Obstet Gynecol Scand* 2000;79:331–335.

16 Kihlstrand M, Stenman B, Nilsson S, et al. Water-gymnastics reduced the intensity of back/low back pain in pregnant women. *Acta Obstet Gynecol Scand* 1999;78:180–185.

17 Dumas GA, Reid JG, Wolfe LA, et al. Exercise, posture, and back pain during pregnancy. Part II: exercise and back pain. *Clin Biomech* 1995;10:104–109.

18 Freedman FB, Hall D. *Yoga for Pregnancy.* London: Sterling, 1998.

19 Schatz MP. *Back Care Basics.* Berkeley: Rodmell Press, 1992.

20 Balaskas J. *Preparing for Birth with Yoga.* Rockport: Element Books, 1994.

21 Ostgaard HC, Andersson G, Wennergren M. The impact of low back and pelvic pain in pregnancy on the pregnancy outcome. *Acta Obstet Gynecol Scand* 1991;70:21–24.

22 Breen T, Ransil B, Groves P, et al. Factors associated with back pain after childbirth. *Anesthesiology* 1994;81:29–34.

23 Ostgaard HC, Zetherstrom G, Roos-Hansson E. Back pain in relation to pregnancy: a 6-year follow up. *Spine* 1997;22:2945–2950.

24 Noren L, Ostgaard S, Johansson G, et al. Lumbar back and posterior pelvic pain during pregnancy: a 3-year follow-up. *Eur Spine J* 2002;11:267–271.

25 Brynhildsen J, Hansson A, Persson A, et al. Follow-up of patients with low back pain during pregnancy. *Obstet Gynecol* 1998;91:182–186.

26 Macarthur A, Macarthur C, Weeks S. Epidural anaesthesia and low back pain after delivery: a prospective cohort study. *BMJ* 1995;311: 1336–1339.

27 Macarthur A, Macarthur C, Weeks S. Is epidural anesthesia in labor associated with chronic low back pain? A prospective cohort study. *Anesth Analgesia* 1997;85:1066–1070.

Distinguishing Lupus Renal Flare from Preeclampsia

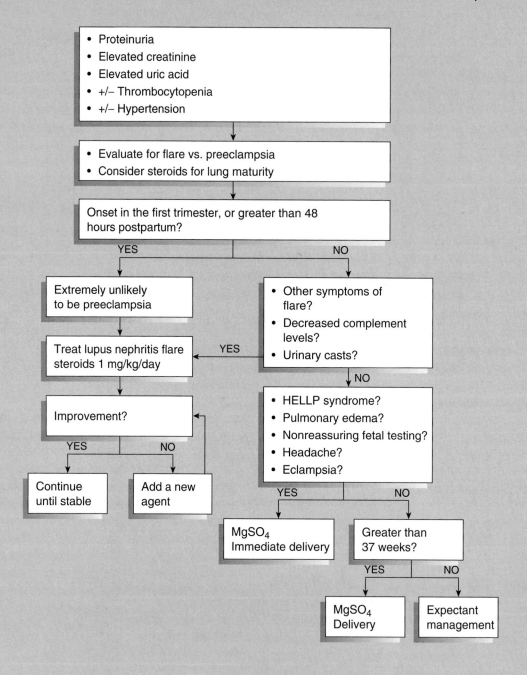

34 Systemic Lupus Erythematosus

Sabrina D. Craigo

Introduction

Systemic lupus erythematosus (SLE) is an autoimmune disease that primarily affects women of childbearing age, with a ratio of nine women affected for every man affected. The disease is characterized by a wide variety of nonspecific symptoms and multiple circulating autoantibodies. Symptoms often wax and wane. The diagnosis is made when at least 4 of 11 criteria described by the American College of Rheumatology are met[1] (Table 34-1). Some patients may have symptoms such as photosensitivity and arthralgia, whereas others may have significant renal or neurologic disease manifestations. Therapy is directed at symptomatic relief and immunosuppression.

SLE is a classic example of a medical condition in which pregnancy can affect the course of the disease, and the disease can affect the course of pregnancy. Pregnancy may be associated with an increased incidence of disease flare and, in rare cases, renal failure or death. In addition, the autoimmune pathophysiology can lead to disease in the fetus or newborn. This chapter reviews SLE in pregnancy, including risks, outcomes, and obstetric and medical management.

KEY POINT

Women with SLE have significantly greater risk of miscarriage, preterm delivery, preeclampsia, fetal growth restriction, and stillbirth.

Effect of Pregnancy on Lupus

Several studies have shown an increase in SLE flares during pregnancy,[2–4] whereas others have not found such an increase.[5–7] Flare rates across studies vary widely, from as low as 15% to as high as 60%.[2,8] Similarly, reports differ with regard to the effect of oral

585

***Table 34-1.* AMERICAN COLLEGE OF RHEUMATOLOGY CRITERIA FOR DIAGNOSIS OF SLE**

Butterfly rash
Discoid lupus
Photosensitivity
Serositis
  Pleuritis
  Pericarditis

Renal disorder
  Proteinuria
  Casts

Oral ulcers
Arthritis involving ≥2 peripheral joints
Neurologic disorder
  Seizures
  Psychosis

Hematologic disorder
  Hemolytic anemia
  Leukopenia
  Lymphopenia
  Thrombocytopenia

Immunologic disorder
  Positive LE prep
  Anti-DNA
  Anti-Sm
  False-positive result of serologic test to syphilis

Antinuclear antibody

LE = lupus erythematosus; SLE = systemic lupus erythematosus; Sm = smooth muscle.

contraceptive pills on flare rate. The lack of consensus may be related to the different populations studied, the difficulty in defining flare, and the variability in the investigators' descriptions of disease activity. Some reports have defined flare as any change requiring a change in therapy, whereas other studies have used the Physician's Global Assessment and a 0–3 scale. Recently, some reports have used the Systemic Lupus Erythematosus Disease Activity Index scale to assess disease activity in a standardized manner.[9,10] There is evidence to suggest the risk of flare is related to disease state at conception; those patients quiescent at conception fare better than do those with active disease.[2,6,11] A correlation between increased anti–double-stranded DNA levels and risk of disease exacerbation has also been reported.[8]

Patients with lupus nephritis are of particular concern because their disease is often more severe and may require more medical therapy. From 15% to 50% of pregnant patients with lupus have preexisting renal disease. The risk of flare during pregnancy among patients with lupus nephritis appears to be related to the presence of active renal disease at conception. In one study, flares occurred in only 5% of a patients in remission at conception but in 36% of patients with active renal disease.[12] Permanent deterioration of renal function during pregnancy has been reported but appears to occur in fewer than 10% of patients with lupus nephritis.[12,13] Of patients with lupus and renal involvement, two thirds will develop preeclampsia.[14] The few maternal deaths reported with lupus in pregnancy have often been associated with lupus nephritis, including two due to opportunistic infections in immunosuppressed patients.[15] Other maternal deaths due to complications of lupus include respiratory insufficiency with multiorgan failure and pulmonary hypertension.[16,17]

What's the Evidence?

Clinical research of SLE in pregnant patients poses particular challenges. Although SLE is diagnosed most commonly in women of childbearing age, only 1 in 300 women are affected. Many are diagnosed after childbearing is completed, some are infertile, and some choose to limit their families after the diagnosis, so general obstetricians may have little, if any, experience caring for SLE patients. In addition to the usual difficulty encountered when studying pregnant women, the different manifestations of the disease make the study of SLE more difficult. The wide spectrum of organ involvement and variation in what constitutes a flare make any research seem ambiguous. The most useful data available on pregnancy and SLE have been taken from case series and case-control studies, usually involving 40–100 pregnancies, collected over many years at several centers around the world. There is one double-blind, placebo-controlled study of hydroxychloroquine use in lupus pregnancy.[18]

Effect of SLE on Pregnancy

Reported rates for miscarriage are 19–26%, and those for stillbirth are 1–8%.[6,7,12,16,19,20] Overall, the risk of fetal loss for patients with lupus is 2.5 times higher than in the general population.[19] Fetal death is often related to placental insufficiency and intrauterine growth retardation (IUGR) and, less commonly, congenital heart block. Several studies have found that those patients with lupus anticoagulant or high levels of anticardiolipin antibodies (ACA) have the highest risk of loss, as do those with a diagnosis of coexistent antiphospholipid antibody syndrome (APAS).[9,19] APAS is diagnosed by the presence of antiphospholipid antibodies (LAC (lupus anticoagulant) and/or significant levels of ACA immunoglobulin G) and clinical complications such as thrombosis or recurrent pregnancy loss. Renal disease has been identified by some groups as a risk factor for pregnancy loss,[20,21] but even in this group of high risk patients late pregnancy loss has been correlated with the presence of LAC.[22,23] Disease activity has also been linked to pregnancy loss.[20,23]

Lupus pregnancies have a significantly high rate of preterm delivery, ranging as high as 20–60%.[10,20,21,25,26] Women with lupus who have low complement levels (C3 and C4) appear to have a stronger chance of delivering prematurely,[8,9] and women with high maternal serum level of α-fetoprotein have an increased risk.[25] Factors that contribute to premature delivery include development of preeclampsia, abruption, and premature rupture of membranes. Data regarding the relation between disease activity and risk of preterm delivery are mixed, with many investigators demonstrating a correlation between disease activity and preterm delivery,[7,10,25] but others showing no correlation.[26] The authors of the negative study noted that differences may have been related to the infrequency of active disease among their patients at conception.

Patients with lupus and hypertension have a particularly high risk of developing preeclampsia, although all patients with lupus are at risk for this condition. Those with renal involvement are at highest risk, and for these patients discerning preeclampsia from a lupus flare can be very difficult. Proteinuria, edema, deteriorating renal function, abnormalities of liver enzymes, and thrombocytopenia can be present in preeclampsia and during flare of lupus nephritis. Decreasing complement levels and red cell casts in urine sediment support a diagnosis of lupus nephritis, as do symptoms consistent with the patient's previous flare symptoms (Table 34-2). The distinction between the two conditions is critical because preeclampsia is treated by delivery, whereas flare is managed with medical therapy. Hypertension contributes significantly to the risk of preterm birth[7,21,25]; the development of severe preeclampsia or HELLP (hemolysis, elevated liver enzymes, and low platelets) syndrome often necessitates premature delivery.

Most series that have reported on pregnant patients with lupus have described an increased risk of 13–30% for IUGR,[7,19,20,27] but some studies have not found this association.[26] Placental effects of the disease are well described and provide a basis for placental insufficiency. These effects include decidual vasculopathy, infarction, thrombosis, chronic villitis, and intervillous fibrin deposition.

Pregnancy carries an increased risk of thromboembolism in well women, and patients with lupus have an even greater risk of venous thromboembolism. This risk appears to be largely related to the presence of LAC, ACA antibodies, or APAS. For women with a history of thromboembolism or a diagnosis of APAS, prophylactic heparin or low-molecular-weight heparin is recommended during pregnancy and 6–8 weeks postpartum.[28]

Overall, pregnant patients with lupus are at risk for many adverse pregnancy outcomes. Hypertension, renal disease, disease activity, complement levels, anti-DNA levels, ACA antibodies,

Table 34-2. **PREECLAMPSIA AND LUPUS NEPHRITIS**

Finding	*Preeclampsia*	*Lupus Nephritis*
Blood pressure	High	Normal or high
Proteinuria	Present	Present
Onset of proteinuria	Sudden	Gradual or sudden
Thrombocytopenia	May be present	May be present
Liver function tests	May be increased	Usually normal
Complement levels	May be low	Low
Anti–double-stranded DNA	Normal, may be mildly increased	High, may show sudden decrease
Urine sediment	Absent	Presents
Response to corticosteroids	No	Yes
Nonrenal lupus symptoms	No	Common

APAS, and LAC are risk factors for adverse outcomes. One of the strongest risk factors for adverse outcome is a previous adverse outcome, with a history of two consecutive adverse outcomes (early miscarriage, late miscarriage, stillbirth, preterm birth, IUGR, or neonatal complication) increasing the risk of adverse outcome fourfold.[29] In view of these fetal and obstetric risks, pregnancy management should include fetal testing (fetal growth assessment by ultrasound and fetal heart rate monitoring), close surveillance for hypertension or preeclampsia, and heparin prophylaxis for those with APAS or previous venous thromboembolism.

Fetal and Neonatal Lupus

KEY POINT

Circulating anti-Ro and anti-La autoantibodies found in some lupus patients can cross the placenta and cause fetal and subsequently, neonatal disease.

Like SLE, neonatal lupus erythematosus (NLE) has a spectrum of manifestations, including skin rash, anemia, thrombocytopenia, leukopenia, increased liver enzymes, and complete congenital heart block (CCHB). The hematologic abnormalities are usually asymptomatic and tend to resolve in the first year of life. The Ro antigen is present in red blood cells and neutrophil membranes contain a Ro cross-reactive protein. Ten percent to 25% of infants born to women with anti-Ro and anti-La antibodies show asymptomatic increases in liver enzymes, but actual liver dysfunction (hepatomegaly or jaundice) is uncommon.[30,31] Up to 16% of children born to mothers with anti-Ro antibodies have the characteristic skin lesions of NLE.[30] The typical skin findings are annular inflammatory lesions or annular erythema. Most often occurring on the face, the skin changes may be misdiagnosed as fungal infections or eczema.

CCHB is the most serious complication of NLE. At one time CCHB was thought to affect a large percentage of offspring of women with SLE, but prospective series have demonstrated that CCHB affects only 1–2% of all fetuses of patients with lupus and anti-Ro(SSA) or anti-La(SSB) antibodies.[30] Dexamethasone has been used in attempt to decrease the antibodies but often has no effect. Third-degree atrioventricular block is easily detected when fetal bradycardia is noted. The condition is irreversible and more than 60% of affected neonates require pacemakers.[32] First- and second-degree heart block has been detected antenatally with fetal echocardiography but may progress postnatally.[33] Although many investigators have suggested serial fetal echocardiography for patients with anti-Ro and anti-La antibodies, this approach has not been well studied. Most cases of CCHB are identified by simple fetal heart rate monitoring in the office, with an obvious persistent bradycardia. Although a few cases of first- and second-degree block have been detected antenatally, these cases are rare, and it is unclear whether early detection changes long-term prognosis. Moreover, because only 1–2% of women with these antibodies will have fetuses that develop CCHB, serial echocardiography would be expensive and likely produce a low yield. If early detection improves response to dexamethasone therapy, such screening may be warranted. A multicenter trial is currently underway to evaluate the utility of a mechanical PR interval measurement in these patients.

Diagnosis

SLE is diagnosed when at least 4 of 11 criteria as described by the American College of Rheumatology are met.[1] Although most patients are aware of their diagnosis when going into a pregnancy, the disease is common enough that a new diagnosis of SLE may be made during pregnancy. New onset cases account for a small percentage of those reported (3–10%),[4,11,26] but in previous studies maternal disease was severe and fetal survival was only 50–65% in this group of patients.[11] The diagnosis should be suspected with new onset of symptoms such as arthritis or unexplained fever, with any unexplained pleuritis or serositis, and when proteinuria is noted outside the setting of preeclampsia. The antinuclear antibody is a sensitive but nonspecific screening test for SLE; 95% of patients with SLE will have a positive antinuclear antibody. One should be aware that many of the criteria are symptoms, so careful history taking is part of the evaluation. Detection of new cases depends to some degree on the health care providers being aware of the condition and criteria for diagnosis.

Pregnancy Management

Women with SLE who become pregnant should be managed by a perinatologist or an obstetrician familiar with the medical and obstetric complications in conjunction with a rheumatologist. Ideally, patients should be seen in the preconception period to review goals, risks, and management recommendations. Medications should be reviewed and optimized for the individual patient with pregnancy issues in mind. Women who require cytotoxic agents should be discouraged from conceiving until their disease is inactive or their disease can be managed with medications with better safety records in pregnancy.

During the first prenatal visit, the patient should be questioned in detail regarding her specific SLE symptoms, and these should be documented in the prenatal chart. Patients tend to have similar symptoms at times of flare. It is also important to assess disease activity at the time of conception and to document which medications have been previously effective. Twenty percent to 35% of patients with lupus have APAS.[34] APAS has implications for pregnancy, with high risk of fetal loss, stillbirth, IUGR, and thrombosis. Coexistence of this condition should be documented or ruled out; treatment with anticoagulation can increase fetal survival to 80%.[34] A first-trimester ultrasound should be obtained to confirm viability and dates because first-trimester loss is common and growth evaluation will be important. A 24-hour urine for protein and creatinine clearance should be obtained in addition to routine laboratory work. An anti–double-stranded DNA level and baseline complement level should be obtained. Patients should be screened for anti-Ro and anti-La antibodies because the presence of these antibodies would trigger counseling with regard to an increased risk of fetal or neonatal disease. Patients with APAS should be given prophylactic heparin and low-dose aspirin.[28]

Prenatal visits should be more frequent than for routine care, and patients should be specifically asked about SLE symptoms at each visit. Blood pressure and urine protein should be monitored at each visit to screen for preeclampsia. Fetal heart tones should be auscultated at each visit, and any bradycardia should be promptly investigated. Antepartum testing with nonstress tests should be planned weekly in the third trimester and possibly twice weekly after 36 weeks. Fetal growth should be evaluated by ultrasound examinations at around 28 and 34 weeks or more often if coexisting conditions further increase the risk of growth restriction (hypertension, APAS, previous IUGR, or abruption).

If flare is suspected at any time, laboratory evaluation may be useful. Complement levels decrease; anti-DNA antibody levels

KEY POINT

All patients should be encouraged to plan conception during a quiescent period and should be using reliable contraception at all other times.

KEY POINT

Management during pregnancy relies on increased maternal and fetal surveillance.

increase during pregnancy but may decrease acutely at time of flare. Alterations in white blood cell count, hematocrit, or platelet count may occur with flare. Proteinuria may signal renal flare, although patients without a history of renal involvement do not commonly develop this complication during pregnancy. Most patients who develop renal flare during pregnancy have a history of lupus nephritis. Nevertheless, distinguishing lupus flare from preeclampsia can be extremely difficult. Both conditions may be associated with hypertension, proteinuria, increasing serum creatinine and uric acid levels, altered platelet counts, elevated transaminases, and headaches. Red blood cells or red cell casts on urinalysis, joint pain, and decreasing complement levels are more consistent with flare. Treatment of flare usually relies on starting or increasing relatively high doses of corticosteroids, but immunosuppressive agents may also be needed. A rheumatologist should be involved when flare is suspected or in cases in which the diagnosis is unclear.

Labor management should be unchanged for patients with SLE. If the patient has been treated with steroids, stress-dose steroids are recommended in labor. Those patients who require prophylactic or therapeutic anticoagulation may have limited anesthetic options, so consultation with an anesthesiologist before delivery is valuable. Those patients at risk for thrombosis have an ongoing increased risk at least 6 weeks postpartum, so continued prophylaxis is warranted.

Effective contraception is a very important issue in the management of patients with lupus because the idea of planning conception at times of disease inactivity is emphasized. Fertility is not affected by SLE. Careful evaluation is recommended before prescribing estrogen-containing contraceptives to any woman with SLE. Estrogens are contraindicated in women with APAS or active lupus nephritis.[35] Progestogen-only contraceptives can be safely used in SLE patients, and intrauterine devices can be used safely in patients who are not severely immunocompromised.

Guiding Questions in Approaching the Patient

- What are the patient's specific lupus symptoms when she has a flare?
- Has the patient ever had nephritis, thromboembolism, or pregnancy complications related to her lupus?

- Is the patient at high risk for fetal or neonatal lupus (previous affected child or anti-Ro and anti-La antibodies)?
- Which medications have been previously effective?
- What was the status of her illness at the time of conception?

Medications

Corticosteroids, specifically prednisone, have been used widely in pregnancy without significant fetal effects. General principles of use include using the lowest effective dose and weaning to the lowest dose that prevents recurrence. Major organ involvement requires larger doses, starting at 1 mg/kg per day. Stress-dose steroids are recommended in labor or at the time of cesarean section for those women who require steroids at any point in the pregnancy. Nonsteroidal anti-inflammatory medications may be used for arthralgias in early pregnancy. Use in later pregnancy is discouraged due to concerns for potential oligohydramnios and constriction of the fetal ductus arteriosis. A chloroquine, such as Plaquenil, is often effective for skin and joint involvement. There are increasing data suggesting a lack of adverse fetal affects.[18] Discontinuation is frequently associated with flare.[36] Cytotoxic agents such as azathioprine and cyclophosphamide should be avoided, if possible. Azathioprine has been widely used for patients with renal transplants with little evidence of teratogenicity, but neonatal immunosuppression can occur. Cyclophosphamide is teratogenic in animal studies and in first-trimester human exposures.[37] Second- and third-trimester exposures are associated with low birth weight. This medication should not be used in pregnancy unless potential benefit to the patient clearly outweighs these risks. Methotrexate is teratogenic and can induce pregnancy loss; it should not be used during pregnancy.

Conclusion

SLE is a complex autoimmune disease with a wide range of clinical manifestations and frequent comorbidities. SLE patients are at risk for many obstetric complications, and although up to 95% will have live births, as many as 30% will deliver prematurely. Rates of stillbirths and early loss are also higher than in the general population. Those at highest risk for complications are women with coexisting APAS, lupus nephritis, a previous child with CCHB, or active disease at conception. Management depends on tailoring of medications and close maternal and fetal surveillance by a care provider familiar with these issues.

Discussion of Cases

CASE 1: PRECONCEPTUAL COUNSELING

A 32-year-old gravida 2, para 2 has a 3-year history of SLE and comes to you for preconceptual counseling. Her previous pregnancies were uncomplicated, but her diagnosis of SLE was made a year after her last delivery.

What questions are important when obtaining a history?

It is important to know about the recent and previous courses of her disease. Medications used should be recorded, including their effectiveness. Her specific lupus symptoms should be reviewed. Specifically review any history of renal disease, thromboembolism, or pregnancy complications.

What laboratory results would be helpful?

A copy of her baseline laboratory values and anti-Ro and anti-La antibody titers should be obtained from her rheumatologist or internist, if possible.

What would you advise her about timing of pregnancy?

Ideally, pregnancy should be planned only when the patient's disease is well controlled, with no evidence of active flare and on no medications or on a regimen thought to be safe in pregnancy. Her risk of flare during pregnancy is likely minimized if she is well controlled at conception.

What would you advise her about prenatal care?

When possible, patients with lupus should be managed by a perinatologist during pregnancy because of the complexity of the disease, multiple potential pregnancy complications, and need for increased surveillance.

CASE 2: HYPERTENSION AND PROTEINURIA IN THE THIRD TRIMESTER

A 30-year-old woman with known SLE presents at 34 weeks of gestation with a blood pressure of 140/90 mm Hg, 1+ proteinuria, and pedal edema. Her pregnancy to date has been uncomplicated. Her lupus usually manifests with joint pain and fatigue. She has never had lupus nephritis. She denies headache or visual changes. Fetal testing is reassuring. The estimated fetal weight is at the 20th percentile for gestational age and the fluid volume is low to normal.

What other information would you like from her history?

It would be important to determine if she has ever had hypertension and if she has any other signs or symptoms of preeclampsia, such as headache, visual changes, or epigastric pain.

What laboratory evaluation would you order?

The workup should include a complete blood cell count, transaminases, lactate dehydrogenase, creatinine and uric acid, complement levels, anti–double-stranded DNA level, 24-hour urine for total protein and creatinine clearance, and urinalysis.

A 24-hour urine shows protein 500 mg, uric acid 7.3 mg/dL, and creatinine 0.9 mg/dL. Liver function tests are mildly increased and the platelet count is 120,000/mm^3.

Do these tests differentiate between lupus nephritis and preeclampsia?

No. Both diagnoses are still possible. It would be important to check the microscopic urinalysis, white blood cell count, complement levels, and anti-DNA levels to better evaluate the possibility of flare.

How does the diagnosis change your plan for management?

A diagnosis of lupus nephritis would prompt aggressive therapy with high-dose corticosteroids. Fetal growth would be monitored every 2 weeks and frequent fetal testing would be recommended. A diagnosis of severe preeclampsia in most instances necessitates delivery.

REFERENCES

1 Tan EM, Cohen AS, Fries JF, et al. The 1982 revised criteria for the classification of systemic lupus erythematosus. *Arthritis Rheum* 1982;25:1271–1277.

2 Petri M, Howard D, Repke J. Frequency of lupus flare in pregnancy: the Hopkins Lupus Pregnancy Center experience. *Arthritis Rheum* 1991;34:1538–1545.

3 Ruiz-Irastorza G, Lima F, Alves J, et al. Increased rate of lupus flare during pregnancy and the puerperium. *Br J Rheumatol* 1996;35: 133–138.

4 Wong KL, Chan FY, Lee CP. Outcome of pregnancy in patients with systemic lupus erythematosus. *Arch Intern Med* 1991;151: 269–273.

5 Lockshin MD, Reinitz E, Druzin ML, et al. Lupus pregnancy, part 1. Case-control prospective study demonstrating absence of lupus exacerbation during or after pregnancy. *Am J Med* 1984;77:893–898.

6 Urowitz MB, Glaedman DD, Farewell VT, et al. Lupus and pregnancy studies. *Arthritis Rheum* 1993;36:1392–1397.

7 Mintz G, Gutierrez G, Garcia-Alonso A, et al. Prospective study of pregnancy in patients with systemic lupus erythematosus. *Arch Intern Med* 1991;151:269–273.

8 Tomer Y, Viegas OAC, Swissa M, et al. Levels of lupus autoantibodies in pregnant SLE patients: correlations with disease activity and pregnancy outcome. *Clin Exp Rheumatol* 1996;14:275–280.

9 Cortes-Hernandez J, Ordi-Ros J,Paredes F, et al. Clinical predictors of fetal and maternal outcome in systemic lupus erythematosus: a prospective study of 103 pregnancies. *Rheumatology* 2002;41: 643–650.

10 Clark CA, Spitzer KA, Nadler JN, Laskin CA. Preterm deliveries in women with systemic lupus erythematosus. *J Rheumatol* 2003;30: 2127–2132.

11 Hayslett JP. The effect of systemic lupus erythematosus on pregnancy and pregnancy outcome. *Am J Reprod Immunol* 1992;28:199–204.

12 Moroni G, Quaglini S, Banfi G, et al. Pregnancy in lupus nephritis. *Am J Kidney Dis* 2002;40:713–720.

13 Oviasu E, Hickes J, Cameron JS. The outcome of pregnancy in women with lupus nephritis. *Lupus* 1999;1:19–25.

14 Nossent HC, Swaak TJG. Systemic lupus erythematosus. VI. Analysis of the interrelationship with pregnancy. *J Rheumatol* 1990;17: 771–776.

15 Huong DLT, Wechsler B, Piette J-C. Pregnancy and its outcome in systemic lupus erythematosus. *Q J Med* 1994;87:721–729.

16 Johns KR, Morand EF, Littlejohn GO. Pregnancy outcome in systemic lupus erythematosus: a review of 54 cases. *Aust N Z J Med* 1998; 28:18–22.

17 Kleinman D, Katz VL, Kuller JA. Perinatal outcomes in women with systemic lupus erythematosus. *J Perinatol* 1998;18:178–182.

18 Levy RA, Lilela VS, Cataldo MJ, et al. Hydroxychloroquine (HCQ) in lupus pregnancy: double blind and placebo-controlled study. *Lupus* 2001;10:401–404.

19 Julkunen H, Jouhikainen T, Kaaja R, et al. Fetal outcome in lupus pregnancies: a retrospective case-control study of 242 pregnancies in 112 patients. *Lupus* 1993;2:125–131.

20 Le Thi Huong D, Wechsler B, Vauthier-Brouzes D, et al. Outcome of planned pregnancies in systemic lupus erythematosus: a prospective study on 62 pregnancies. *Br J Rheumatol* 1997;36:772–777.

21 Rahman P, Gladman DD, Urowitz MB. Clinical predictors of fetal outcome in systemic lupus erythematosus. *J Rheumatol* 1998;25: 1526–1530.

22 Packman DK, Lam SS, Nicholls K, et al. Lupus nephritis and pregnancy. *Q J Med* 1992;83:315–324.

23 Love PE, Santoro SA. Antiphospholipid antibodies: anticardiolipin and the lupus anticoagulant in systemic lupus erythematosus (SLE)

and in non-SLE disorders. Prevalence and clinical significance. *Ann Intern Med* 1990;112:682–698.

24 Petri M, Allbritton J. Fetal outcome of lupus pregnancy: a retrospective case-control study of the Hopkins Lupus Cohort. *J Rheumatol* 1993;20:650–656.

25 Petri M, Howard D, Repke J, Goldman D. The Hopkins Lupus Pregnancy Center: 1987–1991 update. *Am J Reprod Immunol* 1992;28: 188–191.

26 Carmona F, Font J, Cervera R, et al. Obstetrical outcome of pregnancy in patients with systemic lupus erythematosus. A study of 60 cases. *Eur J Obstet Gynecol* 1999;83:137–142.

27 Kobayashi N, Yamada H, Kishid T, et al. Hypocomplementaemia correlates with intrauterine growth retardation in systemic lupus erythematosus. *Am J Reprod Immunol* 1992;28:205–207.

28 American College of Obstetricians and Gynecologists Educational Bulletin. 1998;244:149–158.

29 Ramsey-Goldman R, Kutzer JE, Kuller LH et al. Pregnancy outcome and anti-cardiolipin antibody in women with systemic lupus erythematosus. *Am J Epidemiol* 1993;138:1057–1069.

30 Climaz, R, Spence, D, Hornberger L, Silverman E. Incidence and spectrum of neonatal lupus erythematosus: a prospective study of infants born to mothers with anti-Ro autoantibodies. *J Pediatr* 2003; 142:678–683.

31 Lee LA, Reichlin M, Ruyle SZ, Weston WL. Neonatal lupus liver disease. *Lupus* 1993;5:333–338.

32 Buyon JP, Clancy RM. Neonatal lupus: review of proposed pathogenesis and clinical data from the US-based Research Registry for Neonatal Lupus. *Autoimmunity* 2003;36:41–50.

33 Askanase, AD, Friedman DM, Dische MR, et al. Spectrum and progression of conduction abnormalities in infants born to mothers with anti-SSA/Ro-SSB/La antibodies. *Lupus* 2002;11:145–151.

34 Lockshin MD. Antiphospholipid antibody. *JAMA* 1997;277:1549–1551.

35 Julkunen H. Pregnancy and lupus nephritis. *Scand J Urol Nephrol* 2001;35:319–327.

36 Canadian Hydroxychloroquine Study Group. A randomized study of the effect of withdrawing hydroxychloroquine sulfate in systemic lupus erythematosus. *N Engl J Med* 1991;324:150–154.

37 Janssen NM, Genta MS. The effects of immunosuppressive and anti-inflammatory medications on fertility, pregnancy, and lactation. *Arch Intern Med* 2000;160:610–619.

Management of Rheumatoid Arthritis in Pregnancy

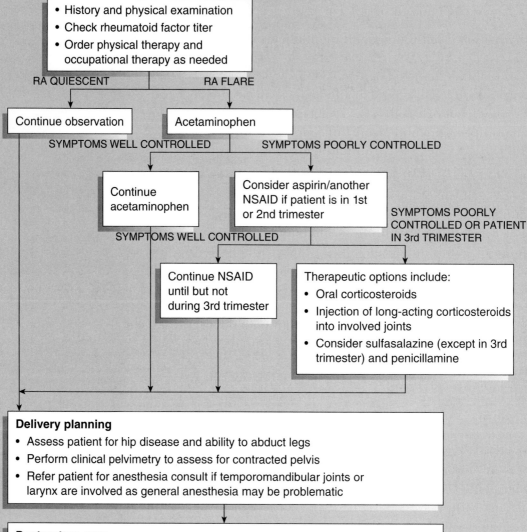

35 Rheumatoid Arthritis

Karen O'Brien

Introduction

A chronic multisystem disease characterized by a variety of systemic manifestations, rheumatoid arthritis is the most common systemic rheumatic disease. Although its exact cause is unknown, its pathogenesis is immunologically mediated by infiltrating T cells that secrete inflammatory cytokines. The prevalence of rheumatoid arthritis is 0.8%, and rheumatoid arthritis occurs three times more commonly in women than in men.[1] Rheumatoid arthritis complicates approximately 1 in 1000–2000 pregnancies.[2] This chapter reviews the management of the pregnant patient with rheumatoid arthritis.

Clinical Manifestations of Rheumatoid Arthritis

Rheumatoid arthritis is slowly progressive, with onset usually between 35 and 50 years of age. A classic feature is swelling and pain in one or more of the upper extremity joints, particularly the wrist, metacarpophalangeal joints, and proximal finger joints. Spindle-shaped deformities may result in these affected joints. Involvement of distal finger joints is rare in rheumatoid arthritis. Gradually the arthritis tends to settle symmetrically in joints, with lower extremities becoming involved later.[3]

Cervical vertebrae commonly become involved as the disease progresses, with neck arthritis being a significant cause of disability in patients with rheumatoid arthritis. Lumbar and dorsal vertebral articulations are rarely involved. Of particular concern to the obstetrician is that hip joints may be affected by rheumatoid

601

arthritis, limiting abduction or altering pelvic measurements. However, hip disease in the patient with rheumatoid arthritis is an infrequent and late synovial joint manifestation.[3]

Patients with rheumatoid arthritis may experience fatigue, anorexia, weight loss, and vague musculoskeletal symptoms. Although rheumatoid arthritis primarily remains a synovial process, extra-articular lesions can occur, including rheumatoid nodules in the skin, lungs, and heart; pleurisy; pericarditis; and vasculitis similar to polyarteritis nodosa.[2]

Diagnosis of Rheumatoid Arthritis

There are no absolute diagnostic criteria for rheumatoid arthritis until the disease is far advanced. Within a year of onset of disease, rheumatoid factor should be positive. Rheumatoid factor is usually measured with a latex test, which quantifies antiglobulin antibody-agglutinating latex particles coated with immunoglobulin G. Titers of 1:160 or higher strongly support the diagnosis of rheumatoid arthritis in a patient with a consistent history and physical examination. However, titers of rheumatoid factor may be positive in other inflammatory diseases such as tuberculosis and subacute bacterial endocarditis. Other rheumatic diseases such as systemic lupus erythematosus are also commonly associated with positive titers of rheumatoid factor.[2,3]

In 1987, the American Rheumatism Association formulated revised criteria for the classification of rheumatoid arthritis. These criteria are (1) morning stiffness in and around joints lasting at least 1 hour before maximal improvement; (2) soft tissue swelling (arthritis) of three or more joint areas observed by a physician; (3) swelling (arthritis) of the proximal interphalangeal, metacarpophalangeal, or wrist joints; (4) symmetric swelling (arthritis); (5) rheumatoid nodules; (6) the presence of rheumatoid factor; and (7) radiographic erosions or periarticular osteopenia in hand or wrist joints. Criteria 1 through 4 must have been present for at least 4 weeks. Rheumatoid arthritis is defined by the presence of four or more criteria, and no further qualifications or list of exclusions are required. In a case control study by Arnett and associates of 262 patients with rheumatoid arthritis and 262 control subjects, these criteria were demonstrated to be 91–94% sensitive and 89% specific for rheumatoid arthritis.[4]

Antepartum Course of Rheumatoid Arthritis

KEY POINT

Rheumatoid arthritis symptoms often improve antepartum.

In 1938, Hench first reported marked improvement in the inflammatory component of rheumatoid arthritis during pregnancy.[5] This observation has been validated by multiple subsequent studies. A retrospective study by Ostensen and coworkers described a 75% remission rate in pregnancy among 31 patients with rheumatoid arthritis.[6] Ostensen and Husby later prospectively studied 12 patients with rheumatoid arthritis in pregnancy and found disease remission in 10 women and disease continuation in two.[7]

Several hypotheses exist to explain pregnancy's apparent ameliorative effect on rheumatoid arthritis. It has been postulated that sex hormones may interfere with cytokine immunoregulation, thus affecting the course of rheumatoid arthritis in pregnancy.

Sex steroids are believed to influence the immune system, although the precise mechanisms are unknown. Gonadal steroids may mediate their effects on the immune system directly by binding to lymphocytes or indirectly through the thymic-hypothalamic-pituitary-gonadal axis.[8]

Unger and colleagues studied 14 patients with rheumatoid arthritis during each month of pregnancy and correlated disease activity with serum concentrations of pregnancy-associated α_2-glycoprotein. Amelioration of disease correlated positively with α_2-glycoprotein levels, suggesting that this protein may play a role in inducing remissions in rheumatoid arthritis during pregnancy. α_2-Glycoprotein has immunoregulatory properties and likely suppresses at least one inflammatory mediator, interleukin-2.[9]

Nelson and associates associated improvement of rheumatoid arthritis symptoms during pregnancy with a disparity in HLA class II antigens between mother and fetus. Significantly more maternofetal disparity in HLA-DR and HLA-DQ antigens was found retrospectively and prospectively in pregnancies characterized by amelioration of rheumatoid arthritis than in pregnancies characterized by active disease. These findings indicate that the maternal immune response to paternal HLA antigens may bring about pregnancy-related amelioration of disease.[10]

Postpartum Course of Rheumatoid Arthritis

Postpartum, rheumatoid arthritis frequently flares. In their retrospective study of patients with rheumatoid arthritis, Ostensen and coworkers found that disease severity commonly increased by 4–10 weeks postpartum. Most patients returned to the same level of disease activity during the year after delivery as that before conception.[6] Disease worsened postpartum in all but one of the 12 patients with rheumatoid arthritis prospectively studied by Ostensen and Husby. Six patients reported a fairly sudden flare 2–3 weeks after delivery, whereas five women noted more gradual exacerbations 6–10 weeks postpartum.[7]

A prospective study by Ostensen and Husby found that the time of disease exacerbation was not associated with duration of lactation, which lasted 2–8 months.[7] However, a prospective study by Barrett and colleagues indicated that breast feeding may increase the risk of postpartum flare, particularly after a first pregnancy.[11] Disease activity was compared during pregnancy and at 6 months postpartum among 49 non–breast feeders, 38 first-time breast feeders, and 50 repeat breast feeders, all of whom had rheumatoid arthritis. After adjusting for possible confounders, increased disease severity was found in patients who breast fed for the first time, with intermediate severity in the other categories. The odds of worsening disease were highest in first-time breast feeders and lowest in women who did not breast feed.[11]

Antepartum Management of Rheumatoid Arthritis

Management of rheumatoid arthritis is intended to relieve pain, decrease inflammation, protect articular structures, and preserve function. Physical and occupational therapies are essential components of a care regimen for affected patients.[2] Outside pregnancy, aspirin or other nonsteroidal anti-inflammatory drugs (NSAIDs) are pivotal to therapy. However, the large doses of aspirin typically used for nonpregnant patients (3–4 g orally daily) may in the pregnant patient result in impaired hemostasis, premature closure of the fetal ductus arteriosus, and prolonged gestation. Therefore, it is recommended that, if a patient requires therapy for rheumatoid arthritis during pregnancy, acetaminophen be tried as a first-line agent. If acetaminophen does not provide relief, aspirin or another NSAID may be tried during the first and second trimesters. If these prove inadequate, oral corticosteroids may be used for relief. Long-acting corticosteroids may also be injected into involved joints; these injections usually provide good symptomatic relief of the affected joint and lasts for several months.[1,2]

If a pregnant patient does not receive sufficient relief with acetaminophen, NSAIDs, and corticosteroids, an alternative agent may need to be considered. Outside pregnancy, different disease-modifying drugs are used for rheumatoid arthritis refractory to NSAIDs and corticosteroids. These include chloroquine, sulfasalazine, methotrexate, gold compounds, azathioprine, and penicillamine. Some of these agents should be completely avoided in pregnancy because of known fetal risks. For instance, gold is not recommended in pregnancy because it causes blood dyscrasias, drug rashes, and nephropathy. Although gold is strongly bound to protein and very little crosses the placenta, theoretically the fetus is also at risk for these complications of therapy.[12] Methotrexate, a folic acid antagonist, is a known teratogen and should not be used in pregnancy. Adverse developmental defects associated with methotrexate use include a "clover-leaf" skull with a large head, swept-back hair, low-set ears, prominent eyes, and a wide nasal bridge; limb defects with absent ossification centers; anencephaly; hydrocephaly; meningomyelocele; mental retardation; and developmental delay.[13]

Careful counseling and reviewing of potential fetal risks of other agents (chloroquine, azathioprine, sulfasalazine, and penicillamine) is essential if these medications are to be considered for therapy. The patient must understand that absolute safety cannot be guaranteed because there are no randomized, controlled trials demonstrating teratogenic effects of these drugs in humans, and results of animal studies may differ from controlled studies in pregnant women. Therefore, reports in the literature regarding the use of these drugs during pregnancy are complex and contradictory.[12]

Animal studies of chloroquine and other quinine-related agents often used to control malaria have shown transplacental transfer with fetotoxicity resulting in anophthalmia, microphthalmia, and growth retardation. A report on the outcome of 169 pregnancies in which antimalarial doses of chloroquine were ingested once weekly throughout gestation described only two anomalous infants, which is not higher than would be expected in this group. One had tetralogy of Fallot and the other had congenital hypothyroidism.[14] There is a growing body of experience with Plaquenil used for control of lupus in pregnancy.

Azathioprine is a purine analog that interferes with the synthesis of adenine and guanine ribonucleosides. The fetal liver lacks the enzyme, inosinate pyrophosphorylase, that converts azathioprine to its active metabolites, and this fetal enzyme deficiency should protect the fetus from adverse effects of azathioprine. Azathioprine has not been associated with specific congenital defects in humans, but sporadic anomalies including preaxial polydactyly have been reported.[14]

Sulfasalazine is a sulfonamide antibiotic often used to manage inflammatory bowel disease. Sulfasalazine binds albumin and theoretically can displace bilirubin, leading to neonatal kernicterus. Two retrospective studies from England and Hungary indicated no increased risk of congenital malformations in patients with Crohn's disease who had taken sulfasalazine throughout pregnancy.[14]

Penicillamine is a heavy metal chelating agent. Animal experiments and a small number of human reports have suggested that congenital connective skin disorders such as lax skin and inguinal hernia may occur in association with maternal penicillamine therapy.[14]

If management of rheumatoid arthritis with acetaminophen, NSAIDs, and corticosteroids has proved inadequate, most authorities recommend that sulfasalazine or penicillamine be considered for further therapy, with appropriate counseling. Because of the risk of neonatal kernicterus with sulfonamide therapy, sulfasalazine should be avoided in the third trimester.[2]

Effect of Rheumatoid Arthritis on Perinatal Outcome

An increased fetal risk during gestation in rheumatoid arthritis has not been conclusively demonstrated. In 1963, Morris and colleagues reported no increase in fetal morbidity or mortality in 34 pregnancies among 17 patients with rheumatoid arthritis.[15] However, Kaplan and coworkers suggested a possible increased rate of pregnancy wastage in patients with rheumatoid arthritis. Their retrospective study compared 96 women older than 40 years with rheumatoid arthritis and previous pregnancies with control subjects and found abortion rates (spontaneous abortions among total pregnancies) to be 25.1% in patients with rheumatoid arthritis and 16.5% in controls.[16]

In contrast, a prospective study by Nelson and associates compared pregnancy outcomes in 144 patients with rheumatoid arthritis and 605 controls and found no significant differences in rates of spontaneous abortion or intrauterine fetal demise.[17] In the prospective study of 12 patients with rheumatoid arthritis by Ostensen and Husby, all patients delivered healthy children. In the control group of 12 patients, one fetal loss occurred at 17 weeks and another at 23 weeks of gestation.[7]

The need for further investigation into the effect of rheumatoid arthritis on perinatal outcome is apparent. Fetal complications during pregnancy are certainly more likely in patients who are receiving aggressive drug therapy. No studies have correlated disease severity with spontaneous abortion rate, which also needs to be investigated.

Planning for Delivery in the Pregnant Patient with Rheumatoid Arthritis

Labor and delivery can pose particular difficulties for patients with preexisting pelvic, hip, or spinal involvement from rheumatoid arthritis. Because contraction of the pelvis is more likely with juvenile onset of rheumatoid arthritis, clinical pelvimetry should be performed in affected patients. Rarely, if severe hip involvement completely precludes abduction of the thighs, a cesarean section may be necessary for delivery.[12]

Involvement of temporomandibular joints and the larynx may complicate intubation, so consultation with an anesthesiologist would be advisable in case general anesthesia is needed. If cervical spine involvement is present, subluxation may occur. Some anesthesiologists use collars in such patients, if intubation and general anesthesia are required, to prevent hyperextension of the neck.[12]

Postpartum Care of the Patient with Rheumatoid Arthritis

For the postpartum patient who desires birth control, combination estrogen and progesterone oral contraceptives are a logical choice because of their efficacy and because of the possibility that they may improve the symptoms of rheumatoid arthritis. The intrauterine device is not recommended for women receiving immunosuppressive therapy. The issue of breast feeding potentially adversely affecting rheumatoid arthritis should be also addressed with the postpartum patient so that she can decide whether or not to breast feed.[2]

If the postpartum patient has decided to breast feed, her medication regimen will need to be assessed in terms of risks to the infant. All drugs taken by the nursing mother will appear to some degree in her milk. The 1988 World Health Organization Working Group on Drugs and Human Lactation recommended against breast feeding while on gold, azathioprine, methotrexate, or aspirin.[18] Acetaminophen, ibuprofen, indomethacin, naproxen, and chloroquine are considered compatible with breast feeding.[19] There are no data on the risks to the breast fed newborn with maternal penicillamine use. The use of sulfasalazine during lactation has been associated with neonatal bloody diarrhea in one case. Other reports have associated 5-aminosalicylic acid, a sulfasalazine metabolite, with neonatal diarrhea. Although this metabolite is excreted in breast milk in small amounts, some newborns cannot tolerate even these minor exposures.[20]

The incidence of depression may be more prevalent in individuals with rheumatoid arthritis than in the general population, with estimates of 17–21%. Patients with rheumatoid arthritis should be assessed closely for signs of postpartum depression.[12]

What's the Evidence?

A good deal of evidence exists from observational data and case series regarding the diagnosis and typical antepartum and postpartum courses for rheumatoid arthritis. Applicable evidence has been reviewed in each pertinent section of this chapter. Although therapeutic options also have been reviewed, there are no evidence-based guidelines for clinicians to rely on when selecting the optimal therapeutic regimen for the pregnant patient with rheumatoid arthritis.

Guiding Questions in Approaching the Patient

Assessing disease extent

- How long has the patient had rheumatoid arthritis?
- Does she have joint or soft tissue swelling? Are these findings symmetric?
- Does she have rheumatoid nodules?

- What is her rheumatoid factor titer?
- Are radiographic erosions or periarticular osteopenia present in hand or wrist joints?
- What therapy has she required before pregnancy?

Antepartum management of rheumatoid arthritis

- Is the patient on any medications considered to be teratogenic or contraindicated in pregnancy?
- Does the patient require medications to control disease severity, or can she be expectantly managed?
- Does the patient have a contracted pelvis or bony hip deformities that might complicate vaginal delivery?
- Does the patient have subluxation of the cervical spine that might complicate general anesthesia if needed?

Postpartum care

- Does the patient wish to breast feed?
- What does she desire for contraception?
- Does she have follow-up care arranged with a rheumatologist because rheumatoid arthritis often flares postpartum?

Conclusion

Because rheumatoid arthritis is the most common systemic rheumatic disease, the obstetrician should be familiar with its usual course and management during pregnancy.

The inflammatory component of rheumatoid arthritis typically improves during pregnancy and worsens postpartum. Acetaminophen, corticosteroids, and NSAIDs are frequently used for pain relief, decrease of inflammation, protection of articular structures, and preservation of function. There has been no conclusive demonstration of increased fetal risk or increased rates of pregnancy loss in patients with rheumatoid arthritis. Delivery planning for the patient with rheumatoid arthritis should include assessment of clinical pelvimetry and ability to abduct hips and consultation with an anesthesiologist. Postpartum, combination estrogen and progesterone contraceptives should be discussed with the patient because they may ameliorate symptoms. In addition, the potential association between breast feeding and postpartum flare should be reviewed. If the patient opts to breast feed, her medications will need to be assessed in terms of their risks to the newborn.

Discussion of Cases

CASE 1: PRECONCEPTION COUNSELING FOR RHEUMATOID ARTHRITIS

A 36-year-old nulligravid woman with a 7-year history of rheumatoid arthritis comes for a pre-pregnancy consultation. She requires methotrexate to control pain, swelling, and stiffness and is followed closely by a rheumatologist.

She asks what she might expect in terms of disease progression if she were to become pregnant.

Her disease severity might improve during the pregnancy and is likely to worsen postpartum.

She asks what she should do in terms of the methotrexate.

Once the patient actively begins attempting to conceive, her medication should be changed, with close surveillance by her rheumatologist.

She should not take methotrexate throughout the pregnancy because it is a known teratogen. Medications to consider as first-line agents include acetaminophen, NSAIDs in the first and second trimesters, and corticosteroids. If other medications are needed, penicillamine and/or sulfasalazine may be considered. Sulfasalazine should not be used in the third trimester because it may predispose the newborn to kernicterus.

The patient is concerned that she may be at increased risk for spontaneous abortion because of her rheumatoid arthritis.

No association between spontaneous abortion and rheumatoid arthritis has been conclusively demonstrated.

CASE 2: DELIVERY PLANS FOR A PATIENT WITH RHEUMATOID ARTHRITIS

You are following a 38-year-old primigravid woman who has had rheumatoid arthritis for 5 years. She is currently at 34 weeks of gestation and you are beginning to plan for her delivery.

She asks you whether she will be able to deliver vaginally.

You will want to perform clinical pelvimetry to assess for a contracted pelvis, which might preclude vaginal delivery. Contracted pelvises are more common in patients with longstanding or juvenile arthritis, so this patient is not likely to have a pelvis that is contracted. You will also want to check that she can abduct her hips sufficiently for delivery. Patients who have had hip replacements or who have significant hip deformities may be unable to abduct their hips significantly.**

The patient asks whether she can have an epidural in labor.

You are concerned that the patient may have specific issues related to obstetric anesthesia,

although an epidural should not be contraindicated. You refer the patient for an anesthesiology consult so that anesthetic options can be discussed in detail. The anesthesiologist will want to review with the patient that general anesthesia, if required, may be difficult if temporomandibular or laryngeal involvement complicates intubation. The anesthesiologist will also need to explain that, if general anesthesia and intubation are required, a collar might be needed to prevent subluxation of the atlantoaxial joint with concomitant hyperextension of the head.

The patient wonders whether she will be able to breast feed.

Breast feeding is a most personal decision, and the patient will need to decide for herself whether she wishes to breast feed or formula feed. The patient should be aware that some studies have associated postpartum rheumatoid arthritis flares with breast feeding. Her medications should be reviewed in terms of compatibility with breast feeding.

The patient is considering various forms of contraception.

Not only are combination oral contraceptives an extremely effective form of birth control, but they also may be beneficial in terms of halting disease progress. Intrauterine devices are not recommended for women on immunosuppressive medications.

REFERENCES

1 Cunningham FG, Gant NF, Leveno KJ, et al. Medical and surgical complications in pregnancy. In: Cunningham FG, Gant NF, Leveno KJ, et al, eds. *Williams Obstetrics,* 21st ed. New York: McGraw-Hill, 2001; p. 1394–1396.

2 De Swiet M. Rheumatologic and connective tissue disorders. In: Creasy RK, Resnick R, eds. *Maternal–Fetal Medicine,* 4th ed. New York: WB Saunders, 1999; p. 1086–1087.

3 Bulmash JM. Rheumatoid arthritis and pregnancy. *Obstet Gynecol Annu* 1979;8:223–276.

4 Arnett FC, Edworthy SM, Bloch DA, et al. The American Rheumatism Association 1987 revised criteria for the classification of rheumatoid arthritis. *Arthrits Rheum* 1988;31:315–324.

5 Hench AB. The ameliorating effect of pregnancy on chronic atrophic (infectious rheumatoid) arthritis; fibrositis and intermittent hydrarthrosis. *Proc Mayo Clin* 1938;13:161–167.

6 Ostensen M, Aune B, Husby G. The effect of pregnancy and hormonal changes on the activity of rheumatoid arthritis. *Scand J Rheumatol* 1983;12:69–72.

7 Ostensen M, Husby G. A prospective clinical study of the effect of pregnancy on rheumatoid arthritis and anyklosing spondylitis. *Arthrits Rheum* 1983;26:1155–1159.

8 Bijlsma JW, Van den Brink HR. Estrogens and rheumatoid arthritis. *Am J Reprod Immunol* 1992;28:231–234.

9 Unger A, Kay A, Griffin A, Panayi GS. Disease activity and pregnancy associated α_2-glycoprotein in rheumatoid arthritis during pregnancy. *Br Med J* 1983;286:750–752.

10 Nelson JL, Hughes KA, Smith AG, et al. Maternal–fetal disparity in HLA class II alloantigens and the pregnancy-induced amelioration of rheumatoid arthritis. *N Eng J Med* 1993;329:466–471.

11 Barrett JH, Brennan P, Fiddler M, Silman A. Breast-feeding and post-partum relapse in women with rheumatoid and inflammatory arthritis. *Arthrits Rheum* 2000;43:1010–1015.

12 Fiddler MA. Rheumatoid arthritis and pregnancy. *Arthrits Care Res* 1997;10:264–272.

13 Buckley LM, Bullaboy CA, Leichtman L, Marquez M. Multiple congenital anomalies associated with weekly low-dose methotrexate treatment of the mother. *Arthrits Rheum* 1997;40:971–973.

14 Ramsey-Goldman R, Schilling E. Immunosuppressive drug use during pregnancy. *Rheum Dis Clin North Am* 1997;23:1–14.

15 Morris WIC. Pregnancy in rheumatoid arthritis and systemic lupus erythematosus. *Aust N Z J Obstet Gynecol* 1969;9:136.

16 Kaplan D. Fetal wastage in patients with rheumatoid arthritis. *J Rheum* 1986;13:875–877.

17 Nelson JL, Voigt LF, Koepsell TD, et al. Pregnancy outcome in women with rheumatoid arthritis before disease onset. *J Rheum* 1992;19:18–21.

18 The WHO Working Group. *Drugs and Human Lactation.* New York: World Health Organization, 1988.

19 Ette EL. Chloroquine in human milk. *J Clin Pharmacol* 1987;27:499–502.

20 Branski D, Kerem E, Gross-Kieselstein E. Bloody diarrhea—a possible complication of sulphasalazine transferred through human breast milk. *J Pediatr Gastroenteral Nutr* 1986;5:316–317.

Approach to Headache in Pregnancy

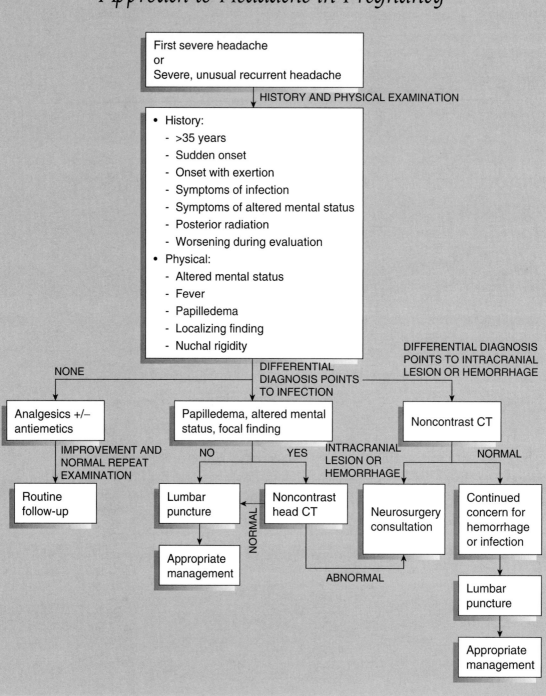

36 Headache

Introduction

Headache is one of the most frequently encountered complaints in clinical practice. More than 80% of women will complain of headaches during their childbearing years; therefore, headaches during pregnancy are quite common.[1] Most of these will be a primary headache syndrome such as tension-type headache (TTH) or migraine. Approximately 10% will have one of the numerous causes of secondary headache, some of which can be life threatening. Although large population-based studies for most types of chronic headaches are lacking or unreliable, migraine headaches currently affect about 18% of American women and approximately 50% of these remain undiagnosed.[2] TTH appears to be more common than migraine and occurs in approximately 42% of women.[3] This chapter includes a discussion of an approach to diagnosing this common and frequently vexing complaint and some recommendations for management.

Because most headaches will fall into one of two diagnoses (TTH or migraine), becoming familiar with the criteria published by the Headache Classification Committee of the International Headache Society for these diagnoses is a high-yield exercise (Tables 36-1 and 36-2). Although knowledge of these criteria can be extremely useful for the clinician, it is important to remember that some of the individual criterion may be missing in a significant proportion of patients who have these types of headaches. In addition, patients can frequently have more than one type of headache, and it is apparent why the diagnosis can be difficult.

Table 36-1. **MIGRAINE WITHOUT AURA**

A. ≥5 attacks fulfilling criteria B–D; migraine <15 d/mo
B. Migraine is defined as episodic attacks of headache lasting 4–72 h
C. With 2 of the following symptoms
Unilateral location
Pulsating quality
Aggravation by or causing avoidance from physical activity
Moderate or severe pain intensity

D. And 1 of the following symptoms
Nausea and/or vomiting
Photophobia and phonophobia

SOURCE: Headache Classification Committee of the International Headache Society. Classification and diagnostic criteria for headache disorders, cranial neuralgias and facial pain. *Cephalagia* 1988;8(suppl 7):1–96.

Because some causes of secondary headache can be life threatening, it is important to have an organized approach to obtaining the history and performing the physical examination of the pregnant woman who complains of headache. A detailed history of the patient's prenatal course, in particular the gestational age, comorbid conditions (such as preexisting hypercoagulable state), and recent trauma or lumbar puncture (LP) are essential historical

---

Table 36-2. **TENSION-TYPE HEADACHE THAT IS INFREQUENT OR EPISODIC**

A. ≥5 previous headache episodes fulfilling criteria B–D; headache <12 d/y (<1/mo)
B. Headache lasting 30 min to 7 d
C. ≥3 of the following pain characteristics
Pressing/tightening (nonpulsating) quality
Mild or moderate intensity (may inhibit but does not prohibit activities)
Bilateral location
No aggravation by walking stairs or similar routine physical activity

D. All of the following
No nausea (anorexia may occur)
No photophobia or phonophobia

E. Not attributed to another disorder

SOURCE: Headache Classification Committee of the International Headache Society. Classification and diagnostic criteria for headache disorders, cranial neuralgias and facial pain. *Cephalagia* 1988;8(suppl 7):1–96.

points that may indicate a specific headache diagnosis. Other important aspects of the history on which to focus include the existence of previous similar headache and whether or not this particular headache represents a change from the patient's customary headache, and onset, duration, location, quality, severity, and presence or absence of associated systemic or neurologic signs or symptoms. One approach to remembering some of these worrisome features of the history and physical examination involves using the SNOOP acronym, which stands for systemic symptoms/ disease, neurologic symptoms or signs, onset sudden, onset after age 40 years, and pattern change (Table 36-3).

Many of the aspects of the historical presentation and physical examination of the patient with headache are suggested by the SNOOP features but should certainly include at least the following: measurement of vital signs including temperature, evaluation for signs of meningeal irritation, evidence of altered sensorium or postictal state, and visual disturbances including evidence of papilledema on funduscopic examination. It is also important for diagnostic accuracy and for the patient's state of mind to palpate the area referred to by the patient as the area of maximal tenderness. This will not only reassure the patient, who is frequently convinced that she have a catastrophic cause for headache, but also disclose the occasional temporomandibular joint syndrome or may suggest temporal arthritis, which is extremely rare in women of childbearing age.

Based on the history and physical examination, some patients will not have a clear diagnosis or will have an increased likelihood

KEY POINT

Key historical points include first or worst headache ever, sudden onset with or without trauma or exertion, and history of altered mental status. Important findings on physical examination include fever, nuchal rigidity, papilledema, focal neurologic abnormality, or apparently altered mental status.

Table 36-3. **WORRISOME FEATURES OF A PARTICULAR HEADACHE (SNOOP)**

Systemic symptoms/signs (fever, myalgias, weight loss)
Systemic disease (hypercoagulable state, malignancy, acquired immunodeficiency syndrome)
Neurologic symptoms or signs
Onset sudden (thunderclap headache)
Onset after age 40 y
Pattern change
    Progressive headache with loss of headache-free periods
    Change in type of headache

SOURCE: Adapted with permission from Dodick DW. Diagnosing headache: clinical clues and clinical rules. *Adv Stud Med* 2003;3:87–92.

of a secondary cause of headache that requires further workup by a laboratory or neuroimaging and require referral to an emergency facility. A normal complete blood cell count, erythrocyte sedimentation rate, and comprehensive metabolic profile (including hepatic and renal function studies) will argue against meningoencephalitis, preeclampsia, or a vasculitic process but should not delay more definitive diagnostic workup in a patient with worrisome signs or symptoms. An increased erythrocyte sedimentation rate is less likely to be useful in pregnancy because it is always elevated.

Patients with papilledema, altered mental status, or focal neurologic findings will receive emergent noncontrast computed tomography (CT) of the brain to rule out hemorrhage or structural lesion. Suspicion of an infectious etiology should prompt empiric antibiotics and the immediate performance of lumbar puncture (LP) unless a CT is indicated (Figure 36-1). In no situation should waiting for laboratory results delay performance of head CT or LP as indicated. An LP should be preceded by plain CT if papilledema, focal neurologic signs, or altered mental signs are present to rule out the possibility of a space-occupying lesion or bleeding. A plain CT of the head exposes the uterus to very small amounts of ionizing radiation in the properly shielded patient and is therefore considered safe. Likewise, an intracranial angiogram is considered quite safe but has largely been replaced by magnetic resonance imaging (MRI) with or without gadolinium

KEY POINT

The patient with a worrisome headache based on history or physical examination should be referred to an emergency facility.

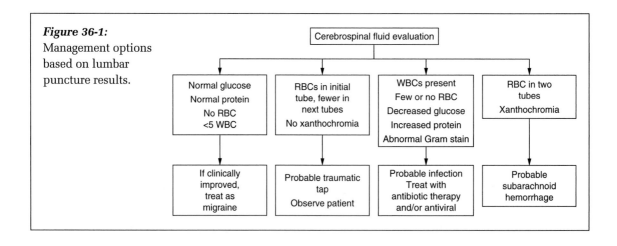

Figure 36-1:
Management options based on lumbar puncture results.

enhancement. MRI has the benefit of using no ionizing radiation and has very few contraindications. Gadolinium does cross the placenta but is excreted through the fetal kidney with no ill effects. MRI angiography has become the standard modality for diagnosing cerebral aneurysms. The gold standard for suspected cerebral venous thrombosis is MRI venography, which can be performed without gadolinium enhancement.

An unusual headache seen only in pregnancy and therefore deserving special attention includes the headache associated with preeclampsia and eclampsia. The complaint of headache in preeclampsia is considered a late finding and will be noted after the widely recognized signs and symptoms of hypertension, proteinuria, and edema. There are many theories as to the pathogenesis of headache in preeclampsia, but the exact cause is not known. These findings typically start in the third trimester or, less frequently, in the late second trimester in a primigravida. The headache is typically diffuse, constant, and mild to severe in intensity. The headache is frequently associated with epigastric pain and visual disturbances. Laboratory abnormalities such thrombocytopenia, increased liver functions, evidence of hemolysis, hyperuricemia, increased creatinine, and proteinuria also suggest preeclampsia. The complaint of headache in preeclampsia and eclampsia was found to be significantly more common (63% vs. 44%) in women who eventually developed seizures in one study of 445 women.[4]

Cerebral venous thrombosis is extremely unusual but is most likely encountered in the older pregnant patient or one with a preexisting hypercoagulable state such as that conferred by one of the genetic thrombophilias (e.g., factor V Leiden mutation, protein S deficiency, or protein C deficiency). One study that examined U.S. hospital discharge data over 12 years, including more than 50,000,000 deliveries, found 5723 cases of intracranial venous thrombosis, indicating an incidence of 11.4 in 100,000 deliveries.[5] Cerebral venous thrombosis causes an unremitting headache and can lead to cerebral vascular hemorrhage that may be associated with other neurologic findings such as seizures, altered mental status, and focal neurologic signs.

The postdural puncture headache (PDPH) is rarely missed because of its temporal relation (usually ≤48 hours) to diagnostic or therapeutic dural puncture. The headache is classically worse when standing or sitting up and is relieved by lying in a supine position. PDPH is rarely associated with tinnitus, nausea, vomiting, and cranial nerve dysfunction. Management of these headaches is discussed below.

Management of headache in pregnancy is not typically a subject of large clinical trials because of ethical concerns. Headache in preeclampsia is usually a late finding and is relieved by delivery. Management also involves control of hypertension and prophylaxis against seizures, which are more common in the patients with preeclampsia or eclampsia and headache. Management of cerebral venous thrombosis involves the use anticoagulants and thrombolytics, most frequently endovascular thrombolytic therapy.[6,7] Because cerebral edema can lead to infarction and intracerebral hemorrhage, with all of the potentially life-threatening complications, comanagement of this condition with a neurosurgeon is advisable. Management of PDPH requires no more than bedrest, hydration, and analgesics, after which the cerebrospinal fluid volume will normalize and the headache will resolve spontaneously. Caffeine has been used orally and intravenously, but recurrence of headache is common.[8,9] The epidural blood patch is the definitive treatment and has essentially replaced the use of caffeine and bedrest with fluid replacement in the control of PDPH. Structural lesions or bleeding will require neurosurgical consultation and specialized monitoring for seizures, electrolyte abnormalities related to the syndrome of inappropriate secretion of andiuretic hormone, and rebleeding. This monitoring should occur in an intensive care unit setting. Infectious etiologies will mandate the use of broad-spectrum antiviral or antibacterial therapy until laboratory testing allows for more specific management of the causative organism. Severe, life-threatening causes of headache are controlled as aggressively as in the nonpregnant patient, and potentially toxic drugs are avoided when possible.

Much more frequently the patient will have one of the primary headaches that make up the vast majority of headache-producing illnesses in this age group. TTH is the most common of these and is usually described as a pressure or band-like constriction around the head. Changes in the criteria for diagnosing TTH by the International Headache Society in 2003 eliminated photophobia and phonophobia as symptoms of TTH, thereby changing many patients' diagnosis from TTH to migraine headache (see Table 36-2). Control of TTH in pregnancy includes the use of acetaminophen as a first-line agent. More severe headaches can be controlled with commercially available combinations of butalbital, caffeine, and codeine. Prolonged use of narcotic analgesics may be associated with habituation and rebound headaches after stopping medication. Nonsteroidal anti-inflammatory medications can also be used but should be prescribed cautiously because of concerns of gastropathy, enhanced bleeding secondary to platelet effects, rebound headaches, and effects on the fetus that might cause premature ductal closure and oligohydramnios. During pregnancy, use of nonsteroidal anti-inflammatory drugs has been limited to very judicious use in the second and early third trimesters. Other therapies that have been tried, are safe, and may be beneficial in selected patients include psychotherapy, massage therapy, acupuncture, and hypnosis. One study has indicated that 80% of pregnant patients develop significant headache decreases by using biofeedback, relaxation therapy, and physical therapy.[10] There is some evidence for the usefulness of nerve blocks for nonpregnant individuals for management of recurrent headaches.[11] Because of low likelihood of complications, it is reasonably likely that they would be helpful for pregnant women.

Migraine headaches have been shown to have a link to estrogen and frequently improve during pregnancy.[12] A few women, approximately 4–8%, will experience worsening of their migraines during pregnancy, and about 10% of migraine headaches occur for the first time during pregnancy.[13] Management of migraine headaches in pregnancy mirrors that of TTH with exceptions related to increased severity, frequency of nausea and vomiting, and potential for prophylaxis. Because migraine headache is typically more severe, the use of narcotic therapy is more frequent. Opioid therapy should be considered second-line therapy with the same precautions described above, and maternal and neonatal addictions are warranted especially in light of the higher-potency opioid analgesics frequently used. The nausea and vomiting that frequently accompany migraine headaches may be controlled with centrally acting antiemetic medications such as chlorpromazine and metoclopramide. Ergot alkaloids have been widely used in migraine management but are absolutely contraindicated in pregnancy because of their potential to produce hypertonic uterine contractions. The most successful drugs for aborting migraine headaches are called triptans and include sumatriptan, naratriptan, rizatriptan, zolmitriptan, almotriptan, frovatriptan, and eletriptan. These drugs are pregnancy category C according to criteria of the U.S. Food and Drug Administration (FDA) because safety in human pregnancies has not been determined, and these medications have known vaso-constrictive properties. Use of these medications should be only under the advice and supervision of a neurologist and/or maternal fetal medicine specialist.

The only drugs approved by the FDA for the prevention of migraine headache are methysergide, propranolol, timolol, divalproex sodium, and divalproex sodium extended release. Topiramate has applied for and will likely receive this indication in early 2004. Methysergide and any other ergot alkaloid are con-traindicated in pregnancy. Divalproex sodium and valproic acid forms are considered FDA category D because of the fetal risk of developing neural tube defects. Many other agents have been used for prophylaxis of migraine headache, and a few are reasonable choices in the pregnant patient. The daily use of antihypertensive medications including β blockers (e.g., timolol and propranolol) or calcium channel blockers (e.g., verapamil) in the smallest effective dose may decrease the frequency and severity of migraine headaches. The most commonly used drugs in these categories have a FDA pregnancy category C. Patients should be carefully monitored to avoid hypotension and significant changes in heart rate, which are recognized side effects of these medications. Antidepressant medications used for migraine prophylaxis include doxepin, amitriptyline, and nortriptyline (FDA category C). Selective sero-tonin reuptake inhibitors and monoamine oxidase inhibitors have also been used as migraine prophylactic agents but are not fre-quently used in pregnancy. Antiepileptic drugs, which are more recently referred to as neurostabilizers, are being increasingly used for migraine prophylaxis and include topiramate and gabapentin (both FDA category C). Because most established migraineurs improve during pregnancy, patients with migraine headaches in pregnancy severe enough to consider prophylactic therapy should be comanaged with a neurologist or the patient's primary care physician if they are comfortable recommending therapy in this situation.

What's the Evidence?

There are no large clinical trials on which to base diagnosis or management of headache in pregnancy nor will the future likely yield any because of ethical considerations. A potentially useful avenue of study would be in the use of nerve blocks and topical lidocaine in aborting acute headaches, especially of the tension and migraine types. Because headaches are so common in the childbearing years and because so many pregnancies are unplanned, exposure to interventions and medications will be inevitable. Most of the manufacturers of the triptans maintain information on patients inadvertently exposed to their products in pregnancy. The Sumatriptan and Naratriptan Pregnancy Registries were the first of these established in 1996 in collaboration with the manufacturer and the Centers for Disease Control and Prevention. The two registries were combined in April 2001. The purpose of the registries is to detect early signals of potential risks in advance of formal epidemiologic studies, supplement animal toxicologic studies, and assist clinicians in weighing risks and benefits of treatment in individual patients. The registry captures data prospectively, includes information only on defects apparent at birth, and is strictly voluntary. These characteristics of the registries are potential weaknesses and, because of the small number of pregnancies included thus far, one should be cautious in using the currently available information. This information in most cases can be obtained from medical support personnel of the companies involved and is typically updated frequently. A registry also exists for use of antiepileptic drugs in pregnancy.

Guiding Questions in Approaching the Patient

- Why is the patient seeking treatment?
- Is this the worst headache of her life?
- Has she had altered mental status?
- Was her headache of sudden onset?
- Was the headache associated with exertion?
- Has she had fever or been feeling unwell?
- Has she had contact with anyone else who is ill?

Discussion of Cases

CASE 1: SEVERE MIGRAINE HEADACHE

A 37-year-old gravida 1, para 0 at 37 weeks of gestation presents with a severe left-side headache associated with photophobia, phonophobia, and nausea for the past 18 hours. The patient has a long personal and family history of migraine headaches but has enjoyed a relatively headache-free pregnancy. It was not unusual for her migraines to last for 2 days before this pregnancy. She had used sumatriptan before becoming pregnant, with good effect, and today took acetaminophen without significant improvement. She denies vomiting, epigastric pain, visual changes, altered mental status, edema, fever, or neck pain. There was no history of diagnosed hypercoagulable state or cerebrovascular disease, deep venous thromboses, or pulmonary emboli.

On physical examination she is squinting in the normal light of the examination room but does not appear ill. Her vital signs are as follows: temperature of 97.8°F, blood pressure of 110/78 mm Hg, pulse of 84 beats/min, and a respiratory rate of 18 breaths/min and unlabored. Examination of the head and neck is normal, including no nuchal rigidity and no tenderness to palpation over the temporal arteries or temporomandibular joints. Neurologic examination is normal. There is no dependent edema, and the remainder of the examination is entirely normal.

What other testing, if any, would you recommend at this point?

Urinalysis.

Urinalysis showed no protein or glucose.

Does she require any further testing to initiate management?

No, any further testing is not recommended.

What is your recommendation for initial management?

Because the patient has tried acetaminophen without benefit, she should try a short-acting narcotic in the hopes of a quick recovery. Reassurance should be given that there is no harm to her or her unborn child with short-term use of narcotic analgesics. If her nausea were to worsen or to progress to vomiting, metoclopramide orally or chlorpromazine orally or rectally may be used.

CASE 2: GRAVIDA WITH WORST HEADACHE OF HER LIFE

A 25-year-old gravida 3, para 2 at 23 weeks of gestation presents with sudden onset of "the worst headache of my life," which started 6 hours before presentation. The headache started immediately on lifting her 40-lb, 4-year-old son. She is not prone to headache and has no personal or family history of migraine headaches or hypercoagulable state. The patient's mother had been diagnosed with a cerebral aneurysm in her 30s.

On physical examination she alert and oriented but is in obvious distress without otherwise appearing ill. Her vital signs are as follows: temperature of 98.8°F, blood pressure of 98/64 mm Hg, pulse of 68 beats/min, and a respiratory rate of 16 breaths/min and unlabored.

Examination of the head and neck is remarkable for nuchal rigidity, but there is no papilledema or tenderness to palpation over the temporal arteries or temporomandibular joints. Neurologic examination is without any focal or lateralizing signs, and the gait is normal. There is no dependent edema, and the remainder of the examination is entirely normal.

What other testing, if any, would you recommend at this point?

This patient should be transported immediately to the nearest emergency facility for further workup. This recommendation is based on the sudden onset of severe headache and the finding of nuchal rigidity on physical examination that raises the concern of hemorrhage from aneurysmal rupture, vascular dissection, or, less likely, infection.

An LP was performed before CT of the brain because there was no papilledema, focal neurologic signs, or altered mental status noted. Cerebrospinal fluid showed no white blood cells but was remarkable for red blood cells and xanthochromia in all tubes despite what was considered an atraumatic procedure. Bacterial studies including Gram's stains and cultures on cerebrospinal fluid showed no organisms.

What is your recommendation for initial management?

The patient should be admitted to an intensive care unit and managed in consultation with the neurosurgical service. Intensive management of blood pressure, vasospasm, hydrocephalus, seizures, electrolyte abnormalities (in particular hyponatremia), cardiac abnormalities, and monitoring for rebleeding are the keys to management of subarachnoid hemorrhage that does not require immediate surgical evacuation, as in this case.

What is the next step in the patient's management?

An MRI angiogram done subsequently showed a saccular (berry) aneurysm. A caesarean section was performed, and a healthy 2,800-g male infant was delivered. The patient then underwent a successful clipping of the aneurysm and recovered uneventfully.

REFERENCES

1 Waters WE, O'Connor PJ. Epidemiology of headache and migraine in women. *J Neurol Psychiatry* 1971;34:148–153.

2 Lipton RB, Stewart WF, Diamond S, et al. Prevalence and burden of migraine in the United States: data from the American Migraine Study II. *Headache* 2001;41:646–657.

3 Schwartz B, Stewart WF, Simon D, Lipton RB. Epidemiology of tension-type headache. *JAMA* 1998;279:381–383.

4 Witlin AG, Saade GR, Mattar F, Sibai BM. Risk factors for abruption placentae and eclampsia: analysis of 445 consecutively managed women with severe preeclampsia and eclampsia. *Am J Obstet Gynecol* 1999;180:1322–1329.

5 Lanska DJ, Kryscio RJ, Stroke and intracranial venous thrombosis during pregnancy and puerperium. *Neurology* 1998;51:1622–1628.

6 Philips MF, Bagley LJ, Sinson GP, et al, Endovascular thrombolysis for symptomatic cerebral venous thrombosis. *J Neurosurg* 1999; 90:65–71.

7 Hsu FP, Kuether T, Nesbit G, Barnwell SL. Dural sinus thrombosis endovascular therapy. *Crit Care Clin* 1999;15:743–753.

8 Morewood GH. A rational approach to the cause, prevention and treatment of postdural puncture headache. *Can Med Assoc J* 1993;149: 1087–1093.

9 Camann WR, Murray RS, Mushlin PS, Lambert DH. Effects of oral caffeine on postdural puncture headache. A double-blind, placebo-controlled trial. *Anesth Analg* 1990;70:181–184.

10 Scharff L, Marcus D, Turk D. Maintenance of effects in the nonmedical treatment of headaches during pregnancy. *Headache* 1996;21: 105–109.

11 Caputi CA. Firetto V. Therapeutic blockade of greater occipital and supraorbital nerves in migraine patients. *Headache* 1997;37:174–179.

12 Marcus DA. Interrelationships of neurochemicals, estrogen, and recurring headache. *Pain* 1995;62;129–139.

13 Aube M. Migraine in pregnancy. *Neurology* 1999;53(suppl 1): S26–S28.

Approach to the Pregnant Woman with Epilepsy

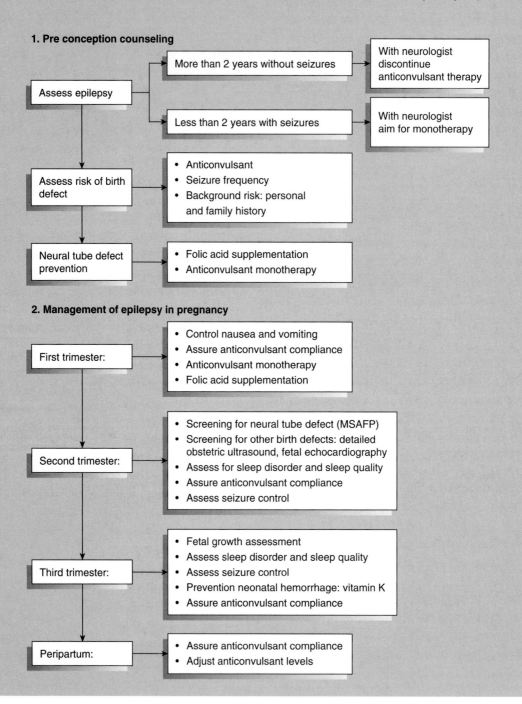

1. Pre conception counseling

Assess epilepsy

→ More than 2 years without seizures → With neurologist discontinue anticonvulsant therapy

→ Less than 2 years with seizures → With neurologist aim for monotherapy

Assess risk of birth defect

- Anticonvulsant
- Seizure frequency
- Background risk: personal and family history

Neural tube defect prevention

- Folic acid supplementation
- Anticonvulsant monotherapy

2. Management of epilepsy in pregnancy

First trimester:

- Control nausea and vomiting
- Assure anticonvulsant compliance
- Anticonvulsant monotherapy
- Folic acid supplementation

Second trimester:

- Screening for neural tube defect (MSAFP)
- Screening for other birth defects: detailed obstetric ultrasound, fetal echocardiography
- Assess for sleep disorder and sleep quality
- Assure anticonvulsant compliance
- Assess seizure control

Third trimester:

- Fetal growth assessment
- Assess sleep disorder and sleep quality
- Assess seizure control
- Prevention neonatal hemorrhage: vitamin K
- Assure anticonvulsant compliance

Peripartum:

- Assure anticonvulsant compliance
- Adjust anticonvulsant levels

37 Management of Epilepsy During Pregnancy

Lucie Morin
Lionel Carmant

Introduction

Epilepsy is defined as the occurrence of two unprovoked seizures that are separated by more than 24 hours. Typical provoking factors that need to be ruled out include drug or alcohol intoxication or withdrawal in adults and fever in children. Epilepsy affects 1–2% of the general population[1] and 0.5% of the women of childbearing age.[2,3] It is the second most common neurologic disorder during pregnancy, after migraine headaches.[4]

Epilepsy and its management have the potential of disrupting the reproductive function of women. Epilepsy and anticonvulsants lead to an increased risk for many complications during pregnancy. Pregnancy can influence the course of the underlying epileptic syndrome, and anticonvulsants can affect the developing fetus and the newborn.

These pregnancies are considered high risk and need careful management by the neurologic and obstetric teams. With proper counseling and monitoring, most women with epilepsy will have a normal pregnancy and delivery, an unchanged seizure frequency, and greater than 90% chance of delivering a normal baby.[5]

Preconception Counseling

EFFECT OF PREGNANCY ON SEIZURE CONTROL Among the topics to be discussed with a woman with epilepsy who is planning a pregnancy is the possibility that seizure frequency may increase; however, for patients who have been free of seizures for longer than 2 years, the need to continue therapy should be reassessed by a neurologist because, after 2 years without a seizure and with a normal electroencephalogram, the risk of seizure recurrence is 20–40%, with more than 90% of the recurrences occurring within 1 year.[6] Withdrawal can be performed over a short period (6 weeks) without increasing the risk of recurrence compared with a longer taper duration.[7]

For those with an active seizure disorder, the frequency of seizures will remain unchanged during pregnancy in about 50% of epileptic women. In 25% of woman, seizure frequency increases,[8] and in a similar percentage of women, seizure frequency will actually decrease. The increased seizure rate during pregnancy is due to three factors. The first factor is the change in anticonvulsant pharmacokinetics that occurs during pregnancy. Increases in plasma volume, renal blood flow, and hepatic metabolism during pregnancy alter the distribution volume and clearance of the anticonvulsant medication. The net result is a decrease in serum drug concentration. At the same time, there is a relative decrease in protein binding sites due to the decrease in plasma albumin in the pregnant state that leads to an increase in free plasma levels of anticonvulsants. This is particularly relevant for drugs that are highly protein bound, such as valproate and phenytoin. For these drugs, it is suggested that, when drug level monitoring is undertaken, free (not protein bound) drug levels should be obtained.[9] Another cause for changes in seizure frequency and drug levels is a decrease in drug absorption. Symptoms caused by pregnancy such as nausea and vomiting during the first trimester and worries over the adverse effects of anticonvulsants on the developing fetus can lead to a loss of compliance by the patient.

The second factor influencing seizure frequency is sleep deprivation induced by pregnancy, labor, and delivery. Sleep deprivation is an important trigger of seizure in all epileptic patients and the sleep debt increases with the duration of pregnancy peaking around delivery. A tonic-clonic seizure occurs during labor in 1–2% of women with epilepsy and within 24 hours of delivery in another 1–2%, which represents a risk of greater than nine times the average probability of a seizure during the rest of the pregnancy.[5] The third factor influencing seizure frequency is the alteration of neuronal excitability induced by hormonal changes.[10]

In practice, it is reasonable to increase the anticonvulsant drug dosage if seizure frequency increases. However, one must first verify compliance and free drug levels to avoid toxic levels, especially during the first trimester.

EFFECT OF EPILEPSY ON PREGNANCY

Women with epilepsy have a slightly increased risk of certain obstetric complications. Most complication rates are at most 2.5 times that of the general population.[11] Hyperemesis gravidarum, anemia, and placental abruption are the most common. Preeclampsia and preterm delivery also tend to occur more frequently. Obstetric interventions such as induction of labor and cesarean section occur twice as often.[11] In general, cesarean sections are performed for obstetric indication but may be indicated in specific circumstances related to epilepsy such unrelenting tonic-clonic seizures during labor.[12]

Perinatal mortality rate is one to two times higher in epileptic pregnancies than in the general population.[13–15] This is believed to be secondary to the effect of anticonvulsant medications, to the hereditary factors associated with epilepsy, and to the association of poor socioeconomic status of women with epilepsy.

EFFECT OF MATERNAL SEIZURES ON THE FETUS Generalized and complex partial seizures can affect the fetal heart rate.[16] This can lead to fetal hypoxia and alterations in the acid-base equilibrium secondary to a decrease in placental blood flow or to maternal hypoventilation after seizures.[16,17] Seizure-induced abdominal trauma can result in fetal injury and placental abruption. There are anecdotal reports of intrauterine deaths after a seizure, although this is a rare event.[15] Although there is no association between maternal tonic-clonic seizures during pregnancy and malformations,[18,19] seizures during the first-trimester have been reported to increase the incidence of congenital malformations when compared with seizures during the rest of the pregnancy (12.3% vs. 4%).[20] One series found an increased risk of developmental delay independent of the drug effect.[21]

EFFECT OF ANTICONVULSANT DRUGS ON THE FETUS Women with epilepsy should be provided with adequate information about the risks and benefits of the drugs to themselves and their offspring. If the woman's epilepsy is well controlled, moving toward monotherapy or even discontinuing all treatment should be discussed with a neurologist in the preconceptual period.

The rate of birth defects is two to three times higher in children born of epileptic mothers than in the general population, with a combined estimated rate of 4–10%.[22–24] This rate can increase three to six times higher than that of the general population in women with a history of congenital malformation and in women using polytherapy. The incidence of the most common birth defects seen in children born to mothers who were taking anticonvulsants during pregnancy are listed in Table 37-1. It is important to note that none of these drugs produce a specific pattern of major malformations. In addition, all the classic anticonvulsants (carbamazepine, phenytoin, valproic acid, and phenobarbital) cause embryopathies but none more than the others. Therefore, it is not recommended to switch from one drug to the other if seizure control is optimal. Few data are available on the newer anticonvulsants. However, preliminary and animal data are reassuring. A registry has been developed in North America to collect data on pregnancies of women with epilepsy[25] (http://neuro-www2.mgh.harvard.edu/aed/registry.nclk).

KEY POINT

Do not change therapy if seizure control is adequate.

It is clearly established that there is an increased risk of minor anomalies in children whose mothers have epilepsy compared with control children.[26] Dysmorphic features, especially epicanthal folds, are noted in children and mothers with epilepsy. However, the incidence of the anticonvulsant embryopathy, defined as major malformations, growth retardation, and/or hypoplasia of the midface and fingers, is the same in women with epilepsy not treated with medication during pregnancy as in the general population.[24] The mechanisms by which anticonvulsant drugs induce teratogenesis are uncertain. They likely

Table 37-1. **INCIDENCE RATE OF THE MAJOR MALFORMATIONS IN CHILDREN BORN FROM TREATED EPILEPTIC MOTHERS**

Cleft lip/cleft palate	1.6%
Gastrointestinal tract defects	0.9%
Urogenital tract defect	0.9%
Neural tube defects	0.8%
Cardiac defects	0.5%

SOURCE: Masnou P, Jami-Ceccomori P. Pregnancy and epilepsy. *Rev Neurol (Paris)* 2001; 157:153–161.

include direct toxic effects and the influence of underlying genetic susceptibility.

Minor malformations are categorized into dysmorphic features listed in Table 37-2. The incidence of these features varies between 1.25% and 11.5% and depends on the type and number of anticonvulsant medications the woman is taking during pregnancy.[27] The use of polytherapy during pregnancy is associated with the highest risk. Nail and phalangeal hypoplasias and craniofacial hypoplasia tend to disappear in infancy, although hypertelorism persists. Parents can be reassured that many of these features become less prominent with age.[28]

The types of major malformation differ according to the anticonvulsant used, but there is a significant amount of overlap. The risk of birth defect is associated with the dose of anticonvulsant. The risk of birth defect increases when polytherapy is used. Table 37-3 lists birth defects according to anticonvulsant medication used in monotherapy. Certain combinations of anticonvulsants such as phenobarbital and phenytoin and the combination of valproic acid with carbamazepine, phenobarbital, or phenytoin particularly increase the rate of birth defects.

Over the past 10 years, eight new anticonvulsants have been available in North America. They are gabapentin, vigabatrin, lamotrigine, topiramate, oxcarbazepine, levetiracetam, tiagabine, and zonisamide (Table 37-4). These are being used more frequently because of their favorable side effect profiles. These newer anticonvulsants are endowed with a low potential for interaction with

Table 37-2. **FETAL ANTICONVULSANT DYSMORPHIC FEATURES**

Craniofacial dysmorphism	Hypoplasia of the midface
	Broad nasal bridge, anteverted nostrils, short nose, long upper lip, maxillary hypoplasia
	Hypertelorism
	Epicanthal folds
	Short neck
	Hypertrichosis
Microcephaly	
Skeletal deformity	Distal phalanx and nail hypoplasia
Transverse palmar crease	

SOURCE: Yerby MS, Leavitt A, Erickson DM, et al. Antiepileptic drugs and the development of congenital anomalies. *Neurology* 1992;42:132–140.

***Table 37-3.*   BIRTH DEFECTS IN ASSOCIATION WITH
TRADITIONAL ANTICONVULSANTS**

ANTICONVULSANT	MOST COMMON BIRTH DEFECTS
Carbamazepine	Cardiac defect
	Craniofacial dysmorphism
	Hip dislocation
	Hypospadias
	Inguinal hernia
	Growth restriction
	Neural tube defect (0.5–1.0%)
Phenobarbital	Cardiac defect
	Cleft lip and palate
	Growth restriction
	Skeletal anomalies
	Urogenital tract defect
Phenytoin	Cardiac defect
	Cleft lip and palate
	Craniofacial dysmorphism
	Growth restriction
	Microcephaly
	Phalangeal and nail hypoplasia
	Skeletal anomalies
	Urogenital tract defects
Valproic acid	Cardiac defect
	Craniofacial dysmorphism
	Hypospadias
	Skeletal defect
	Rib, vertebral, radial hypoplasia
	Spina bifida (1–2%)
	Urogenital tract defect

other drugs, which decreases the risk of production of teratogenic metabolites. Most of them also do not have antifolate properties, which is a potential mechanism of teratogenicity.[29]

Except for topiramate and vigabatrin, the newer anticonvulsants do not appear to be teratogenic in animals when administered in subtoxic doses. Animal reproductive toxicology studies to date have not shown harmful findings for most of the newer anticonvulsants, particularly when compared with the teratogenic potential of established anticonvulsants. The lack of sufficient information about the newer anticonvulsants prevents a general recommendation to their use in women who are planning a pregnancy.[30] Administration of newer anticonvulsants during

Table 37-4. BIRTH DEFECTS REPORTED IN ASSOCIATION WITH THE NEW ANTICONVULSANTS

NEW ANTICONVULSANT	ANIMAL STUDIES	HUMAN STUDIES
Gabapentin[44]	Fetotoxic in rodents Delayed ossification of bones	19 pregnancies No anomalies

Lamotrigine[45]	No anomalies	334 pregnancies
		In monotherapy: 3 cases
		  with birth defects (1.8%)
		Cleft palate, club foot
		In polytherapy: 10 cases
		Cardiac, neural tube,
		  skeletal defects

Levetiracetam[46]	In rodents: skeletal anomalies, growth retardation	
Oxcarbazepine[47]	Hyponatremia	23 pregnancies In monotherapy: 2 cases cardiac, cleft In polytherapy: 3 cases dysmorphism, cleft
Tiagabine[48]		22 pregnancies No anomalies
Topiramate[49]	Digit anomalies in rats Rib anomalies in rabbits	
Vigabatrin[46]	Cleft	9 pregnancies; no case
Zonisamide[50]		26 pregnancies in polytherapy; 2 cases

pregnancy should be limited to those patients who were taking these drugs when their pregnancy started because changing a drug regimen during pregnancy is not advisable.

LONG-TERM EFFECT OF EPILEPSY IN PREGNANCY ON CHILDREN   In the past few years, evidence has suggested that anticonvulsants given in utero may result in intellectual disability and behavioral change in the offspring in later life.[31,32] There is a slight increase in the risk of cognitive impairment among children born to mothers with epilepsy compared with those of nonepileptic mothers. The possibility of later intellectual or behavioral difficulties should be raised, but it should be emphasized that currently the risk is not quantifiable.

ASSESSMENT AND RECOMMENDATION BEFORE CONCEPTION   ***REEVALUATING THE NEED FOR ANTICONVULSANT THERAPY***   It is necessary to decide whether treatment is indicated at all. This will depend on an assessment of the balance between the risks of drug therapy versus those of the untreated epilepsy. The risk of seizure recurrence depends on the time since the previous seizure. In seizure-free patients, a 2-year interval is judged sufficient to taper off therapy. All decisions about tapering need to be individualized and made in conjunction with a neurologist.

AIM FOR MONOTHERAPY For women with active epilepsy, it is ideal to identify the best single agent that could achieve seizure control because the incidence of birth defect clearly increases with polytherapy. It is not recommended to switch from one to the other if seizure control is adequate. If a patient is using one of the newer anticonvulsants, and this therapy maintains ideal seizure control, continuing that medication during pregnancy is reasonable.

KEY POINT

Monotherapy, if possible, is preferred.

PREVENTION OF NEURAL TUBE DEFECTS Folate has been clearly shown to decrease the frequency of neural tube defects in the general population. Because some antiepileptic drugs decrease folate levels (e.g., phenytoin, phenobarbital, and carbamazepine), and because neural tube defects are increased by therapy with some drugs, namely valproate and carbamazepine,[33,34] supplemental folate should taken by pregnant women with epilepsy, even though few studies have assessed the effect of supplementation. It is reasonable to administer folate at higher doses (4 mg/day) than in nonmedicated women owing to the diminished absorption and increased metabolism of folate in patients on hepatic enzyme-inducing antiepileptic drug. It is optimal to begin supplementation 3 months before conception and until 12 weeks of gestation.

KEY POINT

Folic acid should be started before conception.

Pregnancy Care

HABITS AND NUTRITION

Women with nausea and vomiting of pregnancy should receive nutritional advice to minimize vomiting. When dietary measures are not sufficient, the use of an antiemetic agent is required. Pregnant women should also make sure to adopt a lifestyle conducive to satisfactory sleep routine. The importance of compliance to medication should be reinforced at every prenatal visit.

ANTICONVULSANT MONITORING

There is no evidence to support changing medications after the tenth completed week of gestation. Changing medical therapy may increase the patient's seizure frequency and should be avoided if the first trimester has passed. Monotherapy with the lowest efficacious dose is the goal for all women of reproductive age. Weaning to a single anticonvulsant medication is best carried out before conception. If the patient is free of seizure on the current medication regimen, anticonvulsant monitoring should be performed only if seizures recur or if signs of toxicity appear. If the woman is not seizure free, it is recommended to monitor free serum levels and adjust medication doses as needed.

SCREENING FOR BIRTH DEFECTS   Women with epilepsy should be offered antenatal screening for neural tube defects through maternal serum α-fetoprotein screening. The sensitivity of such screening for detecting an open neural tube defect is 85%.[35] This screening is optimally performed between 16 and 18 weeks of gestation but can be performed between 15 and 22 weeks. A targeted ultrasound should also be performed between 16 and 20 weeks to screen for neural tube defects and other anomalies. This scan has a sensitivity of 90% for detecting neural tube defects and, in some specialized centers, can approach 95% sensitivity. If indicated, amniocentesis should be offered for evaluation of amniotic fluid α-fetoprotein and acetylcholinesterase levels and for karyotype. The sensitivity of amniotic fluid α-fetoprotein and acetylcholinesterase screening for the detection of neural tube defects is greater than 99%.[35] A fetal echocardiogram should be performed at 18–22 weeks of gestation to evaluate for congenital heart defects. Serial ultrasound examinations for the assessment of fetal growth are indicated because the risk of intrauterine growth restriction is increased.

Peripartum Care

PREVENTION OF HEMORRHAGE IN THE NEWBORN   Neonates who were exposed to anticonvulsant medications, mostly those that induce the microsomal enzyme system in utero, are at increased risk of postnatal hemorrhage due to a deficiency of vitamin K–dependent clotting factors.[36] More than 40 cases of neonatal bleeding associated with maternal anticonvulsant therapy have been published.[37] However, there are no data establishing decreased incidence of bleeding in women who received vitamin K supplementation. In addition to the routine prophylaxis commonly given to all newborns, the prenatal administration of vitamin K is therefore advocated at a dose of 10 to 20 mg orally daily for the last month of gestation.[38]

ANTICONVULSANT MONITORING During labor, sleep deprivation and failure to administer or absorb anticonvulsants lead to a potential increase in seizure activity. If tonic-clonic seizures occur during labor, the differential diagnosis of eclampsia needs to be considered. The management of eclampsia is done with magnesium sulfate, whereas the tonic-clonic seizures of epilepsy are best controlled with intravenous benzodiazepines. If epileptic seizures occur in the peripartum period, a short-acting benzodiazepine will limit neonatal side effects. A typical regimen used for acute treatment of seizures is lorazepam 10 mg as an intravenous bolus to be repeated every 20 minutes for recurrence. After the administration of benzodiazepine, adjustment of the baseline anticonvulsant medication should be undertaken depending on the drug level.

After delivery, there is a return toward normal metabolism that occurs progressively over the ensuing month. When an increase in dosage has been necessary during pregnancy, one should monitor drugs levels postpartum with the intention to return to prepregnancy levels over the ensuing month.

BREAST FEEDING Exposure to anticonvulsants will continue after birth in infants of breast-feeding mothers. Most infants will breast feed successfully, and the benefits of breast feeding are believed to outweigh the small risk of anticonvulsant exposure.[39] Anticonvulsants cross into breast milk in inverse proportion to protein binding and in direct relation to the plasma concentration. The infant's serum concentration is proportional to the amount excreted in breast milk and to the drug's half-life in neonates, which is more variable and can be more prolonged than in adults.[39,40] The ratio of anticonvulsants in breast milk to that in maternal blood is 0.01–0.93, depending on the drug, except for levetiracetam, which has an unusually high excretion into breast milk.[41] Vigabatrin and gabapentin are excreted mainly in the urine, thus making accumulation unlikely. Lamotrigine can accumulate in breast milk especially in association with valproate.[42] Breast feeding is compatible with carbamazepine, phenytoin, and valproate intake. In general, discontinuation of breast feeding should be considered if sedation, poor feeding, or irritability occurs.[40]

EPILEPSY IN THE OFFSPRING Women with epilepsy should be counseled concerning the risk of epilepsy in their offspring. Most epileptic syndromes are associated with a complex inheritance, and the risk for a child born of a mother with idiopathic epilepsy is 2–4%, which is significantly above the general population risk of idiopathic epilepsy estimated at 0.5–1%. Paternal epilepsy does not appear to influence these numbers.[43]

Guiding Questions in Approaching the Patient

Pregnancy care: assessing seizure control during pregnancy

- When was the last seizure? What is the seizure frequency?
- What anticonvulsant(s) is the patient taking?
- Is the patient suffering from nausea and vomiting?
- Is the patient taking her anticonvulsant as prescribed?
- Is the patient waking up often at night or enduring insomnia and excessive daytime drowsiness?

Preconception assessment: assessing risk of congenital malformation in the epileptic patient

- What are the type and dosage of anticonvulsant(s)?
- Is she using monotherapy or polytherapy?
- Could she have her medication discontinued or could one anticonvulsant be effective in achieving seizure control?
- Does she have a personal or family history of congenital birth defects?

Conclusion

The management of pregnancy in an epileptic woman requires close monitoring and counseling that begin before conception. This requires a team approach involving the epileptologist, obstetrician, and nursing team. However, efforts are motivated by the fact that most of these woman with optimal care will go on to have a normal pregnancy and deliver a normal baby.

Discussion of Cases

CASE 1: PRIMIPARA WITH CHRONIC EPILEPSY

You are evaluating a 20-year-old gravida 1 at 10 weeks of gestation. She is treated with valproic acid 500 mg three times daily. She had a grand mal seizure the previous week. Her last visit with her neurologist was 6 months ago. She complains of nausea and vomiting of 3 weeks' duration. She was not able to use her medication prescribed due to her nausea.

What other testing would you recommend at this point?

Office urine analysis, viability ultrasound, and serum-free valproate.

Urine analysis showed 1+ ketones, viability ultrasound displays a live fetus at 10 weeks of gestation, and serum-free valproate is 100 µmol/L.

What is your recommendation for initial management?

Control nausea and vomiting by hydration, nutritional advice, and antiemetics. Reinforce compliance for anticonvulsant intake. Valproic acid should be adjusted and neurology consultation should be arranged. An office follow-up visit in 1 week should be scheduled.
    Seizure activity can increase in pregnancy due to the physiologic changes of pregnancy that lead to change in the bioavailability of the anticonvulsant. However, nausea and vomiting and noncompliance are also very important causes
of increased seizure activity. The patient must understand that seizure activity in itself may be detrimental to the developing fetus. There is no need to change anticonvulsant therapy because all are potentially teratogenic. Screening for birth defects and use of folic acid are in order.

The nausea and vomiting symptoms for this patient slowly subsided. She understood the importance of taking her anticonvulsant and followed your recommendations. At 32 weeks her valproate level is 200 µ/mL (therapeutic level 300–830 µmol/L). She has had no seizure since she increased compliance.

What would you recommend? When was her last seizure? What is the frequency of the seizure?

None since her first trimester.

Does she take her medication as prescribed?

She tells you she is compliant.

Does she have nausea or vomiting?

No. Therefore, there is no need to increase her medication level. When a patient is asymptomatic, there is no need to increase the level of anticonvulsant to achieve a laboratory therapeutic level. Hemodilution is the most likely explanation in the compliant patient. Free levels of valproate should be ordered.

CASE 2: EVALUATION OF CHOICE OF SEIZURE MEDICATION

You are evaluating a woman at 14 weeks of gestation who is taking topiramate for refractory partial seizures. This is the only medication that was able to achieve seizure control. Her pregnancy has been uneventful.

What is your plan?

Assess background risk for congenital birth defect, inquire about the periconceptional use of folic acid, and assess epilepsy control.

The patient has a negative history for congenital birth defects, she has been taking a multivitamin supplement every day that contains folic acid 0.4 mg, and her most recent seizure occurred 1 year previously.

Topiramate is a new anticonvulsant. The only data available are from animal studies that showed digit and rib anomalies. There are no human data available. If epilepsy is best controlled by this anticonvulsant, it is preferable not to change to a traditional anticonvulsant. All traditional anticonvulsants have teratogenic potential. Changing to a traditional anticonvulsant may precipitate increased seizure activity. Seizure activity in itself is potentially detrimental for the developing fetus, although, with partial seizure, the effect may be not as significant as for grand mal seizure.

REFERENCES

1 Hauser WA, Hesdorffer DC. *Epilepsy: Frequency, Causes, and Consequences.* Landover: Epilepsy Foundation of America, 1990; p. 1.

2 Hiilesman VD, Teramo K, Bardy AH. Social class, complications, and perinatal deaths in pregnancies of epileptic women: preliminary results of the prospective Helsinki study. In: Janz D, Brossi L, Dam M, et al, eds. *Epilepsy, Pregnancy, and the Child.* New York: Raven Press, 1982; p. 87.

3 Brackley K, Rubin P. Maternal illness in pregnancy. In: Renni JM, Robertson NRC, eds. *Textbook of Neonatology,* 3rd ed. Edinburgh: Chuchill Livingstone, 1999; p. 179.

4 Swartjes JM, van Geijn HP. Pregnancy and epilepsy. *Eur J Obstet Gynecol Reprod Biol* 1998;79:3–11.

5 Crawford P. Epilepsy and pregnancy. *Seizure* 2001;10:212–219.

6 Chadwick D. Randomized study of AED withdrawal in patients in remission. Medical Research Council. AED withdrawal study group. *Lancet* 1991;337:1175–1180.

7 Tennison M, Greenwood R, Lewis D, Thorn M. Discontinuing antiepileptic drugs in children with epilepsy. A comparison of a six-week and a nine-month taper period. *N Engl J Med* 1994;330:1407–1410.

8 Yerby MS. Pregnancy and epilepsy. *Epilepsia* 1991;32(suppl 6): S51–S59.

9 Yerby MS, Friel PN, McCormick K. Antiepileptic drug disposition during pregnancy. *Neurology* 1992;42(suppl 5):12–16.

10 Morrel MJ. Hormones and epilepsy through the lifetime. *Epilepsia* 1992;33:S49–S61.

11 Yerby M, Koepsell T, Daling J. Pregnancy complications and outcomes in a cohort of women with epilepsy. *Epilepsia* 1985;26:631–635.

12 Hiilesmaa VK. Pregnancy and birth in women with epilepsy. *Neurology* 1992;42(suppl 5):8–11.

13 Andermann E, Dansky L, Kinch RA. Complications of pregnancy, labour and delivery in epileptic women. In: Janz D, Brossi L, Dam M, et al, eds. *Epilepsy, Pregnancy, and the Child.* New York: Raven Press, 1982; p. 61.

14 Annegers JF, Baumgartner KB, Hauser WA, Kurland LT. Epilepsy, antiepileptic drugs, and the risk of spontaneous abortion. *Epilepsia* 1988;29:451–458.

15 Crawford P. Epilepsy and pregnancy. *Seizure* 2001;10:212–219.

16 Nei M, Daly S, Liporace J. A maternal complex partial seizure in labor can affect fetal heart rate. *Neurology* 1998;51:904–906.

17 Teramo K, Hiilesmaa V, Bardy A, et al. Fetal heart rate during a maternal grand mal epileptic seizure. *J Perinat Med* 1979;7:3–6.

18 Samren EB, van Duijn CM, Christiaens GC, et al. Antiepileptic drug regimens and major congenital abnormalities in the offspring. *Ann Neurol* 1999;46:739–746.

19 Canger R, Battino D, Canevini MP, et al. Malformations in offspring of women with epilepsy: a prospective study. *Epilepsia* 1999;40: 1231–1236.

20 Lindhout D, Meinardi H, Meijer JW, et al. Antiepileptic drugs and teratogenesis in two consecutive cohorts: changes in prescription policy paralleled by changes in pattern of malformation. *Neurology* 1992; 42(suppl 5):94–110.

21 Leonard G, Andermann E, Ptito A, et al. Cognitive effects of antiepileptic drug therapy during pregnancy on school-age offspring (abstract). *Epilepsia* 1997;38(suppl 3):S170.

22 Samren EB, Van Duijn CM, Koch S, et al. Maternal use of antiepileptic drugs and the risk of major congenital malformations: a joint European prospective study of human teratogenesis associated with maternal epilepsy. *Epilepsia* 1997;38:981–990.

23 Kaneko S, Battino D, Andermann E, et al. Congenital malformations due to antiepileptic drugs. *Epilepsy Res* 1999;33:145–158.

24 Holmes LB, Harvey EA, Coull BA, et al. The teratogenicity of anticonvulsant drugs. *N Engl J Med* 2001;344:1132–1138.

25 Beghi E, Annegers F. Pregnancy registries in epilepsy. *Epilepsia* 2001;42:1422–1425.

26 Dravet C, Julian C, Legras C, et al. Epilepsy, antiepileptic drugs, and malformations in children of women with epilepsy: a French prospective cohort study. *Neurology* 1992;42(suppl 5):75–82.

27 Gaily E, Granstrom ML, Hiilesmaa V, et al. Minor anomalies in off-spring of epileptic mothers. *J Pediatr* 1988;12:520–529.

28 Koch S, Losche G, Jager-Roman E, et al. Major and minor birth mal-formations and antiepileptic drugs. *Neurology* 1992;42(suppl 5): 83–88.

29 Finnell RH, Nau H, Yerby MS. Teratogenicity of antiepileptic drugs. In: RH Levy, RH Mattson, RS Meldrum, eds. *Antiepileptic Drugs.* New York: Raven Press, 1995.

30 Palmieri C, Canger R. Teratogenic potential of the newer antiepileptic drugs. What is known and how should this influence prescribing? *CNS Drugs* 2002;16:755–764.

31 Nelson KB, Ellenberg JH. Maternal seizure disorder outcomes of pregnancy and neurologic abnormalities in the children. *Neurology* 1982;32:1247–1254.

32 Speidel BD, Meadow SR. Maternal epilepsy and abnormalities of the fetus and newborn. *Lancet* 1972;2:839–843.

33 Lindhout D, Schmidt D. In utero exposure to valproate and neural tube defects. *Lancet* 1986;1:1392–1393.

34 Yerby MS. Management issues for women with epilepsy. Neural tube defects and folic acid supplementation. *Neurology* 2003;61(suppl 2): S23–S26.

35 Clinical management guidelines for obstetrician-gynecologists. Neural Tube Defects ACOG Practice Bulletin, number 44, July 2003. *Obstet Gynecol* 2002;102:203–213.

36 Hey E. Effect of maternal anticonvulsant treatment on neonatal blood coagulation. *Arch Dis Child* 1999;81:208–210.

37 Moslet U, Hansen ES. A review of vitamin K, epilepsy and pregnancy. *Acta Neurol Scand* 1992;85:39–43.

38 Zahn C. Neurologic care of pregnant women with epilepsy. *Epilepsia* 1998;39 (suppl 8):S26–S31.

39 Quality Standards Subcommittee of the Americans Academy of Neurology. Management issues for women with epilepsy (summary statement). *Neurology* 1998;51:944–948.

40 American Academy of Pediatrics, Committee on Drugs. The transfer of drugs and other chemicals into human milk. *Pediatrics* 1994;93: 137–150.

41 Pennell PB. Antiepileptic drug pharmacokinetics during pregnancy and lactation. *Neurology* 2003;61(suppl 2):S35–S42.

42 Tomson T, Ohman I, Vitols S. Lamotrigine in pregnancy and lactation. *Epilepsia* 1997;38:1039–1041.

43 Annegers JF, Hauser WA, Elveback LR, et al. Seizure disorders in offspring of parents with a history of seizures—a maternal–paternal difference? *Epilepsia* 1976;17:1–9.

44 McLean MJ. Gabapentin in the management of convulsive disorders. *Epilepsia* 1999;40(suppl 6):539–550.

45 Tennis P, Eldridge RR, and the International lamotrigine pregnancy registry scientific advisory committee. Preliminary results on pregnancy outcomes in women using lamotrigine. *Epilepsia* 2002;43:1161–1167.

46 Palmieri C, Canger R. Teratogenic potential of the newer antiepileptic drugs. What is known and how should this influence prescribing? *CNS Drugs* 2002;26:755–764.

47 Friis ML, Kristensen O, Boas J, et al. Therapeutic experiences with 947 epileptic out-patients in oxcarbazepine treatment. *Acta Neurol Scand* 1993;87:224–227.

48 Leppik IE, Gram L, Deaton R. et al. Safety of Tiagabine: summary of 53 trials. *Epilepsy Res* 1999;33:235–246.

49 Glauser TA. Topiramate. *Epilepsia* 1999;40(suppl 5):571–580.

50 Kondo T, Kaneko S, Amanoy et al. Preliminary report of teratogenic effects of zonisamide in the offspring of treated women with epilepsy. *Epilepsia* 1996;37:1242–1244.

Aneurysm and Mode of Delivery Pathway

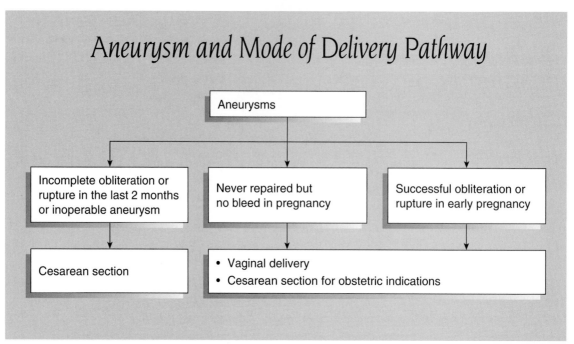

Aneurysms

- Incomplete obliteration or rupture in the last 2 months or inoperable aneurysm → Cesarean section

- Never repaired but no bleed in pregnancy
- Successful obliteration or rupture in early pregnancy
  - Vaginal delivery
  - Cesarean section for obstetric indications

AVM and Mode of Delivery Pathway

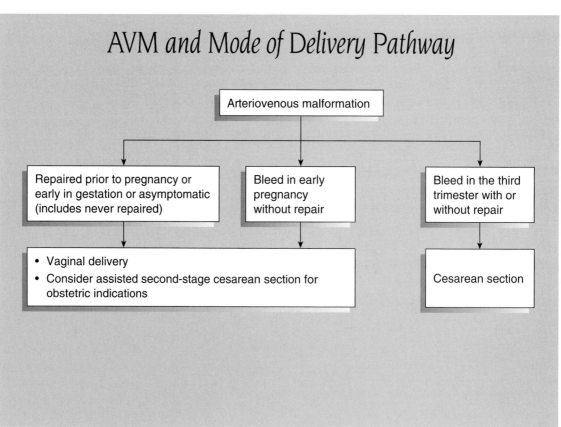

Arteriovenous malformation

- Repaired prior to pregnancy or early in gestation or asymptomatic (includes never repaired)
  - Vaginal delivery
  - Consider assisted second-stage cesarean section for obstetric indications
- Bleed in early pregnancy without repair
- Bleed in the third trimester with or without repair → Cesarean section

38 Intracranial Hemorrhage in Pregnancy

Teresa Marino

Introduction

Cerebrovascular disorders in pregnancy can occur secondary to arterial or venous occlusive disease or from vascular anomalies such as aneurysms and arteriovenous malformations. Pregnancy has been associated with an increased risk of stroke, and stroke related to pregnancy is associated with significant morbidity and mortality rates.[1] Risk factors for occlusive disease include hypertension, diabetes, hypercoagulable conditions, emboli, and drugs such as cocaine. Although rare, emboli secondary to ischemic heart disease, rheumatic disease, or endocarditis have also been reported.[2]

Hemorrhagic cerebrovascular disorders are a rare but serious complication of pregnancy. Anatomically, intracranial bleeds can be classified as intracerebral (ICH) or subarachnoid (SAH). Of the various types of nontraumatic intracranial hemorrhage, SAH has been most frequently associated with pregnancy. When SAH is identified in pregnancy, the mechanism of hemorrhage is most often the result of a ruptured aneurysm or bleeding from an arteriovenous malformation (AVM) (Table 38.1).[3] In contrast, intracerebral hemorrhage is most often secondary to complications of hypertension, including preeclampsia and eclampsia. Intracerebral bleeding is the most common cause of death in the eclamptic patient.[2,4]

The incidence of ICH from aneurysmal or AVM rupture is difficult to assess, but based on review articles and case series this

***Table 38-1.* CAUSES OF INTRACRANIAL HEMORRHAGE IN PREGNANCY**

Aneurysms
Arteriovenous malformations
Hypertension
Severe preeclampsia/eclampsia
Anticoagulation/coagulopathy
Trauma
Cocaine abuse
Tumors

complication appears to occur in 0.05% of all pregnancies.[3–5] ICH is the third most frequent cause of maternal death from nonobstetric causes and accounts for 5–14% of all maternal deaths in pregnancy.[3,4,6,7] The immediate mortality rate after an ICH has been reported as high as 50%.[3] As maternal mortality from other causes has decreased, intracranial hemorrhage has become a relatively more significant cause of maternal death.

Because ICH remains a rare event, no definitive guidelines have been established to counsel and manage pregnant women. The incidence, pathophysiology, and management of ICH secondary to aneurysms and AVM are reviewed from the current obstetric, neurosurgical, and anesthesia literature.

What's the Evidence?

The data on the natural history of aneurysms and AVM are incomplete, controversial, and mostly based on retrospective studies. A few prospective studies have followed these lesions in the general population with respect to their incidence of rupture and outcome, thus allowing extrapolation to the pregnant patient. There are no randomized trials comparing treated with untreated women with intracranial lesions with respect to their risks in pregnancy or pregnancy outcomes. There are no evidence-based studies to guide us through the therapeutic options for aneurysms and AVMs in pregnancy. As such, treatment relies on clinical management derived from the nonpregnant population. Information regarding the potential complications of intracranial hemorrhage and possible prevention and treatment options is derived from case series and prospective studies in the nonpregnant general population.

Natural History and Pathophysiology of Aneurysms and Arteriovenous Malformations

There are several considerations that may influence the natural history of intracranial aneurysms and AVM including genetic and systemic factors and unique anatomic and pathophysiologic disturbances directly attributable to the lesion.

ANEURYSMS

KEY POINT

Aneurysms are generally located at sites of vessel bifurcation in or near the circle of Willis.

There are three most common types of aneurysms: saccular or berry, fusiform, and dissecting. Most recent evidence has suggested that the etiology of aneurysms is consistent with hemodynamically induced degenerative vascular injury. Ninety-five percent of intracranial aneurysms are asymptomatic lesion; the advent of more sophisticated neuroimaging techniques has resulted in a larger number of incidental asymptomatic vascular anomalies being identified. Asymptomatic lesions rupture at a rate of 1–3% per year; this risk rises to 6.25% for symptomatic lesions.[6,9,10] Rebleeding occurs in 10–20% of cases during the first month; if left untreated, the annual risk of rebleed may be 2–3% after the first year.[6,9] Sudden death occurs in 10–15% of patients who develop aneurysmal rupture and may be as high as 13–35% in pregnancy.[6,9,10] Maternal mortality is directly associated with clinical grade (Table 38-2). Approximately 50% of women who develop a ruptured aneurysm in pregnancy previously underwent a successful pregnancy without difficulty.[4,6]

Widespread screening for cerebral aneurysms is not warranted. Numerous medical conditions including autosomal dominant

Table 38-2. **CLINICAL GRADING SCALE FOR INTRACRANIAL ANEURYSMS**

GRADE	CLINICAL CONDITION
0	Unruptured
I	Asymptomatic or minimal headache, nuchal rigidity
II	Moderate to severe headache, nuchal rigidity, no neurologic deficit other than cranial nerve palsy
III	Drowsiness, confusion, mild focal deficit
IV	Stupor, moderate to severe hemiparesis, possible early decerebrate rigidity and vegetative disturbances
V	Deep coma, decerebrate rigidity, moribund appearance
+1 grade	For vasospasm or systemic disease

Source: Hunt WE, Hess RM. Surgical risk as related to time of intervention in the repair of intracranial aneurysms. *J Neurosurg* 1968;28:14–19.

polycystic kidney disease, coarctation of the aorta, and collagen diseases such as Marfan's and Ehlers-Danlos syndromes have been associated with intracranial aneurysms. In these cases and in patients with a first-degree relative with a cerebral aneurysm, screening may be considered with computed tomography (CT) of the head.

ARTERIOVENOUS
MALFORMATIONS

KEY POINT

AVMs are the most dangerous of the congenital defects in the cerebral vasculature and can be located anywhere between the frontal region and the brainstem and the spinal cord.

Supratentorial lesions account for almost 90% of AVMs; the remaining 10% are located in the posterior fossa.[11] AVMs occur in about 0.1% of the population, or one-tenth the incidence of aneurysms. These lesions are formed from dilated arteries and veins without intervening capillary beds. Gliotic tissue may be mixed with the vascular tangle. This high-flow arteriovenous communication potentiates several flow-related phenomena. Aneurysms may form within the AVM and are thought to worsen the prognosis. The size of these lesions can vary extensively from millimeters to several centimeters. The vast majority are solitary lesions, but multiple lesions can be seen in association with syndromes, such as Rendu-Osler-Weber and Wyburn-Mason.[12]

A study evaluating the natural history of unruptured AVM in nonpregnant patients prospectively followed over an average of 8 years reported an annual rupture rate of 2.2% and average annual morbidity and mortality rates of 2.8% and 0.7 % respectively.[13] The peak age of onset of symptoms associated with AVM is 20–40 years. By age 40 years, 40% of all AVMs have bled at least once. In a comparison of aneurysmal with angiomatous rupture in pregnancy, the mean maternal age of rupture of an AVM was younger than the age of those bleeding from aneurysmal rupture, reflecting the congenital nature of the lesion.[4,9,12,14] Bleeding from an AVM, like aneurysmal bleeding, may be intraparenchymal, intraventricular, or subarachnoid.

Presenting symptoms and subsequent management influence outcomes of patients with AVMs. If left untreated, the rate of rebleeding is highest during the first year after initial hemorrhage at a rate of 6–7% and then remains relatively constant with a mortality rate of 1% per year.[9,12,14,15]

Physiologic Changes of Pregnancy and the Effect on Intracranial Lesions

The normal physiologic changes in pregnancy may affect the risk of hemorrhage from an aneurysm or AVM. Blood volume, stroke volume, and cardiac output increase in pregnancy, the latter by almost 50%, peaking at 32 weeks of gestation. Plasma volume also increases by 1300 mL, whereas red blood cell mass increases by only 400 mL, resulting in dilutional anemia. Vascular resistance decreases with a resulting decrease in systemic blood pressure until midpregnancy and returns to normal at term. Human cerebral blood flow averages approximately 50 mL/min per 100 g of brain tissue and is normally regulated to maintain constant flow over a wide range of systemic blood pressures. Levels of systemic oxygen and carbon dioxide markedly affect this autoregulation of cerebral blood flow.[2]

Pregnancy is a relatively hypercoagulable state with an increase in all clotting factors except factors XI and XIII. Levels of several hormones including estrogen, progesterone, and relaxin, which have been found to affect blood vasculature and connective tissue, also increase in pregnancy. These hemodynamic and endocrine changes associated with pregnancy may predispose to aneurysm enlargement, disruption, and rupture. There has been some suggestion that cerebral aneurysms and AVMs may increase in size during pregnancy because of laxity of vascular walls.[1,16,17]

Effects of Pregnancy on Risk of Intracranial Bleed

For women of childbearing age with a cerebral aneurysm or AVM, one of the most important questions is whether pregnancy will increase the risk of ICH. The available information in pregnancy is obtained from population-based and retrospective studies and is presented below. All of these studies are limited by size of the series and selection bias due to referral populations. Some studies have suggested that there is no association between pregnancy and delivery and intracranial hemorrhage, whereas others have noted an increased risk of bleeding in pregnancy.[1,3,18] Many women with an aneurysm or AVM have been advised not to become pregnant because of concerns of rupture, which may further bias the data toward favorable outcomes.

The incidence of aneurysmal rupture during pregnancy in a referral population has been estimated to be about five times that seen in the same age group of nonpregnant women.[3] However, in a well-defined population study in Rochester, Minnesota between 1955 and 1979, there were no cases of intracranial hemorrhage among over 26,000 pregnancies.[18]

Another retrospective review of 154 cases of intracranial hemorrhage confirmed by imaging, autopsy, lumbar puncture, or surgical findings found aneurysms to be responsible for 77% of hemorrhages that occurred in pregnancy and AVMs for 23%. Ruptured aneurysms accounted for 75% of antepartum hemorrhages and all postpartum hemorrhages. When assessing for risk factors possibly associated with an increased chance of hemorrhage in pregnancy, 49 patients had an increased blood pressure and most of these were diagnosed with aneurysms.[19]

Kittner and coworkers identified 31 women ages 15–44 years who had been discharged from all area hospitals in central Maryland and Washington, D.C. between 1988 and 1991.[20] Seventeen of these women had a cerebral infarction and the major causes were severe preeclampsia and eclampsia followed by central nervous system vasculopathy. The relative risk for cerebral infarction during pregnancy was 0.7, which is not different from the general population risk; however, the relative risk increased to 8.7 in the postpartum period. In the same study, 14 women were identified with intracranial hemorrhages from aneurysmal or AVM rupture. About two thirds of the bleeds secondary to an AVM occurred in the second trimester.[20]

Numerous investigators have reported a trend toward increased intracranial bleed secondary to AVM rupture in the latter half of gestation and the postpartum period.[14,20–22] Eclampsia as a cause of intracranial bleed has been reported in 14–44% of cases.[20] In a widely quoted study, women younger than 45 years, diagnosed with an AVM, and pregnant within 2 years of diagnosis were compared with a group also diagnosed with AVM but who did not have a pregnancy. The incidence of SAH in the pregnancy group was 85% compared with 10% in the nonpregnancy group.[14] Horton and associates retrospectively reviewed 451 women who had an AVM and altogether 540 pregnancies and who had been referred for stereotactic radiation.[22] Seventeen hemorrhages occurred for a rate of 0.036 per person year, and the risk of hemorrhage from a previously unruptured AVM during pregnancy was estimated to be 3.5% , which was not different from the annual rupture rate in the general population. Of 375 vaginal deliveries, none was complicated by intracranial hemorrhage during labor and delivery, suggesting no increased risk of first hemorrhage among women with previously unruptured AVM in pregnancy. However, this risk applies only to women with no previous bleed; those with a previous hemorrhage were noted to have a risk of 5.8% during subsequent pregnancies, with the highest risk during the first year after rupture. This review was limited by selection bias because women were referred for treatment and the review did not include those women who presented with a fatal hemorrhage or a poor neurologic grade.[22] Forester and colleagues reviewed 191 women of childbearing age who presented for stereotactic radiosurgery, 116 of whom had pregnancies.[21] Of these women, 35 had never bled at the time of presentation, 67 had bled but never in pregnancy, and 14 women bled for the first time in pregnancy. These 14 women experienced 15 hemorrhages, three in the first and third trimesters and nine in the second trimester, which suggested an increased risk of rupture in the second trimester. Theoretically, this may reflect the hemodynamic changes that occur at this time, including increases in cardiac output and blood volume.[21] This increased tendency of AVMs to bleed in the second trimester and a higher tendency to rebleed than aneurysms suggests that shunting through the intracranial AVM may increase during pregnancy and thus predispose to rupture and focal ischemic events from AVM.[14,19-22] The clinical significance of these hemodynamic changes in promoting hemorrhage is unclear because adverse effects of labor and delivery on the rate of AVM rupture remains unproved.[22]

CLINICAL MANIFESTATIONS

KEY POINT

Signs and symptoms of aneurysmal and AVM bleeding are indistinguishable. Pregnancy does not significantly alter the clinical presentation of SAH.

Intracerebral bleeding secondary to preeclampsia or eclampsia may also present in the same fashion. SAH is the most common presentation of aneurysms. Blood is released directly into the cerebrospinal fluid under arterial pressure and increases intracranial pressure. Consistent with the bleeding, SAH typically presents abruptly with sudden onset of severe headache. The headache may be associated with loss of consciousness, nausea and vomiting, or seizures. Meningism and low back pain may develop several hours later. Focal neurologic deficits may occur from intraparenchymal bleeding or mass effects. Bleeding typically lasts a few seconds, but rebleeding is common and the highest risk remains within the first day. Complications in patients with intracranial hemorrhage include vasospasm, seizures, hyponatremia, hydrocephalus, cardiac abnormalities such as arrhythmias, and death.

EVALUATION

The first step is to determine the presence of an ICH and then to evaluate the etiology. Head CT with or without contrast remains the cornerstone for evaluation of an ICH. In the acute phase, CT can differentiate SAH from intraparenchymal hemorrhage. Radiation exposure lower than 5 rad has not been shown to be teratogenic. In general, with abdominal shielding, CT of the head is associated with almost zero radiation exposure to the fetus.

Lumbar puncture is mandatory if there is a strong suspicion of SAH and the CT is normal or inconclusive but has ruled out a mass lesion. Immediate centrifugation of the cerebrospinal fluid helps differentiate true SAH from a traumatic tap. Cerebral angiography is not contraindicated in pregnancy and should be considered if diagnostic doubt remains. The morbidity rate of angiography remains low. In a meta-analysis combining the risks of permanent or transient neurologic complications, reviewers found a significantly lower risk of angiographic complications in patients with SAH compared with those with transient ischemic episodes or strokes (1.8% vs. 3.7%).[23] It is the most definitive procedure available for the diagnosis and localization of an AVM. Anatomic and physiologic information such as nidus configuration, relation to surrounding vessels, and draining portions of the AVM can be obtained. Iodinated contrast agents are physiologically inert and pose little risk to the fetus. Angiography may be delayed in patients with profound alteration of consciousness with or without focal neurologic signs because of the associated guarded prognosis and a mortality rate approaching 80% in the first week. CT angiography and magnetic resonance angiography are noninvasive tests that are useful for screening and presurgical planning but do not achieve the resolution of traditional angiography.

Guiding Questions in Approaching the Patient

- Which diagnostic tests are safe in pregnancy?
- Is the patient a surgical candidate?
- What are the anesthetic considerations in the pregnant atient?
- What are the possible complications of a subarachnoid bleed?

Management and Treatment Options

Surgery remains the mainstay of therapy for SAH secondary to aneurysmal rupture. The surgical option of choice remains clip placement across the neck of the aneurysm. Recently, endovascular techniques using biopolymers and image chain devices have been performed. These intraluminal approaches to the cerebral aneurysm have emerged as safe alternatives. Endovascular detachable balloons and coil embolization are techniques that offer an alternative treatment option in selected patients, in particular those whose lesions are surgically inaccessible.[24] However, experience in pregnancy is limited to case reports and there is some concern regarding exposure to fluoroscopic contrast material.[25]

The timing of intervention is also controversial. The risk of rebleed and prevention of vasospasm have led to a practice of early surgical intervention within 48–72 hours of initial presentation.[26,27] Appropriateness of early intervention also depends on the grade at presentation (see Table 38-2). Patients with grades IV and V are less likely to undergo early intervention due to clinical instability, presence of cerebral edema, or a clot and up to 25% develop a fatal initial hemorrhage.[13]

An international cooperative study on the timing of aneurysmal surgery noted worst outcomes in patients whose surgery was performed 7–10 days after bleeding with vasospasm and rebleed as the leading causes of morbidity and mortality.[26] Younger patients seem to have a higher risk of developing vasospasm, and early surgical clipping with minimal manipulation of blood vessels has been advocated to prevent rebleed and vasospasm.[26,27]

The anesthetic management of pregnant women undergoing craniotomy can be difficult and requires knowledge of the hemodynamic, cardiac, and pulmonary changes that occur during pregnancy. Exposure to anesthesia during even during the first trimester is not associated with an increased incidence of fetal malformations above the baseline risk for the general population.[28] Failed intubation remains the most serious complication and has been reported to increase up to 10-fold in pregnant patients.[29] Regional anesthesia is not contraindicated for use in labor or delivery in patients who have previously undergone a craniotomy for intracranial bleeding.

Several case series have been reported in pregnant women. In 1979, Minielly and colleagues reported on eight pregnant women with ruptured aneurysms treated between 1967 and 1977, seven of whom underwent surgical intervention.[30] No maternal mortality was reported and only one patient had a permanent neurologic deficit.[30] Dias and Sekhar reported on a series of 106 women with antepartum aneurysmal hemorrhage; 55 were treated surgically and 51 were managed expectantly.[19] After adjusting for several covariants, including grade, maternal and fetal mortality rates were lower in the operative group. Maternal mortality rate was 11% in the operative group compared with 63% in expectant management group. Although the researchers concluded that the surgical treatment group had a better outcome, this series spanned over two decades when surgical treatment was not always offered and initial neurologic status was not described.[19] In the same case series 35 women had intracranial bleed secondary to AVMs; 13 women underwent surgical management and 22 women were treated conservatively. Maternal mortality rates were 23% and 32%, respectively, for these two groups, which was not statistically different.[19] Because no clear benefit of surgery has been found with AVMs, some surgeons advocate operative intervention to remove only significant hematomas that cause midline shift or mass effect. These patients may have additional vascular abnormalities such as aneurysms or feeding vessels associated with the AVM, which further increases the complexity of surgery.

Complications of Intracranial Hemorrhage

Cerebral vasospasm is a devastating complication of SAH that is associated with high morbidity and mortality rates. Ischemic events in the brain secondary to vasospasm may occur as soon as 3 days after initial bleeding, and the incidence usually peaks at 4–10 days.[25,31] Vasospasm occurs in 10% of all patients and leads to symptomatic cerebral ischemia or infarcts in more than half of these cases. The most significant consequence remains delayed ischemic neurologic deficits. Cerebral vasospasm seems to be related to the presence of blood in the subarachnoid space, which may cause production of free radicals, endothelins, ferrous hemoglobin, decreased nitric oxide, and other macromolecules that cause an abnormal state of inflammation and vasoconstriction.[27] The incidence of vasospasm after surgical clipping or endovascular techniques is comparable at approximately 23%.[26,27]

Clinical manifestations such as altered consciousness and focal neurologic signs should prompt investigation with imaging studies. Transcranial Doppler velocimetry study is a noninvasive technique that may be useful to assess the presence of vasospasm and may show increased blood flow velocity in the vessels, presumably due to narrowing of the vessel lumen. CT can differentiate hydrocephalus from new bleeding. Angiography remains the gold standard for the diagnosis of vasospasm.

Although few randomized, controlled trials have been performed, "triple-H therapy," which consists of hypervolemia, hemodilution, and hypertension, represents the mainstay of therapy for cerebral vasospasm and has been shown to improve patient neurologic outcome and survival in the nonpregnant population.[26,27,29,31] It is assumed that, in the presence of vasospasm, cerebral blood flow is impaired and becomes pressure dependent. The practice of providing volume expansion with colloid is based on observations that local cerebral blood flow in an ischemic brain area changes directly with cardiac output. Further, hypovolemia seems to develop after SAH, and as such the goals to improve cerebral perfusion include initially restoring and then expanding intravascular volume. Hemodilution decreases blood viscosity, thereby decreasing peripheral resistance and in theory improving microcirculation.[30] Despite treatment, 34% of patients will develop symptomatic vasospasm. Complications of triple-H treatment include pulmonary edema, myocardial ischemia, hyponatremia, renal washout, and hemorrhagic infarcts.[31]

Hypertension also worsens SAH. The use of calcium antagonists such as nimodipine has been found to have neuroprotective and vasodilator effects. Nimodipine has been shown to decrease the incidence of cerebral infarction and poor outcome by 33%.[32] Nimodipine has become standard care in patients with SAH, is well tolerated, and can be given in doses of 60 mg four times per day. Although not contraindicated in pregnancy, nimodipine has not been well studied in pregnant women. Lowering blood pressure may decrease the risk of rebleeding, but this benefit may be offset by an increased risk of infarction.[32,33] Despite a lack of randomized control trials, the Stroke Council of the American Heart Association has recommended avoiding hypovolemia and maintaining a mean arterial blood pressure of 10–20 mm Hg higher than baseline.[34]

Seizures may occur in patients with SAH and unsecured aneurysms or AVMs. The use of antiepileptic agents in pregnancy is well established. Although there has been an association with teratogenicity in the first trimester, the risks of withholding treatment and benefits of administration must be considered. Agents such as Dilantin and Tegretol are typically used. Although no guidelines are set, in general, these drugs are continued for 6 months in patients who have suffered a bleed.[35]

Numerous other treatment modalities such as antifibrinolytic therapy, antioxidants, free radical scavengers, and immunosuppression have been investigated. Further clinical trials are necessary to determine the overall effects on morbidity and mortality.[27,31]

Guiding Questions in Approaching the Patient

- When did the intracranial bleed occur and has it been surgically controlled?
- What is the safest mode of delivery for this patient?
- Is there an obstetric indication for cesarean delivery?

Labor and Delivery in Patients With an Intracranial Bleed in Pregnancy

There are few outcome studies available for the pregnant population; as such, each case must be managed individually, taking into account the patient's neurologic status in consultation with a materal fetal medicine specialist, neurosurgeon, and anesthesiologist. In general, pregnant patients should be treated the same as the nonpregnant population. Pathway 2 shows the delivery protocol for patients who have developed an intracranial bleed during the current pregnancy.[2,3,19] In the past, cesarean section delivery was advocated for all women with an uncontrolled vascular anomaly that had bled during pregnancy to avoid hemodynamic changes associated with labor and vaginal delivery. For women who have had surgical clipping or repair of an aneurysm or AVM before pregnancy or early in pregnancy, labor and delivery should be allowed to proceed normally and cesarean delivery should be reserved for the usual obstetric indications. Current recommendations suggest that, if bleeding occurred in the first trimester or early second trimester, consideration should be given to an early epidural, shortened second stage, and assisted vaginal delivery. Consultation with the anesthesiologist should be made before the patient arrives in labor or early in labor because special considerations including avoidance of maternal hypotension or hypertension must be addressed. Although there are few guidelines regarding patients who have had a late third trimester intracranial hemorrhage or who have incomplete obliteration of the vascular anomaly, cesarean section appears to be a safe option. Difficult ethical dilemmas arise when the mother is in the late third trimester and comatose because the question of fetal salvage becomes paramount.

Conclusion

Intracranial hemorrhage in pregnancy remains a rare but life-threatening condition. There are very few well-designed studies to dictate counseling and management in pregnancy. As a result, the available data from the general population, including that from observational cohorts and case series, are used to establish guidelines in pregnancy. Diagnosis and treatment should not be delayed secondary to pregnancy. Complications remain frequent even with appropriate treatment. Mode of delivery is dictated by the course in pregnancy.

Discussion of Cases

CASE 1: INTRACRANIAL HEMORRHAGE IN PREGNANCY

A 22-year-old gravida 1 presented to the emergency department at 16 weeks of gestation complaining of a severe headache with nausea and vomiting. Neurologic and laboratory evaluations were normal. Her blood pressure was normal.

What is the next step?

Due to persistence of the severe headache, a CT scan was ordered and the patient was counseled regarding the negligible risk of radiation exposure to the fetus. The CT scan demonstrated subarachnoid hemorrhage without evidence of an intracranial mass.

When would a lumbar puncture be indicated?

Lumbar puncture is mandatory if there is a strong suspicion of SAH and the CT is normal or inconclusive but has ruled out a mass lesion.

She was managed expectantly and returned at 22 weeks of gestation with recurrent severe headache, confusion, and focal neurologic deficit.

What are the options at this time?

A repeat CT scan showed recurrence of the subarachnoid bleed and the patient was counseled

and consented for a surgical procedure by the neurosurgeon. The patient was counseled regarding the small risk of anesthesia and preterm labor associated with surgery in the second trimester. A fetal ultrasound evaluation noted a live fetus corresponding to 22 weeks of gestation without abnormalities. She underwent an uncomplicated craniotomy and an uncomplicated postoperative course. She received seizure prophylaxis. After a short rehabilitation, she was sent home. She went into labor at 39 weeks and had a spontaneous vaginal delivery.

CASE 2: *AVM* IN *PREGNANCY*

A 35-year-old gravida 2 presents to prenatal clinic for routine obstetric care at 15 weeks of gestation. She has a known 7-cm AVM in the frontal lobe. She has been asymptomatic for 5 years. She is concerned regarding pregnancy outcome and mode of delivery.

What are your recommendations?

Although there are no studies specifically addressing the natural history of an AVM in pregnancy, she has been asymptomatic longer than 5 years, and it would be reasonable to continue with expectant management. If her pregnancy remains uneventful, a vaginal delivery could be considered.

REFERENCES

1 Jaigobin C, Silver F. Stroke in pregnancy. *Stroke* 2000;31:2948–2951.

2 Intracranial hemorrhage. In: Clark SL, Cotton DD, Hankins GDV, Phelan JP, eds. *Critical Care Obstetrics,* 3rd ed. Massachusetts: Blackwell Science, 1997; p. 577–589.

3 Wiebers DO. Subarachnoid hemorrhage in pregnancy. *Semin Neurol* 1998;3:226–229.

4 Dias MS. Neurovascular emergencies in pregnancy. *Clin Obstet Gynecol* 1994;37:337–354.

5 Maymon R, Fejgin M. Intracranial hemorrhage during pregnancy and puerperium. *Obstet Gynecol Surv* 1990;45:157–159.

6 Stoodley MA, MacDonald L, Weir BKA. Pregnancy and intracranial aneurysms. *Neurosurg Clin North Am* 1998;9:549–556.

7 Sadasivan B, Malik GM, Lee C et al: Vascular malformations in pregnancy. *Surg Neurol* 1990;33:305–313.

8 Barno A, Freeman DW. Maternal deaths due to spontaneous subarachnoid hemorrhage. *Am J Obstet Gynecol* 1976;125:384–392.

9 Barrow DL, Reisner A. Natural history of intracranial aneurysms and vascular malformations. *Clin Neurosurg* 1993;40:3–39.

10 Barrett JM, Van Hooydonk JE, Boehm FH. Pregnancy-related rupture of arterial aneurysms. *Obstet Gynecol Surv* 1982;37:557–566.

11 Al-Shahi R, Warlow C. A systematic review of the frequency and prognosis of arteriovenous malformations of the brain in adults. *Brain* 2001;124:1900–1926.

12 Ondra SL, Troupp H, George ED et al. The natural history of symptomatic arteriovenous malformations of the brain: a 24-year follow-up assessment. *J Neurosurg* 1990;73:387–391.

13 Brown RD Jr, Weibers DO, Forbes G et al. The natural history of unruptured intracranial arteriovenous malformations. *J Neurosurg* 1988;68:352–357.

14 Robinson JL, Hall CJ, Sedzimir CB. Arteriovenous malformation, aneurysms and pregnancy. *J Neurosurg* 1974;41:63–70.

15 Wilkins RH. Natural history of intracranial vascular malformations: a review. *Neurosurgery* 1985;16:421–430.

16 Ortiz O, Voelker J, Eneorji F. Transient enlargement of an intracranial aneurysm in pregnancy: case report. *Surg Neurol* 1997;47:527–531.

17 Weir BK, Drake CG. Rapid growth of residual aneurysm neck in pregnancy. *J Neurosurg* 1991;75:780–782.

18 Wiebers DO, Whisnat JP. The incidence of stroke among pregnant women in Rochester, Minn 1955 through 1979. *JAMA* 1975;254:3055–3057.

19 Dias, MS, Sekhar, LN. Intracranial hemorrhage from aneurysms and arteriovenous malformations during pregnancy and the puerperium. *Neurosurgery* 1990;27:855–866.

20 Kittner SJ, Stern BJ, Feeser BR, et al. Pregnancy and the risk of stroke. *N Engl J Med* 1996;335:768–774.

21 Forster DMC, Kunkler IH, Hartland P. Risk of cerebral bleeding from arteriovenous malformations in pregnancy: the Sheffield experience. *Stereotact Funct Neurosurg* 1993;61(supp 1):20–22.

22 Horton JC, Chambers WA, Lyons SL et al. Pregnancy and the risk of hemorrhage from cerebral arteriovenous malformation. *Neurosurgery* 1990;27:867–872.

23 Cloft HJ, Joseph GJ, Dion JE. Risk of cerebral angiography in patients with subarachnoid hemorrhage, cerebral aneurysm, and arteriovenous malformation: a meta-analysis. *Stoke* 1999;30:317–320.

24 Brilstra EH, Rinkel GJE, van der Graaf Y, et al. Treatment of intracranial aneurysms by embolization with coils: a systematic review. *Stroke* 1999;30:470–476.

25 Piotin M, Filho CBA, Kothimbakam R, et al. Endovascular treatment of acutely ruptured intracranial aneurysms in pregnancy. *Am J Obstet Gynecol* 2001;185:1261–1262.

26 Kassell NF, Torner JC, Haley EC Jr, et al. The International Cooperative Study on timing of aneursymal surgery: Part I-overall management results. *J Neurosurg* 1990;73:18–36.

27 Janjua N, Mayer S. Cerebral vasospasm after subarachnoid hemorrhage. *Curr Opin Crit Care* 2003;9:113–119.

28 Duncan PG, Pope DW, Cohen MM, et al. Fetal risk of anesthesia during pregnancy. *Anesthesia* 1986;64:790–794.

29 Hawkins JL, Koonin LM, Palmer SK, Gibbs CP. Anesthesia-related deaths during obstetric delivery in the United States, 1979–1990. *Anesthesiology* 1997;86:277–284.

30 Minielly R. Yuzpe AA, Drake CG. Subarachnoid hemorrhage secondary to ruptured cerebral aneurysm in pregnancy. *Obstet Gynecol* 1979;53:64–70.

31 Treggiari-Venzi M, Suter P, Romand JA. Review of medical prevention of vasospasm after aneurysmal subarachnoid hemorrhage: a problem of neurointensive care. *Neurosurgery* 2001;48:249–262.

32 Pickard JD, Murray GD, Illingworth R et al. Effect of oral nimodipine on cerebral infarction and outcome after subarachnoid hemorrhage: British Aneurysm Nimodipine trial. *BMJ* 1989;298:636–462.

33 Wijdicks EF, Vermeulen M, Murray GD, et al. The effects of hypertension following aneurysmal subarachnoid hemorrhage. *Clin Neurol Neurosurg* 1990;92:111–117.

34 Mayberg MR, Batjer HH, Dacey R, et al. Guidelines for management of aneurysmal subarachnoid hemorrhage: a statement for health care professionals from a special writing group of the Stroke Council, American Heart Association. *Circulation* 1994;90:2592–2602.

35 Crowell Rm, Grss DR, Olivy CS, et al. Ruptured cerebral aneurysms: perioperative manangement. In: Ratcheson RA, Wirth FP, eds. *Concepts in Neurosurgery, Vol. 6.* Baltimore: Williams & Wilkins, 1994; p. 59–76.

Approach to Dermatologic Issues in Pregnancy

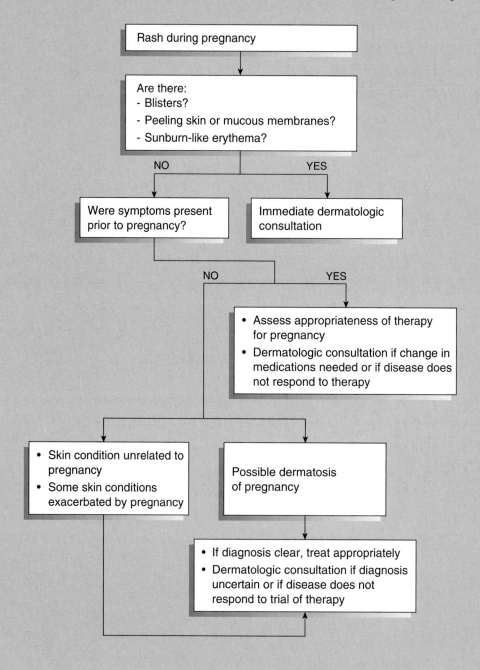

39 Dermatoses in Pregnancy

Kathryn Schwarzenberger

Introduction

Skin problems are common during pregnancy. Most of these are common skin conditions that also affect nonpregnant women; however, there are several, well-characterized dermatoses that occur only during pregnancy. Because some of these conditions may affect the course or outcome of the pregnancy, it is essential when initially evaluating a pregnant woman with a skin problem to determine whether the problem is related directly or indirectly to the pregnancy.

Physiologic Skin Changes During Pregnancy

Pregnancy is a dynamic state with many immunologic, hormonal, metabolic, and vascular changes. In pregnancy, as in other conditions, the skin provides visible evidence of these changes. Predictable skin changes during pregnancy that may affect any woman include pigmentary alterations, most commonly melasma (chloasma) and darkening of the linea alba and areola. Increased levels of melanocyte-stimulating hormone, estrogen, and possibly progesterone are thought to be the cause of these pigmentary changes. Mild to moderate hirsutism is relatively common during pregnancy. Changes in the hair cycle during pregnancy may result in increased retention of the actively growing, or anagen, hairs, which makes the hair feel especially thick and lush during gestation. Unfortunately, this is often followed several months postpartum by diffuse hair shedding from telogen effluvium. Striae distensae on the abdomen and occasionally on the breasts, thighs, and buttocks occur in most pregnant women, and many develop skin tags around the neck and axillae. Physiologic hyperemia with palmar erythema and spider angiomas are some of the vascular changes that may arise during pregnancy.

Most of these changes are of cosmetic concern only and require no treatment during pregnancy. Some conditions, such as hirsutism and hyperemia, usually resolve postpartum without treatment. Persistent facial hair can be controlled with regular twice-daily application of topical eflornithine 13.9% cream (Vaniqa). This product, which inhibits ornithine decarboxylase in hair follicles, has no depilatory effect and must usually be used continuously for at least 6 months for best results. Continued use is then required to maintain the hair loss. "Bleaching creams" that contain hydroquinone or α-hydroxy acids may hasten the resolution of melasma postpartum, particularly when used in conjunction with aggressive sun protection. Commercially available products include a variety of hydroquinone 4% products, many of which contain sunscreen and some of which also include acids (e.g., glycolic or lactic acid) to enhance penetration. These products should be applied topically twice daily to areas of hyperpigmentation for up to 2 months. A combination product that includes hydroquinone, tretinoin, and a topical corticosteroid (Tri-Luma) is also available for control of moderate to severe facial hyperpigmentation.

Postpartum hair loss from telogen effluvium usually resolves gradually, with regrowth within 1 year. In exceptional cases, shedding can continue for longer periods, and women with a genetic propensity to androgenetic or pattern hair loss may have persistent thinning on the anterior or frontal scalp. There is no effective therapy for telogen effluvium, and affected women should be reassured that most will have complete regrowth. Because metabolic abnormalities including thyroid disease and iron deficiency anemia can also cause diffuse hair loss, evaluation for these should be considered if hair loss persists.

The management of striae distensae remains suboptimal, although some investigators have reported anecdotal success using pulsed dye laser[1] and intense pulsed light.[2] Tretinoin cream has been used with variable success in the management of stretch marks.[3]

Effect of Pregnancy on Preexisting Skin Conditions

Pregnancy may affect the expression of skin conditions that existed before the pregnancy. Inflammatory diseases, including atopic dermatitis, psoriasis, acne vulgaris, and urticaria, may worsen or improve. The altered immune status during pregnancy may affect certain infections, such as condyloma acuminata, which often worsen. Autoimmune diseases may flare and, in some cases, affect the outcome of the pregnancy. The effects of pregnancy on different skin diseases have been reviewed recently.[4]

Melanocytic nevi may arise, enlarge, or darken during pregnancy, possibly related to an increased expression of estrogen and progesterone receptors on their surface. However, not all studies have demonstrated any consistent "normal" change in nevi during pregnancy, so evaluation of any changing or atypical-appearing pigmented lesion is essential. Melanomas during pregnancy are often diagnosed at a more advanced stage during pregnancy than are melanomas in nonpregnant women,[5] although it is not clear whether this is due to a delay in diagnosis or some intrinsic biologic difference between the two states. Pregnancy itself does not appear to adversely affect the outcome of melanoma.[6] Some dermatologists may hesitate to perform skin biopsies on pregnant women, so communication and appropriate education of the consultant is essential. In 2002, melanoma was the most frequently diagnosed malignancy in U.S. women ages 25–29 years.[7] For many of these otherwise healthy women, their obstetrician may be their primary and, in some cases, only health care provider. A complete skin examination at the initial visit and attention to skin changes that arise during pregnancy are warranted.

KEY POINT

Pigmented lesions that undergo change during pregnancy or have an atypical appearance must be evaluated, including possible biopsy.

Dermatologic Therapies During Pregnancy

Because the use of some common dermatologic therapies is problematic during pregnancy, it is important to ask patients if they are being treated for any skin conditions (Table 39-1). Patients may fail to identify dermatologic treatments, particularly topical products, as medications and may neglect to mention their use. Oral antibiotics, in particular the tetracyclines (pregnancy category D), are frequently prescribed for skin problems such as acne, rosacea, and hidradenitis suppurativa and for less common

Table 39-1. **COMMON DERMATOLOGIC MEDICATIONS**

MEDICATION	*TRADE NAME*	*COMMON USE*	*PREGNANCY CATEGORY*
Acne and rosacea preparations			
Topical			
Erythromycin 2% topical	Various	Acne	B
Clindamycin 1% topical	Various	Acne	B
Benzoyl peroxide	Various	Acne	C
Erythromycin in-benzoyl peroxide	Benzamycin	Acne	C
Clindamycin-benzoyl peroxide	BenzaClin, Duac	Acne	C
Metronidazole 0.75% and 1%	MetroGel, Noritate, others	Rosacea	B
Azelaic acid 15% and 20%	Azelex, Finevin, Finacea	Acne, rosacea	B
Tretinoin	Retin-A and others	Acne, photoaging	C
Adapalene 0.1%, 1%	Differin	Acne	C
Tazarotene 0.05%, 1%	Tazorac	Psoriasis, acne	X
Oral			
Tetracycline, doxycycline, minocycline	Various	Acne, folliculitis, hidradenitis, rosacea	D
Isotretinoin	Accutane	Cystic acne	X
Anti-infectives			
Topical			
Mupirocin 2%	Bactroban	Impetigo	B
Permethrin 5%	Elimite, others	Scabies	B
Lindane 1%	Kwell, others	Scabies	B
Azole antifungals	Various	Dermatophyte infections, yeast	B and C
Penciclovir 1%	Denavir	Herpes simplex	B
Oral			
Acyclovir	Zovirax	Herpes infections	B
Valacyclovir	Valtrex	Herpes infections	B
Famciclovir	Famvir	Herpes infections	B
Anti-inflammatory			
Topical			
Corticosteroids	Various	Inflammatory dermatoses	C
Tacrolimus 0.03%, 0.1%	Protopic	Atopic dermatitis, other conditions	C
Pimecrolimus 1%	Elidel	Atopic dermatitis, other conditions	C
Oral			
Corticosteroids	Various	Inflammatory dermatoses	C

(Continued)

Table 39-1. **COMMON DERMATOLOGIC MEDICATIONS (*CONTINUED*)**

MEDICATION	*TRADE NAME*	*COMMON USE*	*PREGNANCY CATEGORY*
Antipsoriatic			
Topical			
Calcipotriene 0.005%	Dovonex	Psoriasis	C
Tazarotene 0.05%, 1%	Tazorac	Psoriasis, acne	X
Oral			
Acitretin	Soriatane	Psoriasis	X
Methotrexate sodium		Psoriasis	X
Cyclosporin A	Neoral	Psoriasis	C
Miscellaneous			
Topical			
Imiquimod 5%	Aldara	Warts, molluscum, keratoses	B
Hydroquinone 4%	Various	Hyperpigmentation	C
Fluorouracil	Efudex, Carac	Actinic keratoses	X
Eflornithine HCl 13.9%	Vaniqa	Hirsutism	C
Minoxidil 2%	Rogaine	Androgenetic alopecia	Unknown

SOURCE: Physicians Desk Reference 2003.

conditions such as some autoimmune blistering diseases. The oral retinoids isotretinoin (Accutane) and acitretin (Soriatane) are extremely potent teratogens. Acitretin, used to control psoriasis and various other skin conditions, should be used with caution in women of childbearing potential because it has a particularly long half-life. Pregnancy should be avoided for at least 3 years after its discontinuation. At least 1 month should elapse before considering pregnancy after completing of a course of isotretinoin. Since its return to the U.S. market in the past decade, dermatologists have prescribed thalidomide for the management of a number of dermatologic conditions. Because of the risk of teratogenicity, comprehensive pregnancy prevention programs have been created and participation is required of any physician who wishes to prescribe isotretinoin or thalidomide.

Topical retinoids, including tretinoin (marketed as Retin-A and other products) and adapalene (Differin) are used primarily for the control of acne vulgaris and chronic sun damage. Although they are designated as pregnancy category C drugs, their use is not generally advised during pregnancy. Another topical retinoic acid derivative, tazarotene (Tazorac or Avage) deserves special mention because it is a pregnancy category X drug. Originally approved for the management of plaque-type psoriasis, tazarotene is currently marketed for the management of comedonal acne and chronic sun damage. Strict contraception and pregnancy testing before prescribing tazarotene are indicated in the package labeling.

Other, more commonly used dermatologic therapies may require special consideration during pregnancy. Use of hydroxyzine, a commonly prescribed H_1 antihistamine, is contraindicated (pregnancy category X) during the first trimester of pregnancy but is a category C drug thereafter. Corticosteroids, systemic and topical, are pregnancy category C. Because most topical corticosteroids are minimally absorbed, they can generally be used safely during pregnancy, although their potential for thinning the skin and causing stretch marks, particularly in areas of occlusion such as the axillae, groin, and under the breasts, should be remembered. Ultrapotent, class 1 topical corticosteroids, including clobetasol propionate 0.05%, can cause reversible hypopituitary axis suppression even from topical use; their use should be limited to no more than 50 g/week for up to 2 consecutive weeks.

KEY POINT

Each patient should be questioned about the use of topical medication and whether she is being treated for a skin condition.

Dermatoses of Pregnancy: Introduction

There are several, relatively rare, dermatoses whose onset and etiology relate directly to pregnancy: pruritic and urticarial papules and plaques of pregnancy (PUPPP), prurigo of pregnancy, pruritic folliculitis of pregnancy (PFP), gestational pemphigoid, and intrahepatic cholestasis of pregnancy (ICP). Impetigo herpetiformis, a form of pustular psoriasis in pregnancy, is often included in this group. Some investigators believe that PFP and prurigo of pregnancy are forms of PUPPP.

What's the Evidence?

Unfortunately, the relative rarity of the dermatoses of pregnancy has made their study under controlled conditions impossible. Information about the clinical features and prognosis of these dermatoses has been obtained from a number of case reports, retrospective, and cohort studies. An excellent evidence-based systematic review was recently published.[8]

Guiding Questions in Approaching the Patient

- Did the skin condition exist before the pregnancy?
- Has the pregnancy caused or contributed to worsening of the skin condition?
- Is the patient using any dermatologic medications, and, if so, are they safe for use during pregnancy?
- Are there blisters, diffuse sunburn-like erythema, mucosal lesions, or peeling of the skin that necessitate immediate dermatologic consultation?
- Could the skin condition be a drug reaction?
- If topical therapies are prescribed, can the patient comply with the regimen?

Dermatoses of Pregnancy

PRURITIC URTICARIAL PAPULES AND PLAQUES OF PREGNANCY

PUPPP (Figure 39-1) is one of the most common dermatoses of pregnancy and occur as frequently as 1 in 130 pregnancies.[9] The etiology of PUPPP remains unknown. Although the condition is not associated with any specific pregnancy complications, the itching it causes can be quite severe. PUPPP characteristically

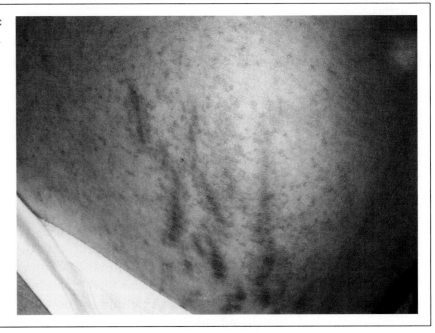

Figure 39-1: Pruritic urticarial papules and plaques of pregnancy. Itchy papules arise within striae.

affect primigravidas in the third trimester. Some investigators have reported an increased incidence in multiple gestations, and it has been suggested that rapid or excessive weight gain and the resultant stretching of the skin may trigger the onset of this condition. The eruption generally starts as small, itchy bumps in the abdominal striae. Skin around the umbilicus is usually spared. The rash spreads over several days to involve the thighs, buttocks, breasts, and arms. The face, palms, and soles are spared, as are mucosae. As the name of the condition suggests, the skin lesions usually are erythematous papules (small bumps <5–10 mm in diameter) and plaques (larger skin lesions measuring up to several centimeters in diameter); however, there can also be microvesicles, hive-like wheals, and target lesions. Another term for this condition is *polymorphic eruption of pregnancy.*

KEY POINT

PUPPP is a very common disorder that has no effect on the pregnancy outcome but can cause significant disability from pruritus.

PUPPP has no associated systemic signs or symptoms. The diagnosis is usually made on clinical findings. The histologic findings of PUPPP are nonspecific, and there are no characteristic laboratory abnormalities, making the diagnosis one of exclusion. A skin biopsy may help distinguish PUPPP from other dermatoses; in particular, a biopsy for immunofluorescence testing may be necessary to distinguish this from gestational pemphigoid if there are associated vesicles or blisters.

Management of PUPPP consists of regular and frequent applications of topical corticosteroids. Mid- to high-potency corticosteroids, such as triamcinolone 0.1% or fluocinonide 0.5%, can be applied to affected areas up to three to four times a day. Creams may be cosmetically preferable to ointments. An appropriate amount of topical corticosteroids must be prescribed because failure to apply adequate amounts may result in treatment failure. An estimated 30 g of a topical preparation is needed to cover the skin of an "average" adult once. Systemic corticosteroids may be considered in prolonged or particularly severe cases. The use of topical antihistamines such as diphenhydramine (Benadryl and Caladryl) and doxepin (Zonalon) has been complicated by development of allergic contact dermatitis, and because the two conditions may share similar features, use of these antihistamines is not recommended. Anecdotal response to ultraviolet B phototherapy, useful in the management of other pruritic dermatoses, has been reported.[4]

Recurrence of PUPPP during successive pregnancies is exceptional, and subsequent use of oral contraceptives is not associated with exacerbation of the condition. PUPPP must be clinically distinguished from eczematous dermatoses, including atopic dermatitis (which frequently affects skin on the antecubital and popliteal fossae and may involve the face), allergic contact dermatitis, scabies (which may involve the finger webs, skin around the wrists, areola and umbilicus, and genitalia), drug reactions, and viral exanthems. A thorough medical history will often help distinguish between PUPPP from any of the above conditions. Patients should be asked about a personal or family history of atopic conditions (allergies, asthma, hay fever, or history of childhood eczema). Any associated symptoms, particularly those that might suggest an infectious etiology, make the diagnosis of PUPPP unlikely and should prompt further evaluation. A dermatologist should be consulted immediately in the presence of blistering skin lesions, if there is mucosal involvement, or if there is skin tenderness, fragility, or peeling.

PRURIGO OF PREGNANCY

Prurigo of pregnancy (Figure 39-2) consists of itchy, erythematous nodules and papules that resemble those of prurigo nodularis in nonpregnant women. The lesions, found mostly on the extremities but rarely on the abdomen, are thought to result from repeated scratching. The finding of increased serum immunoglobulin E

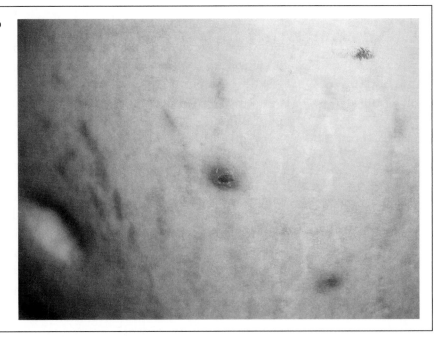

Figure 39-2: Prurigo of pregnancy. Excoriated, scattered itchy papules on the abdomen are visible.

levels in some affected patients suggests that the condition may arise from pruritus gravidarum in women with underlying atopy.[10] This condition, which may be relatively common, occurs variably during the course of gestation, persists throughout pregnancy, and resolves postpartum. Other than itching associated with the lesions themselves, there is no associated maternal or fetal morbidity or increased mortality. Lesions should be distinguished from arthropod bites, scabies, allergic contact dermatitis, or folliculitis. Symptomatic treatment with mid-potency topical corticosteroids, such as triamcinolone 0.1% cream, is usually sufficient to control the itching.

PRURITIC FOLLICULITIS OF PREGNANCY

PFP has also been described in a very small number of pregnancies.[11] PFP consists of a generalized eruption of sterile, erythematous, follicular pustules and papules that develop in the second or third trimester. Lesions resolve postpartum and are not associated with any increased maternal or fetal risk. The condition must be distinguished from acne and other forms of folliculitis, including bacterial folliculitis, usually from *Staphylococcus aureus* or *Pseudomonas aeruginosa* ("hot tub folliculitis"), fungal folliculitis (*Pityrosporum* spp. or *Candida*), or mechanical forms of folliculitis, such as might result from heat or occlusion. Many patients with PFP are asymptomatic, and no treatment is needed. Topical corticosteroids, ultraviolet B phototherapy, and benzoyl peroxide have been used with some success.

GESTATIONAL PEMPHIGOID

Gestational pemphigoid (Figures 39-3 and 39-4) has historically been known by other names, including "herpes gestationis" and "pemphigoid gestationis." Because this is an autoimmune blistering disease with absolutely no relation to herpesvirus infections, many investigators believe the name "herpes gestationis" is misleading and should be abandoned.

Gestational pemphigoid appears to be caused primarily by immunoglobulin G autoantibodies that bind to a specific molecule in the basement membrane zone of the skin called *bullous pemphigoid antigen 2*. These antibodies activate complement by the classic pathway, which causes a loss of adhesion of basal layer keratinocytes and leads to development of tense skin blisters. The diagnosis of gestational pemphigoid is confirmed by the finding

Figure 39-3:
Gestational
pemphigoid. Itchy,
urticarial papules
have crusts at sites of
previous blisters
(courtesy Kenneth E.
Greer, MD).

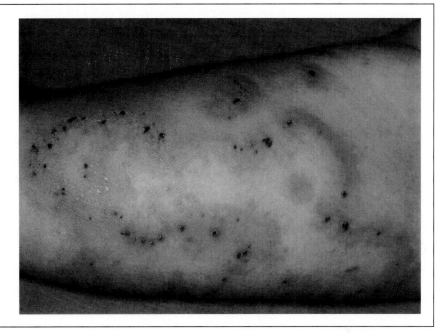

Figure 39-4:
Gestational
pemphigoid. Small,
tense blisters overlie
itchy plaques.

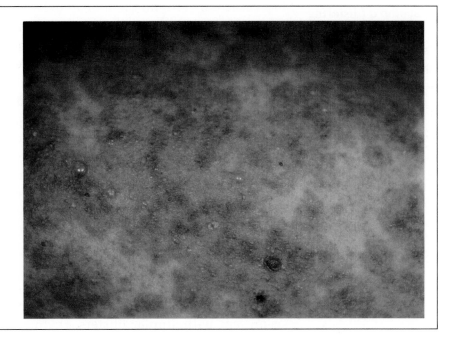

of C3 deposition along the base of the epidermis with immuno-fluorescence studies. The exact etiology of gestational pemphigoid remains unclear. It has been hypothesized that the disease results from an immunologic response directed against MHC class II antigens of paternal haplotype at the placental basement membrane zone, which then cross-react with maternal skin.

Gestational pemphigoid occurs less frequently than does PUPPP, affecting approximately 1 in 50,000 pregnancies. Most cases begin in the second or third trimester (mean 21 weeks), although it can begin as soon as in the first trimester or be delayed until the immediate postpartum period.[12] Skin lesions usually start as itchy plaques or hive-like lesions on the abdomen before spreading to involve the trunk and extremities. Periumbilical skin is involved in most cases. Straw-colored, fluid-filled vesicles or blisters, which may be up to several centimeters in diameter, arise on an erythematous base. Because the skin splits at the level of the basement membrane zone, the blister is relatively deep and tense. The face, palms, soles, and mucosal membranes are spared.

Patients with gestational pemphigoid itch but should have no other associated symptoms. The course of the disease during pregnancy varies. After onset, the symptoms may initially decrease. Most cases flare around the time of delivery, after which the disease gradually remits over a period of weeks or months.[13] In rare cases, the disease persists and may "transform" into bullous pemphigoid. Some women experience recurrences with menses or with use of oral contraceptives. Unlike PUPPP, gestational pemphigoid commonly recurs with subsequent pregnancies, often at an earlier stage of gestation. Subsequent pregnancies, however, may be spared. The intensity of symptoms may vary during successive pregnancies and cannot be predicted.

The presence of blisters should prompt dermatologic consultation, and skin biopsies with immunofluorescence studies should be obtained to confirm the diagnosis. Although PUPPP may cause microvesicles on the skin, it should not cause large blisters. Relatively common skin diseases that may be considered in differential diagnosis include allergic contact dermatitis and blistering drug reactions. Other autoimmune bullous disorders including pemphigus vulgaris and bullous systemic lupus erythematosus can present with similar blisters. Erythema multiforme, which

KEY POINT

All pregnant women who develop a blistering skin eruption should be referred to a dermatologist.

can be associated with herpes simplex infections, can cause widespread erythematous-based blisters or target lesions but it can be clinically distinguished from gestational pemphigoid by the presence of mucosal involvement and lesions on the palms and/or soles. Scabies infestations occasionally cause blisters.

Mild or limited cases of gestational pemphigoid may respond to regular application of mid- to high-potency topical corticosteroids. Antihistamines may help alleviate itching. Most patients require systemic corticosteroids and usually respond to prednisone up to 0.5 mg/kg daily. Recalcitrant cases may require larger doses, although only rarely are doses exceeding 80 mg/day needed. Once the disease is controlled, the corticosteroid dose should be decreased to the smallest amount that will prevent blistering. Because the disease tends to flare around the time of delivery and postpartum, it may be necessary to temporarily increase the dose at that time. Women who have been on corticosteroids for prolonged periods may be at risk of adrenal suppression, and the need for "stress-dose" steroids at time of delivery should be considered. Different immunosuppressant therapies have been used with variable success for the postpartum management of gestational pemphigoid in nonlactating women; in most cases, their toxicities prevent their use during pregnancy.

Gestational pemphigoid is not associated with any increased maternal risk, although women with a history of the disease may have an increased incidence of Grave's disease or other autoimmune diseases.[14] Placental insufficiency may result in small-for-gestational-age infants and preterm delivery; however, there is no increased fetal mortality attributed to gestational pemphigoid.[15] Transplacental transfer of antibodies may cause transient blistering in a small percentage of infants.[16] Affected infants require no specific therapy because the skin lesions resolve with antibody clearance.

INTRAHEPATIC CHOLESTASIS OF PREGNANCY

Although no primary skin lesions are associated with ICP, the intense, intractable pruritus it causes may result in skin excoriations from repeated scratching. "Physiologic" itching (pruritus gravidarum) is not uncommon early in pregnancy; however, ICP usually does not occur before the third trimester. Scratching may cause skin excoriations and/or bruising; if left unattended, open areas of skin may become secondarily infected. Overt jaundice develops in a minority of cases, and it may follow the onset of itching by a matter of weeks.[17]

The diagnosis of ICP is suggested clinically by the presence of itching without specific skin lesions. Most affected women have increase serum levels of bile salt acids, and some have mildly increased liver transaminases. A thorough skin examination should be done to look for primary skin lesions (i.e., papules, pustules, wheals, burrows, and blisters) that suggest other dermatologic conditions.

Other causes of hepatic injury, including infections and drug toxicity, must be considered in the presence of jaundice or significantly increased liver transaminases. Systemic conditions that can also cause itching without primary skin lesions include thyroid disease (hypothyroidism or hyperthyroidism), iron deficiency anemia, and renal disease. Evaluation for these should be undertaken when clinically indicated. The diagnosis and management of ICP is covered in detail in Chap. 17.

IMPETIGO HERPETIFORMIS

Impetigo herpetiformis is an extremely rare pustular eruption that occurs during pregnancy. Because of clinical and histologic similarities, it has been called a form of pustular psoriasis,[18] and some researchers have argued that this is not a specific dermatosis of pregnancy. In contrast, others feel that this is a separate entity, particularly because most affected women have no history of psoriasis. Skin lesions erupt usually during the third trimester and consist of erythematous plaques or patches in the groin, axillae, and on the neck. Small, superficial pustules stud the edge of the lesions, which tend to spread by peripheral extension, that leave behind yellowish crusts. Large areas of the body may be involved, although the face, palms, and soles are usually spared. Mucous membranes are occasionally involved, and pustules under the nails may cause their separation from the underlying nail bed.

Women with impetigo herpetiformis may be systemically ill, with fever, chills, nausea, vomiting, and diarrhea. Evaluation for systemic infection is appropriate. Open areas of skin can become secondarily infected. Symptomatic hypocalcemia is a potential complication of impetigo herpetiformis, although whether the hypocalcemia is a cause or consequence of the condition remains a subject of debate.

The term *impetigo herpetiformis* reflects the clinical appearance and, like the term *herpes gestationis*, incorrectly suggests an infectious cause for this noninfectious condition. The diagnosis of this condition is confirmed with a skin biopsy, which shows histologic changes similar to those of pustular psoriasis. Bacterial cultures may help rule out secondary infection; however, intact pustules of impetigo herpetiformis are sterile. Systemic corticosteroids are the primary therapy for this condition, and most women respond to prednisone 30–60 mg/day. Therapy must be continued until the skin lesions are controlled, after which the corticosteroids can be slowly tapered off. Successful anecdotal use of cyclosporine has been reported.[19] The disease usually remits after delivery, although cases of recurrence with subsequent pregnancies have been reported.

Conclusion

Skin disorders are common in pregnancy. There are a number of physiologic changes in pregnancy about which clinicians can be reassuring to their patients. Some skin disorders are diseases exclusively present in pregnancy such as pruritic and urticarial papules and plaques of pregnancy. Many, but not all, topical medications are acceptable in pregnancy. Many skin disorders can be treated by the obstetrical care provider, but a pregnant patient with a blistering skin eruption must be referred urgently to a dermatologist.

Discussion of Cases

CASE 1: THIRD TRIMESTER PRURITIC RASH

A 23-year-old primigravida presents at 36 weeks of gestation complaining of an intensely itchy rash on her abdomen and thighs. The rash started on her abdomen and is spreading. She otherwise feels well and has no associated systemic complaints. Pregnancy to date has been uncomplicated, although she has gained close to 45 lb. Medications include only prenatal vitamins, and she denies use of over-the-counter medications or herbal products. Her medical history is notable for environmental allergies to ragweed and some pollens, and she may have had eczema as a child. She did use a new body lotion in the preceding weeks.

Physical examination shows a healthy-appearing, gravid woman with prominent abdominal striae. There are numerous 2- to 3-mm red papules prominently and symmetrically located in the abdominal striae and grouped along the lateral thighs. Few scattered lesions are present on the breasts. The face, palms, soles, and mucosal membranes are spared. There are no blisters.

What is the most likely diagnosis at this point?

PUPPP. Features consistent with this include occurrence during first pregnancy, onset during third trimester, itchy lesions that start in abdominal striae, an association with excessive or rapid weight gain, and the patient is otherwise well.

What else should be considered in the differential diagnosis?

Atopic dermatitis can flare during pregnancy, but the distribution in this case is not characteristic. Atopic dermatitis often involves the skin on the antecubital and popliteal fossae and may involve the face. An allergic reaction to the body lotion or other topical products is possible, but it is unlikely to involve the skin within striae and spare the skin in between. Allergic contact dermatitis should be considered if the pattern of the rash is linear (suggesting trauma or scratching, as one might experience from contact with plants such as poison ivy) or if it has a pattern consistent with the exposure. It may also have small vesicles or blisters and crusts, which would be unusual in PUPPP. The presence of blisters should necessitate evaluation for gestational pemphigoid. Drug eruptions, viral exanthems, and infestations such as scabies can present with itchy papules on the torso and extremities.

What should be done to confirm the diagnosis?

Most cases of PUPPP are sufficiently characteristic that a clinical diagnosis can be made at the initial presentation.

Are additional tests needed?

Skin biopsy findings in PUPPP are not specific, but they may help identify alternative diagnoses. Biopsy should be considered if the diagnosis is unclear. Blood work is not helpful because there are no expected abnormalities. A scabies preparation, which can be done in the office, may be considered if this is in the differential diagnosis.

How would you treat this woman?

Most cases of PUPPP will respond to frequent application of a mid-potency topical corticosteroid such as triamcinolone 0.1% cream. A sufficient amount of cream should be prescribed; an 80-g tube is often a reasonable amount with which to begin. The cream can be applied up to three to four times a day. The patient should be cautioned not to apply much in the axillae, under the breasts, or in the groin folds because thinning of the skin and striae are particularly likely to develop in these areas. Oral antihistamines such as diphenhydramine or hydroxyzine may provide help provide some relief from itching, although sedation can be a problem. The nonsedating antihistamines may be less effective at relieving itch. If symptoms do not decrease after several days of this regimen, a stronger topical corticosteroid such as fluocinonide 0.05% cream may be tried, or systemic corticosteroids can be started. Symptoms should resolve after delivery.

When should a dermatologist be consulted?

A dermatologist should be involved whenever there are blisters (to rule out gestational pemphigoid or other autoimmune blistering disease) or whenever there is mucosal involvement, a sunburn-like erythema, or peeling of the skin. The latter could indicate a serious drug eruption, Stevens-Johnson syndrome, toxic shock syndrome, or toxic epidermal necrolysis. Consultation is also reasonable anytime the diagnosis is uncertain, or whenever the condition does not respond to a reasonable course of treatment.

Should the patient worry about recurrences during successive pregnancies?

As a rule, PUPPP occurs only during first pregnancies. Recurrences during menses, with use of oral contraceptives, or during subsequent pregnancies are not anticipated.

CASE 2: RASH WITH BLISTERS AT 23 WEEKS

A 27-year-old primigravida presents at 23 weeks of gestation complaining of skin lesions. In the past several weeks, she has developed what she initially thought were hives on her abdomen. The lesions, however, have spread to involve other areas of her trunk and extremities, and she recently developed blisters within some of the lesions. The lesions itch, but she has no associated systemic symptoms. She is otherwise healthy, and pregnancy to date has been uncomplicated. She has no history of skin problems. Her only medications are prenatal vitamins. She is not aware of exposure to any others with skin problems.

Examination shows a well-appearing gravid woman. There are multiple red papules and plaques, some measuring up to several centimeters in diameter, on the abdomen, involving periumbilical skin, and on other areas of the torso and extremities. Many have a tense, fluid-filled blister overlying them. The blisters do not rupture when pressure is applied. There are no lesions on the face, palms, or soles. Mucous membranes, including the lips, are spared.

What diagnoses should immediately be considered?

Gestational pemphigoid should be suspected in this woman with hive-like lesions and blisters arising in the second trimester. The differential includes other autoimmune blistering diseases

(e.g., pemphigus vulgaris and bullous lupus erythematosus), bullous erythema multiforme (usually involves mucosal membranes, palm, and sole), allergic or severe irritant contact dermatitis, and bullous drug eruptions. PUPPP can cause tiny vesicles but should not cause large bullae. Urticaria should not blister. If the blisters are small, and/or if they are located in a dermatomal pattern, herpes simplex, varicella, and/or herpes zoster may be considered. The bullous form of impetigo causes blisters, but these are usually superficial and rupture when touched.

What testing should be done to confirm the diagnosis?

Skin biopsies with immunofluorescence studies are needed to confirm the diagnosis. A biopsy of one of the blisters would be expected to show subepidermal blistering on routine (hematoxylin and eosin) staining. An additional biopsy of nonlesional skin should be sent in special medium for direct immunofluorescence staining. Not all pathology laboratories are equipped to do skin immunofluorescence studies, and tissue may need to be sent to a special reference laboratory.

What about other laboratory work?

There are no specific abnormalities that would be expected on routine studies. Serum can be sent with the skin for indirect immuno-fluorescence studies to look for antibodies to pemphigus and pemphigoid and the "HG" (herpes gestationis) factor, which may be present in some cases of gestational pemphigoid. Fluid from an intact blister should be submitted for bacterial culture if there is concern about bullous impetigo.

Once the biopsies are done, what should be done for initial management?

Very mild cases of gestational pemphigoid can be managed with topical corticosteroids and antihistamines. However, most cases will require therapy with systemic corticosteroids. Unless contraindicated for other reasons, a reasonable starting dose would be prednisone 0.5 mg/kg daily. Because immunofluorescence studies may take several days to weeks to be returned, treatment should be initiated once a presumptive diagnosis is made.

The diagnosis of gestational pemphigoid is confirmed, and the patient has improved after taking prednisone for several weeks.

What now?

Taper the dose of prednisone until the smallest dose needed to control blistering and symptoms is reached. Many women have a flare around the time of delivery, so a peripartum increase in dose may be needed. The corticosteroids can then be tapered gradually after delivery. Some women may have a protracted postpartum course; in these cases, use of alternative immunosuppressant therapies may be considered to minimize the long-term use of systemic corticosteroids.

When should a dermatologist be involved?

Dermatologic consultation is appropriate whenever there are blisters on the skin. Other findings that should prompt dermatologic consultation include mucosal lesions, a sunburn-like redness of the skin, or peeling of the skin. These could suggest a severe drug reaction, such as toxic epidermal necrolysis, erythema multiforme, toxic shock syndrome, or other serious skin conditions.

All dermatologists should be familiar with blistering skin disorders, and any should be able to perform the appropriate testing. However, because gestational pemphigoid is a relatively rare condition, referral to a dermatologist with a special interest or expertise in managing autoimmune skin conditions may be necessary, particularly for the management of severe or recalcitrant cases.

REFERENCES

1 McDaniel DH. Laser therapy of stretch marks. *Dermatol Clin* 2002;20:67–76.

2 Hernandez-Perez E, Colombo-Charrier E, Valencia-Ibiett E. Intense pulsed light in the treatment of striae distensae. *Dermatol Surg* 2002;28:1124–1130.

3 Pribanich S, Simpson FG, Held B, et al. Low-dose tretinoin does not improve striae distensae: a double-blind, placebo-controlled study. *Cutis* 1994;54:121–124.

4 Kroumpouzos G, Cohen LM. Dermatoses of pregnancy. *J Am Acad Dermatol* 2001;45:1–22.

5 Travers RL, Sober AJ, Berwick M, et al. Increased thickness of pregnancy-associated melanoma. *Br J Dermatol* 1995;132:876–883.

6 Daryanani D, Plokker JT, Dettollo JA, et al. Pregnancy and early-stage melanoma. *Cancer* 2003;97:2248–2253.

7 Surveillance, Epidemiology, and End Results (SEER) Program. SEER*Stat database: incidence—SEER 9 regs public use, November 2002 submission (1973–2000). National Cancer Institute, DCCPS, Surveillance Research Program, Cancer Statistics Branch, released April 2003, based on the November 2002 submission. Available at: www.seer.cancer.gov

8 Kroumpouzos G, Cohen LM. Specific dermatoses of pregnancy: an evidence-based systematic review. *Am J Obstet Gynecol* 2003;188: 1083–1092.

9 Roger D, et al. Specific pruritic diseases of pregnancy. A prospective study of 3192 pregnant women. *Arch Dermatol* 1994;130:734–739.

10 Vaughan Jones SA, et al. A prospective study of 200 women with dermatoses of pregnancy correlating clinical findings with hormonal and immunopathological profiles. *Br J Dermatol* 1999;141:71–81.

11 Kroumpouzos G, Cohen LM. Pruritic folliculitis of pregnancy. *J Am Acad Dermatol* 2000;43(1 pt 1):132–134.

12 Jenkins RE, Hern S, Black MM. Clinical features and management of 87 patients with pemphigoid gestationis. *Clin Exp Dermatol* 1999;24: 255–259.

13 Shornick JK. Dermatoses of pregnancy. *Semin Cutan Med Surg* 1998;17:172–181.

14 Shornick JK, Black MM. Secondary autoimmune diseases in herpes gestationis (pemphigoid gestationis). *J Am Acad Dermatol* 1992;26: 563–566.

15 Shornick JK, Black MM. Fetal risks in herpes gestationis. *J Am Acad Dermatol* 1992;26:63–68.

16 Chen SH, Chopra K, Evans TY, et al. Herpes gestationis in a mother and child. *J Am Acad Dermatol* 1999;40(5 pt 2):847–849.

17 Lammert F, Marschall Hu, Glantz A, Matern S, et al. Intrahepatic cholestasis of pregnancy: molecular pathogenesis, diagnosis and management. *J Hepatol* 2000;33:1012–1021.

18 Breier-Maly J, Wantanabe R, Fujiwara H, et al. Generalized pustular psoriasis of pregnancy (impetigo herpetiformis). *Dermatology* 1999; 198:61–64.

19 Imai N, et al. Successful treatment of impetigo herpetiformis with oral cyclosporine during pregnancy. *Arch Dermatol* 2002;138:128–129.

Screening and Management of Substance Abuse in Pregnancy

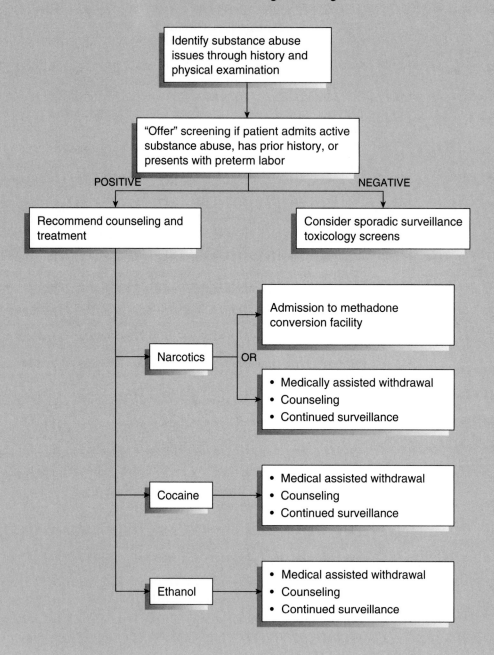

40 *Substance Abuse in Pregnancy*

Gary E. Kaufman

Introduction

Substance abuse affects as many as 30% of pregnancies in some centers—substantially more than preeclampsia, gestational diabetes mellitus, or preterm labor. A small percentage of women who abuse drugs receive regular prenatal care. Infections with hepatitis B, hepatitis C, human immunodeficiency virus (HIV), and syphilis are far more common in addicted women.

It is a difficult matter to assess the obstetric and medical complications associated with substance abuse. Confounding variables including medical complications, inadequate prenatal care, smoking, poor nutrition, and poverty are common among substance abusers. A large proportion of women with substance abuse problems are unmarried, on public assistance, and poorly educated. Many are homeless. Many of the women were children of substance abusers and victims of physical or sexual abuse as children themselves.[1] The care and management of women with substance abuse problems must involve a team approach and reflect the complexity of the entire family and social situation. Despite the association of substance abuse with poverty and poor prenatal care, abuse is seen among all populations. The observant obstetrician should be aware of signs of substance abuse in all patients.

This chapter focuses on the three primary substances of abuse that most obstetricians will encounter in practice, namely ethanol, cocaine, and opioids. The goal of each section is to give a summary of the background, teratogenicity, effects on pregnancy, management options, and outcomes with each agent.

Ethanol

HISTORY AND BACKGROUND	Ethanol has been produced and consumed by humans longer than 12,000 years, making it perhaps the oldest known substance of abuse. Abuse has been described in writings of ancient Egypt, Greece, and the Old Testament. Ethanol has a clear influence on family violence, accidental injury, and violent crime. Except for a brief trial of prohibition from 1919 to 1933, ethanol is the only substance of abuse discussed here that is legal in the United States for general consumption and usage. The per-capita consumption of ethanol in the United States exceeds 2 gallons per individual. Fetal alcohol syndrome (FAS) is estimated to affect 1 in 500 to 1 in 3000 children.[2]

TERATOGENICITY

The teratogenicity of ethanol is well established. The syndrome of effects seen with ethanol abuse during pregnancy (FAS) includes prenatal and postnatal growth restriction, a pattern of facial features, and an increased incidence of other malformations. Facial features include short palpebral fissures, absent philtrum, hypoplastic midface, low nasal bridge, and flattening of the maxilla. An increased incidence of cleft lip and palate has been suggested. Poor dental development, hearing loss, poor vision, and scoliosis have been reported. An increased incidence of childhood leukemia has been reported, especially with late pregnancy exposures.

The incidence of FAS reported is 4–35% in women who drink at least 5 oz of ethanol daily. The risk of binge drinking and more moderate levels of ethanol consumption is difficult to assess because of self-reporting errors and confounding variables. Beer drinkers may be at greater risk than other ethanol consumers.[3]

EFFECTS ON PREGNANCY

There are multiple medical risks to the mother from ethanol ingestion including poor nutrition, pancreatitis, hepatitis, and cirrhosis. Ethanol exposure causes a symmetrical growth restriction in the fetus.

WITHDRAWAL

Withdrawal from ethanol can last 2–10 days, with the most severe symptoms during the first 72 hours. The onset of withdrawal

KEY POINT

Ethanol withdrawal can be life threatening and requires therapy during pregnancy.

occurs 6–48 hours after the last ingestion of ethanol. Patients develop restlessness, agitation, tremor, tachycardia, nausea, vomiting, insomnia, and anorexia. Occasionally, more severe symptoms can develop, including delirium, hallucinations, paranoid delusions, and grand mal seizures. Withdrawal can be life threatening. Progression from mild to severe symptoms does not always occur, and the first sign of withdrawal may be grand mal seizures.

TREATMENT OPTIONS

Counseling and group support are the primary options to avoid maternal use of alcohol. Screening for other substance of abuse and sexually transmitted diseases is suggested. Admission for withdrawal is suggested if there have been any previous withdrawal symptoms to ethanol. Initial laboratory data including complete blood cell count (CBC), electrolytes, liver function tests, magnesium level, and blood alcohol level should be obtained. The typical elimination of alcohol is 30 mg/dL per hour. This may be increased during pregnancy or longer in a person with active hepatic disease. Blood alcohol level can be used to calculate the expected time for full withdrawal. Supplementation with thiamine, folic acid, prenatal vitamins, and iron should begin at admission. Parenteral multivitamins in intravenous fluids may be needed.

Benzodiazepines including lorazepam (Ativan), chlordiazepoxide (Librium), and diazepam (Valium) control the major symptoms of withdrawal. Typical dose schedules for chlordiazepoxide are 25–50 mg daily for the first 2 days and then decreased gradually over 10 days. Diazepam can be used alternatively at 10 mg daily and decreased by 20–25% over approximately 5 days. Phenobarbital can also be used to control minor symptoms, with 15–60 mg every 4–6 hours as needed on the first 2 days and then decreased gradually.

Disulfiram (Antabuse) should not be used during pregnancy because of an association with clubfoot, VACTERL syndrome, and phocomelia of the lower extremities.[4]

OUTCOMES

Growth and development of FAS children is often abnormal, with short stature, microcephaly, and persistent learning difficulties being commonly reported. Hyperactivity and attention deficit disorders are more common among the offspring of heavy alcohol users. FAS is the leading cause of mental retardation in the United States.

BREAST FEEDING   Ethanol levels in breast milk are similar to levels in maternal blood. At a maternal level of 100 mg/dL, the newborn would receive approximately 164 mg of ethanol per feeding. The effects of regular moderate intakes of ethanol may result in changes in the composition of milk and the newborn feeding pattern. Ethanol impairs milk ejection, which may cause additional difficulties with breast feeding.

Cocaine

HISTORY AND BACKGROUND   Cocaine use dates back to AD 1100–1500 in South America. It was prized by the Peruvian Indians and used by the ruling class. The Europeans became increasingly interested in cocaine during the latter half of the 19th century. Albert Niemann separated cocaine from the coca leaf in 1860. One of the founders of John Hopkins University School of Medicine, William Halsted, injected purified cocaine under the skin for anesthesia in the 1880s. Sigmund Freud used cocaine on patients with various ailments and published a paper entitled "On Coca." Cocaine was also included in many patent medications. The Harrison Narcotic Act of 1914 prohibited the use of cocaine in medicine and other products.

TERATOGENICITY   There appears to be a roughly fourfold increase in urogenital abnormalities among the offspring of women addicted to cocaine in pregnancy. Multiple other anomalies have been described in cocaine abusing women; however, many of these affects may be due to confounding lifestyle issues. The anomalies that have been associated with maternal cocaine abuse include anomalies of the gastrointestinal system (especially atresias), limb reduction anomalies, and cardiac anomalies. Of note, however, one meta-analysis of 45 studies concluded that when users of multiple other non-cocaine drugs were used as controls, the adverse outcomes did not appear to be related to cocaine use.[3]

EFFECTS ON PREGNANCY   Cocaine has dramatic hemodynamic effects including transient hypertension and vasoconstriction. These are probably due to cocaine's ability to block uptake and breakdown of norepinephrine at adrenergic nerve endings. Animal models have demonstrated decreased uterine and placental blood flow after cocaine use. This results in decreased oxygen delivery to the fetus. Cocaine's low molecular weight and high solubility in lipids and water allow it to cross the placenta quickly. The vasoconstriction caused by cocaine may slow some of the transfer of cocaine from mother to fetus. Amniotic fluid may accumulate cocaine and metabolites.

Cocaine has been linked in humans to uterine rupture, placental abruption, stroke, and fetal death. In the first trimester cocaine leads to increased rates of pregnancy loss. Cocaine increases the contractile activity of myometrium. Premature birth is increased with cocaine use. Meconium passage is more common. Premature birth has been reported in up to 50% of cocaine abusing women not receiving prenatal care.

The medical complications seen with cocaine use in nonpregnant individuals also can play a role in pregnancy. Myocardial infarction, cardiac arrhythmias, stroke, and seizures are seen in pregnancy. Acute cocaine intoxication may initially present with a syndrome that mimics preeclampsia or HELLP (hemolysis, elevated liver enzymes and low platelets) syndrome.

WITHDRAWAL

Cocaine withdrawal is described as having three phases. The first "crash" phase that lasts from hours to 4 days is marked by irritability, craving, depression, and sleepiness. The second phase is a depression lasting 1–10 weeks. The third phase is marked by cravings and a gradual return of normal emotions. This third phase may last months.

TREATMENT OPTIONS

Simple observation is possible as many women withdraw from cocaine. Acute toxicity or agitation may be controlled with chlordiazepoxide (Librium) 25 mg orally daily, diazepam (Valium), or lorazepam (Ativan). Marked hypertension can be managed by labetalol or nitroprusside in severe cases. Depression may be ameliorated by short courses of doxepin (Sinequan) 25 mg orally twice daily or desipramine (Norpramin). Bromocriptine (Parlodel) may provide relief from cocaine cravings but is contraindicated with hypertension and should be used with caution in pregnancy.[4]

OUTCOMES

Neonatal growth restriction has been associated with cocaine use during pregnancy. This appears to be substantiated even with controlling for background characteristics, cigarette use, and alcohol exposure.[2] After controlling for other exposures, children at 7 years who had been exposed to cocaine in utero were twice as likely to be below the 10th percentile in. Children born to women older than 30 years and exposed to cocaine were four times more likely to have clinically significant height deficits at age 7 years.[5] A link between cocaine abuse and sudden infant death syndrome has been reported in some studies, but controversy exists.

BREAST FEEDING   Cocaine is excreted into human breast milk. Cocaine use is not compatible with breast feeding.

Heroin and Narcotics

HISTORY AND BACKGROUND

The medical use of opiates dates back more than 6000 years to the Egyptians and Mesopotamians. Natural opiates are derived from the opium poppy *Papaver somniferum*, which means "sleep-inducing." Thomas de Quincey first described opium addiction in 1822 in *Confessions of an English Opium Eater*, his autobiographical account. Morphine was derived from opium around 1810 and was quickly appreciated as a way of relieving the pain of injuries or surgery. The name *morphine* was derived from the Greek god of dreams, Morpheus. In 1827 E. Merck & Company of Darmstadt, Germany began commercial manufacturing of morphine.

Morphine became available in the United States in the 1850s and was widely used during the Civil War. Morphine addiction quickly followed. By the late 1800s opium use had become popular in the United States. The exposure to opium was stimulated by the drug being brought in to the country by Chinese immigrants who arrived to work on the railroads. Codeine was first extracted from opium in 1832. By 1843 the injection of morphine by syringe was described by Alexander Wood of Edinburgh. The increased potency and quicker onset were noted.

Heroin is a semisynthetic opiate that was developed in 1874. Ironically, it was promoted as a morphine substitute that was felt to produce less risk of dependency. By 1898 the Bayer Corporation of Elberfeld, Germany began production of diacetylmorphine and coined the name *heroin*. There was no regulation of opiates in the United States until 1914, when Congress passed the Harrison

Narcotics Act. This required doctors who prescribe narcotics to register and pay a tax. In 1923 the Narcotics Division of the U.S. Treasury Department restricted all narcotic sales. In 1924 the Heroin Act made possession or manufacture of heroin illegal in the United States. Heroin has had an impressive effect on modern culture, and the list of writers, musicians, and actors who became involved could occupy many pages.[6]

Heroin in its a pure form is a bitter-tasting white powder. Street heroin can vary from white to dark brown, depending on impurities and additives. A traditional "bag" of heroin measures approximately 100 mg and sells for approximately $10. Some areas of the country have seen decreased cost of heroin, which has resulted in increased use. Purity has been increasing over the past decade, which in turn has decreased injection as a primary route and replaced it with snorting. This has the additional appeal of decreasing the risks of HIV and avoiding some of the stigma associated with intravenous heroin use. Unfortunately, it is also accompanied by the untrue assumption that heroin is less addictive when snorted. The rapidity of addiction varies by type of narcotic ingested. Some of the narcotics available to health care workers including the short-acting narcotics result in addiction with a more limited exposure than to heroin or to oral prescription narcotics.

Methadone was first synthesized before World War II in Germany. Isbell and Vogel demonstrated in 1949 that methadone was an effective medication for addicts withdrawing from heroin. Methadone maintenance was researched at Rockefeller University in 1964.

Prescription narcotic analgesics also have become a significant source of addiction. In addition to direct prescription from a physician, these are readily available for illicit purchase. The more potent preparations, including extended-release oxycodone (e.g., OxyContin), are particularly desired by narcotic addicts. The combinations of narcotics with acetaminophen are dangerous from the standpoint of hepatic damage with indiscriminate use. Anecdotally, there is an increased prevalence of individuals who are addicted to prescription narcotics and turn to heroin for a less expensive source of drug.

TERATOGENICITY

No clear teratogenicity pattern has been described with heroin and other narcotics.[3]

EFFECTS ON PREGNANCY

Many of the maternal medical risks of narcotic abuse are the result of lifestyle factors. Poor nutrition is common, as are iron deficiency anemia and folic acid deficiency. There may be an increased exposure to sexually transmitted diseases from indiscriminate sexual activity and exchange of sex for drugs. Contaminated needles may result in bacterial endocarditis, hepatitides B and C, HIV infection, abscesses, and ulcers.

Heroin has been associated with pregnancy complications including intrauterine fetal growth restriction, passage of meconium, preterm premature rupture of membranes, preterm delivery, and fetal demise. Neonates born to narcotic users go through a withdrawal syndrome similar to that seen in adults. This can include sleep abnormalities, hyperactivity, diarrhea, fever, and convulsions.

Tolerance to narcotics develops rapidly, specifically to produce euphoria or sedation. Cross-tolerance to narcotics also occurs, varying only with the specific potency and pharmacokinetics of the opiate used. A withdrawal syndrome can occur quickly, and a mild withdrawal syndrome has been reported after as few as 5 days of morphine use.

WITHDRAWAL

Opioid withdrawal produces painful physical symptoms in the mother but are not typically life threatening to an adult. Mild to moderate symptoms include opioid craving, anxiety, restlessness, muscle aching, dilated pupils, mild insomnia, anorexia, rhinorrhea, chills, yawning, piloerection ("goose flesh"), tachycardia, and hypertension. More severe symptoms can include diarrhea, vomiting, tremors, tachycardia, stomach cramps, kicking movements, and low-grade fever. During pregnancy, uterine irritability and increased fetal activity can be seen. Acute withdrawal may present an increased risk of intrauterine death.

TREATMENT OPTIONS

Methadone stabilization and medical withdrawal are the primary therapeutic options during pregnancy. Methadone stabilization is generally preferred, but there may be circumstances that require medical withdrawal because of unavailability of methadone programs.

METHADONE STABILIZATION

Methadone use in pregnancy has been studied since the late 1960s. It has proved effective in decreasing heroin use and dependency on other legal and illegal drugs. It is most effective in improving pregnancy outcome when it is used as part of a multidisciplinary program that includes counseling, prenatal care, nutritional counseling, and social services. Establishing a stable fetal environment and avoiding fluctuations in serum narcotic levels decreases the likelihood of neonatal narcotic abstinence syndrome and fetal stress.

Methadone stabilization is done with the goal of reversing any signs of withdrawal as promptly as possible. An initial oral dose of 10–40 mg is given. An additional dose of 5–10 mg is given every 3–4 hours as need to control objective signs of withdrawal. The dose required in a 24-hour period can then be combined into a single oral daily dose. The goal is to decrease narcotic cravings and symptoms of withdrawal without producing sedation. Objective scoring systems have been developed to assess presence and severity of withdrawal manifestations.

Methadone is well absorbed orally and has a half-life of 24–36 hours. This is far longer than the approximately 2-hour half-life of heroin. Methadone allows once-daily dosage for most patients. Split (twice daily) dosing may offer some benefits to women who have withdrawal symptoms before daily dosing. The logistics of this prevent widespread use.[7]

Parenteral methadone (Dolophine) represents a quicker option for titration and may be preferable. Because of increased bioavailability the parenteral doses are half the necessary oral doses. An initial dosage of 10 mg intramuscularly can be followed by additional 5–10 mg intramuscularly every 2–3 hours as needed to control withdrawal. When conversion to oral dosing occurs, the parenteral dosage will need to be doubled. For example, a patient who requires 45 mg intramuscularly over 24 hours will most likely require 90 mg orally as a maintenance dose.

Daily oral doses of methadone 50–150 mg are typically required to decrease narcotic cravings and desire for illegal opioid use. Dosages of methadone often require increases by approximately 20% as pregnancy advances to prevent withdrawal symptoms. This is most noticeable in the third trimester. This is explained by the increased plasma volume and renal blood flow that occurs with the later stages of pregnancy. After delivery, methadone doses are decreased by one third to maintain the same effects on the mother without intoxication.[8]

Women taking methadone should be cautioned against the use of opioid agonist-antagonist medications such as pentazocine (Talwin), nalbuphine (Nubain), or butorphanol (Stadol) because they can precipitate acute withdrawal. Use of opioid antagonists such as naloxone (Narcan) should be used only as a last resort with severe narcotic overdose. Administration of these to pregnant women who are opioid dependent can result in spontaneous abortion, premature labor, or stillbirth.

Careful coordination with pediatric care is essential. Neonates born to mothers enrolled in methadone maintenance programs typically experience some form of withdrawal within 24–72 hours of birth. Early discharge from the hospital should be avoided. There is little correlation between maternal methadone dose and neonatal abstinence syndrome. Neonatal abstinence syndrome can be more severe than adult withdrawal, and treatment is recommended. Withdrawal symptoms can be managed with paregoric, narcotics, or phenobarbital. When seizures do result from untreated withdrawal in the newborn, they seem to have a good prognosis long term. Most newborns have normalization of any electroencephalographic changes within the first year of life.[8]

MEDICAL WITHDRAWAL

Medical withdrawal from opioids is not recommended during pregnancy but may be a necessary process when methadone stabilization is not available or acceptable to the patient. There appears to be no significant benefit to withdrawal at any particular time in pregnancy. Withdrawal from methadone should be done slowly and should not be initiated until a stable dose of methadone is identified. Ideally, the weekly decrease in dosage should be 2.5–5 mg maximum. As the remaining dosage becomes smaller, the weekly taper should also be slower. Fetal surveillance of fetuses that are potentially viable is suggested. Fetal demise has been observed even with close fetal monitoring. Clonidine has been used to decrease symptoms of withdrawal and may be a useful adjunctive therapy.

Buprenorphine (Subutex) is a schedule III semisynthetic mixed opiate agonist-antagonist that prevents opioid withdrawal and has a "ceiling effect." This carries a lower risk of abuse and side effects than the full agonist opioids. It is poorly available orally, but sublingual tablets provide an easy route of administration. It is also marketed in combination with naloxone as Suboxone. Although buprenorphine is listed as a category C medication, there are few published data on use during pregnancy. No significant problems have been reported in the limited case report data available. Some studies have demonstrated the possibility of less severe neonatal withdrawal syndrome. Methadone remains the current standard of care for opioid-dependent women.[4]

OUTCOMES

Methadone maintenance substantially decreases the incidence of obstetric complications seen in heroin abusers. No chronic conditions have been identified in children who have been exposed to methadone in utero.

BREAST-FEEDING

Heroin use is contraindicated during breast feeding according to the American Academy of Pediatrics.

Methadone reaches breast milk at a milk:plasma ratio of 0.83. Thus, a mother on methadone would expose her infant to a very small amount of methadone compared with the dose received in utero. In evaluating the risk of breast feeding in a mother on methadone, it is necessary to consider if the mother is well controlled on a stable dose of methadone, has had no evidence of other substance abuse, and has been participating in a supervised treatment program. The mother's HIV status should be known. The methadone that reaches breast milk may help prevent withdrawal in the addicted infant. The American Academy of Pediatrics and the World Health Organization Working Group on Human Lactation consider methadone compatible with breast feeding.

What's the Evidence

There is little prospective research published on substance abuse during pregnancy. The Center for Substance Abuse Treatment, U.S. Department of Health and Human Services has prepared an online document, Pregnant, Substance-Using Women, Treatment Improvement Protocol Series 2 (http://www.health.org/govpubs/bkd107/2h.aspx), that has a very comprehensive set of protocols and guidelines available[4] based on expert panel opinion.

Guiding Questions in Approaching the Patient

As a provider approaches a pregnant patient with a substance abuse problem, it is helpful to ask the following questions:

- What services are available in the community to assist with treatment?
- What other providers can be involved so that a multispecialty approach can be developed?
- Are there financial and social issues that also need to be addressed, including domestic abuse, housing, additional children at risk, and transportation?
- Can care be provided in a sensitive and supportive manner to avoid additional guilt?
- What is the best medical approach to assist the patient in avoiding active substance abuse and in continuing prenatal care?

Conclusion

Management issues for pregnancies complicated by substance abuse vary by the type or types of substances abused. These women are at high risk for having significant psychosocial complicating factors such as poverty, low education status, low socioeconomic status including homelessness, prior incarceration, psychiatric illness, and being victims of intimate partner and family abuse. To the extent that resources allow, a team approach is likely to be most beneficial. Substance abuse crosses all socioeconomic strata, however. Each patient should be screened for substance abuse by medical history taking at least once in a pregnancy. Evaluation should also be undertaken for signs or symptoms suggestive of substance abuse.

Discussion of Cases

CASE 1: METHADONE MAINTENANCE IN PREGNANCY

A 28-year-old gravida 4, para 0121 presents to an emergency room seeking detoxification from heroin. She reports that she is pregnant and uses 12 bags a day. She is living on the street. Her previous delivery was an emergency cesarean section at 33 weeks of gestaion with no prenatal care. The last menstrual period is uncertain. She is complaining of joint aches and muscle cramps. On examination she has "goose flesh." Blood pressure is 140/90 mm Hg with a heart rate of 9 beats/min. Her uterine size consistent with a 12-week pregnancy. Fetal heart rate is auscultated.

What should your initial evaluation include?

Prenatal blood work including blood type and screen, rapid plasma reagin, hepatitides B and C screening, CBC, and HIV screening; Papanicolaou's smear with cultures for gonorrhea and *Chlamydia*; urinalysis; urine for toxicology; ultrasound to confirm intrauterine pregnancy and dating; and screen for tuberculosis (purified protein derivative). You are fortunate because there is a local program that will dispense methadone in pregnancy. You review the options of methadone maintenance with the patient and she agrees to participate and enroll in methadone maintenance, counseling, and prenatal care.

How do you adjust her initial dose?

Admit the patient to a facility where she can be observed during titration. At this early gestational age, no fetal surveillance is required. An initial dose of methadone 20 mg orally or 10 mg intramuscularly should be given in an attempt to reverse withdrawal symptoms as quickly as possible. Additional doses of 5–10 mg orally or 5 mg intramuscularly can be given every 3 hours until symptoms resolve.

How is a daily dosage determined?

After 24 hours of titration, the total dosage given can be used as an approximation of a daily
maintenance dosage. **For example, if the patient required 20 mg orally initially and then received three additional doses of 10 mg orally over 24 hours, a reasonable initial dose would be 50 mg orally daily. Because the oral bioavailability of methadone is approximately half that of parenteral methadone, the patient who received 10 mg intramuscularly initially and then three additional doses of 5 mg intramuscularly would receive a daily dose of 50 mg orally.**

The patient is adjusted to a daily dose of 80 mg daily and continues with prenatal care and daily methadone administration. At 30 weeks of gestation, the patient begins to complain of withdrawal symptoms, particularly in the early morning.

How should her dosage be adjusted?

Increased requirements of 20% are commonly seen in the third trimester. Increase the dosage by 5 mg daily to see if symptoms decrease. This can be done every 3–4 days as an outpatient. If symptoms persist, you can consider readmitting the patient for dosage adjustment under observation.

The patient delivers vaginally at 39 weeks, and the newborn is admitted to the nursery for observation. The patient's daily methadone dose is 105 mg orally daily at the time of delivery.

How should the maternal dose be adjusted after delivery?

A decrease of 30% is typical after delivery.

The patient's dose is decreased to 75 mg daily, and she tolerates this dose well.

CASE 2: HYPERTENSION AND TACHYCARDIA IN PATIENT WITH NO PRENATAL CARE

A 32-year-old gravida 4, para 0030 is brought to labor and delivery. She has had no prenatal care. Her fundal height measures 32 cm and fetal heart tones at 136 beats/min are heard with a Doptone. She is agitated, and her blood pressure measures 150/92 mm Hg with a heart rate of 110 beats/min. Regular contractions are noted on the monitor. The fetal heart rate pattern is reassuring. No useful history can be obtained from the patient. Your intern suggests the diagnosis of preeclampsia and asks the nurse to prepare a magnesium bolus.

What steps are appropriate during the initial evaluation?

Place the patient on a fetal heart rate monitor to assess fetal well-being. Obtain blood for liver function tests, serum urea nitrogen, creatinine, blood type and screen, rapid plasma reagin, hepatitides B and C screening, CBC, and platelet count. Obtain urine for toxicology and protein. If the patient is stable, perform a targeted ultrasound to estimate dating, fetal weight, and position.

The patient's toxicology returns positive for cocaine metabolites. The patient has mild increases in liver function tests, but the remainder of her blood work is normal. Ultrasound suggests a fetus at approximately 34 weeks of gestation with normal amniotic fluid volume. There is no evidence of abruption. There is no proteinuria.

The patient's blood pressure normalizes over the next 2 hours, and her agitation decreases. She appears sleepy but responds appropriately to questions. Magnesium sulfate is discontinued because the presumptive diagnosis of preeclampsia appears wrong.

What is the next step in managing the pregnancy?

Because the patient's agitation is decreasing, there is little need for medication during cocaine withdrawal. If the patient demonstrates symptoms of depression, doxepin or desipramine may be helpful. The patient should be referred to drug treatment services and encouraged to begin prenatal care.

REFERENCES

1 Kaltenbach KA. Effects of in utero opiate exposure: new paradigms for old questions. *Drug Alcohol Depend* 1994;36.

2 Nordstrom-Klee B, Delaney-Black V, Covington C, et al. Growth from birth onwards of children prenatally exposed to drugs: a literature review. *Neurotoxicol Teratol* 2002;24:481–488.

3 REPROTOX Database, Reproductive Toxicology Center.

4 Mitchell JL, et al. *Pregnant, Substance-Using Women Treatment Improvement Protocol Series 2.* Substance Abuse and Mental Health Administration DHHS Publication No. (SMA) 95-3056. Washington, DC: US Department of Health and Human Services, 1995.

5 Covington C, Nordstrom-Klee B, Anger J, et al. Birth to age 7 growth of children prenatally exposed to drugs: a prospective cohort study. *Neurotoxicol Teratol* 2002;24.

6 Hoegerman G, Schnoll S. Narcotic use in pregnancy. *Clin Perinatol* 1991;18:1.

7 Wittmann BK, Segal S. A comparison of the effects of single- and split-dose methadone administration on the fetus: ultrasound evaluation. *Int J Addict* 1991;26:2.

8 Herman J, Stancliff S, Langrod J. Methadone maintenance treatment (MMT): a review of historical and clinical issues. *Mount Sinai J Med* 2000;67:5–6.

Approach to Obesity in Pregnancy

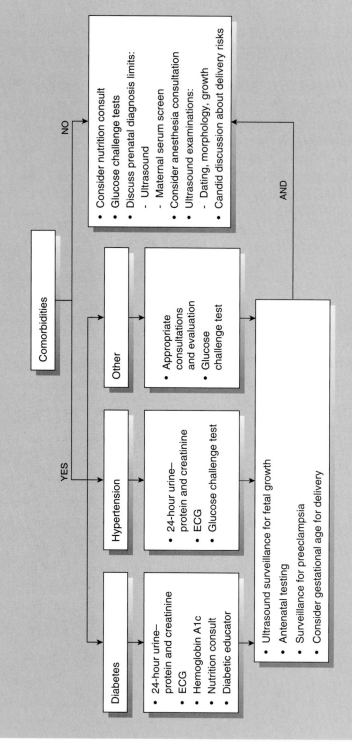

41 Management of the Obese Pregnant Patient

Emily R. Baker

Introduction

Obesity is rapidly becoming the primary health risk in the United States. Sadly, being overweight or obese is currently more prevalent than being of normal weight. Sixty-four percent of the population is overweight or obese, and 30% of the population is obese.[1] The prevalence of obesity differs by subcategories of the population. Obesity is more common in women who are African American or Hispanic and in older, multiparous women. Various definitions and categorizations for obesity have been proposed. At present, the most common uses body mass index (BMI) as the primary descriptor of appropriateness of body weight. The formula for BMI is:

$$BMI = \frac{weight\ (lb)}{height\ (in.) \times height\ (in.)} \times 703$$

Criteria have been set for the definitions of underweight, normal weight, overweight, and obese. Obesity is defined as a BMI of at least 30 kg/m² and overweight as a BMI of 25–29 kg/m². Many have set BMI levels to describe degrees of obesity. A BMI of at least 40 kg/m² has been called extreme obesity or class III obesity. A weight greater than 300 lb has been defined as massive obesity. Table 41-1 provides the ranges of weight for a given height for each BMI category.

Obesity affects the general health of women in a multitude of ways. Each of these can have an effect on a woman's risk for adverse pregnancy outcome and her risk of chronic disease. Data have suggested that obesity has a greater effect on health than

Table 41-1.   **OBESITY**

	BODY WEIGHT (LB)			
	NORMAL	*OVERWEIGHT*	*OBESE*	*EXTREME OBESITY*
BMI (kg/m²)	19–24	25–29	30–39	40–54
Height				
4 ft 10 in.	91–115	119–138	143–186	191–258
4 ft 11 in.	94–119	124–143	148–193	198–267
5 ft 0 in.	97–123	128–148	153–199	204–276
5 ft 1 in.	100–127	132–153	158–206	211–285
5 ft 2 in.	104–131	136–158	164–213	218–295
5 ft 3 in.	107–135	141–163	169–220	225–304
5 ft 4 in.	110–140	145–169	174–227	232–314
5 ft 5 in.	114–144	150–174	180–234	240–324
5 ft 6 in.	118–148	155–179	186–241	247–334
5 ft 7 in.	121–153	159–185	191–249	255–344
5 ft 8 in.	125–158	164–190	197–256	262–354
5 ft 9 in.	128–162	169–196	203–263	270–365
5 ft 10 in.	132–167	174–202	209–271	278–376
5 ft 11 in.	136–172	179–208	215–279	286–386
6 ft 0 in.	140–177	184–213	221–287	294–397

BMI = body mass index.

KEY POINT

Identifying the degree of obesity can help guide the level of concern for adverse outcome.

does smoking or poverty.[2] The strongest links are with diabetes and hypertension, which clearly have an influence on pregnancy outcomes. Obese women have rates of pregestational diabetes and pregestational hypertension that are 3–10 times higher than for normal-weight women. Other health problems associated with obesity include hypertension, hyperinsulinemia, dyslipidemia, coronary artery disease, cerebrovascular accident, osteoarthritis, gallbladder disease, sleep apnea, and some cancers including colon and breast.[3] In addition, obesity, illness, and sedentary lifestyle have substantial negative effects on mental health.

Effect of Obesity on Maternal and Perinatal Outcomes

Several studies have documented the magnitude of risks for adverse maternal outcome in women with obesity.[4–6] Risks are related to the degree of obesity. Even overweight status poses a risk of adverse outcome. Obesity and overweight status are independent risk factors for development of preeclampsia.[7,8] One large study demonstrated significant increases in risk for preeclampsia with odds ratios (OR) of 2.4 for overweight women and 5.2 for obese women.[5] Obese women have a three- to fivefold increased risk of gestational diabetes. The literature has suggested that obese pregnant women have a 14–25% risk of preeclampsia and 6–14% incidence of gestational diabetes.[9]

Little evidence exists about the effect of weight on respiratory function in pregnancy. Obesity is associated with increased prevalence of asthma and sleep apnea.[10] Pregnant obese women have a higher likelihood of sleep apnea.[11] Obesity decreases chest wall compliance and increases airway resistance. This leads to decreased total lung capacity, forced vital capacity, forced expiratory volumes, and functional residual capacity. Pregnant women have decreased residual volume and functional residual capacity.[12] A clinical significance is that pregnant women have precipitous development of hypoxia with apnea that is further enhanced by obesity.

Patients with sleep apnea should be carefully assessed. The settings for a home continuous positive airway pressure devices should be known. Women should bring their home device with them during labor and delivery because a home device tends to be better tolerated than a different hospital system. Somnolence or hypotension in this setting should raise suspicion of carbon dioxide retention or incipient right heart failure.

KEY POINT

Preexisting morbidities are strong predictors of adverse outcome.

Alterations in cardiovascular functioning have an effect on pregnancy. Morbid obesity is characterized by an increase in total blood volume, decreased systemic vascular resistance, and increased resting cardiac output, which may be additive with similar pregnancy changes. There is an increase in mean oxygen consumption to meet the metabolic requirements of the adipose tissue. Many severely obese patients have impaired left ventricular contractility, diastolic dysfunction, and a depressed ejection fraction some with left ventricular dilatation and hypertrophy. Sudden increases in intravascular volume may not be tolerated well. Assessment of cardiac function is important for women with massive obesity. Changes in physical examination such as new wheezes, gallops, or increased jugular venous distention may be difficult to detect. More invasive strategies, such as invasive pressure monitoring or arterial blood gas measurements, are warranted when a patient deteriorates and the etiology is unclear.

An increased likelihood of thromboembolism has been associated with obesity and pregnancy.[13,14] Other risk factors include preeclampsia, multiple births, and cesarean delivery; however, most pregnancies complicated by thromboembolism do not have an identified risk factor. It is likely that inherited thrombophilias play a large role in determining risk for thromboembolism and that this knowledge will allow more precise recommendations with regard to prophylaxis. At present, no specific guidelines have been set for routine prophylaxis in pregnancy. It seems quite reasonable based on what it currently known that obese pregnant women have enough risk during delivery that some prophylaxis should be given, particularly if there has been a cesarean delivery.

Most studies have found an increased risk of cesarean delivery. Influences for this outcome due to obesity include macrosomia, induction of labor, preeclampsia, and concern for logistic difficulty with an emergency cesarean delivery. One of the larger studies found rates of cesarean delivery to be 32% for the obese, 23% for the overweight, and 16% for normal-weight women.[7] One study found the risk of emergency cesarean section to be increased, with an OR of 1.83.[5] The likelihood of a successful vaginal birth after cesarean is as low as 15%, with a 50% risk of infectious morbidity.[15] Even in one study with a high likelihood of successful vaginal birth after cesarean and low rates of infectious morbidity, no decrease in costs could be attributed to a trial of labor in obese women.[16]

The risks of all infectious morbidities are increased. A study of more than 280,000 pregnancies found that obese women have increased risks for genital tract infection (OR 1.24), urinary tract infection (OR 1.39), and wound infection (OR 2.24).[5] These investigators found a modest increase in the likelihood of postpartum hemorrhage (OR 1.39).[5]

Perinatal outcomes are affected by obesity. Macrosomia is significantly more common in obese women, with a two- to threefold higher likelihood.[5] Inadequate evidence exists to predict a specific effect due to obesity on risk of shoulder dystocia. The significant difficulty in estimating fetal weight in obese women adds to the difficulty of assessing risk for shoulder dystocia. The concern for an adverse effect of macrosomia also includes the risk of resultant childhood and adult obesity.

The chance for a small-for-gestational-age baby is less for obese than for a woman with normal weight.[4,9] No consistent finding has been seen regarding the likelihood of premature birth. There does appear to be evidence of an increased risk for fetal death (OR 2–3).[17–19] The estimated stillbirth rate for women with obesity is 1.5–2.0 in 1,000 births.

Controversy exists as to whether obesity is a significant risk factor for congenital structural abnormalities, especially neural tube defects. Many but not all studies have demonstrated an association. The evidence seems most compelling for spina bifida.[20] Insulin resistance and abnormalities in metabolism including folic acid have been considered possible mediators of teratogenesis. A recent population based case-control study of 40,000 births demonstrated an increased likelihood of different structural abnormalities in obese women, including spina bifida, structural heart abnormalities, omphalocele, and multiple abnormalities.[21]

Because of the increasing prevalence of morbid obesity and bariatric surgery, reports of outcomes after bariatric surgery are being published.[22,23] Uncomplicated pregnancies are common. There is some evidence that the likelihood of gestational diabetes, macrosomia, and cesarean section is decreased. Some women who have gastric banding have to undergo adjustment to manage nausea and vomiting. There are case reports of women with gastric bypass or biliopancreatic diversion surgery having severe iron, vitamin A, and vitamin B_{12} deficiencies. In these women, particular attention needs to be given to vitamin supplementation. Some women may require parenteral iron or vitamin B_{12}. Some women who have had bypass surgery experience a "dumping syndrome" after carbohydrate administration and will require an diabetes screening other than the oral glucose challenge test.

KEY POINT

Question patients about symptoms of a dumping syndrome before a glucose challenge test.

Pregnancy Management

ANTEPARTUM CARE

Consultation with a registered dietitian will be helpful to obese women for management of weight gain and appropriate supplementation of vitamins and minerals. Not every community has an abundance of access to nutritionists, and consultation may need to be allocated to women with severe obesity. Consultation would be especially important in women who have had bariatric surgery. Each woman should have her initial BMI recorded on her chart.

Weight loss before pregnancy is the ideal nutritional intervention. Failing that, limitation of weight gain will improve perinatal outcome. Weight gain of more than 25 lb is associated with macrosomia. Even for obese women, weight gain less than 6 kg or weight loss is associated with low birth weight. For obese women, a modest weight gain is best. An additional rationale for limiting weight gain is the effect on prevalence and worsening of obesity. No characteristic has been identified to target women at greatest risk of weight retention. Currently, the Institute of Medicine recommends weight gains of 28–40 lb for underweight, 25–35 lb for normal, 15–25 lb for overweight, and 15 lb for obese women. An exercise program must also be encouraged for obese pregnant women.

Obesity presents some logistic issues in the outpatient clinic. One such issue is that many scales do not register above 290 lb. Often additional weights can be hung on clinic scales. Hospital bed scales may register greater weights than clinic scales. It is best to avoid the humiliation of weighing women on a hospital freight scale. Likewise, appropriately sized sheets and gowns should be used. It may be difficult to auscultate fetal heart tones. The patient (or other staff members) can lift the abdominal panniculus to allow placement of the Doppler at the base of the panniculus.

Recommendations with regard to screening for diabetes vary. A common recommendation is for screening in each trimester. The American Diabetes Association recommends screening as soon as feasible, with a repeat glucose challenge test at 24–28 weeks.[24] The screening and diagnostic criteria are the same for obese as for normal-weight women. A glucose challenge test cannot be done in women with a dumping syndrome. Home fingerstick blood glucose monitoring is the most reliable alternative.

KEY POINT

Be vigilant to detect gestational diabetes and hypertension.

All women should be offered prenatal diagnosis testing, especially in light of the evidence that obesity itself may increase the risk of congenital abnormalities. Maternal serum screening for neural tube defect and trisomy 21 must take into account the patient's weight. A second-trimester ultrasound is very difficult to accomplish with obesity and should be put off until at least 18 weeks. The sonographer may need the help of the patient or an assistant to retract the abdominal panniculus to place the transducer where there is relatively less adipose tissue. An earlier transvaginal study could be considered, but this study has a lower detection rate.

Close surveillance must be maintained for chronic hypertension, gestational hypertension, and preeclampsia. Use of an appropriately sized cuff is necessary. A thigh cuff can be used on the arm. Assessment of fetal weight is very difficult by palpation, ultrasound examination, or maternal self-assessment. Despite its limitations, serial ultrasound examinations should be done as a screen for appropriate fetal growth. Antenatal testing with non-stress tests or biophysical profiles is essential for women with diabetes or hypertension, particularly in light of the risk of still-birth associated with obesity.

INTRAPARTUM CARE   It is essential to involve an anesthesiologist at the beginning of delivery management and preferably before admission. Substantial anesthetic risks are posed by the ventilatory and cardiovascular complications of obesity and the patients' comorbidities. The majority of anesthesia-related maternal mortality is associated with obesity. The anesthesiologist will face the challenges of difficulty with intravenous access, intubation, and regional block. Reliable intravenous access is critical and should be secured at the beginning of labor.

Obesity and pregnancy can make standard tracheal intubation difficult. An obese patient with a difficult airway will not be a candidate for emergency general anesthesia. Consultation with an anesthesiologist is warranted to formulate and prepare for a backup plan if an emergency arises. Preparation for fiberoptic intubation while the patient is awake could be considered. Early placement of epidural or intrathecal catheters is recommended for logistical reasons to decrease maternal morbidity and decrease the ventilatory and cardiac work associated with labor. The obstetrician must keep in mind that the initiation of anesthesia will take a longer period for an obese woman than for a normal-weight woman.

Extubation of obese patients can also be difficult and should not be considered routine. Causes of decreased drive to breathe (e.g., narcotics), decreased ability to breathe (e.g., magnesium toxicity), and decreased oxygen exchange (e.g., pulmonary edema) should be sought and controlled.

Several equipment issues need to be addressed. An appropriately sized bed is important for patient comfort and for allowing mobility within the bed. Most hospitals now stock these. A bed trapeze will facilitate the patient's mobility. Likewise, it is important

KEY POINT

Obtain consultation with an anesthesiologist before delivery.

to make sure before admission that the hospital has an appropriately sized operating table. Lateral extenders are available for some tables. Elastic bandages may need to be added to monitor belts if increased length is needed. A metal bedpan may be needed because plastic ones can collapse. It may be necessary to place blocks under a wall-mounted toilet to support the weight of the patient. Appropriately sized gowns should be made available. If needed, two staff members can use draw sheets around the thighs to lift and displace thigh fat for examinations and delivery.

Women should labor in the lateral position with elevation of the head and chest. Some obese women cannot tolerate lying in the supine position. No oral intake should be given. Careful assessment of intake and output is needed, especially in women with cardiac dysfunction. It may be necessary to use bladder catheterization, but care then needs to be taken to encourage patient mobility. Selected patients may benefit from continuous pulse oximetry. Preparation for the possibility of cesarean section includes identifying additional staff members to assist with transfer. Be aware that it will take much longer time from decision to delivery for these women. Similarly, remaining cognizant of the risk for shoulder dystocia and the need for additional support is prudent.

Despite the logistical issues of an urgent or emergent cesarean delivery, it is best for women to try to deliver vaginally because of the substantially increased risks of morbidity from thromboembolism, puerperal infection, wound dehiscence, and hemorrhage.

However, cesarean delivery is common and poses several challenges. It is prudent to have a frank discussion with the patient about the logistics of her delivery, the risk of adverse fetal outcome based on difficulty in managing fetal distress, and the risk of maternal morbidity.

KEY POINT

Developing hospital and clinic guidelines and identifying facility requirements will improve ability to provide care.

The site of incision for a cesarean section needs to be individualized because the distribution of weight is quite variable. Several case series or small controlled series have been published about different approaches. One approach is retraction of the panniculus with tape to the mother's shoulders. The advantages of transverse incisions below the panniculus are a thinner layer of adipose tissue, a more secure closure, less postoperative pain, and potentially shorter duration from skin incision to delivery. The disadvantages are placement in a moist area that is difficult to keep clean and inability to explore the upper abdomen. In addition, the panniculus may not be retracted in a fashion as to compromise the airway. A supraumbilical approach has also been used. For women with severe abdominal obesity, the relative location of the umbilicus to the uterus is more inferior. This approach allows a less deep incision than standard midline incisions but most often requires a fundal uterine incision. The decision to use this approach must take into consideration the patient's plans as to whether to have more pregnancies.

The technical difficulty relates to the depth of the wound. It is helpful to plan to have additional assistants for retraction. Long instruments should be available. Closure of the fascia should be done with a delayed absorbable suture such as polydioxanone or with permanent suture. Use of subfascial and subcutaneous drains can allow detection of bleeding and decrease the likelihood of wound separation. Likewise, many surgeons place intermittent subcutaneous sutures with absorbable suture to decrease the likelihood of wound separation. Use of prophylactic antibiotics is essential.

Currently, the American College of Obstetricians and Gynecologists recommends consideration of cesarean delivery if estimated fetal weights are above 4500 g in a woman with diabetes and 5000 g in a woman without diabetes.[25] A midpelvic vaginal delivery should be done only with great caution. Strong consideration should be given to perioperative venous thrombosis prophylaxis with heparin or with sequential compression stockings. Care should be taken that the patient moves in bed every 2 hours. Likewise, early ambulation is important.

POSTPARTUM CARE Many women will require prolonged postpartum hospitalization due to complications or logistic issues. Breast feeding should be encouraged because it decreases the likelihood of childhood obesity and it may enhance maternal weight loss. All women with insulin-requiring gestational diabetes should have a 75-g oral glucose tolerance test at least 6 weeks postpartum. A discussion about contraception should take into account the effect of obesity on efficacy of the method.

What's the Evidence?

There is ample evidence for the increasing prevalence of obesity in the United States. The National Health and Nutrition Examination Survey (http://www.cdc.gov/nchs/nhanes.htm)

administered by the National Center for Health Statistics provides a reliable estimation of the prevalence of obesity. Cohort studies have demonstrated the effect of obesity on pregnancy outcomes. There have not been trials of interventions intended to decrease risks in obese women other than those of secondary morbidities such as diabetes and hypertension. Unfortunately, other than these interventions, improvement in outcomes will rely on prevention of obesity and success in weight reduction before pregnancy.

Guiding Questions in Approaching the Patient

- What is the patient's BMI?
- Does the patient have comorbidities such as hypertension or diabetes?
- Does she have a history of surgical or anesthesia complications?
- Does my clinic and hospital have the necessary equipment and facilities to care for obese women?
- Has the patient had bariatric surgery?

Conclusion

The increasing prevalence of obesity complicates current obstetrical care. Obese gravidas are much more likely to have comorbidities including hypertension and diabetes. There is an increased risk of developing gestational diabetes and hypertension during a pregnancy. Risks of adverse maternal and neonatal outcomes such as cesarean birth, infectious morbidity, thromboembolism, macrosomia, and fetal death are increased. Prenatal management should be guided to allow early detection of diabetes and hypertension, and to minimize weight gain to 15 pounds. Planning for intrapartum care should include anesthesiology consultation and confirmation that the hospital has appropriate equipment and staff

Discussion of Cases

CASE 1: OBESE MULTIPARA WITHOUT COMORBIDITIES

A 28-year-old gravida 3, para 2 woman presents for prenatal care at 8 weeks of gestation. Her weight is 200 lb and her height is 5 ft 4 in., for a BMI of 36 kg/m². She has no history of chronic hypertension or obesity. Her two other children were born at term and weighed 8 lbs.

What evaluation do you recommend at this point?

A discussion of dietary choices and weight gain target. Nutrition consultation if resources are available. Discussion of prenatal diagnosis options and limitations. Ultrasound examination for dating. Glucose challenge test.

Her glucose challenge test, maternal serum screen, and ultrasound examination are normal. Her pregnancy remains uncomplicated.

What evaluation do you recommend in the third trimester?

Glucose challenge test at 24–28 weeks and ultrasound examination for growth at 32 weeks. Ultrasound examination should be repeated later if you are unable to assess fundal height growth clinically.

She develops hypertension and proteinuria at 37 weeks.

What preparations need to be made for her delivery?

Anesthesiology consultation. Be sure that the hospital has appropriate equipment. At this weight, she is unlikely to need special equipment.

CASE 2: OBESE PRIMIGRAVIDA DELIVERED BY CESAREAN SECTION

A 40-year-old primigravida presents for care at 24 weeks of gestation. Her weight is 330 lb, height is 5 ft 4 in., and BMI is 58.6 kg/m². She has not had medical care for many years.

What evaluation do you recommend at this point?

Ultrasound examination to confirm dates and for morphology screen, glucose challenge test, electrocardiogram, and nutritional consultation.

Results of her glucose challenge test and 3-hour glucose tolerance test are abnormal.

Insulin is initiated at 26 weeks. Antenatal testing is reassuring. Weekly visits are started at 32 weeks. An ultrasound examination at 38 weeks shows an estimated fetal weight of 4000 g.

What are appropriate next steps?

Confirm that the hospital has all needed equipment, anesthesiology consultation, and discussion with patient about delivery management.

She goes on to have an induction of labor. She has failure to progress at 4 cm and is recommended to have a cesarean section.

Are there any specific plans for her delivery that needs to be made?

Arrange for an appropriate number of assistants and long instruments, thromboprophylaxis with sequential compression stockings or heparin, and use delayed absorbable or permanent suture on the rectus fascia. Use of drains should be considered.

She has an uncomplicated delivery and postpartum course. She will need a 75-g glucose tolerance test 6 weeks postpartum.

REFERENCES

1 Flegal KM, Carroll MD, Ogden CL, Johnson CL. Prevalence and trends in obesity among US adults, 1999–2000. *JAMA* 2002;288:1723–1727.

2 Sturm R. Wells KB. Does obesity contribute as much to morbidity as poverty or smoking? *Public Health* 2001;115:229–235.

3 Manson JE. Skerrett PJ. Greenland P. VanItallie TB. The escalating pandemics of obesity and sedentary lifestyle. A call to action for clinicians. *Arch Intern Med* 2004;164:249–258.

4 Castro LC, Avina RL. Maternal obesity and pregnancy outcomes. *Curr Opin Obstet Gynecol* 2002;14:601–606.

5 Sebire NJ, Jolly M, Harris JP, et al. Maternal obesity and pregnancy outcome: a study of 287,213 pregnancies in London. *International Journal of Obesity and Related Metabolic Disorders. Journal of the International Association for the Study of Obesity* 2001;25(8): 1175–1182.

6 Lu GC, Rouse DJ, DuBard M, et al. The effect of increasing prevalence of maternal obesity on perinatal morbidity. *Am J Obstet Gynecol* 2001;185:845–890.

7 Baeten JM, Bukusi EA, Lambe M. Pregnancy complications and outcomes among overweight and obese nulliparous women. *Am J Public Health* 2001;91:436–440.

8 Sibai BM, Gordon T, Thom E, et al. Risk factors for preeclampsia in healthy nulliparous women: a prospective, multicenter study. *Am J Obstet Gynecol* 1995;172:642–648.

9 Baeten JM, Bukusi EA, Lambe M. Pregnancy complications and outcomes among overweight and obese nulliparous women. *Am J Public Health* 2001;91:436–440.

10 Ebbeling CB, Pawlak DB, Ludwig DS. Childhood obesity: public health crisis, common sense cure. *Lancet* 2002;360:473–482.

11 Maasilta P, Bachour A, Teramo K, et al. Sleep-related disordered breathing during pregnancy in obese women. *Chest* 2001;120: 1448–1454.

12 Unterborn J. Pulmonary function testing in obesity, pregnancy and extremes of body habitus. *Clin Chest Med* 2001;22:759–767.

13 Lindqvist PG, Kublikas M, Dahlback B. Individual risk assessment of thrombosis in pregnancy. *Acta Obstet Gynecol Scand* 2002;81: 412–416.

14 Ros HS, Lichtenstein P, Bellocco R, et al. Pulmonary embolism and stroke in relation to pregnancy: how can high risk women be identified? *Am J Obstet Gynecol* 2002;186:198–203.

15 Barrilleaux PS, Scardo JA, Martin JN. Mode of delivery for the morbidly obese with prior cesarean delivery: vaginal versus repeat cesarean section. *Am J Obstet Gynecol* 2001;185:349–354.

16 Edwards RK, Harnsberger DS, Johnson IM, et al. Deciding on route of delivery for obese women with a prior cesarean delivery. *Am J Obstet Gynecol* 2003;189385–390.

17 Cnattinguis S, Bergstrom R, Lipworth L, Kramer MS. Prepregnancy weight and the risk of adverse pregnancy outcome. *N Engl J Med* 1998;338: 147–152.

18 Simpson LL. Maternal medical disease: risk of antepartum fetal death. *Semin Perinatol* 2002;26:42–50.

19 Froen JF, Arnestad M, Frey K, et al. Risk factors for sudden intrauterine unexplained deaths: epidemiologic characteristics of singleton cases in Oslo, Norway, 1986–1995. *Am J Obstet Gynecol* 2001;184: 694–702.

20 Frey L, Hausler WA. Epidemiology of neural tube defects. *Epilepsia* 2003;44(suppl 3):4–13.

21 Watkins ML, Rasmussen SA, Honein MA, et al. Maternal obesity and risk for birth defects. *Pediatrics* 2003;111:1152–1158.

22 Wittgrove AC, Jester L, Wittgrove P, Clark GW. Pregnancy following gastric bypass for morbid obesity. *Obesity Surg* 1998;8:461–464.

23 Martin LF, Finigan KM, Nolan TE. Pregnancy after adjustable gastric banding. *Obstet Gynecol* 2000;95:927–930.

24 Diagnosis and classification of diabetes mellitus. American Diabetes Association. *Diabetes Care* 2004;27(suppl 1): S5–S10.

25 Fetal macrosomia. *ACOG Pract Bull* 2000;22.

Index